US Army Psychiatry *in the* Vietnam War

New Challenges in Extended Counterinsurgency Warfare

NORMAN M CAMP, MD

Colonel, Medical Corps,

US Army (Retired)

BORDEN INSTITUTE
US ARMY MEDICAL DEPARTMENT CENTER AND SCHOOL
Fort Sam Houston, Texas

Daniel E. Banks, MD, MS, MACP | LTC MC USA | *Director and Editor in Chief, Borden Institute*

Linette Sparacino | *Volume Editor*

Christine Gamboa-Onrubia, MBA | *Creative Director & Production Manager, Fineline Graphics, LLC*

Published by the Office of The Surgeon General

Borden Institute, US Army Medical Department Center & School, Fort Sam Houston, Texas

Library of Congress Cataloging-in-Publication Data

Camp, Norman M., author.
    US army psychiatry in the Vietnam war : new challenges in extended
counterinsurgency warfare / Norman M. Camp.
        p. ; cm.
United States army psychiatry in the Vietnam war
Includes bibliographical references and index.
I. Borden Institute (U.S.), issuing body. II. Title. III. Title: United
States army psychiatry in the Vietnam war.
[DNLM: 1. Mental Disorders—therapy—United States. 2. Military
Psychiatry—methods—United States. 3. Military Personnel—psychology—United
States. 4. Vietnam Conflict—United States. WM 110]
RC550
616.85'212—dc23
                        2014030696

PRINTED IN THE UNITED STATES OF AMERICA

For sale by the Superintendent of Documents, U.S. Government Printing Office
Internet: bookstore.gpo.gov   Phone: toll free (866) 512-1800;   DC area (202) 512-1800
Fax: (202) 512-2104 Mail: Stop IDCC, Washington, DC 20402-0001

ISBN 978-0-16-092550-4

Contents

Note to the readers. This volume utilizes some materials that are not available either in print or online. Several colleagues gave me access to their personal journals kept during their tours in Vietnam. Other colleagues shared papers they had written either during their tours in Vietnam or after their return home, but had never published. Other unpublished sources of information include handouts or other materials I received at various times during my Army career: when I attended Officer Basic Course, when I completed my residency, when I deployed to Vietnam, and after my return. None of these materials are considered "sensitive" by the military. I have included some of these materials as exhibits in the chapters, attachments to the chapters, or appendices to the volume. They are also listed in the references for each chapter, followed by a note that the document is available as indicated in this volume.

Physicians serving in Vietnam were provided a wide array of psychotropic medications, especially including newer neuroleptic and anxiolytic tranquilizing medications and the tricyclic antidepressants, for use with soldiers with psychiatric symptoms. In the field these were most often referred to by their brand names and not their generic names. I have followed suit in this book, only indicating the generic names when physicians used those names.

There were very few female military personnel in Vietnam, most of whom were assigned as nurses. Thus, unless noted otherwise, the experiences and observations chronicled in this book are those of men, and the use of pronouns reflects this reality.

There are references in this work to many important and timely articles that appeared during the war in the *USARV Medical Bulletin*, which was published from 1966 to 1971 to provide useful information for Army Medical Department personnel throughout the theater. This collection is archived at the US Army Academy of Health Sciences, Stimson Library, Fort Sam Houston, Texas. Complete PDF versions of articles can be accessed via the Internet at http://cdm15290.contentdm.oclc.org/cdm/landingpage/collection/p15290coll4. Individual articles can be searched using the author's last name. —Norman M Camp

About the Author

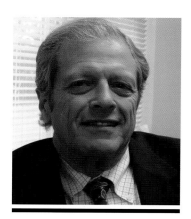

Norman M Camp, MD
Colonel, Medical Corps,
US Army (Retired)

DURING THE CREATION AND COMPLETION of this volume, Norman M Camp, MD brought a unique blend of training and experience to the task of making sense of the many political, environmental, institutional, social, and psychological strands that interacted to ultimately create a morale and mental health crisis among US ground forces in Vietnam. Pivotal was his service as psychiatrist and commanding officer of the 98th Neuropsychiatric Medical Specialty Detachment (KO) in Vietnam from October 1970 to October 1971—the period of greatest demoralization and dissent—for which he received the Bronze Star for Meritorious Achievement. Before going to Vietnam he completed his general medical internship at Letterman Army Hospital in San Francisco, California, and his general psychiatry residency at Walter Reed General Hospital in Washington, DC. After his return he completed child and adolescent psychiatry fellowship training at Letterman Army Hospital/University of California, San Francisco and psychoanalytic training with the Baltimore-Washington Institute for Psychoanalysis.

Additional familiarity with social sciences research came through his assignment as research investigator with the Department of Military Psychiatry, Walter Reed Army Institute of Research (WRAIR) in Washington, DC, from 1980 to 1985, where he had the opportunity to conduct a survey of veteran Army psychiatrists who served in Vietnam regarding their professional activities in the theater. His WRAIR assignment also resulted in his publishing (with Stretch and Marshall) an annotated bibliography of the psychiatric and social sciences literature pertaining to the effects of the war on troops serving in Vietnam, and later a long overdue exploration of the potential confusion of military psychiatric ethics arising during war. Practical augmentation of these experiences came through Dr Camp's assignments as Chief of Psychiatry of an Army hospital in Germany, Chief of the Community Mental Health Activity at a post in the United States, and as a member of the teaching faculty at Walter Reed Army Medical Center.

Dr Camp retired as a colonel from active service in 1988. He was awarded the Army Surgeon General's "A" Proficiency Designator as having attained the highest level of professional achievement recognized by the Army Medical Department. After his military retirement, Dr Camp relocated to Richmond, Virginia, where, in addition to maintaining an active clinical practice of psychiatry and psychoanalysis, he steadfastly directed his professional energies to the education and training of the next generation of psychiatrists. As Clinical Professor of Psychiatry at the Medical College of Virginia/Virginia Commonwealth University, he served for almost two decades as the Director of Psychotherapy Training for the psychiatry residency-training program.

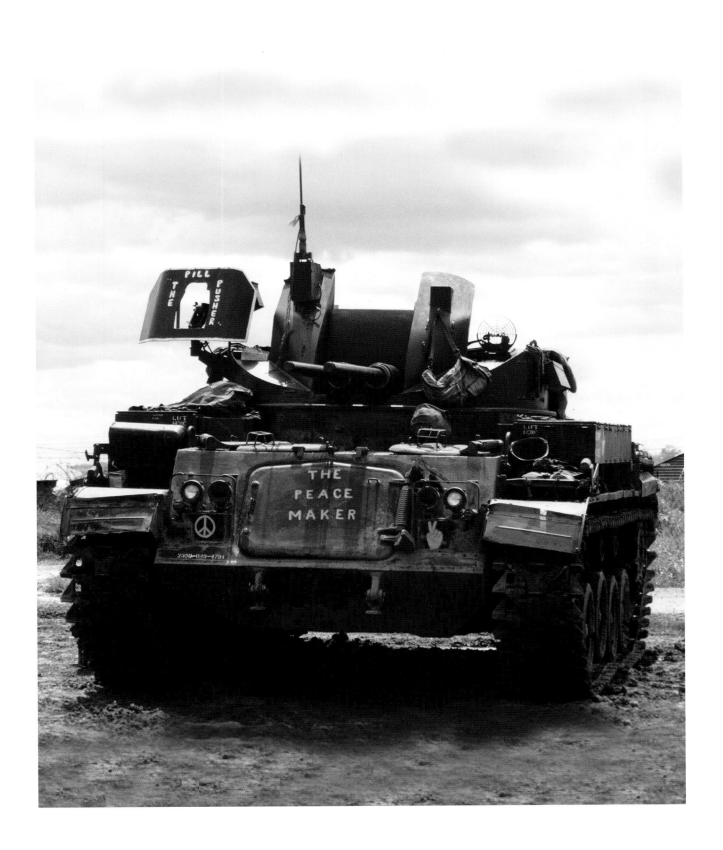

Foreword

[Opposite] M42 Duster self-propelled antiaircraft gun, "The Peace Maker." The name given this particular M42 Duster by its crew apparently associates its formidable firepower to the iconic Army Colt .45 Peacemaker revolver from the late 1800s. However, in this photograph, taken in 1970 during the second half of the war, there are decorations flanking the name, that is, the international peace symbol and the hand sign for peace, which were emblems that had been adopted by the Vietnam War protest movement in the United States. These markings are consistent with the growing confusion of values among the replacement troops sent to fight in Vietnam as the war lengthened, which in turn appears to be linked to the morale, discipline, and mental health crisis that developed.

When this war is over it will be a brighter day.
When this war is over it will be a brighter day.
But it won't bring back those poor boys in the grave.

JJ Cale and Eric Clapton

FIFTY EIGHT THOUSAND DEAD, 300,000 wounded, and $189 billion spent to process the Vietnam War from 1965 to 1972. America went into this war incrementally, sliding down a slippery slope. Our decision to become involved and our strategy to win the war were flawed. Looking out on a post–World War II landscape, we saw communism running rampant and the Cold War heating up. Vietnam presented an opportunity to stem the "Red Tide," so we came to the aid of our South Vietnamese allies. Unfortunately, the South Vietnamese government was weak, autocratic, and corrupt. It represented the last vestiges of three centuries of colonialism.

Our initial strategy was to fight a short war with overwhelming force. The enemy strategy was to conduct a prolonged, low-intensity counterinsurgency regardless of casualties. We misunderstood and underestimated the resolve of our enemy. As many times before and since, we did not heed the lessons of history. Domestic issues of the day influenced overall strategy. During the 1960s, our government was focusing on large social programs and wanted our intrusion into Southeast Asia to have minimal impact on the American public—a "guns and butter" policy. Crucial strategic decisions that would ultimately affect the conduct of the war were made with domestic policy in mind.

The National Guard and Reserves were not mobilized. A selective draft was initiated, which targeted poor and disadvantaged single males in rural and urban areas, and was echoed in pop culture—Creedence Clearwater Revival's "I ain't no Senator's son. . . ."

Troops were sent to Vietnam under a 1-year rotation policy. This approach ultimately led to a breakdown in unit cohesion and disrupted continuity of leadership. Further breakdown of morale, discipline, and effectiveness occurred during the rise of social unrest at home with the civil rights movement and the counterculture youth movement. Soldiers were keenly aware of these events and of the public's ever increasing feelings against the war and the troops themselves—the "baby killers." All these events played out on television. The war was conducted in the living rooms of America night after night, ultimately leading to a decline in the national will to support the war.

To further add to the US military's problems in country, our South Vietnamese allies introduced readily available heroin, and a drug epidemic ensued among the troops. With the culmination of these many forces swirling about, it should be no surprise that our soldiers' behavior was affected in a negative manner manifested by low morale, disobedience, antimilitary aggressive behavior, distrust, and a lack of respect for leaders and the "Green Machine" in general.

To make sense out of psychiatry in the Vietnam War is a daunting proposition. Mental health personnel were caught up in the same environment as the troops. Very few of the 135 psychiatrists deployed to Vietnam were unaffected by the war. Many had strong conflicting emotions surrounding the war. Some psychiatrists were overwhelmed, had a sense of helplessness, and felt they were being used as a trash bin for ineffective soldiers. They too felt victimized by the Green Machine.

Meanwhile in America, the psychiatric community was extremely polarized, with large numbers strongly against the war. Many stateside physicians openly criticized their colleagues serving in Vietnam for supporting the Army Medical Department's primary mission—to conserve the fighting strength. Feelings ran high and active duty physicians were in effect told by their colleagues, "Don't treat the wounded to send them back to their units; medevacuate as many as possible out of the country." As a newly minted psychiatrist serving in Vietnam with the 1st Cavalry Division, I felt betrayed by my own specialty, but their feelings did mirror those of the American public, which ultimately lost all national will to conduct the war. No war can be won if your citizens are against it.

In the aftermath of the war the American public, the military, and civilian leadership collectively breathed a sigh of relief to see Vietnam recede in the rear view mirror. Our first counterinsurgency war in the 20th century was an embarrassment and a failure.

People just wanted to forget it, particularly the behavioral issues. It is interesting that the psychiatric literature pertaining to the war is often contradictory and misleading. The psychiatric records and data that came out of Vietnam were very spotty, fragmented, and incomplete. The Army eventually "lost" most of the primary source material. There has never been a study of "what went wrong" or an official history written of Army psychiatry in the Vietnam War.

Colonel Mike Camp, US Army (Retired), is to be commended for undertaking the daunting task of collecting a composite of published and unpublished articles, reports, and survey Army documents pertaining to mental health issues during the Vietnam War. Dr. Camp had boots on the ground as commander of one of two neuropsychiatric teams (KO) and has walked the walk. The culmination of his efforts is a highly readable, interesting, and valuable account of troop behavior, leadership issues, and historical events ultimately leading to our failure in Vietnam. He divides the war into two phases: 1965–1968, an idealistic time, and 1968–1972, a war inexorably careening awry; as you read you will understand why.

This history is a virtual goldmine of material pertinent to mental health issues in counterinsurgency warfare. Important lessons learned then are as pertinent today as they were 40 years ago.

It is a must read for civilian and military leadership as well as mental health professionals. Since Vietnam, the United States has fought two counterinsurgency wars in the Middle East. Some problematic issues have been addressed, and support of our military is very positive. However, today, even with an all-volunteer Army, there are challenges to be met—discipline problems, suicides, domestic issues, and multiple rotations.

In the end, mental health must be recognized as a command issue from the very top down. Leaders involved with strategic and operational planning must always keep in mind the effects of their decisions on troops placed in harm's way. Colonel Camp's worthy efforts to construct a history of mental health during the Vietnam War fill an important gap that is long overdue. It is an insightful and valuable archive of the many lessons learned relative to our present and future.

Major General Richard D Cameron
US Army (Retired)

Preface

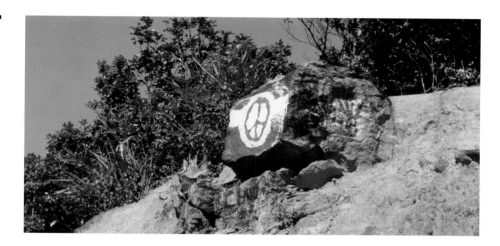

THE AMERICAN GROUND WAR IN VIETNAM (1965–1973) was a "low intensity," "irregular," counterinsurgency/guerrilla war that became prolonged, socially condemned, and ultimately produced great national agony and incalculable cultural aftereffects. Even now, four decades after the last troops were withdrawn, arguments still remain as to whether America was defeated, failed to achieve its military and political objectives, or withdrew prematurely because a liberal media convinced the public that the war could not be won at any reasonable cost. Regardless of the position one chooses, the war was extremely costly in terms of casualties—including psychiatric casualties—and the loss of American resources and international prestige.

Also indisputable, the US Army suffered a severe breakdown in soldier morale and discipline in Vietnam—matters that are at the heart of military leadership and overlap with the mission of Army psychiatry. More specific to psychiatry, the psychosocial strain affecting the troops and their leaders in Vietnam produced a wide array of individual and group pathologies that thoroughly tested the deployed psychiatrists and their mental health colleagues.

No single statistic can reasonably characterize the Army's shifting, as well as accelerating, psychiatric and behavioral challenge in Vietnam. Psychiatric attrition through the course of the war—the incidence of soldiers hospitalized or excused from duty status—ranged between 12 per 1,000 per year and 16.5 per 1,000 per year.[1–3] Although this record appears very favorable compared to rates for the Korean War (73/1,000/year)[4] and World War II (28–101/1,000/year),[4] it is misleading. Not only does this rate address only one measure of soldier psychological and behavioral dysfunction, but in averaging 8 years of experience it also minimizes the fourfold increase in the last few years of the war and disguises the problems that ultimately emerged. In fact, if the increases in psychiatric conditions through the second half of the war are combined with similar increases in behavioral problems (skyrocketing rates for judicial and nonjudicial punishments, racial incidents, combat refusals, attacks on officers and noncommissioned officers, and casual heroin use)—problems that are mostly not included in psychiatric statistics—an incontrovertible truth emerges: the US military ultimately sustained a debilitating psychosocial crisis in Vietnam that, in addition to its humanitarian costs, jeopardized combat readiness. When there is acknowledgment of the extensive morale and discipline problems, there is a tendency to dismiss them as consequences of the emergent drug culture of the times as if the Army, especially in Vietnam, did not unravel from within but was literally infected by a toxic agent that has since been eradicated.[5] Most important, and quite surprising, there has been no official history written about Army psychiatric and behavior problems in Vietnam nor has there been a systematic study by the Army of what happened.

The Army mental health personnel who served in Vietnam brought with them a confidence in principles of combat psychiatry derived from hard-fought pragmatic experiences in World War I, World War II, and Korea. These were handed down by those who served in those wars through systematic efforts at reconstruction and analysis. For example, following both world wars, veteran psychiatrists worked with the US Army Medical Department's historical unit to elaborate a review of the structure and role of Army psychiatry in support of the nation's combat activities.[6–8] The results were an exceptionally thorough and scholarly series that became classics in military psychiatry.

The Army evidently planned to sponsor publication of a similar history of psychiatry after the Korean War. Regrettably, this effort was suspended in 1983 because of the death of the principle author, Colonel (Retired) Albert J Glass. In the late 1990s, his colleague, Colonel (Retired) Franklin Del Jones, took steps to salvage the progress that Glass had made, and the results of this collaboration reside on the server at the Uniformed Services University of the Health Sciences (http://www.lrc.usuhs.edu/Archivex/pdf/CombatPsych.pdf). A partial history of psychiatry in the Korean War also exists in Glass's publications,[9–12] which are augmented by those of other psychiatrists who either served in Korea,[13–15] conducted investigations there,[16,17] or sought to review the record years later.[18]

Taken together, these accounts summarize the psychiatric dimensions of those wars and document the evolution and utility of combat psychiatry. They highlight the considerable challenges faced by Army psychiatrists and the limits of their available psychiatric resources, their achievements, and at times their failures. They also reveal how the changing circumstances within each war altered clinical presentations, treatment approaches, and therapeutic results, as well as led to changes in the preparation and training of mental health personnel who followed. Most importantly, they underscore the necessity that Army psychiatry work closely with military planners regarding potential threats to morale, cohesion, and force resiliency.

However, with regard to the experience in Vietnam, the record has remained fragmented and confused. In the immediate aftermath of the Vietnam War, the Army Medical Department apparently intended to sponsor the creation of a history of Army psychiatry in the war along with other medical specialties,[19] but that project was never begun. The Walter Reed Army Institute of Research (WRAIR) made a tentative effort in the early 1980s under the leadership of Jones. Although WRAIR convened a group of representative psychiatrists who had served during the war, they abandoned the project, evidently because of how much time had lapsed since their service in Vietnam and because the documentation that could have served as primary source material could not be located by the Army (Figure 1).

There have been a few publications that provide summaries of Army psychiatry in Vietnam, but they are limited because they primarily focus on observations from the advisor period and the first half of the war.[4,20–22] In 1975, after the withdrawal of US forces, Jones and Colonel Arnold W Johnson Jr. published a preliminary overview of Army psychiatry in Vietnam when Johnson was serving as the Psychiatry and Neurology Consultant to the Office of The Surgeon General, US Army.[1] They described common clinical entities and provided gross data demonstrating rising prevalence patterns in the theater, which they associated with changing military circumstances and policy features of the war. However, they left greater detail and synthesis for other accounts, which unfortunately were never published—a blind spot repeated even in Jones' otherwise excellent later reviews of the history of military psychiatry.[23,24]

FIGURE 1. Letter to Dr David Marlow

DEPARTMENT OF THE ARMY
THE CHIEF OF MILITARY HISTORY AND THE CENTER OF
MILITARY HISTORY
WASHINGTON, DC 20314

REPLY TO
ATTENTION OF

Clinical History

March 31, 1983

Dr. David H. Marlowe
Chief, Department of Military Psychiatry
ATTN: SGRD-UWI-A
Walter Reed Army Institute of Research
Washington, D.C. 20012

Dear Dr. Marlowe:

Regretfully, I must inform you that despite several
promising leads, I have been unable to locate the records
you requested for a history of psychiatry in Vietnam. As
you suspected, except for a few, it seems they have been
destroyed.

I believe, therefore, that I must make a basic decision
about the future of the project. If these records were
essential for a good clinical history, it would seem I have
no choice but to reluctantly cancel the volume. On the
other hand, if you believe something of value might be produced without them, I would, of course, be willing to continue.

I would very much appreciate the advice of you and your
colleagues on this matter before I reach my decision.

Sincerely,

Jeffrey Greenhut, Ph. D.
Director, Clinical History

Other circumstances also help explain the absence of a more complete Vietnam military psychiatry history. Until it was forced to study heroin use among soldiers late in the war,[25-27] the Army undertook relatively little formal psychiatric research in Vietnam after regular forces were committed in 1965. Notable exceptions were the study of physiologic, psychological, and social correlates of stress by Major Peter Bourne and his WRAIR colleagues conducted in 1965 and 1966,[28] and the surveys of illegal drug use in 1967 by Captains Roger A Roffman and Ely Sapol,[29] and in 1969 by Captain M Duncan Stanton.[30] Also, there were visits to Vietnam late in the war to investigate the drug abuse epidemic by Colonel Stewart L Baker Jr[31] and Colonel Harry C Holloway,[32] senior military psychiatrists, as well as Norman Zinberg, MD,[33] a civilian psychiatrist, which produced informative reports.

Anecdotal accounts published by psychiatrists who served in the war are also a useful source of information.[34] Regrettably, considerable skew is introduced because, of the 28 psychiatrists who served with the Army and who published accounts, 23 (82%) were assigned there during the first half of the war. The few articles by psychiatrists that served during the drawdown phase of the war, when psychiatric attrition rates were highest, are limited descriptions of local patterns of drug abuse or drug treatment programs. Also, of 46 publications from the entire group, half appeared only in the *US Army Vietnam Medical Bulletin*—a nonjuried publication that was produced and circulated in Vietnam and discontinued in early 1971.

Thus, it was with these features in mind—the rampant psychiatric and behavioral disturbances in the second half of the war, followed by decades of institutional disregard for this unprecedented, dangerous state of affairs—that the author set out to create *US Army Psychiatry in the Vietnam War*. The methodology utilized was that of assembling and synthesizing information drawn from a wide variety of available sources to document the successes and failures of the deployed Army psychiatrists and allied mental health and medical personnel. This approach was augmented by data from the author's 1982 survey of the veteran psychiatrists who served with the Army in Vietnam.[35,36] Whereas this review was intended to serve as a historical record, it is not the comprehensive history that should have been developed by the Army. Nonetheless, it does define many of the most salient "lessons learned" with respect to the variables that affected the morale, discipline, mental health, and performance of the troops deployed in Vietnam, as well as those bearing on the mental health specialists sent to support them.

This work will undoubtedly evoke questions that cannot be readily answered; but hopefully it will help shape thought and discovery by others regarding future conflicts. Certain features of the Vietnam theater, that is, a counterinsurgency/guerrilla war that became protracted and politically contentious at home, may more be the nature of US wars in the future than the relatively popular, main force warfare that characterized the earlier wars of the 20th century.[37]

It should be acknowledged from the outset that this work has favored data actually observed in Vietnam or as proximate to the experience there as possible. For a variety of reasons, time and distance from a combat theater are notorious in producing revisions of memory. Furthermore, apart from various exceptions, this review only nominally mentions the other Army mental health professionals (nurses, social workers, psychologists) and paraprofessionals (enlisted specialists) who served side by side with Army psychiatrists in Vietnam throughout the war. It also does not do justice to the considerable numbers of nonpsychiatrist physicians who found themselves in Vietnam bearing the full weight of the psychiatric challenge in their area. In addition, the work also omits discussion of the many psychiatrists and allied personnel in the military evacuation network beyond Vietnam who received (and were challenged by) the most seriously affected soldier-patients from the war. The essential roles these groups played and the sacrifices they made are worthy of their own historical record.

Regrettably, because of the absence of data, this review does not specifically address additional stressors that may have been associated with serving in specific assignment types or situations in Vietnam (eg, officers and noncommissioned officers, elite troops such as Rangers and Special Forces, Army aviators, helicopter crewmen, scouts, tankers, healthcare professionals and paraprofessionals, chaplains, graves registration personnel, explosive ordnance disposal personnel, long-range reconnaissance patrol personnel, advisors, snipers, so-called tunnel rats). On the other hand, although there was extensive study of POWs following their release,[38] the findings pertaining to psychiatric effects of captivity were felt to be tangential to this review. The work also does not include the psychiatric experience of allied military forces in Vietnam or attempt a systematic comparison of the Army with other branches of the US military. Regarding the latter, in selected instances references to the published works addressing the experiences of Navy physicians, including psychiatrists, who provided care for the Marines serving in Vietnam are utilized because of the overlapping nature of the Marine mission with that of the Army.

This account also does not address neurological problems specifically or the deployment of neurologists in Vietnam, although the medical specialties of neurology and psychiatry share a developmental history, and "neuropsychiatry" was commonly used as a synonym for psychiatry throughout the war. In fact, a position for one neurologist was included in the Table of Organization and Equipment of the two Army neuropsychiatry specialty medical detachments that were deployed in Vietnam beginning in 1965; however, by 1970 that connection had been dissolved.

A full review of the important matter of postwar psychosocial effects on those who accepted America's call to service in Vietnam is well beyond the scope of this work. Because, by policy, the majority of personnel assigned there served a single deployment, typically 12 to 13 months in length, concern for long-term psychological effects was of secondary importance among the active service branches during the war. However, during the latter years of the war and the decades to follow, growing evidence of an apparently high prevalence of delayed psychiatric and behavior symptoms among veterans brought increasing clinical and research interest in the negative effects associated with service in Vietnam.[34]

Finally, the reader should view the psychiatric treatment philosophy and clinical approaches represented in this work through the lens of the Army medical and psychiatric doctrine of the 1960s and early 1970s and the applicable civilian standards of care of the times. In this respect it is notable that following the war, the American Psychiatric Association's diagnostic nomenclature, the *Diagnostic and Statistical Manual of Mental Disorders*, 3rd edition (DSM-III [1980]), underwent a radical and controversial revision that, for the first time, required explicit phenomenological criteria for the diagnosis of psychiatric conditions. In time this sea change in the field of psychiatry powerfully affected how society viewed mental health.[39] It also generated a dominant, empirically grounded, biobehavioral psychiatry that in many respects supplanted the decades-old model favoring intrapsychic and psychosocially based etiologic assumptions for psychiatric conditions that had prevailed throughout the war. Within the military, the combination of this paradigm shift and the postwar establishment of the new diagnostic entity, posttraumatic stress disorder (PTSD), redefined levels of acceptable risk for soldiers exposed to the psychological hazards of combat deployment in more conservative terms. This in turn lowered the tolerance levels for psychological risk for combat soldiers within military medicine and psychiatry (This will be discussed in Chapter 12, Exhibit 12-1, concerning post-Vietnam challenges to the forward treatment doctrine.)

REFERENCES

1. Jones FD, Johnson AW Jr. Medical and psychiatric treatment policy and practice in Vietnam. *J Soc Issues*. 1975;31(4):49–65.

2. Baker SL Jr. Traumatic war disorders. In: Kaplan HI, Freedman AM, Sadock BJ, eds. *Comprehensive Textbook of Psychiatry*. 3rd ed. Baltimore, Md: Williams & Wilkins; 1980: 1829–1842.

3. Datel WE. *A Summary of Source Data in Military Psychiatric Epidemiology*. Alexandria, Va: Defense Technical Information Center; 1976. Document No. AD A021265.

4. Tiffany WJ Jr. The mental health of Army troops in Vietnam. *Am J Psychiatry*. 1967;123:1585–1586.

5. Kuzmarov J. *The Myth of the Addicted Army: Vietnam and the Modern War on Drugs*. Boston, Mass: University of Massachusetts Press; 2009.

6. Bailey P, Williams FE, Komara PO, Salmon TW, Fenton N, eds. *Neuropsychiatry*. In: *The Medical Department of the United States Army in the World War*. Vol 10. Washington, DC: Office of The Surgeon General, US Army; 1929.

7. Glass AJ, Bernucci R, eds. *Neuropsychiatry in World War II*. Vol 1. *Zone of the Interior*. Washington, DC: Medical Department, US Army; 1966.

8. Glass AJ, ed. *Neuropsychiatry in World War II*. Vol 2. *Overseas Theaters*. Washington, DC: Medical Department, US Army; 1973.

9. Glass AJ. Psychiatry in the Korean Campaign: a historical review, 1. *US Armed Forces Med J*. 1953;4(10):1387–1401.

10. Glass AJ. Psychiatry in the Korean Campaign: a historical review, 2. *US Armed Forces Med J*. 1953;4(11):1563–1583.

11. Glass AJ. Psychotherapy in the combat zone. *Am J Psychiatry*. 1954;110:725–731.

12. Glass AJ. History and organization of theater psychiatric services before and after June 30, 1951. In: *Recent Advances in Medicine and Surgery*, 19–30 April 1954. Washington, DC: Army Medical Service Graduate School; 1954: 358–372.

13. Kolansky H, Cole RK. Field hospital neuropsychiatric service. *US Armed Forces Med J*. 1951;2(10):1539–1545.

14. Peterson DB. The psychiatric operation, Army Forces, Far East, 1950–1953, with statistical analysis. *Am J Psychiatry*. 1958;112(1):23–28.

15. Marren JJ. Psychiatric problems in troops in Korea during and following combat. *US Armed*

Forces Med J. 1956;7(5):715–726.

16. Rioch DM. *Problems of Preventive Psychiatry in War.* Washington, DC: Army Medical Service Graduate School; October 1954. Project 6-60-015, Subtask No. 6.

17. Harris FG. *Experiences in the Study of Combat in the Korean Theater, II: Comments on a Concept of Psychiatry for a Combat Zone.* Washington DC: Walter Reed Army Institute of Research; October 1956.

18. Ritchie EC. Psychiatry in the Korean War: perils, PIES, and prisoners of war. *Mil Med.* 2002;167(11):898–903.

19. Neel S. *Medical Support of the US Army in Vietnam 1965–1970.* Washington, DC: US Government Printing Office; 1973.

20. Colbach EM, Parrish MD. Army mental health activities in Vietnam: 1965–1970. *Bull Menninger Clin.* 1970;34(6):333–342.

21. Johnson AW Jr. Combat psychiatry, I: A historical review. *Med Bull US Army Europe.* 1969;26(10):305–308.

22. Johnson AW Jr. Combat psychiatry, II: The US Army in Vietnam. *Med Bull US Army Europe.* 1969;26(11):335–339.

23. Jones FD. Psychiatric lessons of war. In: Jones FD, Sparacino LR, Wilcox VL, Rothberg JM, Stokes JW, eds. *War Psychiatry.* In: Zajtchuk R, Bellamy RF, eds. *Textbooks of Military Medicine.* Washington, DC: Department of the Army, Office of The Surgeon General, Borden Institute; 1995: 3–33.

24. Jones FD. Disorders of frustration and loneliness. In: Jones FD, Sparacino LR, Wilcox VL, Rothberg JM, Stokes JW, eds. *War Psychiatry.* In: Zajtchuk R, Bellamy RF, eds. *Textbooks of Military Medicine.* Washington, DC: Department of the Army, Office of The Surgeon General, Borden Institute; 1995: 63–83.

25. Holloway HC, Sodetz FJ, Elsmore TF, and the members of Work Unit 102. Heroin dependence and withdrawal in the military heroin user in the US Army, Vietnam. In: *Annual Progress Report, 1973.* Washington, DC: Walter Reed Army Institute of Research; 1973: 1244–1246.

26. Howe RC, Hegge FW, Phillips JL. Acute heroin abstinence in man, I: Changes in behavior and sleep. *Drug Alcohol Depend.* 1980;5(5):341–356.

27. Howe RC, Hegge FW, Phillips JL. Acute heroin abstinence in man, II: Alterations in rapid eye movement (REM) sleep. *Drug Alcohol Depend.* 1980;6(3):149–161.

28. Bourne PG, ed. *The Psychology and Physiology of Stress: With Reference to Special Studies of the Viet Nam War.* New York, NY: Academic Press; 1969.

29. Roffman RA, Sapol E. Marijuana in Vietnam: a survey of use among Army enlisted men in two southern Corps. *Int J Addict.* 1970;5(1):1–42.

30. Stanton MD. Drug use in Vietnam. A survey among Army personnel in the two northern corps. *Arch Gen Psychiatry.* 1972;26(3):279–286.

31. Baker SL Jr. US Army heroin abuse identification program in Vietnam: implications for a methadone program. *Am J Public Health.* 1972;62(6):857–860.

32. Holloway HC. Epidemiology of heroin dependency among soldiers in Vietnam. *Mil Med.* 1974;139(2):108–113.

33. Zinberg NE. Rehabilitation of heroin users in Vietnam. Contemp Drug Problems. 1972;1(2):263–294.

34. Camp NM, Stretch RH, Marshall WC. *Stress, Strain, and Vietnam: An Annotated Bibliography of Two Decades of Psychiatric and Social Sciences Literature Reflecting the Effect of the War on the American Soldier.* Westport, Conn: Greenwood Press; 1988.

35. Camp NM, Carney CM. US Army psychiatry in Vietnam: Preliminary findings of a survey: I. Background and method. *Bull Menninger Clin.* 1987;51:6–18.

36. Camp NM, Carney CM. US Army psychiatry in Vietnam: preliminary findings of a survey, II: Results and discussion. *Bull Menninger Clin.* 1987; 51(1):19–37.

37. Spector RH. *After Tet: The Bloodiest Year in Vietnam.* New York, NY: The Free Press; 1993.

38. Sonnenberg SM, Blank AS Jr, Talbott JA. *The Trauma of War: Stress and Recovery in Viet Nam Veterans.* Washington, DC: American Psychiatric Press; 1985.

39. Mayes R, Horwitz AV. DSM-III and the revolution in the classification of mental illness. *J Hist Behav Sci.* 2005;41:249–267.

Acknowledgments

ANY THANKS FOR THE HELP I RECEIVED in developing and writing this book has to begin by my paying tribute to my two psychiatrist colleagues at the 98th Neuropsychiatry Medical Specialty Detachment (KO) in Vietnam, Drs. Nathan and Barbara Cohen. Not only did they perform their military medical duties tirelessly, unselfishly, and unflinchingly—despite our year being one of the most difficult in the war—but their friendship, counsel, and moral support were crucial in my maintaining my own poise there, both professionally and personally.

Also high on my list of those deserving thanks are Ronald Bellamy, MD, the former Managing Editor of the Borden Institute, three successive directors of the Borden Institute—Dave Lounsbury, MD; Martha Lenhart, MD, PhD; and Daniel Banks, MS, MD—and, more generally, the editorial staff of the Borden Institute. Their enthusiastic belief in me and my vision for this project reaches back a decade and has served as a core element in my perseverance despite many obstacles. Furthermore, it was my good fortune to have been assigned Linette Sparacino, who has edited in the field of military psychiatry for more than 25 years, as my volume editor. Ms. Sparacino not only offered the ideal combination of personal warmth and thoughtfulness, editorial wisdom, and technical expertise, but she also brought to the task a unique grasp of the historical literature on military psychiatry and awareness of the psychosocial complexity of the Vietnam War for America and those in military service.

I also need to acknowledge and thank the many kind souls—too numerous to list individually—who have tolerated reading and commenting on, usually with good humor, earlier parts of my manuscript. Their earnestness and indulgence has surely helped me avoid getting sidetracked by my personal reflections. However, I have to explicitly acknowledge three individuals by name because of their hard work on behalf of this project and their sustained and generous support of me in the process.

Richard D Cameron, MD, MHA, CPE, an Army psychiatrist, was the commander of the 98th Neuropsychiatric Medical Specialty Detachment (KO) for the first half of his tour in Vietnam followed by service as the division psychiatrist with the 1st Cavalry Division. His distinguished military career, which included his being promoted to the rank of major general, led to assignments as hospital commander, both in Germany and in the United States; Division Surgeon; Corps Surgeon; Commander of Walter Reed Army Medical Center; Commander of Health Services Command; and Deputy Assistant Secretary of Defense for Medical Readiness. My work was undoubtedly greatly enhanced by Major General Cameron generously sharing his comprehension of the psychiatric challenges faced in the Vietnam theater, especially from the standpoint of the division psychiatrist, and his deep background in military medical administration and leadership.

H Spencer Bloch, MD, a civilian-trained psychiatrist and a Vietnam veteran, served his tour in-country as Director, Inpatient Psychiatry Service for the 935th Neuropsychiatric Medical Specialty Detachment (KO). Following his return to civilian life he sought further training in child and adolescent psychiatry, adult psychoanalysis, and child/adolescent psychoanalysis, ultimately publishing *Adolescent Development, Psychopathology, and Treatment*. Dr Bloch's extensive experience in Vietnam in the treatment of serious psychiatric conditions, combined with his in-depth psychiatric and psychoanalytic education and training, made him invaluable in deepening my understanding of the wide variety of clinical presentations in Vietnam and the challenges associated with their treatment.

Finally, the counsel of James E McCarroll, PhD, MPH, an Army psychologist, was sought because of his professional background in both research methodology and clinical practice. In the course of his very accomplished military career, Colonel McCarroll served in a series of assignments in the United States and overseas, including at Walter Reed Army Institute of Research in Silver Spring, Maryland. Upon his retirement he joined the Center for the Study of Traumatic Stress of the Uniformed Services University of the Health Sciences in nearby Bethesda, Maryland. His numerous publications address effects of exposure to traumatic events and stress associated with military deployment, including the secondary effects on military families. Because of his unique and specialized background, Colonel McCarroll's advice across a broad spectrum of issues has been invaluable, especially in the work's combination of qualitative and quantitative data.

Last, but anything but least, I wish to extend my eternal gratitude to my wife, Sydney—not only for her love, interest, and forbearance through the long and sometimes difficult task of writing this book, but especially for being my unflagging emotional base 40 years ago when I served in Vietnam.

A Psychiatrist's Experience During The Drawdown in Vietnam: Coping With Epidemic Demoralization, Dissent, and Dysfunction at the Tipping Point

Change-of-command ceremony for the 95th Evacuation Hospital in the winter of 1970. Such a demonstration of military order and purpose was intended to inspire the medical personnel assigned to the hospital as well as US military and Vietnamese patients who were observing from the adjacent wards. Photograph courtesy of Richard D Cameron, Major General, US Army (Retired).

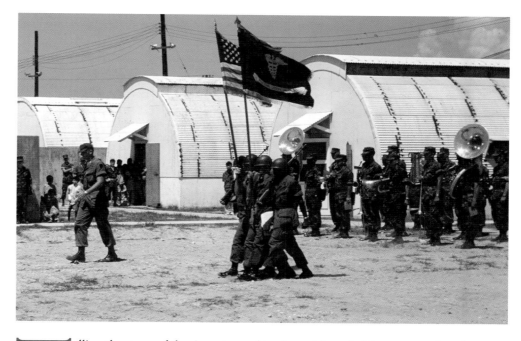

Telling the story of the Army's psychiatric problems in Vietnam requires that one start at the end so that the beginning and middle have context. As for the bitter end, the war in Vietnam came to a dramatic close on 30 April 1975, when America's ally, the government of South Vietnam, surrendered to the overwhelming military force of North Vietnam. For the United States this represented a resounding strategic failure, if not a tactical one. Although American combat personnel had been completely withdrawn 2 years earlier, it must be acknowledged that this was in response to great opposition to the war at home[1]; widespread demoralization in the theater, which was often expressed in psychiatric conditions and behavioral problems (see Chapter 2, Figure 2-2 and Chapter 8, Figure 8-1); and a military leadership that was on its heels. This degradation of military order and discipline, as well as a general compromise of the mental health of the force, was unprecedented and mostly unanticipated because American troop strength had been dropping steadily since mid-1969, and the numbers of US combat casualties had been falling proportionally.

In an effort to document the psychiatric dimensions associated with these calamitous circumstances, I begin here with selected recollections and impressions from my service from October 1970 to October 1971, roughly year 6 of the 8 years of the ground war, as psychiatrist and commanding officer of the 98th Neuropsychiatric Medical Detachment (KO), one of the US Army's two specialized psychiatric treatment and referral centers in Vietnam. Most of what follows was written during the decade after I returned from Vietnam. It was augmented with my official Report of Activities of the 98th Medical [Psychiatric] Detachment (KO) covering the last quarter of l970 (Appendix 1 to this volume) and recently cross-validated with my psychiatric colleagues who served with me at the 98th KO Team. Inclusion of my subjective reactions is consistent with psychiatry's time-honored recognition of the value of the participant-observer approach to data gathering and interpretation.

PREDEPLOYMENT PSYCHIATRIC TRAINING AND PREPARATION

American ground forces were committed in the Republic of South Vietnam in March 1965,[1] in opposition to a communist takeover of that country by indigenous guerrilla forces (Viet Cong) and regular units from the North Vietnam Army (NVA). When I arrived in the fall of 1970, midway through the drawdown years of the war (1969–1973), peace negotiations were being haltingly pursued with North Vietnam, and the earlier US offensive strategy of attrition had been replaced with a defensive one that sought area security and "Vietnamization" of the fighting (ie, turning the fighting over to the South Vietnamese). Still, we were very much at war in Southeast Asia, casualties continued to mount, and public opposition had become impatient and strident.[2]

Despite having many reservations, I volunteered to serve in Vietnam as my next assignment after residency training in psychiatry at the US Army's Walter Reed General Hospital in Washington, DC. Early in 1970, at the time I agreed to an assignment to Vietnam, over 400,000 US troops were still there[3] (from a peak of 538,700 in mid-1969[3]), and I felt it was the right thing to do. However, I also thought I was destined to be sent

anyway because I was one of only two in my graduating class of eight without children.

Overall, my education and training in psychiatry at Walter Reed was excellent. Yet, as far as preparing me specifically to serve as a military psychiatrist in Vietnam, it fell short in three important regards. First, there is the matter of military identity and indoctrination. Like most of my classmates, before beginning the program in psychiatry in 1967 I had completed 5 weeks of Medical Corps Officer Basic Training at the Medical Field Service School at Fort Sam Houston in San Antonio, Texas. However, this was quickly overshadowed by the clinical experience at Walter Reed, a large, busy medical center located in the midst of a densely populated urban area and geographically isolated from the larger Army. Even though my classmates and I wore Army uniforms beneath our white clinical coats, and many of our patients were casualties from Vietnam, we preferred to believe that our training (3 years) would outlast the war, and that we were serving as neutral caregivers who were functioning on the sidelines. This is even more remarkable considering that we were training in the nation's capital and directly exposed to the wrenching social tumult of the late 1960s, especially events associated with the increasingly bitter struggle over the war.

As for the specialized training in psychiatry, our didactic curriculum at Walter Reed did include specific references to combat's high potential to be psychologically traumatic. It also addressed more generally the uniquely stressful influences associated with military environments and circumstances (social as well as physical). However, as I only appreciated after serving in Vietnam, the training was biased in favor of forms of psychological disturbance *within* the individual patient, including soldiers engaged in combat. This training provided only limited practical experience regarding pathogenic group dynamics that can form within military populations and that warrant a "community psychiatry" model. This shortcoming was despite programmatic intentions to the contrary.[4] We mostly studied the principles of prevention and treatment of combat breakdown among soldiers exposed to sustained combat as was seen in earlier wars. And quite strikingly, there was no evident feedback loop to our training program from the Vietnam theater that could have alerted us to the accelerating social, psychiatric, and behavioral problems there—problems not primarily linked to combat exposure. In short, we literally prepared to fight the last war.

Finally, totally absent from our curricula at Walter Reed was acknowledgment of the combat psychiatrist's potential, and most exquisite, ethical dilemma. This refers to situations when clinical decisions become burdened by a clash between military priorities (centered on ostensible collective values) and those of the individual soldier (centered on ostensible individualist values). Although this is not unique to military psychiatry, it ultimately became very pointed in Vietnam and greatly complicated the deployed military psychiatrists' role requirements with implications both for the individual soldier and military force conservation and preparedness.[5,6] This subject will be explored in Chapter 11.

In the spring of 1970 my training at Walter Reed concluded, my assignment in Vietnam loomed, my denial of the personal relevance of the war dissolved, and I felt increasingly unsettled as I made my way to Travis Air Force Base in California for my flight to Southeast Asia. As circumstance would have it, this was a period of reintensification of the war protests in the United States in response to the May incursion into Cambodia by US forces and its allies and the associated riots and student shootings at Kent State (four deaths) and Jackson State University (two deaths) by National Guard troops.[2] It also roughly coincided with an upsurge in alienation of draft-eligible men as a consequence of the Nixon Administration's revision of the selective service procedures eliminating draft deferments and the introduction of a draft lottery system that would be implemented in calendar year 1970.[7,8] These events only served to further heighten opposition, or at least doubt, among the soldiers who were sent to Vietnam as replacements. After 5 years of this war, most Americans had become thoroughly disheartened, impatient with the peace negotiations and the pace of troop withdrawal, and mistrustful of the government and the military.[2] And the mental health of the Army appeared to be unraveling as a consequence,[9,10] especially in Vietnam.[11(p96)] Worst of all, the public seemed to condemn anyone connected with the war, including those whose duty it was to serve there—as if the only honorable attitude for the soldier would be one of opposition and avoidance.[12]

Nonetheless, when I joined the plane full of other replacements on their way to Vietnam on 4 October 1970, my training at Walter Reed had led me to assume that for each individual soldier whose fate it would be to face (directly or indirectly) his counterpart in combat, his reservations or hesitancy could result in his becoming a casualty, physical or psychiatric. If such misgivings were shared by enough of his comrades, the potential also existed for entire units to fail. More specifically, I had confidence in combat psychiatry's doctrine of forward treatment I'd been taught: that brief, simple treatments applied in the vicinity of the soldier's unit and accompanied by the clear expectation that he will soon resume his military duties serve to limit his disability, and, by extension, protect his unit from associated reduction in its combat effectiveness.[13,14]

In other words, as I saw it, a vital part of my job in Vietnam was to support the soldier's inclination to see his military duty through and to oppose the natural aversion of soldiers to combat risks—the "loss of the will to fight" that had been posited to be at the heart of combat stress reactions.[15] However, as I learned soon enough, I was operating under a flawed assumption. By fall 1970, most of the soldiers sent to Vietnam—the majority of whom were either draftees or volunteered to join the Army because they were told it would lower their chances of facing combat—had little sense of duty about serving there. I was not able to anticipate the corrosive psychosocial impact that society's opposition to the war in Vietnam would have on the thousands of soldiers who shared America's war weariness yet still would be sent as replacements to defend its cause under circumstances of increasing moral ambiguity.

THE MISSION, STAFFING, AND STRUCTURE OF THE 98th MEDICAL (PSYCHIATRIC) DETACHMENT

I was assigned to serve as commander of one of two specialized US Army psychiatric referral and treatment centers in Vietnam. Throughout my year the 98th Psychiatric Detachment was attached to the 95th Evacuation Hospital, which was located along the northern coast of South Vietnam near the city of Da Nang. The 95th Evacuation Hospital consisted of a 320-bed "general" hospital and five outlying dispensaries. It was staffed with 65 physicians, representing all medical specialties; 65 nurses; and over 300 enlisted corpsmen. Its mission was to provide a broad range of medical services to the 50,000 to 60,000 American military and civilian personnel in the surrounding area as well those of allied forces. Because the Da Nang Airfield was located on the other side of the city from the hospital and was heavily used by US aircraft, the 1st Marine Division and innumerable smaller US military units (primarily combat support) provided security for the region and a safe haven for our hospital compound, even though the hospital itself was surrounded by a large population of displaced Vietnamese. The 98th Psychiatric Detachment was configured and equipped to be "semimobile" and theoretically could have moved elsewhere to meet changing psychiatric needs; however, it remained physically and organizationally attached to the 95th Evacuation Hospital throughout the year.

Our detachment had a professional complement of four fully trained psychiatrists—one more than we were authorized (in addition to myself, Majors Nathan and Barbara Cohen [married], and Henry [Gene] Robinson—all of whom had just completed their psychiatry training in civilian programs). They likewise remained assigned to the 98th Psychiatric Detachment for the entire year. Later in the year Captain Leslie Secrest, a partially trained psychiatrist, transferred in from his previous assignment near the demilitarized zone with the 1st Brigade, 5th Mechanized Infantry Division. We also had one social work officer assigned (one less than authorized), as well as several psychiatric nurses (one was authorized) who staffed our 15-bed inpatient ward. Although also authorized, we did not have a psychologist assigned. Finally, exceedingly important were the 15 to 20 enlisted corpsmen (neuropsychiatric specialists) who were assigned and who had Army training in social work or clinical psychology.

The mission of the 98th Psychiatric Detachment was to provide specialized hospital-level treatment (up to 30 days) for troops evacuated from all Army units in the northern half of South Vietnam as well as to serve as one of two out-of-country evacuation staging centers for patients needing additional care. The 98th KO Team also provided mental hygiene consultation service (MHCS) capabilities for the large number of nondivisional units from the Da Nang area and scattered along the northern coast of South Vietnam. In effect, our clinical assets were organized around provision of three primary services: (1) definitive inpatient care, (2) assessment and treatment of outpatients, and (3) administrative and forensic evaluations. We also offered psychiatric consultation to the other medical and surgical services of the 95th Evacuation Hospital and its outlying dispensaries as

well as provided on-site consultation and staff training within the Da Nang Stockade. Episodically we provided consultation to command elements of units that came to our attention as referring an inordinately high number of soldiers or whom we learned had sustained some unusual event, for example, a suicide, racial incident, or a "fragging" (term adopted to refer to incidents of soldiers assassinating other service members, including superiors, using fragmentation grenades or claymore mines).

THE INFREQUENCY OF CLASSIC COMBAT EXHAUSTION

Regrettably I did not collect and retain numerical data on the types of patients we evaluated and treated at the 98th Psychiatric Detachment during the year. It was Army policy that all medical records (inpatient and outpatient) remain at the medical treatment facility and in the soldier's personal health record. US Army Republic of Vietnam (USARV) headquarters did collect monthly counts of psychiatric inpatients within a limited taxonomy: psychotic disorders, psychoneurotic disorders, character and behavior disorders (ie, personality disorders), stress reaction, combat exhaustion, and observation-no psychiatric diagnosis.[16] (This is detailed in USARV Regulation 40-34, *Mental Health and Neuropsychiatry*, a complete copy of which is provided in Appendix 2 to this volume.) However, evidently these records were not brought back to the United States or, if they were, they were not archived after the war.

With regard to classic combat exhaustion cases—combat soldiers disabled by psychophysiological reactions to combat—those were seen only occasionally. By design, this should have been the case. As will be explained in Chapter 7, the majority of the combat-generated cases should have been treated at lower medical treatment echelons by each division's medical and psychiatric personnel and returned to duty. As a referral facility, the 98th Psychiatric Detachment was structured to mostly provide extended care for refractory cases (so-called 3rd echelon care).

In fact, throughout the war and throughout the theater, there was a lower incidence of psychiatric and behavior problems generated by combat exposure and risk than had been anticipated from earlier wars. This was attributed to a collection of stress-mitigating factors in the Vietnam theater such as sporadic combat, tours typically limited to 1 year, and various technological advantages held by US troops. Additionally, by 1970 the Army of the Republic of Vietnam (ARVN) was more likely to do the fighting ("Vietnamization" of the war). The enemy had also reduced the overall pace of the fighting.[11(p97)] Furthermore, in the last few years of the war, American troops seemed quite willing to avoid contact with the enemy when possible, even to the point of faking patrols.[11]

However, we, along with other medical personnel assigned to the 95th Evacuation Hospital, did treat many outpatients with less dramatic stress symptoms stemming from combat exposure, or from anticipation of combat. These ranged from psychological symptoms such as anxiety, depression, or aggressive outbursts; to psychophysiologic symptoms such as gastrointestinal irritability or insomnia; to psychosomatic conversion symptoms such as "helmet headache" or "rucksack paralysis" (exaggerated complaints of numbness, tingling, or weakness of the arms from the weight of the pack).

I recall particularly well two soldiers who had acute, disabling reactions to combat. The first I saw within the first few months of my tour. He resembled many of the reactions reported in earlier wars:

CASE 1: Sergeant With Acute Combat Stress Reaction and Partial Paralysis

---

Identifying information: Sergeant (SGT) Alpha was a single, white, E-5 who was evacuated by helicopter to the 95th Evacuation Hospital with other casualties following a nearby firefight.

History of present illness: He complained of numbness and paralysis from the waist down following a near miss by an enemy rocket.

Past history: None obtained.

Examination: Within a relatively brief period of time and in the setting of the hospital's receiving area, I confirmed that he was not otherwise psychiatrically impaired and that there was no physical explanation for his symptoms.

Clinical course: After I listened to his rather bland account of becoming overwhelmed by the combat

situation, I told SGT Alpha that he was suffering with an expectable and temporary reaction from the stress of his ordeal and that soon the numbness of his legs would wear off and the strength in his legs would recover. Although he claimed he could not sit, with effort and my assistance he was able to sit on a stool. I gave him a pair of sawhorses to hold on to for balance and reassured him that he could return to his unit when he felt ready to walk. I also instructed him to seek help from his battalion aid station if his symptoms recurred after he left the 95th Evacuation Hospital. I further instructed the nurses on duty to be matter-of-fact about his imminent recovery and resumption of duty function and to express curiosity about how the rest of the members of his platoon had fared—a group to which he clearly felt committed. When I checked back later I learned that he had walked out of the hospital after about an hour.

Discharge diagnosis: Conversion reaction—paraparesis (ie, a form of combat-induced, acute stress disorder).

Disposition: Returned to duty to be followed by his battalion surgeon.

Source: Case drawn from memory of author in 1980.

I learned no more about SGT Alpha except that he was not returned to us for further psychiatric attention. At the time I was satisfied that this rapidly applied management of conversion symptomatology was effective and in keeping with the previously mentioned forward treatment doctrine for fresh combat-generated psychiatric conditions. The other combat-related case I saw in my last month in Vietnam, and it was different in some important respects.

CASE 2: Private With Disabling Anxiety During His First Firefight

---

Identifying information: Private (PVT) E-2 Bravo was a young, white, first-term enlisted soldier who was new to Vietnam, had never before been in a firefight, and was brought to me by the military police after he had been arrested for desertion under fire.

History of present illness: While he was being processed into the stockade, he complained of acute anxiety and demanded to see a psychiatrist.

Past history: None obtained.

Examination: PVT Bravo was found to have no wounds or other physical problems. He was intelligent and without cognitive impairment. He became agitated as he described how scared and panicked he had become when the fighting erupted, his opposition to the war, and how, naturally, he had boarded the medevac helicopter that had darted in to retrieve the seriously wounded. Even though he was clearly quite afraid—initially of the fighting, and now of confinement and prosecution—he did not demonstrate a psychiatric disorder. It was especially notable that the patient indicated little or no affiliation with members of his unit or commitment to their military mission (compared to SGT Alpha, Case 1).

Clinical course: I felt I had little to provide him other than compassion and reassurance that he did not have a mental disorder. I acknowledged his courage in acting on his convictions but stated that I believed he would probably pay some price for it.

Discharge diagnosis: No disease found.

Disposition: PVT Bravo was psychiatrically cleared and released back to the military police authority.

Source: Case drawn from memory of author in 1980.

PVT Bravo left me with a vivid and uncomfortable memory because he was so direct and naïve in expecting me to save him from the consequences of having made a seemingly rational choice, at least to him, in a seemingly irrational situation. He evidently stirred an ethical conflict within me. However, I felt some consolation in knowing that at least the price he would pay would not include death or becoming wounded, nor the guilt of participating in a war to which he felt morally opposed. Parenthetically, I also wondered how I would have handled his situation.

DRAWDOWN PHASE
DEMORALIZATION AND ALIENATION

Far more demanding of our unit's professional time and energy was the deluge of referrals for whom combat exposure was not a central factor and who expressed symptoms and behaviors associated with disillusionment, despair, dissent, and dysfunction. In that the 98th Psychiatric Detachment was the psychiatric treatment facility of last resort for soldiers from units throughout the northern half of South Vietnam, we were in a unique position to appreciate the bigger picture. What was striking was that most of the soldiers we saw had been previously functional in the United States. This strongly suggested that in becoming symptomatic in Vietnam, especially in such large numbers, significant pathogenic influences were operating at the group or social level. In other words, they had become overwhelmed by a complex interaction of circumstantial stressors and individual characteristics. Whereas our soldier-patients were the more symptomatic individuals, they were the leading edge of a far wider and more ominous demoralization and alienation that was distorting the US Army in Vietnam—a social breakdown of the military organization itself.

Demoralization and Alienation
Beyond the Clinic

Demoralization was glaringly evident with practically every encounter with a service member we had, in or out of clinical settings, and mostly irrespective of rank. Depression and depressive equivalents were ubiquitous. Signs and symptoms included sleeping and eating disorders, irritability, inefficiency, social withdrawal, and psychosomatic symptoms, as well as various regressive behaviors that were attempts to ease these painful feelings, for example, covert or passive antiauthority behaviors, self-medication with drugs or alcohol, and sexual hyperactivity.

In 1967, early in my training at Walter Reed, I had periodically heard soldier-patients repeat a boast they had adopted in Vietnam, "Yea though I walk through the valley of the shadow of death, I will fear no evil—For I am the meanest son of a bitch in the valley." (This play on the 23rd Psalm of David derives from the "infamous Special Forces prayer."[17(p251)]) As time passed and Americans became increasingly opposed to the war, this was replaced with "It's not much of a war, but it's the only war we have." By the time I had arrived in Vietnam in the fall of 1970, cynicism among the replacement troops was even more evident in their "Who wants to be the last man killed in Vietnam?" When I left at the end of my year there, it had become frankly despairing in "If I ever look like I give a fuck, call a medic!"

Especially conspicuous were the provocative behaviors of the younger black enlisted soldiers who would congregate in large clusters and seemed to relish the considerable commotion generated by their prolonged, ritualized handshakes (the "dap"). When passing one another they would exchange the "black power" salute (a raised fist), and many wore black pride jewelry, modified their uniform (eg, having "Bro" embroidered in front of their last name), or wrote slogans on their helmet (ie, "No gook ever called me Nigger"[18(p66)]). Whereas in one sense these were understandable expressions of black pride and solidarity consistent with the rising civil rights movement in the United States, they also easily edged over the line in conveying dissent, and in some cases menace, in the racially charged context of Vietnam. In earlier years the military in Vietnam sought to suppress such group expressions of solidarity among black soldiers through regulations, but these had subsequently been dropped as racial tensions had become increasingly incendiary.[19] Open expressions of racial provocation were not as prominent among the white soldiers, but it was not uncommon to see the Confederate battle flag on display. Although this may have been intended as an expression of regional pride, it was universally interpreted by the black soldiers as racist.

More critically, there existed a spirit of solidarity among lower-ranking soldiers, irrespective of race, centered on strong antimilitary sentiment. Personalized, nonregulation decorations of hair or uniform by enlisted members (EM) openly declared these attitudes. ("Penciled on helmet camouflage bands and chalked elsewhere were such graffiti as peace symbols, slogans such as 'Re-up? I'd rather throw up,' 'Power to the people,' 'Kill a noncom for Christ,' . . . and 'The Army [or Westmorland, or some selected person or outfit] sucks.'"[18(p66)]) Furthermore the challenges to military authority seemed implicitly enforced by the weapons that they carried (or to which they had easy access).

The reciprocal for this spirit of provocation by the enlisted soldier was the apathetic or indifferent reaction of the noncommissioned officer (NCO) or officer. His resigned, inattentive attitude apparently reflected his reaction to intimidation and the uncertain authority that characterized the Army in Vietnam at that time.

Demoralization and Alienation on the 95th Evacuation Hospital Compound

The world of the 95th Evacuation Hospital compound seemed to be a microcosm of the theater. Upon my arrival in Vietnam I was informed by the senior Army psychiatrist in Vietnam, the USARV Psychiatry and Neurology Consultant, Colonel Clotilde Bowen, that I would be assuming command of the 98th Psychiatric Detachment because my psychiatry training had taken place in an Army medical center, and I was presumed to be loyal to military goals and authority. She considered this necessary because the 95th Evacuation Hospital commander, Colonel Jerome Weiner, had threatened to evict the 98th KO Team because some members of its professional staff had been encouraging antimilitary attitudes among the hospital's personnel and patients. (I only came to fully appreciate a decade later why Colonel Weiner was so negative toward the mental health team when I read Shad Meshad's published account of his antiwar, antimilitary advocacy when he was assigned to the 98th Psychiatric Detachment as a social work officer before I arrived.[20])

Upon arriving at the 95th Evacuation Hospital, I learned that it was not uncommon for the Army doctors there to be threatened by patients if the doctors did not agree to evacuate them out of Vietnam. In fact, I was told that shortly before I arrived, our unit's neurologist had been stalked by an armed patient and was required to go into hiding until the soldier was apprehended. (I have not seen further documentation of this particular application to military doctors of the intimidation that enlisted soldiers used against authority figures at that time in Vietnam. However, in an unpublished thesis, David J Kruzich, a social work officer with the 1st Cavalry Division in Vietnam the same year, provided examples of fraggings [or attempts] and included: "A soldier attempted to frag the division psychiatrist who refused to remove him from duty status for psychiatric reasons. The frag bounced off of a screen covering the clinic window and detonated outside."[21(p34)])

On the other side of the issue, however, many of the physicians I came to know at the 95th Evacuation Hospital strongly sympathized with the soldier-patient's wish to have a medical excuse to leave Vietnam. As a matter of practice, these doctors would exaggerate the diagnosis as far as they thought they could to justify the soldier's medical evacuation and felt satisfied that they were contributing to ending the war. (I have not seen further documentation of this either; however, in *365 Days*, RJ Glasser's fictionalized reflections from his service as an Army doctor at an Army evacuation hospital in Japan in 1969, this perspective was echoed. Chapter 1 centered on moral and ethical conflicts in a drafted doctor who sought to manipulate the Army return-to-duty rules so that his recovering patient did not have to resume his tour of duty in Vietnam.[22])

I also learned upon my arrival that one of the 95th Evacuation Hospital's barracks had been claimed as the exclusive territory of the black enlisted soldiers and was barred to others. Periodically Colonel Weiner and his staff would cautiously stage a "health and welfare" inspection of this barracks in search of unauthorized weapons and soldiers who were absent without leave (AWOL). Furthermore, although we were aware of fragging incidents among the nearby support units, several days after my arrival, matters became more personal when a grenade, which apparently had either failed to explode or was intended to serve as a warning to someone, was discovered laying near the doctors' quarters.

Clinical Expressions of Demoralization and Alienation

The enormous volume of psychiatric referrals we saw who had debilitating demoralization and smoldering animosity toward military authority indicated to us that the US Army in Vietnam was indeed at war with itself. Regardless of presenting symptoms, whether it was bitterness and drug use by the younger soldier or depression and alcohol abuse by the older NCO, the reciprocal hatreds and resentments across the superior–subordinate line were easily surfaced (officers were seen less commonly by us, often because of their worry that it could damage their military career).

Modal Presentation for the Enlisted Soldier Seen at the 98th Psychiatric Detachment

Identifying features:
- Lowest ranks, white, drafted, 18 to 22 years old
- Between 5 and 7 months into his 12-month tour
- Not usually assigned to a combat unit—may have seen some action

Impetus for referral:
- Command-referred: either for psychiatric clearance in conjunction with processing the soldier for administrative separation from the Army for repeated discipline problems, or regarding court-martial proceedings for UCMJ (Uniform Code of Military Justice) violations
- Self-referred: seeking rescue from military authority while insinuating threats of loss of impulse control (with weapon used against NCO, injure himself, or by getting "hooked" on drugs)

Background:
- From small town and intact family (happy + or -)
- High school graduate or almost a high school graduate
- Preservice history of social drug use, pre-Vietnam service record was satisfactory
- Has, or had, a girlfriend at home (waning contact)

Clinical observations:
- Quite self-preoccupied, especially regarding release from Vietnam
- Not too disturbed about having been drafted
- Not too passionate about the morality of the war
- Quite passionate in blaming the "lifers" (immediate superiors) and wanting to be free of military control
- Casual about admitting to drug use in Vietnam; references to "close" drug-taking cohorts
- Often fixated/agitated regarding feeling needed at home (eg, to help a sick family member)
- Quite bored and impatient with passage of time
- Painfully aware of unfairness in "the system" (eg, others with safer or more comfortable situations, others leaving Vietnam early as a "drop" [an early release from Vietnam])

Our soldier-patient invariably blamed all of his distress on his circumstance in Vietnam and especially his closest military leaders. The NCO or officer was disdainfully dismissed as a "lifer" or "juicer" (implying alcohol abuse), and was portrayed as an incompetent and malignant authority who was "hassling" him—typically regarding drug use. The soldier-patient, feeling he had nothing to lose, claimed he would not hesitate to destroy his military leader if the warnings went unheeded. Among our caseload, it was extremely common to hear the disgruntled soldier conclude his tirade about his sergeant or officer with "and if he doesn't stop, one of these days somebody's going to frag him!" The allusion was that, if provoked far enough, the disgruntled soldiers in the unit would draw straws for the job of executioner (with a pooled bounty as reward). Furthermore, we knew that fragging could be more than a wishful fantasy as victims from the Da Nang area were brought to our hospital for emergency care. This subject of fragging will be explored more fully in Chapter 2 and Chapter 8. Whereas at this point in time, the US public was not aware of soldier assassinations of their leaders, information we collected informally from nurses who worked in the receiving area of the 95th Evacuation Hospital indicated that such events were not uncommon. It became evident to us that both the prevalence of this defiant threat and the alarming frequency of such acts revealed that lower-ranking soldiers shared extreme feelings of impotence, despair, betrayal, and desperation. Furthermore, the requirement that we assess the level of risk among those we saw was particularly difficult because the threat was often phrased ambiguously.

Modal Presentation for the Noncommissioned Officer Seen at the 98th Psychiatric Detachment

Identifying features:
- White, 30 to 42 years old
- Between 3 and 6 months into second tour in Vietnam
- May have seen some action in first tour but not in this one
- Satisfactory to commendable career performance before this tour

Impetus for referral:
- Self-referred: bitter, depressed, reduced appetite and sleep, acknowledged alcohol abuse
- Command-referred: for ineffectiveness, unreliability, effects of alcohol abuse, low morale

Background:
- Career soldier
- From a small town
- Married with children; no Vietnamese girlfriend
- Waning communications from home

Clinical observations:
- Quite self-preoccupied
- Fearful that he was not needed at home

- Lamenting the absence of military structure and discipline in Vietnam compared to his first tour
- Bitter complaints of lack of support from unit's officers
- Very aware of defiance of enlisted soldiers generally and specifically through heroin use
- Scared to assert authority over oppositional, menacing soldiers (either had been threatened with violence or knew a fellow NCO who had been)
- Evidence of alcohol dependence
- Looking for a (situational) way out; hoping for rescue by the mental health team

The NCO could hardly contain his rage at having his authority challenged by the young soldier and feeling betrayed by his lieutenant who was perceived as too lenient with the restive troops, with the explanation offered that he was closer to their age and typically not a careerist.[18] Furthermore, the NCO feared that attempts at responsible leadership risked his being "blown away" (eg, "fragged").

The Heroin Problem

Coinciding with the bottoming morale, the problem of heroin use by lower-ranking enlisted soldiers also erupted during our year and became enormously disruptive for the military in Vietnam. None of us at the 98th Psychiatric Detachment were surprised to find high drug use among the soldier population during our tour because the rising tide of drug use in the American youth culture was well documented, a very influential phenomenon that will be explored in Chapter 1. What we weren't prepared for, however, was the extremely high proportion of soldiers who were preferentially utilizing heroin (or, in a minority of instances, other drugs with serious addictive potential, such as barbiturates and amphetamines). In early 1970, a few months before my arrival, a very efficient Vietnamese heroin distribution system spread throughout South Vietnam, and our soldiers became eager customers. A carton of cigarettes costing a soldier $1.80 could easily be exchanged for a vial of heroin (250 mg, 95% pure[23]) that would have had hundreds of dollars of American street value. As a consequence of it being available in such a pure and inexpensive form, soldiers commonly used heroin recreationally and socially, usually through smoking with tobacco or snorting.

As heroin use spread, the assessment and management of affected soldiers increasingly dominated our psychiatric team's resources. The information we gained from patients and others suggested that 30% to 40% of the enlisted soldiers in our catchment area, especially noncombat troops, were using heroin, at least sporadically. These informal estimates coincided with those shared by colleagues at our sister unit in the south, the 935th Medical (Psychiatric) Detachment near Saigon. These estimates were collected informally during a psychiatric drug abuse conference held at Cam Rahn Bay in November 1970, which was arranged by Colonel Bowen, the USARV Psychiatric Consultant. For the better part of a year following the beginning of the heroin market, except for monitoring arrests for drug possession, or drug overdose cases, the US military authority in Vietnam could only approximate the extent of heroin use among soldiers, but by any measure it was a rapidly worsening situation.

Drug Rehabilitation/Amnesty Program

In response to rising numbers of soldiers using addicting drugs in Vietnam and an urgent demand for containment of the problem, on 29 December 1970 USARV headquarters published the "Drug Rehabilitation/Amnesty Program"[24] letter (nicknamed the "amnesty program") as a theater adaptation of Army Regulation 600-32.[25] In addition to outlining the procedures and conditions regarding amnesty, the letter directed commanders to provide the following elements for the purpose of drug rehabilitation (as noted in AR 600-32, "for restorable drug abusers, when appropriate, and consistent with the sensitivity of the mission"[25(¶2-5)]). First, the unit commander was to direct any drug-using soldier to the nearest medical facility for whatever acute care medical personnel would determine was necessary. Upon release, the commander was instructed to assess the soldier's potential for successful return to previous duties and responsibilities and, if suitable, enroll him in the unit's Drug Rehabilitation/Amnesty Program. This included informing his direct supervisor of his "key role in the rehabilitation of the soldier"[24(¶6C (4))] and linking the rehabilitee with a counseling "buddy"—a peer who could "act as a positive influence, and . . . provide counseling and supportive assistance in the soldier's endeavors to remain free of drugs."[24(¶6C(2)a(2))] The program was also to provide the soldier with group therapy "wherein [he] may receive support from ex-drug abusers, associate with others who are attempting to stop using drugs; and receive professional counseling from the unit surgeon, chaplain or qualified visiting professionals."[24(¶6C(3))] Finally, the commander was to destroy all records of the soldier's participation in these programs (ie, amnesty and rehabilitation) when the soldier departed the unit.

Unfortunately, establishing an effective drug treatment and rehabilitation program turned out to be far harder than drafting a policy. During the 9 or so months between when the heroin market began to thrive and the implementation and standardization of the urine drug-screening procedures, there was great confusion as to how to identify drug-using soldiers, how to manage (medical, administrative, or judicial) their drug use or drug-related misbehavior, and how to ultimately decide if they were fit for further duty, in Vietnam or elsewhere. Furthermore, word-of-mouth dissemination of news of an "amnesty program," which initially seemed to exist in name alone, implied judicial carte blanche to soldiers and promises of medical magic to commanders.

The urgency of the problem meant that major Army units were forced to draw upon the resources at hand to improvise facilities and programs intended to offer drug treatment and rehabilitation. These typically had whimsical, unmilitary names (ie, "Sky House," "Highland House," "Operation Guts," "Head Quarters," "Pioneer House," "Crossroads," and so forth), were spawned from the imaginations of those involved, usually individuals with little or no experience treating substance abuse, and often were staffed with counselors who claimed to have kicked the habit themselves.

With rare exception, these programs achieved only marginal success in keeping enrollees from returning to heroin use (unless the soldier was within a few weeks of the end of his tour in Vietnam) and often faded away because of discouragement in the staff or the unit's command, exposure of drug dealing or use by the staff, or the departure of key staff members who were rotated home from Vietnam. Finally, in June 1971, over halfway through my tour, reliable urine drug-screening technology came on line in Vietnam and allowed the US military to identify drug users (but for the first 5 months this was limited to soldiers departing Vietnam) and monitor detoxification in controlled centers; but it had only a modest effect on soldier use (see Chapter 9).

Throughout this stormy period, the 98th Psychiatric Detachment was often at cross purposes with those commanders who chose to interpret the USARV Drug Rehabilitation/Amnesty Program to mean that the management of these soldiers was to be solely in a hospital-based, medical program. Typically with no notice and little or no documentation, soldiers by the truck full arrived at our hospital, often after a trip of many hours and without having received any prior medical attention, for hospitalization, (presumably) detoxification, and rehabilitation or evacuation out of Vietnam. Furthermore, the soldiers themselves were eager to be hospitalized by us—they hoped indefinitely—to get relief from duty and military authority. In innumerable instances, the soldier had waited until he was in legal jeopardy before demanding that he be admitted to the amnesty program—in clear contradiction to the regulation.

Our assessments often utilized a narcotic antagonist to measure the extent of physical dependency. This approach was recommended in a Technical Guidance Letter (see Appendix 3)—"for battalion surgeons, division surgeons and psychiatrists, and MEDCOM (Medical Command) physicians/psychiatrists in the evaluation, treatment, and processing of patients suspected of narcotic addiction"—distributed by the 67th Medical Group (21 October 1970), the command authority over Army medical units in the northern half of South Vietnam. This medically supervised challenge test consisted of the subcutaneous administration of increasing doses of Nalline [N-allyl-normorphine] to suspected opiate-dependent soldiers to bring out objective signs of withdrawal (which, if induced, would then be treated supportively).[26] This test was only positive for about one out of every 10 soldiers,[27] primarily those who had resorted to intravenous use or snorting. For the remainder, we assumed that their continued use of heroin should, in large part, be considered volitional (ie, misconduct), and we returned them back to their units for further rehabilitative, judicial, or administrative considerations—to be medically monitored by their dispensary physician. In our estimation, this manner of triage was consistent with USARV Regulation 40-34[16] (*Medical Services: Mental Health and Neuropsychiatry*), which stipulated that outpatient management should be emphasized over inpatient, and hospitalization was to be avoided when possible, especially in the case of soldiers who primarily needed custodial care; but it did make us unpopular with the drug-using soldiers and with many commanders.

By way of a case example, the following material (disguised) is from the record of a psychiatric contact at the 95th Evacuation Hospital.

CASE 3: Attempted Murder Suspect Seeking Exoneration Through the Drug Amnesty Program

Identifying information: PVT Charlie was a 25-year-old, single, black E-2 who was assigned as a sentry dog handler and who was in the process of being charged with intent to commit murder.

History of present illness: He was brought to the 98th Psychiatric Detachment by his first sergeant prior to pretrial confinement because he complained that he was addicted to heroin ("snorting two caps per day") and was demanding to be admitted to "the amnesty program." According to accompanying documents, the patient shot another soldier in the stomach after he had confronted the patient with his failure to stand guard duty earlier. The patient's excuse at the time was that he could not perform guard because he had ingested four capsules of Binoctal (a French barbiturate), snorted heroin, and smoked marijuana. As he chased the other soldier and shot him with his pistol, he was heard screaming, "I'm going to kill you, you white bastard!"

Past history: PVT Charlie was raised in Alabama as the youngest of three sons. His parents separated about the time of his birth and he rarely saw his father. His mother died of a heart condition when he was 12. At 15, he was sent to a juvenile confinement facility for burglary. Upon release 2 years later he lived briefly with his father, produced an erratic employment record, and then enlisted in the Army. During a prior tour in Vietnam he received two Article 15s (for AWOL and failure to obey an order). During his current assignment he received three Article 15s (for AWOL), and a bar to reenlistment.

Examination: In the receiving ward of the 95th Evacuation Hospital, the patient presented as a tall, thin, young man who was calm, fully alert, oriented, and in no distress. His manner was provocatively unmilitary, punctuated with gestures and phrases of the black culture. His mood and thought processes were normal. He appeared of average intelligence, and his judgment and insight were fair. He was blasé about the interview and blamed his shooting of the other soldier on his drug habit.

Clinical course: Monitored administration of Nalline failed to demonstrate physical dependence to opiates.

Discharge diagnosis: The examining psychiatrist concluded that the patient did not warrant a psychiatric diagnosis but should be considered to have strong antisocial tendencies. He also expressed the opinion that PVT Charlie should be considered fully accountable for his behavior regarding the shooting incident, but that his apparent heavy drug use, if substantiated, could be considered a mitigating circumstance.

Disposition: The patient was cleared for duty and for administrative or judicial proceedings.

Source: Report of psychiatric evaluation prepared for the Office of the Staff Judge Advocate.

Given the circumstances, it is not surprising that PVT Charlie was not seen subsequently at the 98th Psychiatric Detachment.

CHALLENGES FOR THE 98th PSYCHIATRIC DETACHMENT

As the year progressed our clinical resources and stamina were increasingly taxed by such referrals. The following review of the professional components of the 98th Psychiatric Detachment and the 95th Evacuation Hospital will be illustrative.

The Inpatient Service

Our inpatient facility and staff permitted us to offer a level of care equivalent to a stateside military psychiatric unit, and we were typically very busy delivering milieu-centered care and pharmacotherapy for soldiers who manifested a broad range of psychiatric disorders. Our relatively low rate of admission compared to the extensive prevalence of maladjustment among the troops was in large part a consequence of our intention to distinguish medically treatable illness from command issues of morale and discipline. In compliance with USARV Regulation 40-34, we applied the principles of combat psychiatry, that is, returning the soldier back to duty as soon as medical treatment issues subsided. However, we were frequently challenged by commanders who insisted we admit soldiers who, by our assessment, did not have a psychiatric disorder. These soldiers did possess the capacity to perform their duties (or discontinue drug use, or conform to properly executed military orders, etc) and consequently warranted a custodial setting instead. We often lost these battles and, to our distress, our ward's treatment milieu became predictably disrupted by these soldiers.

In the cases of those we did admit for detoxification, our program results were often uncertain because, despite our best efforts, it was impossible to keep our psychiatric ward drug-free, and, for most of the year, we had no reliable laboratory capacity to monitor withdrawal. Vietnamese boys stood patiently outside the hospital's barbed-wire perimeter day or night ready to supply the demand for drugs, and emptied plastic heroin containers were commonly found among our hospital's waste. Probably the most disconcerting element for us was that the majority of soldiers we saw did not agree they had a problem. They typically rationalized their habit by either denying that the use of heroin was disabling or dangerous, or by blaming the Army for forcing them to serve in such an impossible situation as Vietnam, or both.

The Outpatient Service

In our outpatient clinic, we did see a very small proportion of soldiers who genuinely sought treatment for their inability to adjust, that is, those who did not blame something outside of themselves for their difficulties and wanted assistance in shoring up flagging personal resources. More commonly, we performed an endless series of evaluations of discontented, dysfunctional soldiers for whom command sought either administrative separation from the Army or counseling in conjunction with the USARV Drug Rehabilitation/ Amnesty Program. These soldiers were often sullen, resentful, and obstreperous. The majority of them were determined to manipulate the system so as to obtain relief from their discontent through being eliminated from the Army (and presumably sent home from Vietnam) as quickly as possible, even if it meant they would receive a prejudicial discharge.

In October a change to AR 635-212,[28,29] the Army regulation for underperforming soldiers who were being processed for discharge from the Army, eliminated the requirement that a psychiatrist evaluate every soldier for whom a commander recommended administrative separation from the service (see Appendix 4). However, the flow of these referrals continued to accelerate because if the commander was in a hurry to get rid of a contentious soldier who was failing to perform, he could bypass a lengthy process requiring documentation of failed rehabilitation efforts if he could get an Army psychiatrist to label the soldier a "character and behavior disorder" (ie, a sustained, especially preservice, pattern of maladjustment). This was very trying work for us because we, too, often felt caught in the middle. We sought to execute our duties responsibly and felt loyal to the Army, even while we were eager for the war to end (and even more eager for our year in Vietnam to end).

More palpable, however, was our commitment to the relief of suffering in our soldier-patients. We felt empathetic with their antiwar feelings, if not their antimilitary ones. We also were respectful of their self-protective instincts. However, in the majority of cases they did not manifest a psychiatric condition, including a character and behavior disorder, and we believed that administrative or judicial Army agencies, and not medical authorities, held primary responsibility for their disposition. In this regard, we attempted to reduce the numbers of inappropriate referrals of soldiers for simple insubordination and indiscipline through the dissemination of a memo to local commanders reiterating the specifics of the Army regulation for administrative separations for unfitness and unsuitability (Appendix 5, 98th Medical Detachment (KO) Memo: "Requirements for Psychiatric Evaluation as Part of Elimination of Enlisted Personnel Under the Provisions of AR 635-212").

(After I left Vietnam I read that just across Da Nang harbor from us, Lieutenant Commander HW Fisher, Navy psychiatrist, was having similar difficulties with the command referrals from the 1st Marine Division.[30] According to Fisher's report, of 1,000 consecutive referrals, he diagnosed 96% having character and behavior disorders. [See Chapters 2 and 9 for a further discussion of his referrals.])

Technically we had the option of offering psychiatric treatment or proposing other rehabilitative steps that the commander might implement. However, in the majority of instances these soldiers reacted to us as if we were agents of a persecuting Army and would not cooperate. Also, by this time, commanders had little spirit for attempting further rehabilitative efforts as well. They were having their own morale crisis.[10,31] This can be illustrated in the memo to all subordinate commands from Brigadier General Hixon, Chief of Staff, XXIV

Corps, some time in the spring of 1971 (Appendix 6, "Administrative Elimination Under Provisions of AR 635-212"). XXIV Corps was a major component command of Headquarters, US Army Republic of Vietnam (USARV) and controlled all US ground forces in I Corps Tactical Zone, which comprised the five northernmost provinces of South Vietnam. In the memo General Hixon commended the leadership for reducing the numbers of soldiers with drug abuse patterns who were inappropriately recommended for Honorable or General Discharge and urged commanders to further shorten the time lag in the administrative processing of undesirable or unfit soldiers. Remarkably, however, he also commented that,

> [I]t has been noted with concern that in several cases referred to this headquarters for elimination . . . a well documented record is provided of shirking and/or frequent incidents of flagrant disregard of orders and regulations, to include contemptuous behavior toward superiors. In these same cases, however, the unit commander reported without comment that no disciplinary action had been taken or was pending. . . .

As the year progressed there was increasing emphasis through the Army chain of command in Vietnam on communicating leadership principles to commanders and urging them to take a moderate stance toward troop complaints and provocations. Guidance letters came regularly from USARV headquarters instructing commanders and their staffs how to participate in "rap sessions" with unit Human Relations Councils. One example, dated 10 February 1971 (Subject: Human Relations),[32] which offered advice regarding how to lead seminars with soldier groups, encouraged commanders to: relinquish traditional symbols of authority, such as entering the room last or using a speaker stand or stage; "Be prepared to admit that error or injustice has occurred"; "recognize the fact that [it] may be a result of your own ignorance or misinformation"; and share "some intimate, personal experience . . . in order to become a member of the group."[32]

Finally, it is not possible to overemphasize how valuable our enlisted corpsmen (neuropsychiatric specialists, commonly referred to as "psych techs" or simply as "techs") were in the assessment and treatment of this difficult population. They served as the primary counselors for approximately 80% of referrals. Not only did these corpsmen prove to be extraordinarily capable and committed to the mission and the soldier-patients they saw, but they also had an enormous advantage over the professional staff in working with soldiers because, being comparable in age and rank, they were more likely to be trusted.

Command Consultation

Primary prevention outreach activity in military psychiatry (eg, providing advice to commanders regarding matters that may be negatively affecting soldier morale and psychological fitness) falls under the heading of command consultation and has a rich professional heritage dating back to World War II and the Korean War. Psychiatric support in the military context also insinuates that clinical assistance includes efforts to mediate between the symptomatic soldier and his primary group, that is, the small unit to which he is, or should be, a member (secondary prevention). "Group" refers to his enlisted cohorts as well as to his more immediate military leaders (NCOs, officers) and presumes the primacy of the military mission. However, during our year, the psychiatrists with the 98th Psychiatric Detachment had limited success with these social psychiatry activities for several reasons.

First and most obvious, our time and energies were consumed with performing evaluations and providing care for the huge volume of referrals. Also, the units with whom we might liaise—typically nondivisional, noncombat units—were scattered widely across the northern half of South Vietnam, and we faced formidable transportation and communication obstacles to interact with them. In addition, because I was the only one of the four psychiatrists with the 98th KO Team with any pre-Vietnam military experience, the others were far less confident leaving the clinical setting to deal with line commanders and NCOs. Furthermore, on those occasions when I sought to provide consultation to a unit that was referring unusually high numbers of solders to us, I more often than not came away discouraged. I either encountered despondency among leadership elements similar to what we saw in our soldier-patients, or found my interest and expertise to be unwelcome. I was treated as an outsider by both officers and NCOs, and I had the strong impression that they feared I was there to expose their failures.

One consultation I do recall took place on the USS *Oriskany*, an aircraft carrier. I probably remember it because it was dramatic in nature and because I was invited to intervene and not treated as a threat.

Example of Command Consultation (Secondary Prevention)

In March 1971, I was flown offshore to the USS *Oriskany* at the invitation of the senior medical officer who wanted my help in responding to a suicide pact made by six sailors who worked in the boiler room. These men complained that requiring them to work in the extreme heat there was inhumane, and they had threatened to jump overboard if they weren't relieved of that duty. Once aboard, I conducted clinical interviews with each of them in the boiler room (140°F —disturbingly hot) and then met collectively with them to listen to their grievances. Not surprisingly, many were diffuse complaints about authoritarian military regulations and so forth. I also had an extensive interchange with the medical staff and the sailors' supervisors. I concluded that these were not cases of clinical depression but of dispirited sailors. I supported command in keeping these sailors at their jobs but encouraged command to devise a system of special incentives (eg, shorter shifts, more breaks, additional perks) that could compensate for those elements of the boiler room environment that were beyond the stress level of other jobs aboard the ship. I also suggested that if there was a suicide attempt, that it be regarded as misconduct rather than as a symptom of mental illness, and that these sailors be informed of that before the fact.

Later I informally heard that one of the sailors had jumped off the stern of the carrier, in the daylight, in front of witnesses. The sailor was safely retrieved, held in sickbay for a day for observation, and ultimately placed in the brig to await administrative proceedings. There were no subsequent incidents of this nature afterward, and command was satisfied with this outcome. I had no information as to how the men experienced it.

REDEPLOYMENT

Consequent to nothing more momentous than months, weeks, hours, and minutes ticking by, I packed up my things and left Vietnam on 4 October 1971, exactly 1 year after I arrived. By then, US forces still numbered over 200,000 and soldiers were still dying or becoming wounded in combat, even if at a reduced rate. The end of the war was promised but not yet in sight. By then, all three of my original psychiatrist colleagues had rotated home after their year was over, and I was involved in orienting replacement staff for the 98th. As an aside, my physical safety was never in serious jeopardy in the course of the year, but that is the sort of thing one dared not acknowledge until your DEROS flight left the tarmac. I don't regret that I went to Vietnam, and I am very proud to have served my country. However, I left Vietnam deeply troubled by what my psychiatric unit faced during our year.

Clearly the long drawdown from the protracted, stalemated, and bitterly controversial war had substantially and negatively affected the US Army in Vietnam. By the time we arrived late in 1970, the requisite military culture of commitment and cohesion had retrogressed into a pathological, antimilitary one with features suggesting a class war between lower ranks and their superiors—an inversion of military morale. From our vantage point, the consequent psychiatric challenges were truly staggering—with respect to our stamina and resources, and regarding our feelings about the work. In other words, we had our own demoralization with which to contend. Instead of providing a therapeutic function for our soldier-patients, or an educational/consultation one for their leaders, we were far more often relegated by circumstances to serving as sorters, medicators, processors, and too often custodians for the psychological casualties of a seriously dysfunctional military organization.

Consequently, perhaps with the exception of our inpatient service, the 98th Psychiatric Detachment served a limited and, more often than not, quite unsatisfying role—unsatisfying to the majority of soldiers who sought relief through us, unsatisfying to the commanders who referred them, and unsatisfying to ourselves. As for our patients, we listened to a flood of anguish and made our best efforts to provide empathy, support, and occasionally antianxiety or antidepressant medication. We ultimately, necessarily, returned the soldier, or the NCO, to the same situation from which he came and were powerless to alter him or it. For a series of reasons our attempts at primary and secondary prevention through command consultation were equally unsatisfying: we could not influence the social pathology affecting our soldier-patients and their leaders as the greater strain was at the "macro" level; our psychiatric detachment was organizationally only adjunctive to the military units we were responsible for serving; and we

favored the individual model of psychopathology that had been the basis of our training.

Despite all this, I did derive some consolation from the knowledge that the deterioration of morale, discipline, and mental health in the theater did not exceed the tipping point, that is, widespread institutional failure, riots, mutiny, dereliction of duty, or outright sabotage, and American combat preparedness was not seriously tested by the enemy. Furthermore, when I recalled specific soldiers who were clearly better off because we were there, I felt some satisfaction as well.

POST-VIETNAM SYNTHESIS

In the decade that followed my service in Vietnam, I found myself increasingly frustrated with the Army's failure, including that of Army psychiatry, to study the serious, and in many respects disabling, morale and mental health problems that became so widespread in the theater. Fortunately in 1980 I was assigned to Walter Reed Army Institute of Research (WRAIR) and had an opportunity to explore these matters in more depth. Following an exhaustive review of the psychiatric and social science literature surrounding the war[33] and extensive discussions with colleagues, including FD Jones, who served in Vietnam during the buildup phase, I delineated the following set of socio-environmental features that I believed were so corrosive to the troops serving in the drawdown in Vietnam.

PATHOGENIC PSYCHOSOCIAL STRESSORS AMONG LOWER RANKS DURING THE DRAWDOWN

Summary of the Demoralizing Stressors Borne by the Replacement Soldiers of 1970 and 1971

Encounters with enlisted soldiers at the 98th Psychiatric Detachment and elsewhere taught us a great deal about the stressors that led them to feel so dispirited, angry, and desperate. They can be divided into the following six categories. Because there is considerable overlap, and in that it is difficult to distinguish cause from effect, there is no assumption of order of importance. It is again underscored that it was our sense that these psychosocial stressors affected all service members in Vietnam to varying degrees in 1970 and 1971, not just our patients.

Feeling Purposeless

There was a predictable morale-depleting effect when the US switched from a more active, offensive strategy in Vietnam to a defensive one ("Vietnamization"). This left the soldier feeling little purpose in his risk and sacrifice. Instead, according to the soldiers we saw, they felt they were only marking time while waiting for America to carefully extricate itself from the region. Such deterioration in military espirit and conduct during a withdrawal has been seen in previous American wars.[34] Apparently, as long as the military objective has been perceived as still having meaning, the austere, regimented, and dangerous living and working conditions, including the combat itself, have been mostly tolerable. But following even a clear victory or negotiated truce, much less an ambiguous conclusion like in Vietnam, reactions associated with demobilization arose. It was our impression that in drawdown Vietnam, military personnel, especially those who were not careerists, demonstrated through behaviors and, at times, psychiatric symptoms, their reluctance to take risks and make further personal sacrifices, especially forced remoteness from loved ones and from previous social roles.

Feelings of Shame

The soldier assigned in Vietnam in the drawdown phase also had to contend with the sense of being blamed by Americans at home. As the war progressed it was increasingly common for returning soldiers to be greeted by war protesters with jeers and taunts like "baby killers,"[35,36] and even allegedly spit on.[11,37] By 1970, much of the stateside media as well as sentiments from loved ones[38] seemed of one voice—that participation in the war was dishonorable and that true patriots were individuals who avoided service there or openly opposed the military. Although he wanted to believe that his activities in Vietnam "don't mean nothing!" because "the World" was only what existed outside of Vietnam, it was our impression that the soldier serving late in the war was nonetheless deeply troubled by the condemnation he personally sustained by cooperating, no matter how passively or partially, with the US military effort. Some have argued[39,40] that the personnel who fought in Vietnam were unaffected by the controversy because they were apolitical; however, from our experience, many clearly struggled with contradictory feelings—for example, opposed to the war yet critical of war protesters in the United States.[12]

Feeling Increasingly Vulnerable

As soldiers experienced a diminishment of the shared, combat-centered goals, there was a rising concern for personal safety. In Vietnam in 1970 and 1971, every soldier we spoke to was reassured to learn of the declining troop numbers and casualty rate. However, he perceived that the US resolve for fighting the war was dissipating and that the original rationale was questionable at best. He might have found it tolerable to be there if he could believe his war might end soon—safely for him—through a negotiated truce and a troop withdrawal; but this prospect remained elusive and distant. He felt especially tormented when he heard of other soldiers who suddenly—seemingly randomly—received a "drop" (early return to the United States), or of whole units that left on short notice. This would be especially hard for the soldier who remained behind and was assigned to combat duty because, although everyone seemed to agree that a ceasefire was imminent, he and his buddies were still sent on missions. To him, therefore, these were meaningless missions that could lead to contact with enemy forces. Thus, there was little impetus to be a bold warrior, and his attention necessarily became focused around trying to influence factors that might reduce his exposure and increase his survival odds.

Feeling Excessive Hardship

Soldiers had to make do with less in the culture of "(relative) deprivation."[41,42] The late Vietnam soldier morale also seemed eroded by the prevailing attitude among US forces centered on the attainment of individual status and comfort, which had replaced an earlier one of collective purpose and individual sacrifice.[43] Upon his arrival in Vietnam, the new soldier rapidly became aware that various individuals, usually those with the opportunities of rank or position, seemed to suffer appreciably less with respect to hardships, deprivations, or risk than others in this retrograding circumstance. The traditionally disadvantaged, that is, racial minorities and the underclasses, were the ones most likely to have to get along with less[43]—the men with the most to risk and the least to gain. Perceived disparities especially included who was most likely to become a combat casualty or suffer greater exposure to the inhospitable environment. Particularly vexing was to be deprived of otherwise quite ordinary, but precious, commodities (air-conditioners, flush toilets, etc) and opportunities (to socialize with Western women or freely transport oneself to post exchanges, recreational areas, or other facilities, etc). Furthermore, we saw that the soldier that was new to Vietnam was quickly warned by his fellow soldiers that those with rank and seniority had status, comfort (relative), and limited risk. Even worse, any tendency for these leaders to promote their careers through combat enthusiasm could result in unnecessary casualties.[31]

The Effects of Prolonged Confinement, Boredom, and Isolation

It is impossible to exaggerate the combined longing for home and loved ones and the search for a justifying meaning for his risk and sacrifice that preoccupies a soldier sent to fight in a foreign setting. The soldiers we treated in Vietnam repeatedly shared these same kinds of yearnings and concerns with us. Thus, adding to his feeling impotent, exploited, and shamed was the soldier's boredom in reaction to inactivity and isolation. In the Saigon area many US personnel found ways to have judicious, off-duty contact with the Vietnamese outside of military boundaries despite the lack of authorization, and in so doing some may have found opportunities to learn about the Vietnamese and their culture and discover meaning in their experience. However, for most soldiers South Vietnam outside military compounds was "off limits,"[44] and contact with the indigenous Vietnamese was through limited interactions with day laborers hired by the military to perform menial jobs on the bases or brief, mutually exploitive transactions with prostitutes when the opportunity arose.[44,45] The week of rest and recuperation ("R & R") leave, which was enjoyed by all personnel at some point in their tour, served as a highly valued form of psychological decompression; but in the long run it represented a minor exception. As a result, thousands of American troops were sequestered in small, isolated, and heavily guarded compounds or firebases. The only way to venture out for any reason, such as a trip to the post exchange or even to an appointment at the hospital, was in one of a very limited number of military vehicles or aircraft. Consequently, opportunities to escape the embrace of the immediate military setting and authority were rare. This predictably fueled "island fever" (ie, heightened interpersonal conflicts and intolerance) among the troops stuck in these small cantonments.

Feeling Debased and Oppressed by Military Authority

Many a soldier recounted to us how his initial willingness to serve out his military obligation in Vietnam, despite hardship and risk, was quickly replaced by a bitter disillusionment as he experienced the actual conditions in the theater. Apparently this conversion arose once he was fully cut off from previous ties and identities. He then became a participant—no matter how indirectly or passively—in the socially condemned war. He was immersed in the inverted and adversarial culture of the Army in Vietnam, surrounded by the antimilitary attitudes of his peers. Although it was not likely that someone with rank would openly debase a soldier in Vietnam, the prevalent status and privilege system in a culture of relative deprivation and risk powerfully implied stigmatization and devaluation. Throughout the war, soldiers who faced little or no combat risk were referred to by the combat-exposed troops by the disdainful term REMF—*rear echelon mother f--ker.*" Furthermore, by this point in the war, this distinction was greatly heightened because the troops challenged most combat objectives. The prospect of cohorts risking being killed or wounded signified the most explicit form of debasement possible in their eyes. Reactions of those feeling victimized readily fueled latent tensions between other subgroups (ie, racial minority vs white, disadvantaged vs social mainstream, and younger vs older), which periodically clashed as a displacement for anti-institutional passions. Especially prevalent were tensions between enlisted soldiers and military leaders regarding drug use and possession.

Soldier Shame, Despair, and "UUUU"

The stressors outlined above were compounded by many others such as:

- the impairment of pre-Vietnam bonding with fellow soldiers, leaders, and the military mission (so-called commitment and cohesion) because of the random, individualized, 1-year tours in Vietnam;
- disruption of ties between soldiers and their small unit officers because of the theater policy of rotating officers from command to staff positions after 6 months (to increase opportunities to command);
- racial and "generation gap" tensions brought to the combat theater from the increasingly fractious stateside culture;
- the extremely inexpensive heroin that was efficiently marketed by the Vietnamese almost no matter where a unit was located;

- popular press publications exposing corruption by high-ranking Vietnamese and opportunistic Americans,[18(p150),43,46] as well as allegations of combat atrocities, a subject that will be explored in Chapter 6; and
- the persistent possibility of attack by an enemy who might become bolder as the US troop strength declined and defenses thinned.

As a consequence, lower-ranking soldiers bonded around antimilitary sentiments as if victims of a tyrannical regime. The resultant collective state of mind was especially reflected in the popular graffiti "UUUU" (which stood for: "We are the unwilling, led by the unqualified, doing the unnecessary, for the ungrateful").[18(pp44,111),46,47(p10)] This slogan expressed the collection of elements that comprised the soldier's acute sense of moral conflict and betrayal. Referring to himself as the "unwilling" alluded to a sense of impotence and of feeling coerced. "Led by the unqualified" referred to feeling misled by his most immediate leaders, as well as insinuates the danger he faced in combat. "Doing the unnecessary" condemned the war's rationale and, by implication, those with ultimate authority (civilian and military). And, "for the ungrateful" revealed his feelings of alienation from fellow Americans and his consequent disdain. This soldier's lament included no specific reference to feeling blamed and stigmatized, but such feelings were in fact the source of the slogan's paradoxical components, that is, it was a collection of psychological efforts that served to proclaim his innocence and find others more deserving of blame and shame.

Soldier Adaptations and Symptoms

The projections and rationalizations noted above apparently provided only limited relief because we saw many types of individual and group efforts, some more adaptive than others, to reduce this painful state. The most common of these are what sociologist Erving Goffman called "removal activities" and "release binge fantasies," that is, activities useful at killing time or awareness of circumstance that have been described in settings of forced confinement such as prisons or mental institutions.[48] The soldier in late Vietnam ritualistically marked his "short-timer's calendar," searched the sky to sight "freedom bird" flights to the United States, and generally had prolonged and rapturous discussions with peers about desires to be fulfilled in abundance once he was released from "Nam" back to "the World." Whether through legitimate activities, such as shopping at the post exchange, watching movies, attending USO (United Service Organizations) shows, or recording cassette tapes to send home, or more questionable ones, such as drug and alcohol use or frequenting prostitutes, the pursuit of such avenues was obviously highly valued. It takes little additional data to understand the degree to which the soldier experienced himself as miserable and isolated from life and the living, and, like the prison inmate, felt that time had to be "done."

Soldiers also chose to relieve pent-up tensions through various "counterauthority" behaviors. These consisted of episodic, peer-group-sanctioned, passive but inherently aggressive behaviors that were designed to preserve a sense of individual autonomy through some form of forbidden activity that would frustrate military authorities yet avoid real risk. Behaviors such as "search and avoid" combat missions[11]; "shamming," that is, the pretense of activity but without productivity; and especially, habitually getting "stoned" (intoxicated, but with illegal drugs) served this end. The great popularity of heroin use by soldiers in Vietnam can be explained on the basis that it allowed the maximal fulfillment not only of the goals of "removal" (from place and circumstance) and "counterauthority" (the sense of thwarting the institution and its authorities), but also of two other simultaneous goals: submersion in an affirming affinity group and relief of individual psychological tension.

Especially alarming was the growing popularity of the idea of peer group-sanctioned, anonymous assassination of leaders, which at times was a real threat. (Open defiance and threats toward officers and NCOs were far less common but still occurred.) These incidents were more often committed by characterologically predisposed soldiers whose inhibitions were lowered by alcohol or drug use. Desertion and AWOL were a proportionally less common solution because of the alien surrounding environment. Finally, a minority of the enlisted patients we saw, but still an extensive number, became clinically depressed with either agitated or retarded (ie, lethargic) features, usually including preoccupation with concerns of breakthrough of violent impulses (suicidal or homicidal). A much smaller number became totally disabled with psychosis.

PATHOGENIC PSYCHOSOCIAL STRESSORS AMONG OFFICERS AND NONCOMMISSIONED OFFICERS DURING THE DRAWDOWN

Officer/Noncommissioned Officer
Search for Meaning and Motivation

We also learned about the sources of anguish, adaptations, and symptoms among officers and NCOs, but much more came from exchanges outside of the formal clinical setting. Although not disheveled or undisciplined appearing as were many of the young enlisted soldiers, any clinical or social contact with an officer or NCO in 1970 and 1971 revealed him to be equally stressed and miserable in his role of caretaker authority. To a large degree he bore some of the same hardships and deprivations as did everyone who served in Vietnam (risk of attack by the enemy, remoteness from home and loved ones, inhospitable environment, alien cultural surroundings, etc). Like the enlisted soldier, he, too, lacked conviction in an overriding, valid rationale for US military activities in Vietnam. Aspirations for victory shared by those serving earlier in the war had long since been replaced with a simple desire to survive the assignment as safely and as comfortably as possible, and, for the officer/NCO, with as few as possible casualties among his men. To a considerable degree, his sentiments echoed the younger soldier's "UUUU" lament, but he was resigned to his career commitment to the military—right or wrong—and conducted himself accordingly. However, as leader/authority he suffered a sense of corporate impotence regarding military operations in Vietnam (it was a common assumption in 1970–1971 that the South Vietnamese regime could not hold off the communist forces after the US forces departed) and had some appreciation for the decline in the integrity of the military as an institution. Furthermore, having also recently arrived from the midst of American stateside culture, like the lower-ranking enlisted soldiers, he, too, had witnessed its reversal in attitude toward the war in the United States and directly or indirectly felt society's blame of those who served there; but beyond that he had to withstand the stigmatization of his military career. On the other hand, unlike the enlisted soldier (as well as many of the young lieutenants who were just serving out their obligation), the individual with higher rank could at least have some comfort in believing that his career goals might be advanced by service in Vietnam.

Regarding the demoralization and alienation affecting his unit, the officer/NCO believed he was a victim of circumstance (ie, beginning with the bad luck of getting assigned to Vietnam during the drawdown period); had inherited a bad situation from those more truly responsible (such as military and government policymakers or fellow officers who preceded him in Vietnam); and had little enthusiasm for trying to correct the problems related to his angry and undisciplined troops. Nonetheless he was greatly stressed by the hostility and provocation of these soldiers and also morally torn.

Officer/Noncommissioned Officer
Adaptations and Symptoms

As with the young enlisted soldier, the career officer or NCO sought relief from this collection of stressors. However, in his case he had some options only available to those with rank. He also generally wished to avoid confronting his resentful troops. One common and often harmful adaptation was the tendency of many officers to overly defer to their NCOs to enforce that degree of discipline that was unavoidable. This may have been especially true for leaders of platoon-size units where young 2nd lieutenants were more sympathetic with the antiwar, and, to a certain degree, antiauthority values of the soldiers than were their career NCOs. Also, to me and my mental health colleagues it seemed that too often commanders defaulted to medical channels to avoid their own obligation to respond to these pernicious morale and discipline problems. When this happened, our availability for those who more truly needed us was compromised, and more appropriate legal or administrative processes became delayed and confused.

Emotional blunting and escaping time and situation constraints through the use of alcohol was the most commonly used personal relief mechanism for officers and NCOs, similar to the marijuana and heroin use by the enlisted soldiers. However, compared to the enormous attention devoted to drug use among lower-ranking soldiers, alcohol abuse, especially among those with rank, was mostly overlooked in Vietnam until the individual became frankly dysfunctional. From our point of view, alcohol dependency and addiction was as individually disabling as was the use of illegal drugs, but it was much less provocative to the Army, the media, and the public at home.

Of course some officers and NCOs suffered with frank psychopathology, especially variations of depression. This was far more common among the NCOs who had no recourse but to continue to engage with the restive soldiers. Most officers and NCOs seemed to believe that morale was near the flashpoint and elected to bend as far as possible. Some, however, did not and perhaps were targeted for fragging. Likewise the enlisted soldiers noted that they got little or no opposition on most issues, that a minimum was really expected of them, and that open defiance without imperative cause would in all likelihood delay their departure from Vietnam—a most dreaded prospect.[49] Thus, a sort of uneasy stalemate prevailed, but one with many provocative incidents, enormous numbers of psychological casualties, and, perhaps, substantial jeopardy to military preparedness.

THE WALTER REED ARMY INSTITUTE OF RESEARCH VIETNAM PSYCHIATRIST SURVEY

Finally, there are the results from the Walter Reed Army Institute of Research survey of Army psychiatrists who were veterans of the Vietnam War that was mentioned in the Preface and will be more fully described in Chapter 5. This research permitted me to test the generalizability of my experiences, observations, and conclusions, as well as those of other psychiatrists who published their accounts, through the systematic collection of the experiences of all who served. Findings from this survey will be utilized to amplify the subjects covered in Chapters 6 through 11.

In conclusion, despite the late date I believe that through the window of psychiatric experience and sensibilities, important elements explaining the deterioration of morale and mental health in Vietnam can be illuminated with this review. In particular I anticipate that in elaborating and synthesizing this complex history as I have sought to do, the difficulties faced by veterans can be more readily comprehended by those who wish to help and support them. It is also my hope that the results will serve to encourage policymakers and military leaders to appreciate more fully the limitations of human nature under these specific conditions of war and deployment (especially from the standpoint of the social psychology of military groups) and plan accordingly for the future.

REFERENCES

1. Karnow S. *Vietnam: A History*. New York, NY: Viking; 1983.

2. Dougan C, Lipsman E, Doyle E, and the editors of Boston Publishing Co. *The Vietnam Experience: A Nation Divided*. Boston, Mass: Boston Publishing Co; 1984.

3. Department of Defense, OASD (Comptroller). Directorate for Information Operations. US Military Personnel in South Vietnam 1960–1972; 15 March 1974.

4. Tiffany WJ Jr, Allerton WS. Army psychiatry in the mid-'60s. *Am J Psychiatry*. 1967;123(7):810–821.

5. Camp NM. The Vietnam War and the ethics of combat psychiatry. *Am J Psychiatry*. 1993;150(7):1000–1010.

6. Camp NM. Ethical challenges for the psychiatrist during the Vietnam Conflict. In: Jones FD, Sparacino LR, Wilcox VL, Rothberg JM, eds. *Military Psychiatry: Preparing in Peace for War*. In: Zajtchuk R, Bellamy RF, eds. *Textbooks of Military Medicine*. Washington, DC: Department of the Army, Office of The Surgeon General, Borden Institute; 1994: 133–150.

7. Johnston J, Bachman JG. *Young Men Look at Military Service: A Preliminary Report*. Ann Arbor, Mich: University of Michigan, Survey Research Center, Institute for Social Research; 1970.

8. Baskir LM, Strauss WA. *Chance and Circumstance: The Draft, the War, and the Vietnam Generation*. New York, NY: Alfred A Knopf; 1978.

9. Datel WE. *A Summary of Source Data in Military Psychiatric Epidemiology*. Alexandria, Va: Defense Technical Information Center; 1976. Document No. AD A021265.

10. Gabriel RA, Savage PL. *Crisis in Command: Mismanagement in the Army*. New York, NY: Hill and Wang; 1978.

11. Lipsman S, Doyle E, and the editors of Boston Publishing Co. *The Vietnam Experience: Fighting For Time*. Boston, Mass: Boston Publishing Co; 1983.

12. Moskos CC Jr. Military made scapegoat for Vietnam. In: Millett AR, ed. *A Short History of the Vietnam War.* Bloomington, Ind: Indiana University Press; 1978: 67–72.

13. US Department of the Army. *Military Psychiatry.* Washington, DC: HQDA; August 1957. Technical Manual 8-244.

14. Johnson AW Jr. Psychiatric treatment in the combat situation. *US Army Vietnam Med Bull.* 1967;January/February:38–45.

15. Kormos HR. The nature of combat stress. In: Figley CR, ed. *Stress Disorders Among Vietnam Veterans: Theory, Research and Treatment.* New York, NY: Bruner/Mazel; 1978: 3–22.

16. US Department of the Army. *Medical Services: Mental Health and Neuropsychiatry.* APO San Francisco, Calif: Headquarters, US Army Vietnam; March 1966. US Army Republic of Vietnam Regulation 40-34. [Full text available as Appendix 2 to this volume.]

17. Cragg D. Viet-speak. *Maledicta—International J Verbal Aggression.* 1982;6:249–261.

18. Cincinnatus. *Self-Destruction: The Disintegration and Decay of the United States Army During the Vietnam Era.* New York, NY: Norton; 1981.

19. Terry W. The angry blacks in the Army. In: Horowitz D and the editors of Ramparts, *Two, Three . . . Many Vietnams: A Radical Reader on the Wars in Southeast Asia and the Conflicts at Home.* San Francisco, Calif: Canfield Press; 1971: 222–231.

20. Meshad S. *Captain for Dark Mornings: A True Story.* Playa Del Rey, Calif: Creative Image Associate; 1982: Chap 4.

21. Kruzich DJ. Army Drug Use in Vietnam: Origins of the Problem and Official Response. Minneapolis, Minn: University of Minnesota, School of Public Health; May 1979. (Unpublished manuscript; copy provided to author 8 December 1986).

22. Glasser RJ. *365 Days.* New York, NY: G Braziller; 1971.

23. Holloway HC. Epidemiology of heroin dependency among soldiers in Vietnam. *Mil Med.* 1974;139(2):108–113.

24. US Department of the Army. 98th Medical Detachment. APO San Francisco 96349. Subject: Drug Rehabilitation/Amnesty Program. Memo dated 5 April 1971. Reference Headquarters, US Army Vietnam Supplement 1 to AR 600-32, dated 29 December 1970.

25. US Department of the Army. *Drug Abuse Prevention and Control.* Washington, DC: Headquarters, Department of the Army. September 1970. Army Regulation 600-32.

26. Noel PJ Jr, Colonel, Medical Corps, Deputy Surgeon, 67th Medical Group. Procedure for determining narcotic addiction–Technical guidance. 21 October 1970.

27. Camp NM. Report of activities of the 98th Med Det (KO) for the six months ending 31 December 1970 to COL C Bowen, Psychiatric Consultant, USARV. [Full text available as Appendix 1 to this volume.]

28. US Department of the Army. *Personnel Separations: Discharge Unfitness and Unsuitability.* Washington, DC: Headquarters, Department of the Army. 15 July 1966. Army Regulation 635-212. Available at: http://www.whs.mil/library/mildoc/AR672.htm; accessed 21 June 2012.

29. US Department of the Army. Headquarters, US Army Republic of Vietnam. Memo dated 4 June 1971. Subject: Interim changes to AR 635-212 and AR 635-206. Source: DA Message for AGPO, 122117Z.

30. Fisher HW. Vietnam psychiatry. Portrait of anarchy. *Minn Med.* 1972;55(12):1165–1167.

31. Fulghum D, Maitland T, and the editors of Boston Publishing Co. *The Vietnam Experience: South Vietnam on Trial, Mid-1970 to 1972.* Boston, Mass: Boston Publishing Co; 1984.

32. US Department of the Army. Headquarters, US Army Vietnam. APO San Francisco 96375. Subject: Human Relations. Memo dated 10 February 1971.

33. Camp NM, Stretch RH, Marshall WC. *Stress, Strain, and Vietnam: An Annotated Bibliography of Two Decades of Psychiatric and Social Sciences Literature Reflecting the Effect of the War on the American Soldier.* Westport, Conn: Greenwood Press; 1988.

34. Jones FD. Disorders of frustration and loneliness. In: Jones FD, Sparacino LR, Wilcox VL, Rothberg JM, Stokes JW, eds. *War Psychiatry*. In: *Textbooks of Military Medicine*. Washington, DC: Office of The Surgeon General, US Department of the Army, and Borden Institute; 1995: 63–83.

35. Bey D. *Wizard 6: A Combat Psychiatrist in Vietnam*. College Station, Tex: Texas A & M University Military History Series 104; 2006.

36. Lipsman S, Doyle E, and the editors of Boston Publishing Co. *The Vietnam Experience: Fighting For Time*. Boston, Mass: Boston Publishing Co; 1983.

37. Grossman DA. *On Killing: The Psychological Cost of Learning to Kill in War and Society*. New York, NY: Little, Brown; 1995.

38. Tanay E. The Dear John syndrome during the Vietnam War. *Dis Nerv Syst*. 1976;37(3): 165–167.

39. Bourne PG. *Men, Stress, and Vietnam*. Boston, Mass: Little Brown; 1970.

40. Moskos CC Jr. *The American Enlisted Man: The Rank and File In Today's Military*. New York, NY: Russell Sage Foundation; 1970.

41. Stouffer SA. *Studies in Social Psychology in World War II: The American Soldier*. Vol. 1. *Adjustment During Army Life*. Princeton, NJ: Princeton University Press; 1949.

42. Runciman WG. *Relative Deprivation and Social Justice: A Study of Attitudes to Social Inequality in Twentieth-Century England*. London, UK: Routledge; 1966.

43. Spector RH. *After Tet: The Bloodiest Year in Vietnam*. New York, NY: The Free Press; 1993.

44. Doyle E, Weiss S, and the editors of Boston Publishing Co. *The Vietnam Experience: A Collision of Cultures*. Boston, Mass: Boston Publishing Co; 1984.

45. Forrest DV, Bey DR, Bourne PG. The American soldier and Vietnamese women. *Sex Behav*. 1972;2:8–15.

46. Balkind JJ. *Morale Deterioration in the United States Military During the Vietnam Period* [dissertation]. Ann Arbor, Mich: University Microfilms International; 1978: 235. [Available at: *Dissertations Abstracts International*, 39 (1-A), 438. Order No. 78-11, 333.]

47. Eisenhart RW. Flower of the dragon: an example of applied humanistic psychology. *J Hum Psychol*. 1977;17(1):3–24.

48. Goffman E. Characteristics of total institutions. *Symposium on Preventive and Social Psychiatry*. Washington, DC: Walter Reed Army Institute of Research; 15–17 April 1957: 43–84. Expanded as Goffman E. *Asylums: Essays on the Social Situation of Mental Patients and Other Inmates*. New York, NY: Doubleday; 1990.

49. Rose E. The anatomy of a mutiny. *Armed Forces Soc*. 1982;8(4):561–574.

CHAPTER 1

Contexts of the Vietnam War and US Army Psychiatry: A Debilitating War Fought a Long Way From Home

What has been called a strategy of containment is designed to bring about peace and reconciliation in Asia as well as in Europe. In the U.S. view, only if violence is opposed will peace and reconciliation become possible. If aggression succeeds [in Vietnam], the Asian Communists will have shown that [Chinese Communist Chairman] Mao [Tse-tung] is right: The world can only be reshaped by the gun.[1(p5)]

Why We Fight In Viet-Nam
US Department of State Pamphlet
June 1967

A war protest demonstration in Washington, DC, in the spring of 1971. The antiwar movement in the US, which was expressed though increasingly larger and louder protest rallies, marches, and demonstrations, was. For the troops fighting in Vietnam it signified growing opposition to the war and was a prominent if not the overriding contextual factor responsible for their steady demoralization of the troops fighting in Vietnam Photograph courtesy of Sydney Fleischer Camp.

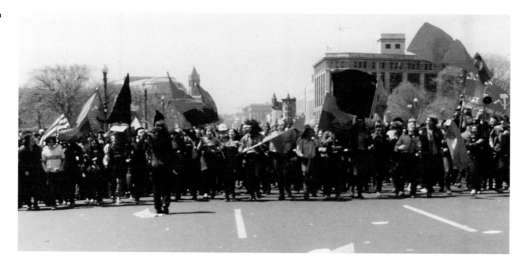

The US ground war in Vietnam (1965–1973) began on 8 March 1965, when over 3,500 men of the 9th Marine Expeditionary Brigade made an unopposed amphibious landing on the northern coast of the Republic of South Vietnam. This was in response to intensification in the fighting between the military forces of South Vietnam—an ally of the United States—and indigenous communist forces as well as those from South Vietnam's neighbor to the north, the Democratic Republic of Vietnam (commonly referred to as North Vietnam). In early May the first US Army ground combat troops, the 173rd Airborne Brigade, arrived in South Vietnam, landing at the mouth of the Saigon River at Vung Tau. In time, service members from all branches of the US military became part of a multinational effort by the United States and other free world allies that sought to block the spread of communism in Southeast Asia.

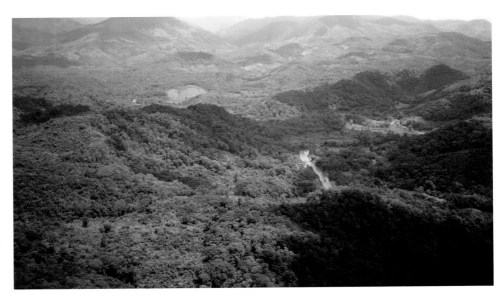

FIGURE 1-1. Arial view of the rugged terrain in Vietnam. Most combat operations in Vietnam occurred away from the urban areas and in the mostly unpopulated four-fifths of the country. In this challenging and unforgiving countryside US troops encountered formidable impediments to movement over the ground, extraordinary heat and humidity, and monsoonal rains for months at a time. Photograph courtesy of Richard D Cameron, Major General, US Army (Retired).

The insertion of American ground forces in Southeast Asia followed a 15-year period of escalating US commitment of financial aid and military advisors whose purpose was to support the government and military of South Vietnam in defending itself against a takeover sponsored by North Vietnam. More than 8 exhausting years of warfare followed. American involvement ended following mounting public protest in the United States, the "Vietnamization" of the allied war effort (assisting South Vietnamese forces to assume the primary combat role), and the drawdown of US military forces and civilian advisors. But just 2 years after the negotiated truce that resulted in the withdrawal of the remaining American military personnel (29 March 1973), North Vietnam violated the truce and overran South Vietnam, which surrendered on 30 April 1975.

The war became far wider, longer, and costlier than predicted—the United States and its allies had become intractably ensnared in Vietnam's simultaneous and protracted social revolution, civil war, and nationalistic opposition to foreign domination. The war also assumed a central role in a decade of social and political upheaval in the United States—a nightmare that threatened its most basic institutions, including the US military. In the second half of the war (1969–1973), as Americans came to disown and denounce the war in Southeast Asia, an increasing and ultimately huge proportion of US troops assigned in Vietnam came to question their purpose there. They expressed in every way short of collective mutiny, including psychiatric conditions, their inability or unwillingness to accept the risks of combat, acknowledge military authority, or tolerate the hardships of an assignment in Vietnam. Yet this all occurred in a setting where combat objectives were still in effect, weapons were ubiquitous, violence was adaptive, and narcotics and other drugs were effectively marketed and widely used by US troops.

This chapter summarizes especially salient aspects of the historical, military, and sociopolitical context of the war that add meaning to the role challenges and ethical issues faced by the Army psychiatrists and allied mental health professionals who served in Vietnam.

VIETNAM: ITS LAND, PEOPLE, CULTURE, AND HISTORY

Throughout the war, it was the rare US soldier who had much understanding of where he was fighting (beyond knowing he was in Southeast Asia) and why (beyond "stopping communism").[2,3] The following offers a condensed description of Vietnam and selected historical features bearing on those questions. Especially useful as sources for this review have been the multivolume series, *The Vietnam Experience*, by The Boston Publishing Company;[4] and *The Vietnam Guidebook*,[5] written by Barbara Cohen, MD, a psychiatrist who served with the Army in Vietnam.

The Land

Located in Southeast Asia and halfway around the world from the United States, Vietnam (a term that will

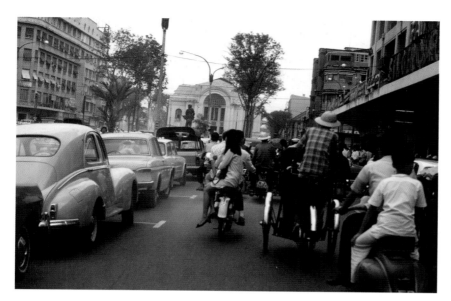

FIGURE 1-2. A street scene in downtown Saigon. Saigon, the capital of the Republic of Vietnam, commonly referred to as South Vietnam, was a large, bustling, urban city during the war. Following the surrender of South Vietnam to North Vietnam in 1975, it was renamed Ho Chi Minh City. Until 1973, when US military personnel were withdrawn from Vietnam, many troops assigned in the Saigon area found ways to interact with the Vietnamese outside of military boundaries, despite the lack of authorization, often for illicit commercial purposes such as prostitution, drug acquisition, and black marketeering. Photograph courtesy of Richard D Cameron, Major General, US Army (Retired).

be used in this section to represent both the northern and southern halves) shares the Indochinese peninsula with the countries of Laos, Cambodia, Thailand, Burma (now Myanmar), and Malaysia. Indochina projects south from the continent of Asia into the South China Sea, and Vietnam hugs its eastern side. Vietnam lies in the tropical zone, its long, thin "S" shape oriented in a north–south direction. Its area approximates that of the state of California, and it extends roughly 1,200 miles from its northern border with China to its southern border on the Gulf of Thailand. Vietnam is a lush country that contains two large, fertile river deltas—the Red River in the north and the Mekong River in the south. These comprise roughly 25% of the country and are linked by a backbone of rugged mountains (Figure 1-1). The northern urban centers of Hanoi and Haiphong lie in the Red River delta, and Ho Chi Minh City (formerly Saigon) is in the Mekong River delta in the south (Figure 1-2). About half of the country is jungle, with roughly 80% covered by tropical vegetation.

The People

Vietnam is one of the world's most densely inhabited countries. During the war the population was estimated to be 40 million people[6]; however, the first scientifically conducted census, which was taken in 1979, 4 years after the fall of the Saigon government, calculated Vietnam's population at 53 million.[5] More than half of the population lives in the coastal plains and the lowlands formed from the two river deltas.

Rural villages are home to 85% of the Vietnamese population[5]; their lives are centered on subsistence farming—mostly rice growing—or fishing. Family life and that of the village are the basic units of Vietnamese culture. As suggested by the name "Indochina," the countries that share the peninsula have arisen from the convergence of the two great civilizations nearby—India and China. Furthermore, because of its geographic circumstance of hugging the coast, Vietnam in particular has served as the crossroads of Southeast Asia.

Over the years of prerecorded history, Indian and Chinese traders, missionaries, and especially immigrants came there and extended their cultures and technologies throughout the area. Its mountainous spine meant that the Chinese influence from the north would eclipse that of India from the west. Most of today's Vietnamese (88%),[5] called the Viet (or Kinh), descended from those who emigrated southward from their ancient homelands in China's southern provinces and mixed with the indigenous people to form the dominant culture. The racial ancestors of the Viet Vietnamese are a mix of Chinese and non-Chinese people of Mongolian descent, as well as those of Indo-nesian and Filipino heritage.[5] At least 54 minority ethnic groups comprise the remaining population,[5] all of which made the American understanding of Vietnam more complicated (Figure 1-3).

The Vietnamese language has elements of Cambodian, Thai, and Chinese and, although it is written in Roman characters, a heritage that dates back to Portuguese missionaries, it is especially challenging for

FIGURE 1-3. A Vietnamese peasant woman from a fishing village on the coast near Nha Trang. At the time of the war roughly 85% of Vietnamese lived in rural villages, and their lives centered on subsistence farming—mostly rice growing—or fishing, and family and village life. The war was not fought as much for territorial control as for the allegiance of these people. Photograph courtesy of Richard D Cameron, Major General, US Army (Retired).

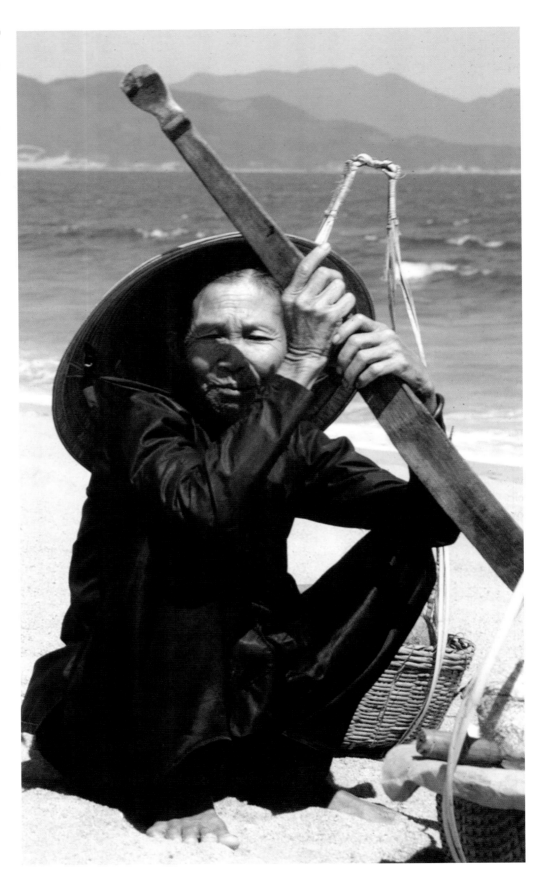

Westerners to speak because it is a tonal language.[6] A syllable may have as many as six inflections, each of which carries a different meaning.

Cultural Identity

Throughout its long history, the national identity of the Vietnamese people has been forged by violent struggles against foreign domination, civil wars, and their own aggressive expansionist ambitions. Indeed, the national borders of Vietnam were not defined until the late 18th century. By then the Vietnamese had incorporated the southernmost areas—the land of the Hindu Cham people who were descended from Hindu and Polynesian cultures.[5] The tumultuous history of the Vietnamese greatly contributed to their tenacity in fighting the United States and its allies in South Vietnam. For them, especially those living in the north, the Vietnam War (1965–1973) merely represented the most recent chapter in a centuries-old resolve to establish territorial claims and self-determination.

Relevant History

China, Vietnam's Colossal Neighbor

The Vietnamese people identify their prehistoric roots as deriving from the ancient, some say legendary, kingdom of Au Lac, a thriving culture that is said to have inhabited land north of Hanoi in the Red River valley. However, between 500 BCE and 300 BCE Chinese emigration into northern Vietnam had begun[6] and, over time, set the stage for almost a thousand years of Chinese rule and assimilation (111 BCE–938 CE).[6] Because of its geographic proximity, Vietnam has always had close political ties with China; moreover, this protracted history of subjugation by the Chinese in the first millennium guaranteed close cultural ties as well. The ultimate defeat of the Chinese in the Battle of the Bach Dang River in 938 CE initiated over 800 years of Vietnamese self-rule before colonization by the French in the mid-19th century.

100 Years of French Colonialism

Western influence in Vietnam began in the middle of the 16th century, when Catholic missionaries arrived from the Portuguese possession of Macao.[5] By the 17th century, French missionaries became even more prominent and helped to open up Vietnam to commerce with the West (French, Portuguese, Dutch). However, these Westerners were regarded with suspicion by Vietnamese emperors as potentially leading to unwelcome foreign influence. Gradually, these nations insinuated themselves in the politics and often violent struggles in Vietnam as they sought to establish exclusive trade rights.

In 1802 Nguyen Anh united by force the southern part of Vietnam with the northern part with the help of a mercenary army raised by the Bishop of Adran, a French missionary.[5] The newly proclaimed emperor named his kingdom Vietnam and established a new capital in Hue. He also granted commercial concessions to French merchants as reward for the military support he had received. Over time, however, the involvement of both native and French Catholic priests in internecine struggles of the Vietnamese led to executions of French priests.[5] These executions stirred the French to intervene through "gunboat diplomacy." The French demanded trade agreements and religious tolerance, but in reality found a pretext for colonization as a means to compete with the British, who were opening up Burma and China to colonial exploitation.[5]

A French naval attack on Da Nang[5] in 1858 began the period of their conquest and colonization of Vietnam, which, except for the period of Japanese control during World War II, continued for almost 100 years. This poorly administered and often brutally governed French colony stirred increasing resistance among the Vietnamese and spawned the formation of the Indochinese Communist Party (1930) by Ho Chi Minh, the revolutionary leader.[5]

America had expressed interest in Vietnam as far back as 1832, when President Andrew Jackson dispatched an envoy,[6] seeking to establish trade agreements. However, they encountered the emperor's policy of isolation with the West and failed to make contact. Fifty years later, when France was pressing its imperialistic ambitions, the United States tried again, this time to broker a peace between France and Vietnam,[6] but France refused to agree to American mediation. Once France had successfully secured its colonial possession, the United States became one of the leading trading partners with French Indochina.

The Period of Japanese Domination

Early in World War II Germany attacked France, and in June 1940 the government of France surrendered to Germany. In September of that year, Japan, Germany's ally, encountered little resistance from the French in Vietnam and began its 5-year occupation.[5] However, over most of that time the French colonial government collaborated with the Japanese and continued to rule the country. Japan mostly exploited the region for labor and materials to supply the war effort, but the occupation intensified opposition against the French and Japanese by Ho Chi Minh and the Viet Minh guerrillas.[5] An ironic note: during this period American representatives met with Ho Chi Minh—the man who would later become an inspirational leader to America's enemy—and offered to provide training and arms to advance their objective of defeating the Japanese.[5]

The surrender of Japan to the Allies in August 1945 created a political vacuum in Vietnam, which led to great instability and fighting. British and Chinese forces sought to take control of the southern and northern halves of Vietnam respectively as stipulated in the post-World War II Potsdam Conference[5]; Ho Chi Minh and the Viet Minh proclaimed their sovereignty over the "Democratic Republic of Vietnam"; and the French attempted to reestablish their colonial system. When the Chinese Communists consolidated their power in China in 1949, they provided weapons and training to the Viet Minh to use against the French.[5]

In 1950, President Truman responded by granting US aid to the French military[7] and sending the first of the American advisors to South Vietnam (which, in time, grew to become US Military Assistance and Advisory Group [MAAG]) to aid the French against the Viet Minh rebels. This was the beginning of the American advisory period. By 1953, the United States was providing 80% of the French military costs in Indochina in the effort to oppose the spread of communism. However, despite this aid, their defeat at Dien Bien Phu ended French claims in Vietnam (7 May 1954).[5]

AMERICA'S SLIDE INTO WAR IN VIETNAM

The Communist Threat and the American Advisor Years

In July 1954, government representatives of France, Britain, the then-Soviet Union, and the United States convened in Geneva and signed an agreement[8] dividing Vietnam at the 17th parallel with the intention of holding national elections in 2 years. The northern part was to be temporarily under the control of Ho Chi Minh and the Viet Minh as a communist regime, and the southern part controlled by Premier Ngo Dinh Diem and his government. However, the Eisenhower Administration soon became convinced that the increasingly repressive and unpopular Diem

regime could not stand up to the combined forces of the communist regime in the north and the indigenous communist opposition in South Vietnam (the National Front for the Liberation of South Vietnam [NLF or Viet Cong]), and their ideological partners, Soviet Russia and Communist China, who indicated their intention to "liberate" the peoples in the south.[1,7] Thus began a US policy of providing direct economic aid and military advisors to train South Vietnamese forces and a decade of escalating tensions, military incursions by both sides, and anticipations of war.

In November 1961, increasing North Vietnam-sponsored guerrilla activities in South Vietnam led President Kennedy to conclude that an even larger commitment would be necessary to bolster the fledgling democracy in South Vietnam. The first official American battlefield casualty was that of Specialist 4th Class James T Davis, who was killed on 22 December 1961, when the Army of the Republic of Vietnam (ARVN) unit he was accompanying drove into a guerrilla ambush a few miles west of Saigon.[5] This policy of increasing troop strengths continued under President Lyndon Johnson, Kennedy's successor. By December 1964, shortly before the first US Marines were inserted into Vietnam, the number of US military personnel had risen to over 23,000.[9]

The War's Rationale and Provocation

To understand how the US government could reach a point where it would expend American lives and resources to fight a counterinsurgency in Vietnam, one must remember that these events arose during the post-World War II Cold War period. World affairs had become extremely tense in the 1950s and 1960s following the defeat of Germany and Japan. Soon after Japan surrendered in 1945, America and its allies found themselves again in an epic struggle against the menace of totalitarianism—this time, Soviet-sponsored communism. Relations between the two ideological camps often approached the flash point, and a catastrophic nuclear war seemed frighteningly possible. For example, between 1950 and 1953 the United States waged a costly war in support of South Korea's defense against a communist takeover by North Korea. Even closer to home, in 1962 the United States came perilously close to nuclear war with the Soviet Union when it learned that the communist regime of Fidel Castro in Cuba was allowing the construction of nuclear missile sites on that nearby Caribbean island.

EXHIBIT 1-1. THE VIET CONG STRATEGY OF TERROR

The terrorism practiced by the Viet Cong [VC] . . . took every conceivable form: harassment, kidnapping, assassination, execution, and massacre. VC terrorists mortared refugee camps, mined village roads, and hurled grenades into crowded city streets. . . . The war that U.S. combat troops encountered when they first arrived in South Vietnam already contained an element of ferocity that few Americans could readily comprehend.

Some of the bloodletting was wholly indiscriminate but much of it was part of a calculated campaign of fear and intimidation. . . . Striking at individuals of authority—hamlet chiefs, religious figures, schoolteachers—the VC eliminated virtually an entire class of Vietnamese villagers. In the process they isolated the peasants from the government that had promised them protection, leaving them only three alternatives: active support of the VC, passive neutrality, or death.

The men and women who carried out such acts were well trained, heavily indoctrinated, highly motivated, and willing to take great risks. . . . [Although they operated in every province in South Vietnam] the infamous F-100 [operating out of a secret base in the jungles of Binh Duong Province] carried the campaign of fear and disruption to Saigon and other urban areas. . . .

When American soldiers began to arrive in South Vietnam in force, the VC turned their strategy of terror on U.S. military personnel and civilians. . . .

But if the Communists were willing to enforce their discipline on defenseless villagers. . . , they found it even more useful to employ the Americans for the same purpose. Their technique was simple, cold-blooded, and chillingly effective: Occupy a village, provoke [an American] attack, then blame the death and destruction on the foreigners. . . .

. . . Communist terror grew more intense as the war went on and was largely directed at civilians without connection to the government. It was often indiscriminate and generally in violation of the principles of military necessity, discrimination, proportionality, and humanity that are the basis of the law of war. The VC strategy of terror, in short, was a systematic, deliberate attack on the civilians of South Vietnam resulting in the death or injury of tens of thousands of noncombatants.

But the Vietnamese were not the only victims. The barbarity of VC terror, the seeming indifference of the enemy to the lives of their own countrymen, had a profound effect on the Americans who came to fight in Vietnam. The cruelty of the VC toward the peasants reinforced the mistaken belief [among US troops] that life was cheap in the countryside. At the same time the inability of the peasants to defend themselves contributed to the contempt with which some GIs regarded them. Their refusal to risk their lives and those of their families by informing on the [Viet Cong] helped nurture the idea that they were themselves the enemy.

Reproduced with permission from Doyle E, Weiss S, and the editors of Boston Publishing Co. *The Vietnam Experience: A Collision of Cultures*. Boston, Mass: Boston Publishing Co; 1984: 156–157.

The growing perception among Americans was that without vigorous opposition by the United States and its allies, democracy could be obliterated by a cascade of communist revolutions (the "domino theory") throughout the developing nations of the world such as those in Southeast Asia.[10] Because the United States was a signatory of the 1954 Southeast Asia Treaty Organization (with France, Great Britain, Thailand, Pakistan, Australia, New Zealand, and the Philippines),[1] South Vietnam's struggle to defend itself against armed aggression from North Vietnam (in violation of the 1954 Geneva Agreement that brought an end to the First Indochina War)[1] presented a compelling opportunity to draw the line with respect to the perceived threat.

Matters coalesced on 2–4 August 1964. South Vietnamese naval commandos had raided two islands in the Gulf of Tonkin claimed by North Vietnam, and in response, North Vietnamese torpedo boats allegedly[8,11,12] attacked two US destroyers—the USS *Maddox* and the USS *Turner Joy*. President Johnson reacted by ordering retaliatory bombing of North Vietnamese gunboats and support facilities. On 7 August, the US Congress approved the Tonkin Gulf Resolution.[8,13] Although not a formal declaration of war, this provided the administration the legal option of committing military forces in Vietnam and set the stage for the war to begin in earnest.[8]

The Marine landing on 8 March 1965 followed a Viet Cong mortar attack in Pleiku in the central highlands, which killed eight and wounded over 100 American advisors, and another attack on the US barracks at Qui Nhon, which killed 21 Americans and wounded 22.[13] President Johnson ordered additional air strikes on targets in North Vietnam, and the objective for the Marines was to provide security for the US warplanes based at Da Nang.

THE SCOPE OF AMERICA'S WAR IN VIETNAM

America's Enemy in South Vietnam

In support of the Republic of South Vietnam and its armed forces, America's enemies in Southeast Asia were twofold: (1) indigenous guerrilla forces (Viet Cong) who operated in South Vietnam and who used the tactics of harassment, terrorism, and ambush in an attempt to destabilize the government of South Vietnam (Exhibit 1-1), and (2) the allies of the Viet Cong, the regular units of the North Vietnam Army (NVA), who staged more conventional attacks on the South Vietnamese military forces and those of its allies in an effort to take over the country.

America's Challenges and Costs

The ground war spanned almost 8 years, and by the time the remaining military personnel were withdrawn in 1973, 3.4 million US military men and women had served in the theater. Between March 1965, when the Marines landed in South Vietnam, and 31 December 1973, 2.6 million service personnel had been deployed within the borders of South Vietnam (including approximately 7,500 women,[14] roughly 85% of whom were nurses[15])—typically for a single, 1-year assignment. Another 50,000 had served there between 1960 and 1965 during the advisor years before the arrival of American ground forces. Finally, approximately 800,000 served in the Southeast Asia theater outside of South Vietnam (in Laos and Cambodia, as well as sailors serving offshore with the US Navy and US Air Force personnel stationed at bases in Thailand and Guam).[15] (See Figure 1-4 comparing military personnel mobilization and casualties through the Vietnam War with earlier American wars.)

To understand the experience of the "typical" serviceman in Vietnam, it is helpful to understand who did the fighting. The reportedly unusually low so-called tooth-to-tail ratio in Vietnam, that is, the proportion of combat troops compared to noncombat troops, has been disputed over the years. According to Spector, a military historian, the official statistics, which indicated that 57.5% of US forces served in combat or combat support units, were inflated. "[The] evidence is overwhelming that only a small minority of servicemen present in Vietnam were engaged in active operations against the enemy."[16(p40)] In his opinion, a more realistic estimate would take into account the percentage of personnel assigned to maneuver battalions. In April 1968, only 29% of soldiers and 34% of Marines were so assigned; but beyond that, the actual figures for those exposed to combat were even lower than what was authorized, that is, because, "the sick, lame, lazy and those on R & R (rest and recuperation), etc." were not among those doing the fighting.[16(p55)] In a more recent review, JJ McGrath, a military historian, indicated that although some claimed a ratio as low as 1:10, by his estimate, at least for the US Army in Vietnam, the ratio of combat to noncombat troops was 1:2, essentially what it was in Korea[17] (see Chapter 3, Exhibit 3-1, "Ratio of Combat Troops to Noncombat/Support Troops in Vietnam"). Thus by these estimates the proportion of Army troops directly exposed to combat risk was somewhere between one-fourth and one-third of the personnel in the theater—roughly half of the official claim.

Because of President Johnson's decision to not utilize Reserve and National Guard units in Vietnam,[16(pp27–28)] the US military, especially the Army, resorted to increased conscription to meet its needs. The result was that an inordinate proportion of those who served were draftees, one-term volunteers (draft-motivated enlistees), "instant NCOs (noncommissioned officers)," and recent graduates of ROTC (Reserve Officers' Training Corps) and OCS (Officer Candidate School)—the so-called "Vietnam-only Army" of mostly citizen-soldiers.[16(p34)] Although draftees comprised only 39% of the Army's overall enlisted and officer force in Vietnam, 70% of the infantry, armor, and artillery were draftees. This is because if one enlisted before being drafted, the odds of serving in a noncombat role were improved. Furthermore, draftees accounted for nearly 55% of those killed and wounded.[4(pp76,78)] The average soldier in the Vietnam War was younger (19 years old) than those who served in World War II (26 years old). They were also better educated than their father's generation of soldiers.

The war in Vietnam is classified as a limited conventional war because there were units larger than 4,000 soldiers operating in the field.[18(p8)] However, more important, it became mostly an irregular, counterinsurgency/guerilla war. According to Shelby Stanton, author of the *Vietnam Order of Battle*:

FIGURE 1-4. Major twentieth century American wars compared by (a) numbers serving worldwide in all branches; (b) theater casualties and (c) hostile deaths.

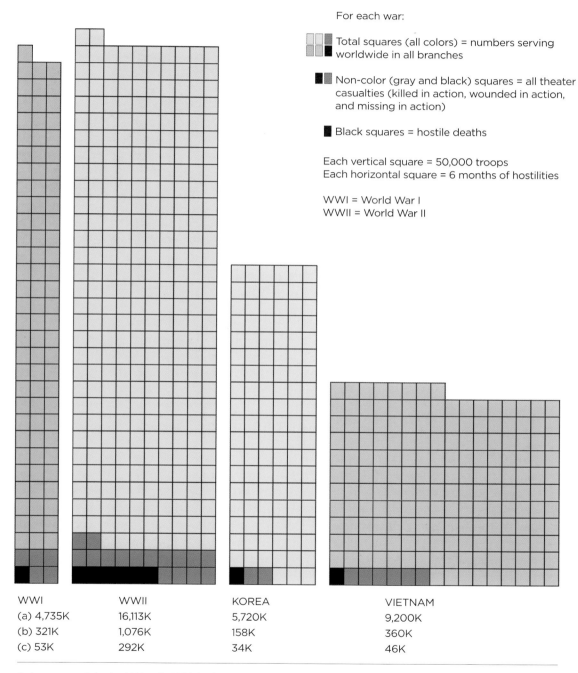

For each war:

Total squares (all colors) = numbers serving worldwide in all branches

Non-color (gray and black) squares = all theater casualties (killed in action, wounded in action, and missing in action)

Black squares = hostile deaths

Each vertical square = 50,000 troops
Each horizontal square = 6 months of hostilities

WWI = World War I
WWII = World War II

WWI	WWII	KOREA	VIETNAM
(a) 4,735K	16,113K	5,720K	9,200K
(b) 321K	1,076K	158K	360K
(c) 53K	292K	34K	46K

Data source: *Principal Wars in Which the United States Participated; US Military Personnel Serving and Casualties*. Washington, DC: Department of Defense, Office of the Assistant Secretary of Defense OASD (Comptroller), Directorate for Information Operations, 15 March 1974: 61.

FIGURE 1-5. US and Army military personnel and Army combat casualties in Vietnam.

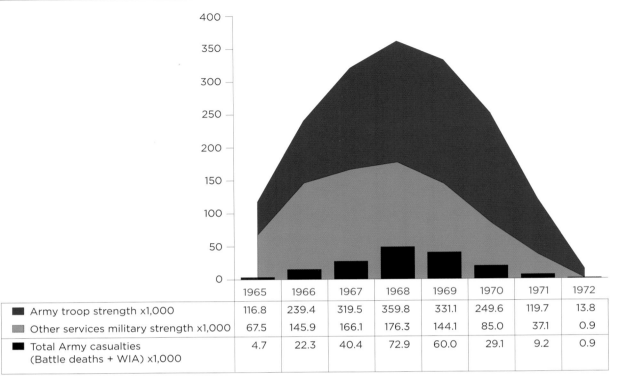

	1965	1966	1967	1968	1969	1970	1971	1972
■ Army troop strength x1,000	116.8	239.4	319.5	359.8	331.1	249.6	119.7	13.8
■ Other services military strength x1,000	67.5	145.9	166.1	176.3	144.1	85.0	37.1	0.9
■ Total Army casualties (Battle deaths + WIA) x1,000	4.7	22.3	40.4	72.9	60.0	29.1	9.2	0.9

Data sources: US and Army troop strength and Army combat fatalities from: Department of Defense, Office of the Assistant Secretary of Defense (Comptroller). *US Military Personnel in South Vietnam 1960–1972*. Washington, DC: Directorate for Information Operations; 15 March 1974. Total Army casualties from: US Army Adjutant General, Casualty Services Division (DAAG-PEC). *Active Duty Army Personnel Battle Casualties and Nonbattle Deaths Vietnam, 1961–1979*. Washington, DC: Office of The Adjutant General Counts. 3 February 1981.

Traditional military doctrine, based on seizing and holding a series of successive terrain objectives, was largely inapplicable. The multidirectional, nonlinear nature of military operations in Vietnam [meant that] . . . goals were redefined [to] . . . adjust to the conflicting demands and novel principles of area warfare.[19(p81)]

The war in Vietnam is also referred to as low intensity because of the low ratio of casualties (killed in action [KIA] and wounded in action [WIA]) to the numbers of personnel deployed compared to previous American wars. For example, a comparison of the peak years of US Army troops' WIA rates during Vietnam (1968 = 120/1,000 troops) and Korea (1950 = 460/1,000 troops) suggests a lower combat intensity in Vietnam.[20(Table1)] However, this could be misleading. According to Spector, in Vietnam:

. . . Men in "maneuver battalions," the units that actually did the fighting, continued to run about the same chance of death or injury as their older relatives who had fought in Korea or in the Pacific [in World War II]. Indeed, during the first half of 1968, the *overall* Vietnam casualty rate exceeded the overall rate for all theaters in World War II, while the casualty rates for Army and Marine maneuver battalions were more than four times as high."[16(p55)]

The data accumulated on the types of wounds sustained in Vietnam are also revealing of the nature of combat there. Many more US casualties were caused by small arms fire or by booby traps and mines than in previous wars, and many fewer were caused by artillery and other explosive projectile fragments.[20]

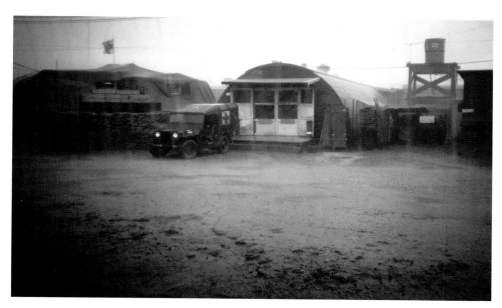

FIGURE 1-6. Monsoonal rains at the 15th Medical Battalion Clearing Station, 1st Cavalry Division base at Phouc Vinh. In addition to the formidable terrain, the long rainy season further hampered operations in the field. Photograph courtesy of Richard D Cameron, Major General, US Army (Retired).

Overall, the pursuit of military objectives in Vietnam by America and its allies became a costly undertaking. Following are some statistics that help to make the point: more than 58,000 US service members were killed in action, missing in action, or died of other causes,[21] and over 300,000 were wounded. Figure 1-5 illustrates overall military personnel strength, Army troop strength, and Army casualties over the course of the war. Because the majority of those sent served in the Army (60%–80%), the majority of the casualties also were from the ranks of the Army (40,132 battle deaths, 96,680 hospitalized wounded in action, 104,605 wounded and returned to duty, and 8,273 died of noncombat causes).[22] At home, an estimated quarter of a million Americans lost an immediate family member to the war. South Vietnam's military casualties numbered over 220,000 killed and almost a half million wounded.

The United States spent $189 billion prosecuting the war and supporting the government of South Vietnam. In 1 year alone, mid-1968 through mid-1969—the peak year of combat activity—America and its allies had over 1.5 million military personnel deployed (543,000 Americans, 819,200 South Vietnamese, and 231,100 from South Korea, Australia, New Zealand, Thailand, and the Philippines combined); US forces staged 1,100 ground attacks of battalion size or larger (compared to only 126 by the communist forces); and there were 400,000 American air attacks, which dropped 1.2 million tons of bombs costing $14 billion.[6]

Ultimately, as noted previously, despite their material and technological inferiority, the enemy's resolve and resilience outlasted the tolerance of the American public, and, under great political pressure at home and internationally, the US government elected to withdraw its ground forces. However, despite this outcome, US forces overall demonstrated great courage and sacrifice in Vietnam, with 246 Americans receiving the Congressional Medal of Honor (154 of which were awarded posthumously).[23]

AMERICA'S TWO VIETNAM WARS: PRE-TET AND POST-TET (1968)

The American story of the ground war in Vietnam should be considered as two Vietnam War stories—starkly different, sequential stories that pivot on the events occurring in 1968. Taken together, these two stories portray a dramatic reversal of fortune for the United States, a reversal that powerfully shaped American culture.

The Buildup Phase: Lyndon Johnson's War (1965-1968)

Lyndon Johnson was sworn into his first full term as President in January 1965, riding the crest of a national political consensus and overall prosperity. It was only, in the words of *Newsweek*, that "[n]agging little war in Vietnam"[4(p58)] that cast a shadow on his ambition to create a "Great Society" of social reforms as his legacy.

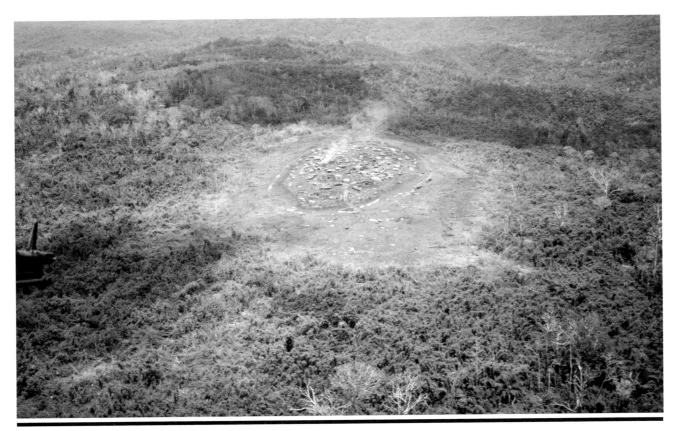

FIGURE 1-7. Aerial view of a 1st Cavalry Division fire support base in 1970. The combat strategy of the US Army in Vietnam through much of the war was that of enemy attrition, which was primarily implemented through "search and destroy" missions. These were commonly initiated from well-defended enclaves such as this one as well as other forward bases. Photograph courtesy of Richard D Cameron, Major General, US Army (Retired).

Nonetheless, the administration was determined to pursue those political agendas as well as ensure that South Vietnam did not fall into the communist sphere. As President Johnson put it bluntly, "I am not going to lose Vietnam . . . I am not going to be the President who saw Southeast Asia go the way China went."[4(p46)]

US combat troop strength expanded rapidly in South Vietnam after the Marine landing in 1965. By June 1966, American troops numbered 285,000, and another 100,000 arrived by the end of the year. The number of inductions into the US military in 1966 alone was almost 320,000 men, a 250% increase over the previous year.[16(p30)]

The US Army, Marine Corps, and Navy (in the Mekong River delta) units committed in South Vietnam typically found themselves operating in a rugged, tropical environment with formidable impediments to movement over the ground, extraordinary heat and humidity, and rains for months at a time (Figure 1-6). Equally important, combat operations conducted 10,000 miles from the United States required a very long logistical network. These troops also operated among an indigenous population of an exotic, Asian culture that spoke an exceptionally difficult language for Americans to learn. The local Vietnamese appeared to tolerate the presence of US troops, but it was common for them to be ambivalent about the government of South Vietnam and to harbor Viet Cong guerrillas. The relationship between the US forces and the South Vietnamese was generally strained; US troops regarded them warily at best.[24,25(p182)]

The combat strategy employed by the US Army in the buildup phase in Vietnam was one of attrition ("body counts" and "kill ratios"),[6] primarily through search-and-destroy missions initiated from well-defended enclaves (Figure 1-7). Guerrilla and terrorist operations by Viet Cong forces and periodic attacks by North Vietnamese regular units were the principle tactics of the communist forces. Consequently, engagement with the enemy more often involved clashes between highly mobile, small tactical units as opposed to battles between major military formations.

More important, US successes were limited as the Viet Cong guerrillas were elusive, dictated the tempo of the fighting, and too often were content to snipe, set booby traps, and ambush American patrols. Their hit-and-run tactics allowed them to fade safely into the jungle or into the local populace if the fight turned against them—tactics ingrained in their culture from centuries of guerrilla warfare against foreign invaders.[18] Consider the following depiction provided by Neller, an Army psychiatrist, who drew upon his experience as a Special Forces medic in Vietnam in 1967:

> The kill zone and ambush scenario is the hallmark of low intensity conflicts and demonstrates that, for the actual combatants, there is no such thing as low intensity when faced with the realities of high-tech warfare. A typical jungle ambush used by US forces in Vietnam, and, in a modified form, also by the enemy would be initiated frequently by a Claymore mine being exploded, and/or each soldier would then throw one grenade. He would then fire one to no more than two magazines from his modern, ultra-light, automatic rifle with well-directed fire. He would finish by throwing the second grenade and initiate his withdrawal while firing his third 20–30 round magazine. A good combat leader would have established a second or even third kill zone and, if available, have on call artillery and air support to protect the withdrawal of his unit. Though the ambush was operational for no more than a couple of minutes, an eleven man rifle squad could have easily used over 1,000 rounds of rifle ammunition, 22 grenades, several Claymore mines, and an assortment of booby traps (explosives) in the kill zone.

> If the goal in antiguerrilla/terrorist warfare is to find, isolate and destroy the enemy, then the order of battle in unconventional warfare is frequently to get the enemy to mass in a predetermined location in sufficient numbers where he can be engaged by a larger, better prepared force. This is similar to the frontier Indian wars of the old West, or back alley street fighting frequently seen in modern ghettos throughout the world. [In Vietnam] this put a lot of stress on small combat units who must be either the bait, the trap, or both.[26(pp36–37)]

US forces were more likely to find themselves in conventional combat engagements against regular North Vietnamese divisions in the northern provinces. However, even these main force units more often than not staged combat initiatives from behind the safety of the 17th parallel demilitarized zone (DMZ) that separated North Vietnam from South Vietnam, thereby eluding pursuit by American units and their allies.[27] Consequently, most combat activity for US forces involved brief encounters between isolated, small units—a war of no fronts. A Joint Chiefs of Staff study reported that of all the US patrols conducted in 1967 and 1968, "less than 1% . . . resulted in contact with the enemy."[18(p60)] Still, when there was contact, the fighting was as bloody and intense as any that occurred in World War II. US forces did periodically stage larger-scale operations during this phase of the war, and some elements of these engagements exacted heavy tolls on the enemy. Notable examples are the Army's battle of the Ia Drang Valley in 1965, the Marines' Operation Hastings in 1966, the Navy's Operation Coronado V in 1967, and, also in 1967, the Army's Operations Cedar Falls and Junction City.[18]

The US military in the late 1960s enjoyed remarkable technological advantages in Vietnam. Weaponry was a prime example. Whether carried with them into the field or employed as tactical support from air strikes or artillery, field commanders could bring to bear formidable firepower on the enemy. If the enemy began to outnumber an allied force in an engagement, close support from the air or from artillery quickly reversed the equation.[18] Another element of US technical superiority in Vietnam was that of air mobility—the ubiquitous helicopter. This was unprecedented in US warfare and allowed reconnaissance and ordnance delivery from the air, heliborne movement of troops for tactical advantage, timely evacuation of the wounded, and frequent resupply. In fact, the first full US Army combat division to be sent to Vietnam was the 1st Cavalry Division (Airmobile). Figure 1-8 shows the firepower that could be delivered quickly onto an enemy.

US Army Medical and Psychiatric Support

Another element in the Vietnam theater that greatly enhanced life for the US combat soldier was the outstanding medical support available. From the outset

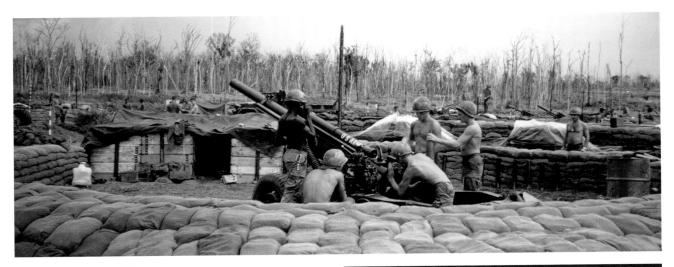

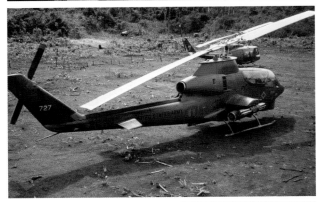

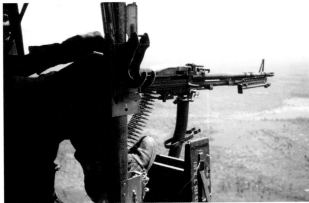

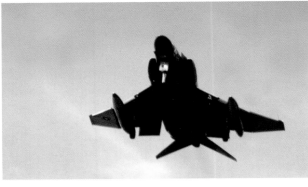

FIGURE 1-8A. (Top) A 105 mm Howitzer artillery piece employed in a fire mission. High on the list of stress-mitigating factors affecting troops was the overall technologic superiority of the US forces, which especially included that of weaponry. If the enemy began to outnumber an allied force in an engagement, field commanders could bring to bear formidable firepower in the form of close support from the air or from artillery. Photograph courtesy of Richard D Cameron, Major General, US Army (Retired).

FIGURE 1-8B. (Top Left) This photograph shows a door gunner's view from a Huey helicopter, the most commonly utilized helicopter for troop transport in Vietnam. US technical superiority in Vietnam included that of air mobility via the expanded use of helicopters. This was unprecedented in US warfare and allowed reconnaissance and ordnance delivery from the air, heliborne movement of troops for tactical advantage, timely evacuation of the wounded, and frequent resupply. Photograph courtesy of Richard D Cameron, Major General, US Army (Retired).

FIGURE 1-8C. (Center Left) An AH-1 Cobra helicopter. The Army used armed helicopters to support ground troops, eventually fielding dedicated helicopter gunships like the Cobra for this purpose. Cobras could be equipped with guns, grenade launchers, rockets, or even guided missiles, and provide rapid and wide-ranging fire against an adversary on the ground. Photograph courtesy of Richard D Cameron, Major General, US Army (Retired).

FIGURE 1-8D. (Bottom Left) An F-4 Phantom in Vietnam. This all-weather, long-range supersonic jet interceptor fighter/fighter-bomber, which was flown by both the Navy and Air Force, was used extensively in the theater to maintain air superiority as well as in the ground attack and in providing reconnaissance. Photograph courtesy of Richard D Cameron, Major General, US Army (Retired).

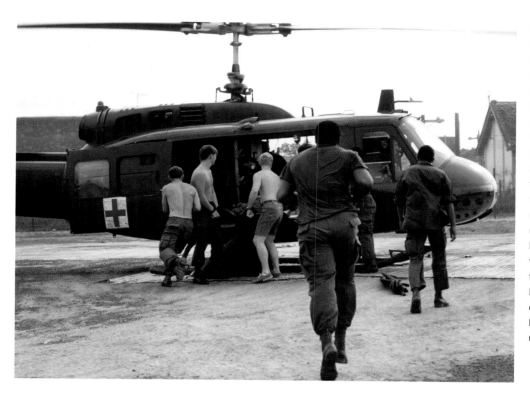

FIGURE 1-9. Medics offloading a casualty from a "dust-off" helicopter at the 15th Medical Battalion clearing station, 1st Cavalry Division at Phouc Vinh. The widespread use of the helicopter as an air ambulance permitted rapid evacuation of wounded soldiers to the most appropriate level of medical care, resulting in a high level of casualty survival among Army troops fighting in Vietnam. Photograph courtesy of Richard D Cameron, Major General, US Army (Retired).

of the war, the US military made every effort to insure that troops received timely, sophisticated medical care, including psychiatric care, despite the hostile physical environment and Vietnam's geographical remoteness.[20] The following is by way of a summary provided by Donald L Custis, a senior Navy surgeon:

> [The medical care provided in Vietnam] was an impressive performance on the part of all three military medical services, epitomizing ideal circumstances for effective integration of casualty evacuation, resuscitation, early definitive treatment, constant resource supply, and electronic communication.
>
> Air superiority with medical helicopters and dedicated fixed-wing ambulance aircraft made possible rapid patient transfer at every echelon of medical care. There were stable, well-established, forward-placed hospitals, comparable with modern stateside urban medical centers, that provided an air-conditioned patient environment, modern operating rooms with piped-in gases, x-ray units, respirators, hypothermia units, orthopedic frames, physiologic monitoring equipment, and sophisticated clinical laboratories. Although occasionally receiving incoming mortar, the

hospitals were fairly secure. All of this, coupled with professional specialists using advanced surgical techniques, created an unprecedented success story in the annals of military surgery. The experience contributed greatly to the birth of today's civilian community life-support rescue squads.[28(p2261)]

The buildup of Army medical units was completed in 1968, when 11 evacuation, five field, and seven surgical hospitals were in place. These facilities, plus the 6th Convalescent Center in Cam Ranh Bay, brought the total bed capacity in South Vietnam to 5,283.[20] Most importantly, the new helicopter ambulance capability also permitted rapid evacuation of the wounded to the most appropriate level of medical care (Figure 1-9). As far as physical casualties, these efforts achieved remarkable success throughout the war. Comparing the ratio of KIA to WIA across wars attests to the superiority of medical care provided in Vietnam (World War II, 1:3.1; Korea, 1:4.1; and Vietnam, 1:5.6).[20]

Once the mobilization was under way, personnel with specialized training in mental healthcare were assigned and widely distributed throughout the theater. This peaked during the 3 full-strength years (1967–1969) when there were approximately 23 Army psychiatrist positions in Vietnam per year, which were supported by a full complement of allied professionals (psychiatric nurses, psychologists, and social workers) and enlisted paraprofessionals.[29] Typically, during those years, one psychiatrist was assigned to each of the seven combat divisions as well as one each to the evacuation and field hospitals, depending on anticipated need and availability. In addition, throughout most of the war, there were two Army Neuropsychiatric Medical Specialty Detachments that were each staffed with up to three psychiatrists.[29] Furthermore, each year of the war a psychiatrist served in a staff position with US Army Vietnam HQ as the Psychiatry and Neurology Consultant to the commanding general and his staff (more specifically, as "Neuropsychiatric Consultant" to the Commanding General, US Army Republic of Vietnam Surgeon).

Finally, the psychiatrists serving in Vietnam brought new tools in the form of antipsychotic (neuroleptic), antianxiety (anxiolytic), and antidepressant (tricyclic) medications—relatively nonsedating psychotropic drugs that had not been available in earlier American wars and that had considerable promise in the management of combat stress reactions and other conditions. A full list of psychotropic medications available in the theater for Army physicians can be found in Datel and Johnson.[30] The structure of Army psychiatric facilities and capabilities will be described in more detail in Chapters 3 and 4.

Special Features of the Psychosocial "Ecology" in the Buildup Phase

During the buildup years of the war, troop morale in Vietnam remained high in general, and attrition due to psychiatric or behavioral problems was exceptionally low compared to previous conflicts.[31] This was somewhat surprising considering the psychologically depleting nature of the remote, exotic, hostile, tropical setting (Southeast Asia) and the enemy's counterinsurgency strategy (politically directed, guerrilla warfare)[32] and resolute tenacity. Furthermore, throughout the war the troops fighting in Vietnam encountered certain novel features that distinguished the theater from those of previous wars and invariably affected morale. For example, the battlefield ecology was powerfully affected by the helicopter mobility of US ground forces; the enemy's elusiveness but lack of a capacity to deliver sustained, precision-guided indirect fire (as with artillery and combat aircraft); and, especially, America's overall strategy of fighting a war of attrition as opposed to one for territorial control.[18] The psychosocial complexion of the "rear" was unique

in that US forces typically staged combat activities from geographically isolated, fixed, relatively secure enclaves that were easily resupplied by helicopter. (Appendix 7 to this volume provides a description of the circumstantial features serving to buoy the overall morale in the 1st Cavalry Division [Airmobile] early in the war by Captain Harold SR Byrdy, division psychiatrist [August 1965–June 1966].) Observations more specific to field conditions are provided in Exhibit 1-2. These observations also suggest high morale during the buildup phase of the war.

On the other hand, one element that was perhaps more insidiously corrosive to troop morale than was realized at the time was that most of South Vietnam outside of American compounds and bases was designated off-limits.[24(pp27–28)] The counterinsurgency/guerrilla warfare necessitated restraints on off-duty troop freedom of movement, but this in turn meant that opportunities for positive interaction between soldiers and the indigenous South Vietnamese were severely limited. Except for his exposure to Vietnamese on-post day laborers, most of whom were suspected of either being thieves or enemy sympathizers, the most profound contact the US soldier was likely to have with a Vietnamese civilian was with a prostitute. According to Allerton, a senior Army psychiatrist, even in Saigon, where American military personnel were allowed some latitude, "Many soldiers believed, and perhaps correctly so, that it was more dangerous in a bar [there] than out in the field in some type of search and destroy mission."[29(p16)]

"Goodwill" contacts under a program of civic action that involved the distribution of food and clothing, the building and repair of community facilities, and the provision of medical assistance—the so-called MEDCAP (Medical Civilian Action Program) missions—were of lower priority than combat activities. Although designed to "win the hearts and minds" of the Vietnamese in the countryside (ie, recruit the loyalty of the villagers by providing for their welfare and security), these efforts brought only qualified success because of inefficiency, cultural obstacles, and misunderstandings.[24(pp36–37)] More favorable contact with the Vietnamese might have encouraged soldiers to develop friendly feelings and compassion for their situation, which would have helped to justify being in a distant land risking one's life. Instead, there was an inevitable rift between the impoverished South Vietnamese villagers and Americans who seemed to be so unapproachable, affluent, and aggressive.

EXHIBIT 1-2. TROOP LIVING CONDITIONS IN THE FIELD

This is Part 1 of a set of observations by Specialist 6th Class Dennis L Menard, an enlisted social work specialist, from his unit consultation visit to a 1st Infantry Division battalion in November 1967. (Part 2, Consultation to a Combat Battalion by a Social Work Specialist, is in Chapter 7.)

Overall, the general appearance of the units was very good, considering field conditions; all of the men and emplacements were dug in well, latrines were well spaced, trash dumps adequate, and there was good organization and tactical set up of the night defensive perimeter. The men wear abbreviated attire, usually no shirts nor pots, and they are cleanshaven each a.m. There are two local barbers on duty everyday, but a few men are still in need of haircuts. Field showers are set up with an adequate water supply. However, not everyone is up to par on personal hygiene, feeling there is no reason to clean up daily. No boots are shined and, of course, none are expected. There is a clothing distribution every two days when the men exchange dirty fatigues, socks, and underwear.

First call is 0530 hours when hot coffee and donuts and pastry are served—very good and in adequate supply. The mess section consists of a few field cooks. There is one hot meal a day, usually in the evening, which is prepared at the base camp and flown out here via resupply helicopter. Most men supplement their breakfast with C-rations, which is also the noon meal. Heating tablets are available for hot C's. The evening is one of the daily highlights. The food is excellent and in ample supply. Meals are served on paper plates with plastic utensils. Chow is consumed in each man's section or assigned area. Most of the men really enjoy the night and act like a group of Sunday School kids on an outing.

Each section (6–8 men) is issued a Sundry Pack every other day which consists of cigarettes, candy, gum, writing paper, shaving gear, soap, and other items. Men lack for little while in the field. Cokes are also in ample supply, each section getting about a case per day for which they have to pay 15 cents a can. Food and rations merit an excellent rating. The battalion supply officer showed that he has a good section and his supplies are adequate. He has no difficulty in getting ammunition, clean clothing every two days, cokes and food. Some of the discrepancies he noted were lack of poncho liners and air mattresses. His biggest headache was lack of ice. Sections get about 10 pounds daily and often drink their cokes warm. Conversation with the EM [enlisted men] in the section revealed high morale, not too many complaints except about the ice and the newly imposed beer restriction. The beer ration had been 2–3 cans per man per day. All men are entitled to one in-country R & R [rest and recuperation], one out-of-country R & R, and one 7-day leave; and the infantry has priority on allocations. When the unit returns from the field, the men are allowed passes in the village. The usual stay is only 1–3 days. No unusual complaints here.

The TO&E [Table of Organization and Equipment] for the battalion stipulates one battalion surgeon, one medical administrative officer, and 36 enlisted medics. Sick call is from 0800 to 1000 hours daily, with a daily average of 10 patients. Usual complaints are rashes, ringworm, boils, and venereal disease. Most referrals are treated in the field. Only those cases which require more sophisticated treatment are sent to the Battalion Aid Station, [for example], fever of unknown origin, eye refraction, broken bones, severe lacerations, and battle wounds.

Source: Menard DL. The social work specialist in a combat division. *US Army Vietnam Med Bull.* 1968;March/April: 53–55.

Efforts to understand soldier stress and resilience in Vietnam have to take into account the draft's influence as well as the military's replacement policy of individualized, 1-year tours. This refers to conscription and assignment policies in which: (*a*) the majority of lower-ranking enlisted soldiers sent to Vietnam were either drafted or "draft-motivated" enlistees (eg, potentially stress-producing), and (*b*) soldiers were rotated into (and out of) Vietnam on an individual basis for 1-year assignments. The 1-year tour—a replacement policy that had its origins during the Korean War—was intended to be stress reducing because these soldiers would perceive their obligation and risk as limited.[3,20]

However, ultimately the churning and depletion of experienced military personnel in the theater (including officers and noncommissioned officers) resulting from the fixed, 1-year rotation system had a hugely negative effect on troop "commitment and cohesion" and, consequently, morale.[10,16] A more specific overview of soldier morale and the psychiatric experience through the course of the war will be elaborated in Chapter 2 and Chapter 8.

1968 and the Enemy Tet Offensives

The year 1968 was America's bloodiest year in Vietnam (16,592 KIA), and events both at home and in Southeast Asia served as the tipping point in reversing US support for pursuing military objectives there. During the 31 days of the month of May, 2,000 Americans were killed—the highest monthly death toll of the war.[33(p147)] June 13th marked the day that Americans had been fighting in Vietnam longer than any war in the 20th century.[34] However, the greatest negative effect arose from the enemy's Tet offensives.

On the morning of 31 January 1968, communist guerrillas broke the Tet, or Lunar New Year, truce and launched coordinated attacks on cities and towns throughout South Vietnam. Although these attacks were ultimately extremely costly to the communist forces and achieved little militarily, their political yield was enormous. Many held the US media accountable for misinterpreting these events as signaling a US defeat and provoking a reversal in public and political support for war.[35] These attacks, as well as the month-long bloody battle to retake Hue and the prolonged siege of the US Marine Corps base of Khe Sanh, created the indelible perception in the United States that the war could not be won. The enemy appeared to defy the Johnson Administration's assurances of imminent defeat, and nowhere in Vietnam seemed secure despite great expenditures of lives and money.

As a consequence, calls for the war to end escalated to such an extent that most other considerations became irrelevant. On 31 March 1968, President Johnson announced that he would halt the bombing over North Vietnam as a prelude to peace negotiations. He also declared that he would not seek reelection in the service of that end. Ten days later he announced that General Creighton Abrams would relieve General William Westmoreland, the original commander of US Military Assistance Command, Vietnam (USMACV).[33] Still, it was not until a year later, mid-1969, before the first Army units pulled out of South Vietnam.[9] America may have begun to disengage in early 1968, but this would become a drawn-out, tortuous drawdown—one which would last 4 years and produce many more casualties.

The Drawdown Phase: Richard Nixon's War (1969–1973)

The second half of the war took on a starkly different character from the first half. By January 1969, when President Nixon succeeded President Johnson, the United States had been at war in Vietnam for 4 years. Nixon promised "peace with honor," negotiations with the enemy, and a gradual drawdown of troops, while confronting extreme impatience and

often violent protest in America.[36] With the change of command in Vietnam, the military strategy of attrition shifted to a defensive one that sought area security and "Vietnamization" of the fighting.[33] Enemy offensive activity also slackened.

Overall US troop strength in Vietnam peaked at 543,400 in mid-1969 and declined through the next 3 years until all combat forces were withdrawn.[9] US operations of battalion size or larger slowly began to decline beginning in mid-1968.[37] Notable exceptions are Operation Dewey Canyon by US Marines (January–March 1969), the US Army's battle for Hamburger Hill (May 1969), and the 1970 Cambodian incursion by combined US Army units and units of the South Vietnamese Army.[37] Still, despite the reduction of combat operations and the peace negotiations, which proceeded erratically, US service personnel continued to die there (from 1969–1972, 15,316 were killed in action and an additional 5,186 died of nonhostile causes).[21]

According to Spector, the evolving stalemate in Vietnam resembled the bloody trench warfare of World War I, a battle in which both sides grossly underestimated the other.

> In the end, the American failure [in Vietnam] was a failure of understanding and imagination. The American leaders did not see that what for them was a limited war for limited ends was, for the Vietnamese, an unlimited war of survival in which all the most basic values—loyalty to ancestors, love of country, resistance to foreigners—were involved.
>
> . . . The result was the bloodletting of 1968. So, caught between an American government that could never make up its mind and a Communist government that refused ever to change its mind, thousands of brave and dedicated men and women gave up their lives to no good purpose.[16(p314)]

The abandonment of hopes for military victory in Vietnam had a powerfully negative effect on the country, the institution of the US Army,[38–40] and especially those whose fate it would be to serve during the drawdown in Vietnam and be required to fight battles of disengagement amid pressures from home to oppose the war and the military.[37] The high esprit and commitment of the soldiers serving in Vietnam in the buildup years had been replaced with sagging morale, alienation, and disaffection by those who replaced them.

New Stressors Affecting the Psychosocial "Ecology" in the Transition and Drawdown Phase

Rapidly deteriorating social and political conditions within American society and in the Vietnam theater deeply affected the successive cohorts of replacement soldiers during the second half of the war. Especially demoralizing were the uncertain combat results in the theater; vacilla-ting, and at times contradictory, government policies and military strategies regarding prosecuting the war and pursuing the peace; and a moral crisis at home that included increasingly radical American politics and a rapidly expanding drug culture.[4] Furthermore, apparently the annualized troop rotation schedules, rapid and wholesale transportation of soldiers and media representatives, and modern technology promoted the accelerated infusion of a growing antiwar, antimilitary sentiment into the ranks of the military there. Similarly, the relative ease of communication with family and loved ones back home meant that deployed military personnel often received disapproving or demoralizing communications regarding their service in the theater. Howard, who served as battalion surgeon with the Marines in Vietnam in 1968, reported that he knew of some suicides that were precipitated by troops receiving a "Dear John" letter. By his description, these letters were often rageful and replete with details of sexual promiscuity as if to punish the Marine for desertion.[41] Tanay, a civilian psychiatrist who visited Vietnam to provide a forensic opinion of a Marine charged with combat atrocities, noted that the accused, who had a commendable combat performance record, murdered four civilian Vietnamese in a displaced rage after receiving a letter from his girlfriend telling him of her new fiancé. He further indicated that "Dear John" letters were greater in frequency from earlier wars and were especially blatantly hostile ones, and he theorized that this was because the widespread hostile or ambivalent attitude toward the Vietnam War meant that the home support that usually helped waiting wives and girlfriends tolerate the absence of their men was missing.[42]

The following observations from Lieutenant Colonel Robert L Pettera, the division psychiatrist with the 9th Infantry Division, give some sense of the war weariness for troops in the field as the war wore on:

> . . . Routine—the never-ending [base camp] routine. If you aren't out on patrol you are filling sandbags, building bunkers or burning trash. You live in a weblock type of tent; it has wooden floors, a canvas roof, and usually no lights.
>
> At night you usually have bunker guard, so no lights in your tent doesn't matter. If you aren't on detail, you are on 30 minute alert, and can't go to the PX [post exchange] or the snack bar, anyway. Your condition in the field is the same old thing. You walk all day and ambush at night; you either sleep in trees or on dykes, or just curl up in the mud with the snakes, mosquitoes and leeches.
>
> . . . [A]nd then the unforeseen happens; not a human wave attack, but your company of 134 men is ambushed by about seven companies of Viet Cong. It's all over in 30 minutes, but other outfits are rushed in to try and save you.[43(p677)]

Soldier demoralization was also fed by seeing the everyday plight of the Vietnamese. Besides witnessing outright collateral damage from the fighting, soldiers assigned in Vietnam could not easily ignore the desperation of the massive numbers of displaced and impoverished refugees produced by the war (Figure 1-10 and Figure 1-11.) The growing demoralization and alienation of soldiers often took the form of psychiatric and behavioral problems, especially drug abuse, racial incidents, and misconduct. These behaviors presented problems for the Army and Army psychiatrists on an unprecedented scale. Paradoxically, these problems apparently arose more often among soldiers serving in the "rear" or in noncombat units.[44] However, even in combat units, troops covertly, and at times overtly, challenged authority, for example, in combat refusal incidents, so-called "search and avoid" missions, and excessive combat aggression (including atrocities, etc).

The extent of soldier dysfunction reached new levels after a Vietnamese-based heroin market began to flourish in the summer of 1970 and large numbers of US soldiers became heroin users.[45] In fact, during the last years in Vietnam the Department of Defense estimated that 60% of deployed personnel were using marijuana and 25% to 30% were using heroin.[37] Equally disturbing to the Army in Vietnam were the incidents of soldiers attacking their superiors, typically with explosives ("fragging"—named after the fragmentation grenade).[37(p101)] Like the widening use of heroin by soldiers, such attacks became increasingly common beginning in 1969 and 1970.

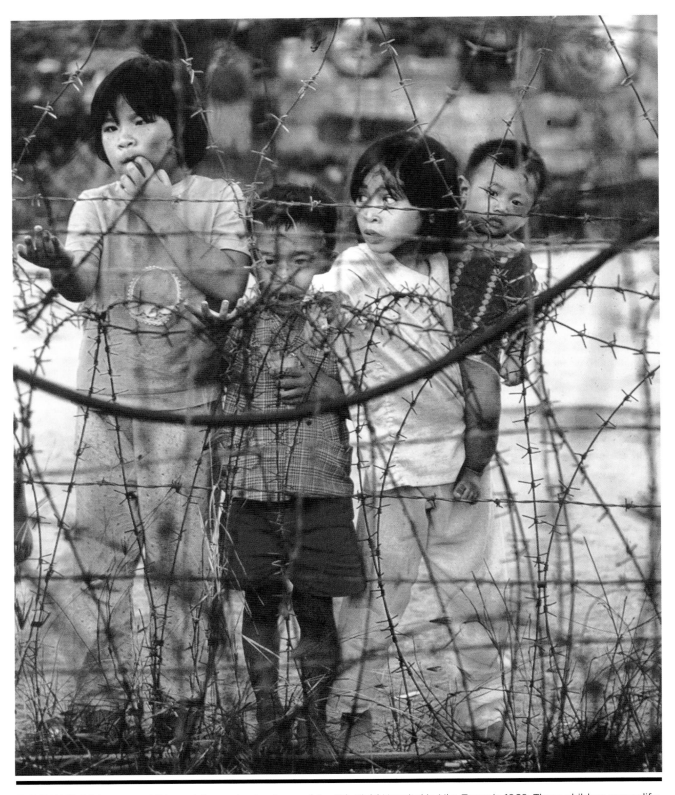

FIGURE 1-10. Vietnamese children at the perimeter fence of the 8th Field Hospital in Nha Trang in 1969. These children exemplify the huge numbers of civilians who were uprooted from their homes and villages by the fighting and forced to congregate for safety near Vietnamese cities and allied military outposts and live a hand-to-mouth existence. Photograph courtesy of Richard D Cameron, Major General, US Army (Retired).

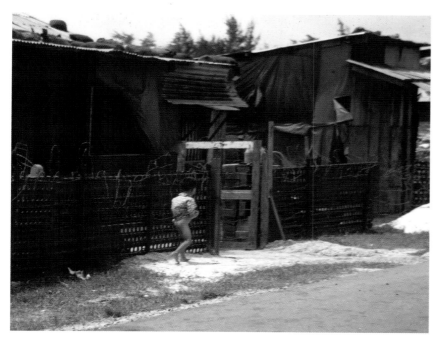

FIGURE 1-11. Improvised Vietnamese shack made from castoff military materials at the entrance to the 95th Evacuation Hospital near Da Nang in 1971. Franklin Del Jones, an Army psychiatrist, reported early in the war that troops reacted negatively to Vietnam's "poverty, prostitution and pestilence." It seems reasonable to assume that a large measure of such reactions came from their witnessing the meager existence of the war's displaced refugees, such as this photograph illustrates. Furthermore, as the antiwar sentiment in the United States increasingly centered on America's responsibility for the war's destructiveness, concern for collateral harm likely increased stress levels for American troops, noncombat as well as combat. Photograph courtesy of Norman M Camp, Colonel, US Army (Retired).

As the war progressed there had been various reports back to the United States suggesting the war effort had become not only costly from the standpoint of American losses, but overly destructive (and thus counterproductive) as well. As a prime example, Jonathan Schell, a journalist, reported on the US Army's "Operation Cedar Falls" near Saigon in January 1967—particularly the struggle to pacify the village of Ben Suc, which was thought to be loyal to the Viet Cong.[46] By Schell's account, the increasingly frustrated American effort, which at times included the provision of food and medical care, led to the total destruction of the village.[46]

Later Schell reported from the field on the extensive damage caused by American military activities in two coastal provinces in South Vietnam in August 1967. Schell observed the ground and air assaults by a collection of brigade-sized units intended to eliminate the enemy's civilian sanctuaries ("Task Force Oregon") and noted the proportion of villages destroyed (70%) and the extent of indigenous population dislocated.[47] He concluded that, although functioning under legitimate authority, most of the US forces are too casual and nonspecific in pursuing their combat goals: "These restraints [rules of engagement] were modified or twisted to such an extent that in practice the restraints evaporated entirely. . . ."[47(p151)] It was his impression that most civil-affairs officials and programs were inadequate to rectify the disintegration of Vietnamese society caused by the American and South Vietnamese military initiatives

in Vietnam. Again, quoting Schell, "the overriding, fantastic fact [is] that we are destroying, seemingly by inadvertence, the very country we are supposedly protecting."[47(p3)]

There also had been scattered reports of frank atrocities by US troops. Then, in November 1969, the American public learned of the massacre of several hundred unarmed Vietnamese civilians by a US Army unit in the hamlet of My Lai, which had taken place in March 1968.[48] The flurry of publicity surrounding this incident and the associated Army investigations and judicial proceedings were compelling to the nation, with the "My Lai massacre" ultimately serving as the rallying point for those insisting that the United States stop all military activities in Vietnam. As it turned out, of the 26 soldiers initially charged with criminal offenses for their actions at My Lai, only 2nd Lieutenant William Calley was convicted.

In time there were increasing accusations from the antiwar movement regarding other war crimes. The "Winter Soldier Investigation," a well-publicized media event sponsored by the Vietnam Veterans Against the War held in Detroit in February 1971, proved especially dramatic. Over 3 days, discharged servicemen from each branch of military service, as well as civilian contractors, medical personnel, and academics, all gave testimony about war crimes they had committed or witnessed during the years of 1963 to 1970.[49] (The subject of excessive combat aggression will be explored in Chapter 6.)

Considerations of the Larger Army During the War

Although the troops in Vietnam—resonant with the restive, antiestablishment sentiments of their peers outside the theater—were more demonstrative, clearly the long and controversial war took a massive toll on the morale and mental health of the US Army more generally.[38–40,50] Specific to mental health, epidemiological data provided by William E Datel regarding the larger Army (by mid-1973) indicated that during the war in Vietnam the worldwide incidence of neuropsychiatric disease among Army personnel rose to near the peak level seen during the Korean War; the psychosis rate for the worldwide active duty Army had never been higher; character and behavior disorder diagnoses (ie, personality disorders[51]) also peaked; and the proportion of Army hospital beds in the United States occupied for all psychiatric causes was greater than it had ever been, including during the so-called psychiatric disaster period of World War II.[52] This is in stark contrast to the exceptionally low Army psychiatric attrition rate of 5 per 1,000 troops per year in the mid-1960s before the start of war in Vietnam.[29]

Finally, on 27 January 1973, the Agreement on Ending the War and Restoring Peace in Vietnam (also known as the Paris Accords) was enacted. This resulted in a temporary ceasefire and ended direct military involvement by the United States in Vietnam following nearly two decades of armed conflict. It stipulated that all US military personnel would be out of Vietnam within 60 days.[5] In compliance the remaining US troops in South Vietnam (there were 24,200 at the beginning of 1973[9]) were rapidly withdrawn, with the last elements departing on 29 March 1973.[8] Also, as stipulated, North Vietnam released 595 prisoners of war.[5] Henry Kissinger, the US Secretary of State, and North Vietnam's Le Duc Tho, a special advisor to the North Vietnamese delegation, were jointly awarded the 1973 Nobel Peace Prize as primary negotiators of the agreement.[53] As mentioned previously, 2 years later North Vietnam violated the truce and overran South Vietnam, which surrendered on 30 April 1975.

CULTURAL POLARIZATION IN AMERICA AND THE VIETNAM WAR

The Social and Political Context of the War

To fully understand the psychosocial forces affecting the soldiers sent to fight in Vietnam, it is important to appreciate the powerful and often clashing cultural crosscurrents in the United States in the 1960s and early 1970s surrounding the war. These social and political phenomena must be viewed against a prehistory that includes the nation's post-World War II experience and subsequent Cold War tensions between the United States and the then-Soviet Union, but also the advent of television coverage of the war, the assassination of President John Kennedy in 1963, and the coming of age of the post-World War II "baby boom" generation.

The years encompassing the Vietnam ground war (1965–1973) represented an excruciatingly volatile period in American life. Intense and often militant challenges to government institutions, especially the military and the war in Vietnam, were increasingly made by: (*a*) the rising civil rights and black-pride movements, (*b*) the emerging "New Left" and a dissenting youth counterculture (the "generation gap"),[54,55] and (*c*) an American public that was becoming progressively disapproving of the war. They, in turn, were opposed by an equally fervent and reactive conservative sector.[4] The prolonged, costly war in Vietnam served as a rallying point, both pro and con, for the passions and ambitions of each group. These three movements, fostered by an expanding drug culture, variously fed on, and were fed by, a widening crisis within the military overall (unprecedented demoralization and alienation), especially in Vietnam. As they synergistically intersected, they generated a groundswell of opposition to military service among draft-eligible men.[4]

It is beyond the scope of this book to offer comprehensive review and analysis of the effects of the war on American life or the influence of the competing political strains in America on the strategy and structure of the military in Vietnam and on those who served there. However, Lang, a sociologist, provided a particularly thoughtful analysis comparing Vietnam with previous American wars as well as similar ones involving the British in South Africa and the French in Algeria. According to Lang, although much of the American troop disaffection, indiscipline, and dysfunction in the last half of the war in Vietnam is familiar in its form as a predictable demoralization reaction to fighting an extended war, what makes Vietnam unique was that it was aggravated by organizational policies and the type of warfare being waged (counterinsurgency); became politicized through rapid contact with the home front; and crystallized along the more visible cleavages of race, risk, and career commitment to the military.[56] For the interested reader, there are numerous additional sources, many of which are poignant and often passionately

FIGURE 1-12. Vietnam War Gallup opinion poll results answering the question: "In view of the developments since we entered the fighting in Vietnam, do you think the US made a mistake sending troops to fight in Vietnam?" by percent of those polled each year (number of data points/year are in parentheses).

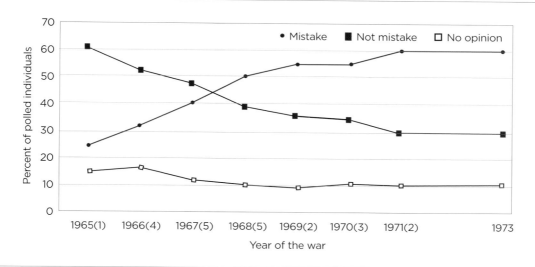

Data source: Gallup GH. *The Gallup Poll: Public Opinion, 1935–1971*. New York, NY: Random House; 1972.

biased as well.[57–73] The following discussion will provide some selective elaboration and amplification.

Increased Public Opposition to the War and Political Activism

Over the course of the war larger and louder antiwar protest rallies, marches, and demonstrations took place in the United States, with some reaching the level of riots.[74] From the outset the Johnson Administration decided not to attempt to squelch public and political opposition to the war or censor the media. This was calculated to foster the impression that it was "business as usual" in America, allowing President Johnson's social programs to continue moving forward.[4] In retrospect, it appears that this strategy backfired.

The new (for this war) television coverage of the war brought the costs and the political turmoil in Vietnam straight into the living rooms of US citizens and most likely accelerated the American public's perception that the war's justification was questionable despite reassurances from the administration. In the words of Laurence Stern, a Vietnam War correspondent, "[Television illuminated the] . . . devastation that was being inflicted on a remote peasant society [and] the spectacle of Americans dying and bleeding in the mountains and paddies."[75(p8)] Stanly Karnow, a Vietnam historian, provided this disturbing analysis of the impact

of TV coverage: "The screen often portrayed human agony in scenes of the wounded and dying on both sides, and the ordeal of civilians trapped by the combat. But mostly it transmitted the grueling reality of the struggle—remote, repetitious, monotonous—punctuated periodically by moments of horror."[8(p523)]

The steadily growing public disapproval of the war in Vietnam can be traced through a series of nationwide Gallup opinion polls (Figure 1-12). As noted, in 1965 only 25% thought US military involvement was a mistake (vs 60% who said "no"); by 1971 these factions had almost completely reversed (60% saying "yes," it was a mistake, and only 30% disagreeing).[76]

Perhaps an equally fateful miscalculation was the administration's decision to rely on conscription and volunteers to fight in Vietnam and to avoid calling up the Reserves and the National Guard. Following the insertion of ground troops in March 1965, the growing manpower requirements in Vietnam resulted in dramatically accelerated draft calls; mass demonstrations and public draft card burnings quickly followed. For example, total inductions in 1965 were about 120,000; those for 1966 and 1967 were 2.5 times the 1965 figure.[16(p30)]

As opposition to the war mounted, the draft became the epicenter of the antiwar protest until the military switched to an all-volunteer force in 1973.[16(p37)]

With each passing year, as the need for more troops became evident, additional criteria for draft exemption were removed to increase the pool of eligible draftees. In December 1969, in an effort to blunt the public's growing concern for unevenness and inconsistency in the Selective Service System, the draft was modified to a lottery system, based on birthdays.[77] Men then knew the likelihood of being drafted based on where their birthdays fell. Ultimately 4 million young men were exempted by high lottery numbers, but more than 200,000 young men were accused of draft avoidance offenses.[77]

The Counterculture and Youth/Student Opposition to the War

Opposition to US involvement in Vietnam began slowly in 1964 on various college campuses as part of a more general rising spirit of student activism. In addition to various liberal causes, "free speech," "free love," "peace," and "do your own thing" were also popular. The means employed to indicate opposition included political advocacy, civil disobedience, "sit-ins," "teach-ins," and generally nonviolent resistance to the status quo. Quoting H. Stuart Hughes, former chair of the Department of History at Harvard University:

. . . [T]he first signs of a new student temper appeared at the turn of the decade with the civil rights demonstrations of the spring of 1960. This third postwar generation among the young . . . alternated protests against racial segregation with activities in the cause of peace. Its heroes were the civil rights workers, white and black, who went into the South in successive summers, a few of whom paid for their devotion with their lives. . . . Commitment to humanity became its imperative, "We Shall Overcome" its anthem, fraternity and good will its modes of moral expression. It sought to refrain from hatred, and its tactics were invariably nonviolent.[78(p23)]

However, a succession of tremendous shocks ushered in a more fervent antiestablishment spirit: the assassination of President Kennedy in the autumn of 1963; the first ghetto uprisings in the summer of 1964; the escalation of the war in Vietnam beginning in 1965 and the impact of the draft; the 1968 assassinations of civil rights leader Reverend Martin Luther King in April and presidential candidate Robert Kennedy in June;

and, also in 1968, the enemy's surprise Tet offensives and other seeming military setbacks in Vietnam. The result was widespread impatience with the prospects for orderly change through more peaceful, passive means, and deep cynicism and mistrust of American institutions and "anyone over 30." The "Woodstock generation," named after the huge rock festival held in upstate New York in August 1969, and its "summer of peace and love" were quickly fading memories as the movement took on a more radical perspective and accepted a more open, and at times violent, revolutionary approach.[4]

Again quoting Hughes:

. . . What has been unusual about the insurgent mood of the past half decade has been its juxtaposition of anarchism and the peremptory silencing of opponents, its peculiar blend of political Puritanism and personal license, and its cult of "confrontation" as a quasi-religious act of witness.[78(p24)]

As one measure, Seligman reviewed more systematic surveys of student attitudes in 1969 and noted that although only 2% of college youth were highly visible activists, roughly 40% of their peers held similar views ("protest prone") and signified a true "generation gap." Among this larger group, approximately one-half endorsed the belief that the United States was a sick society and acknowledged a loss of faith in democratic institutions. Two-thirds endorsed civil disobedience to promote their causes, especially antiwar protests and draft resistance.[55]

Yankelovich surveyed the prevailing mood on American college campuses in 1971 using a national sample and compared results with similar surveys from 1968, 1969, and 1970.[79] He interpreted the earlier student movement as representing the search for a new moral faith, with these students rejecting the dominant mode of thinking in America (eg, faith in technology, rationalism, and traditional middle-class sensibility) and embracing a philosophy that placed a premium on nature and the natural.[79] He also noted that in the 1971 sample, student cynicism and frustration seemed to have replaced much of the earlier commitment to political revolution.[79] In a similar study he compared noncollege youths between 1969 and 1973 and found a dramatic shift away from acceptance of authority and conformity.[80]

Emergent Black-Pride Movement and Racial Tensions

The civil rights movement in the United States has a long, tortured history that reaches back much further than that of student unrest and dissent. More specific to serving in the military, President Harry Truman issued an executive order in 1948 directing the nation's military services to eliminate all vestiges of racial segregation.[81] Since then many positive gains made in the status of black Americans can be directly attributed to the men and women who served in the military. However, the burgeoning civil rights movement in the 1960s heightened black soldiers' awareness of disparities (with accusations of discrimination) in positions and roles for blacks in the military, especially among the younger soldiers and especially regarding combat exposure and risk.[37(p102),82]

For instance, during the initial years in Vietnam, questions were raised as to whether blacks represented an unfair proportion of the combat casualties. In fact, in 1965 and 1966, in each of the deployed combat divisions, the proportion of deaths of African Americans exceeded the proportion of African American soldiers in the division.[16] For example, black soldiers made up 13.4% of the 1st Cavalry Division (AirMobile), but they accounted for 26% of the casualties.[16(p37)] However, as Spector pointed out, closer analysis revealed that overall blacks did not serve in Vietnam out of proportion to their numbers in the general population[16]; and rather than racially driven policies, various other social and cultural factors, for example, levels of education and socioeconomic status, served to select African Americans for greater risk in Vietnam.[16]

Later studies demonstrated that "[what] most determined a man's chances of fighting and dying in Vietnam was not race but class . . . It was the poor who bore the lion's share of the fighting and dying."[16(p338)] Still, beginning in 1967 the military began to reduce the numbers of black soldiers assigned to infantry, armor, and cavalry units in Vietnam, and by mid-1969 the percentage of black casualties was close to the percentage of blacks serving in Vietnam.[82] Official postwar casualty figures include 7,264 deaths among all service branches as "Negro," which is 13% of all deaths in the theater from all causes (58,193).[24]

Racial tensions in America became explosive following the assassination of Reverend Martin Luther King in April 1968. Racial protests and riots erupted at various US military installations worldwide, including those in Vietnam.[16(p249)] The most notorious in Vietnam was in August 1968, when black confinees of the Long Binh stockade, who were protesting alleged discrimination by the Army, seized and held the facility for almost a month.[16(pp253–256)] These sentiments coincided with the rapid evolution of a more radical, "black power" faction that advocated a black pride revolution and rejected assimilation in American culture as a central goal for African Americans. Career military blacks were often caught between their loyalty to the military and the attitudes of the younger, black, enlisted soldiers who were restive and expected solidarity from them regarding their complaints of prejudice and discrimination. As the war wound on, younger blacks increasingly opposed service in a "white man's war," with the accusation being that it was racially inspired (eg, against other people of color) and did not warrant their sacrifices.[83,84]

When Wallace Terry, a correspondent, surveyed soldiers in Vietnam regarding racial perceptions and attitudes in 1970 and compared the results with a similar study he had conducted 3 years earlier, he was disturbed by the depth of the "bitterness" he found[85(p230)] among the new black soldiers. They were averse to fighting in a war they considered to be the white man's folly; had directed their anger primarily toward America; and asserted their intention to return home to take up the fight against repression and racism in America.[85] In a later publication he commented:

[By 1969,] replacing the careerists [who served earlier] were black draftees, many just steps removed from marching in the Civil Rights Movement or rioting in the rebellions that swept the urban ghettos from Harlem to Watts. All were filled with a new sense of black pride and purpose. They spoke loudest against discrimination they encountered on the battlefield in decorations, promotion, and duty assignments. They chose not to overlook racial insults, cross-burnings, and Confederate flags of their white comrades. They called for unity among black brothers on the battlefield to protest these indignities and provide mutual support.

. . . In the last years of the [war] both black soldier and white fought to survive a war they knew they would never win in a conventional sense. And, often, they fought each other. The war, which had bitterly divided America like

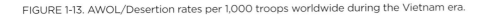

FIGURE 1-13. AWOL/Desertion rates per 1,000 troops worldwide during the Vietnam era.

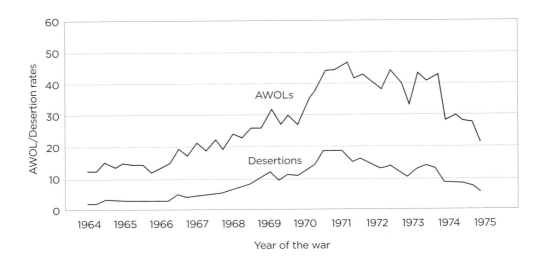

Source: Bell DB. *Characteristics of Army Deserters in the DoD Special Discharge Review Program.* Arlington, Va: US Army Research Institute for the Behavioral and Social Sciences; 1979. Report No. 1229. [Available at: Alexandria, Va: Defense Technical Information Center. Document No. AD A78601.]

no other issue since the Civil War, had become a double battleground, pitting American soldier against American soldier. The spirit of foxhole brotherhood I found in 1967 had evaporated.[84(ppxiv–xv)]

The subject of racial tensions and conflicts in the theater will be discussed further in Chapter 8.

Soldier Resistance and the Underground Movement

Most regrettably, as opposition to the war mounted, public attitudes in the United States toward returning veterans reversed from acceptance to scorn.[86] This apparently left many of those who chose, or were directed, to serve in Vietnam as replacements conflicted as to what represented patriotic, morally justifiable behavior, as well as less tolerant of the inherent risks and hardships they faced there. (Such a clash of values would also invariably complicate the reintegration of returning soldiers and for many may have contributed to chronic psychiatric conditions and serious adjustment difficulties.)

Furthermore, by late 1969, the feeling that one was unlucky in being sent to Vietnam was heightened following the previously mentioned implementation

of the Selective Service System lottery procedure for choosing draft-eligible men that eliminated most draft deferments.[77] Johnston and Bachman compared results of surveys of draft-eligible men conducted in spring 1969, and again in summer 1970, regarding their plans and attitudes toward military service. In that short span of time the majority shifted from identifying with US political and military policies in Vietnam to feeling alienated from the greater society, the government, and US involvement there.[87] The roughly fourfold, Army-wide increases in rates for absent without leave (AWOL) and desertion during the period from 1964 to 1974 provides a measure of the growing opposition to serving over the course of the war (Figure 1-13).[88] Among all the service branches, the number of deserters for the years 1965 to 1974 totaled 380,445, and the desertion rate peaked in 1971 (73.4/1,000 troops), a level exceeding the highest for the Korean War (1953 = 22.3/1,000) and for World War II (1944 = 63/1,000).[39(Table2)] (Perhaps of some interest, Department of Defense statistics indicate that a much higher percentage [36%] of those who left the United States to seek asylum in other countries, such as Canada and Sweden, claimed anti-Vietnam War attitudes as their motive compared to those who did not [9%].[88]) Similarly, administrative discharges from the service for unsuitability, unfitness, or misconduct for all branches rose from approximately 38,000 in 1968 (10.8/1,000 troops/year) to approximately 67,000 in 1972 (28.7/1,000 troops/year), with an average of 40% of these receiving a psychiatric diagnosis of character and behavior disorders.[89]

Organized dissent within the military did not emerge until 1967 and disappeared in 1973 once the troops were out of Vietnam.[25] It apparently was slow in its development because its inspiration required the angst of returning veterans to be combined with draftee resistance. In time a vicious cycle developed in which returning veterans publicly repudiated their Vietnam service record, including joining the war protest movement through organizations such as Vietnam Veterans Against the War, which, in turn, encouraged prospective Vietnam soldiers to oppose service there. In the United States, this essentially first-term enlistee and draftee antiwar resistance movement was especially promulgated through the "alternative culture" coffee houses, underground newspapers (estimated to exist on 300 posts and bases),[25(p234)] antiwar protest petitions, and support from civilian antiwar groups.

An example of an antiwar protest petition is one sent to Congress by 300 sailors aboard the Vietnam-bound USS *Coral Sea*:

As Americans we all have the moral obligation to voice our opinions concerning the Vietnam War. . . . The Coral Sea is scheduled for Vietnam in November. This does not have to be a fact. This ship can be prevented from taking active part in the conflict if we, the majority, voice our opinion that we do not believe in the Vietnam War.[25(p235)]

Two organizations were especially prominent in seeking to organize servicemen to oppose military service: (1) The American Servicemen's Union and (2) the Movement for a Democratic Military.[90] However, as it turned out, most soldiers in Vietnam were not true antiwar protestors and, overall, the resistance "movement" had only limited success.[91] Still, although the antiwar movement within the Vietnam-era military failed to reach revolutionary proportions for several reasons, especially the lack of sympathetic civilians in Vietnam, its emergence was unique in US history and some believed it accelerated withdrawal from the war.[25] Others argue that it emboldened the enemy and thus dragged out the peace negotiations and prolonged the war.[25(p237)] Regardless of which of these views might

be correct, military and government officials were extremely concerned about its progression.

The Spreading Drug Culture and Its Effects on Soldiers Sent to Vietnam

Drug use among teens and young adults in the United States, especially the use of psychedelics and marijuana, rose rapidly in the 1960s in tandem with the emerging dissidence of this group.[45,92,93] Various studies conducted during the Vietnam era comparing drug use among soldiers with their civilian peers demonstrated that the young enlisted soldiers, not surprisingly, brought into the service and into Vietnam their drug use habits from civilian life. Among these studies were the following:

• As the backdrop, a nationwide study of psychoactive drug use among young men conducted at the close of the Vietnam War indicated that the peak of the drug epidemic was 1969 to 1973, and that veterans, regardless of where they served, showed no higher rates than nonveterans.[93]

• Regarding clinical populations in the Army outside of Vietnam, a comparison of 400 psychiatric admissions at Walter Reed General Hospital for each of the years 1962, 1968, and 1969 found that whereas only 1% had drug-related causes in 1962, 20% had drug-related causes for their admission in 1968, and 25% in 1969.[94]

• Regarding measures among nonclinical populations in the military within the United States, surveys of drug use at a stateside military installation conducted in 1970, 1971, and 1972 showed that, over that 3-year time span, the percentage of respondents reporting premilitary drug use increased as did the amount of use and the number of current users.[95] A similar study of patterns of drug use among active duty enlisted men assigned to 56 separate Army units in the United States (N = 5,482), conducted between January 1969 and April 1969, found that one-quarter acknowledged past use of marijuana, amphetamines, lysergic acid diethylamide (LSD), or heroin.[96] Another survey 2 years later (between January 1971 and June 1971) found that almost one-third of new military inductees (N = 19,948) acknowledged drug use as civilians.[97]

• Regarding the scope of the drug abuse problem for US Army personnel in Europe, a study in 1970 and 1971 found the overall incidence of drug abuse in this population was similar to that reported for soldiers in Vietnam and for stateside college students.[98]

- Among soldiers sent to Vietnam specifically, the survey of enlisted soldiers departing Vietnam by Sapol and Roffman in 1967 (N = 584) found that 31.7% reported use of marijuana at least once in their life, but the investigators concluded that the rates were comparable with those reported in published studies among university students.[99] In a survey of soldiers entering or departing Vietnam 2 years later, Stanton found a sizable increase in the reported lifetime use of marijuana among those leaving Vietnam (50.1%) when compared to the 1967 survey, most of which he accounted for by the increase reported by soldiers entering Vietnam.[100] However, Stanton also found a shift toward heavier use among his sample of departing enlisted soldiers (29.6% compared to the 7.4% from the earlier study).[100] Nonetheless, his impression was that the rise in casual marijuana use in Vietnam mostly mirrored rising use patterns among civilian peers.[100]

- Regarding heroin use, a 1972 study simultaneously comparing 1,007 noncombat Army soldiers in Vietnam with 856 counterparts assigned to a stateside post found that 13.5% of Vietnam soldiers and 14.5% of those in the United States reported previous use of heroin.[101] The authors compared their findings with published surveys and concluded that although a heroin epidemic occurred in Vietnam in the early 1970s, assuming that "such an epidemic [w]as 'unique' . . . and 'infected' many average American soldiers appears inaccurate and misleading. Heroin users, regardless of location, appeared demographically and psychosocially more similar than different. . . ."[101(p1154)]

Chapter 2 will provide an overview of Army psychiatric problems in Vietnam, including that of drug use; and Chapter 9 will examine drug and alcohol problems in Vietnam in greater detail.

Disputes About the Ethics of Combat Psychiatry

The shifting social and political zeitgeist in the latter half of the war—particularly the accelerating antiwar and antimilitary sentiment—began to affect psychiatrists and psychiatry and provoked concerns about cooperating with the military. Debates—typically quite passionate—appeared in the literature raising questions regarding the ethics of psychiatrists who performed draft evaluations[102–106] or served with the military, especially in Vietnam.[107–112] Denunciation of military psychiatry came both from psychiatrists and other physicians who had served in Vietnam, as well as from those who had not.[113]

Mental health organizations also sought to take official positions on the war. Even if not specifically questioning the ethics of their colleagues in uniform, they did by implication question the morality of the US military and government. For example, in March 1971, 67% of members responding to a poll of the American Psychiatric Association voted that the United States should terminate all military activity in Vietnam.[114] In July 1972, the American Psychological Association joined seven other mental health associations in attacking the US role in the war.[115] In response, professional support for the US forces was provided by several psychiatrists, most of whom had served in Vietnam.[116–121] Chapter 11 will explore the demoralizing effects of these professional crosscurrents on the psychiatrists sent to Vietnam later in the war and possible effects on their clinical decisions. (In a collateral fashion, the chaplains serving in the Army in Vietnam also underwent condemnation from home because of their cooperation with the military in Vietnam.[122])

SUMMARY AND CONCLUSIONS

This chapter provided an overview of the historical, military, and sociopolitical events associated with America's ground war in Southeast Asia bearing on the challenges faced by Army psychiatry there. America entered the fight in South Vietnam in March 1965 with the intention of blocking the spread of international communism in Southeast Asia. Considering the limited material resources of the enemy, it was anticipated that the United States would quickly prevail. In retrospect, this turned out to be fateful miscalculation. After 8 years of war, 2 years following a negotiated truce and the withdrawal of US combat troops (August 1972) North Vietnam defeated South Vietnam. Thirty years later, Dale Andrade, senior historian at the US Army Center of Military History, and Lieutenant Colonel James Willbanks, Director of Department of Military History, US Command and General Staff College, provided the following summation:

In Vietnam, the U.S. military faced arguably the most complex, effective, lethal insurgency in history. The enemy was no rag-tag band lurking in the jungle, but rather a combination of guerrillas, political cadre, and modern main-force units capable of standing toe to toe with the US military. Any one of these would have been significant, but in combination they presented a formidable threat.[123(p9)]

For America this involved an enormous investment of human and material resources. As the war lengthened the nation lost its resolve, and the preponderance of soldiers sent as replacements—primarily draftees or reluctant volunteers—came to doubt the purpose for their risks and sacrifices, and to oppose service there and military authority in general. These attitudes were strongly encouraged by a growing antiwar sentiment in the United States; a passionate, dissident youth movement; and opposition to military service among black Americans. Facilitative, but also emblematic, this dissenting subculture especially rallied around the burgeoning drug culture of the times. As a consequence, not only did the military in Vietnam show signs of unraveling after 1968, but more generally, the institution of the Army became significantly impaired by this psychosocial malady. More specific to military psychiatry, not surprisingly, these remarkable events and circumstances—this convulsion of life in America—adversely affected the mental health and psychological resilience of a large proportion of the military service members deployed in Vietnam.

In the decades that have followed the Vietnam War, there have been countless publications devoted to describing and analyzing America's failure in Southeast Asia. Although anything close to a proper review of these works is beyond the scope of this volume, a publication by Martin Van Creveld, the distinguished military historian, seems worthy of special note because, besides enumerating an array of evident mistakes made in prosecuting the war, he alluded to the corollary mismanagement of the human element, which has implications for the burgeoning psychiatric and behavioral problems in Vietnam. In his chapter "The Helicopter and the Computer," Van Creveld highlighted data demonstrating the negative effects consequent to the burgeoning weapon systems, electronic communications, and data processing technology in Vietnam. Ubiquitous helicopter mobility, undisciplined use of the tactical field radio, unrepresentative media coverage, and excessive and individualized replacement of personnel, especially commanders, all combined with the torrent of information that was collected to overwhelm the chain of command. Van Creveld argued that "the American command system was enormous, [involved] a heavy additional logistic burden, and in the end collapsed under its own weight . . . and led to one of the least cost-effective wars known to history."[124(p260)] In examining the limitations of the systems analysis approach that was utilized in Vietnam and which provided the rationale for top-level decision making, van Creveld noted that "an approach whose favorite device is number-crunching may be tempted to exclude [all-important] moral and spiritual factors"[124(p240)] and lead to an "information pathology"[124(p248)] that fails to penetrate into the nature of things. He concluded that "to study command as it operated in Vietnam is, indeed, almost enough to make one despair of human reason; we have seen the future, and it does not work."[124(p260)]

The chapter that follows provides a more explicit examination of the emergent trends in psychiatric conditions and behavioral problems that arose during the war and the consequent challenges faced by the deployed US Army leadership and the psychiatric specialists and their mental health colleagues.

REFERENCES

1. US Department of State. *Why We Fight In Viet-Nam*. Washington, DC: Department of State, Office of Media Services; June 1967. Viet-Nam Information Notes (#6).

2. Renner JA Jr. The changing patterns of psychiatric problems in Vietnam. *Compr Psychiatry*. 1973;14(2):169–181.

3. Bourne PG. *Men, Stress, and Vietnam*. Boston, Mass: Little, Brown; 1970.

4. Dougan C, Lipsman S, Doyle E, and the editors of Boston Publishing Co. *The Vietnam Experience: A Nation Divided*. Boston, Mass: Boston Publishing Co; 1984.

5. Cohen B. *The Vietnam Guidebook: The First Comprehensive New Guide to Vietnam With Angkor Wat*. Boston, Mass: Houghton Mifflin; 1991.

6. Doyle E, Lipsman S, and the editors of Boston Publishing Co. *The Vietnam Experience:*

Setting the Stage. Boston, Mass: Boston Publishing Co; 1981.

7.   Doyle E, Lipsman S, Weiss S, and the editors of Boston Publishing Co. *The Vietnam Experience: Passing the Torch.* Boston, Mass: Boston Publishing Co; 1981.

8.   Karnow S. *Vietnam: A History.* New York, NY: Viking; 1983.

9.   Department of Defense, Office of the Assistant Secretary of Defense (Comptroller), Directorate for Information Operations. *US Military Personnel in South Vietnam 1960–1972*; 15 March 1974.

10. Sorley L. *A Better War: The Unexamined Victories and Final Tragedy of America's Last Years in Vietnam.* New York, NY: Harcourt Books; 1999.

11. Ellsberg D. *Secrets: A Memoir of Vietnam and the Pentagon Papers.* New York, NY: Viking; 2002.

12. McNamara RS, with VanDeMark B. *In Retrospect: The Tragedy and Lessons of Vietnam.* New York, NY: Times Books; 1995.

13. Maitland T, Weiss S, and the editors of Boston Publishing Co. *The Vietnam Experience: Raising the Stakes.* Boston, Mass: Boston Publishing Co; 1982.

14. McVicker SJ. Invisible veterans. The women who served in Vietnam. *J Psychosoc Nurs Ment Health Serv.* 1985;23(10):12–19.

15. Kolb RK. Vietnam veteran fact sheet. *Natl Vietnam Veteran Rev.* 1982;November:30–31, 46.

16. Spector RH. *After Tet: The Bloodiest Year in Vietnam.* New York, NY: The Free Press; 1993.

17. McGrath JJ. *The Other End of the Spear: The Tooth-to-Tail Ratio (T3R) in Modern Military Operations.* Fort Leavenworth, Kan: Combat Studies Institute Press; 2007.

18. Doyle E, Lipsman S, and the editors of Boston Publishing Co. *The Vietnam Experience: America Takes Over.* Boston, Mass: Boston Publishing Co; 1982.

19. Stanton SL. *The Rise and Fall of an American Army: US Ground Forces in Vietnam, 1965–1973.* Novato, Calif: Presidio Press; 1985.

20. Neel SH. *Medical Support of the US Army in Vietnam, 1965–1970.* Washington, DC: GPO; 1973.

21. National Archive Records Administration (NARA). *Statistical Information About Casualties of the Vietnam War*: [Southeast Asia] Combat Area Casualties Current File (CACCF), 1998.

22. US Army Adjutant General, Casualty Services Division (DAAG-PEC). *Active Duty Army Personnel Battle Casualties and Nonbattle Deaths Vietnam, 1961–1979, Office of The Adjutant General Counts.* 3 February 1981.

23. Center for Military History. Available at: http://www.history.army.mil/html/moh/mohstats.html; accessed 12 June 2013.

24. Doyle E, Weiss S, and the editors of Boston Publishing Co. *The Vietnam Experience: A Collision of Cultures.* Boston, Mass: Boston Publishing Co; 1984.

25. Balkind JJ. *Morale Deterioration in the United States Military During the Vietnam Period* [dissertation]. Ann Arbor, Mich: University Microfilms International; 1978: 235. [Available at: *Dissertations Abstracts International,* 39 (1-A), 438. Order No. 78-11, 333.]

26. Neller G, Stevens V, Chung R, Devaris D. *Psychological Warfare and Its Effects on Mental Health: Lessons Learned From Vietnam* (unpublished); 1985.

27. Maitland T, McInerney P, and the editors of Boston Publishing Co. *The Vietnam Experience: A Contagion of War.* Boston, Mass: Boston Publishing Co; 1983.

28. Custis DL. Military medicine from World War II to Vietnam. *JAMA.* 1990;264(17):2259–2262.

29. Allerton WS. Army psychiatry in Vietnam. In: Bourne PG, ed. *The Psychology and Physiology of Stress: With Reference to Special Studies of the Viet Nam War.* New York, NY: Academic Press; 1969: 2–17.

30. Datel WE, Johnson AW Jr. *Psychotropic Prescription Medication in Vietnam.* Alexandria, Va: Defense Technical Information Center; 1981. Document No. AD A097610 (or search http://www.dtic.mil/cgi-bin/GetTRDoc?AD=ADA097610&Location=U2&doc=GetTRDoc.pdf).

31. Tiffany WJ Jr. The mental health of Army troops in Viet Nam. *Am J Psychiatry.* 1967;123(12):1585–1586.

32. Moskos CC Jr. Military made scapegoat for Vietnam. In: Millett AR, ed. *A Short History of the Vietnam War.* Bloomington, Ind: Indiana University Press; 1978: 67–72.

33. Dougan C, Weiss S, and the editors of Boston Publishing Co. *The Vietnam Experience: Nineteen Sixty-Eight.* Boston, Mass: Boston Publishing Co; 1983.

34. *Principal Wars in Which the United States Participated; US Military Personnel Serving and Casualties.* Department of Defense, Office of the Assistant Secretary of Defense (Comptroller), Directorate for Information Operations, 15 March 1974.

35. Braestrup P. *Big Story: How the American Press and Television Reported and Interpreted the Crisis of Tet 1968 in Vietnam and Washington.* 2 vols. Boulder, Colo: Westview Press; 1977.

36. Mueller JE. Trends in popular support for the wars in Korea and Vietnam. *Am Polit Sci Rev.* 1971;65:358–375.

37. Lipsman S, Doyle E, and the editors of Boston Publishing Co. *The Vietnam Experience: Fighting For Time.* Boston, Mass: Boston Publishing Co; 1983.

38. Johnson H, Wilson GC. *Army in Anguish.* New York, NY: Pocket Books; 1972.

39. Gabriel RA, Savage PL. *Crisis in Command: Mismanagement in the Army.* New York, NY: Hill and Wang; 1978.

40. Cincinnatus. *Self-Destruction: The Disintegration and Decay of the United States Army During the Vietnam Era.* New York, NY: Norton; 1981.

41. Howard S. The Vietnam warrior: his experience, and implications for psychotherapy. *Am J Psychotherapy.* 1976;30:121–135.

42. Tanay E. The Dear John syndrome during the Vietnam war. *Dis Nerv Syst.* 1976;37:165–167.

43. Pettera RL, Johnson BM, Zimmer R. Psychiatric management of combat reactions with emphasis on a reaction unique to Vietnam. *Mil Med.* 1969;134(9):673–678.

44. Jones FD. Reactions to stress: combat versus combat support troops. Presentation to World Psychiatric Association, Honolulu, Hawaii, 29 August 1977.

45. Baker SL Jr. Drug abuse in the United States Army. *Bull N Y Acad Med.* 1971;47:541–549.

46. Schell J. *The Village of Ben Suc.* New York, NY: Alfred A Knopf; 1967.

47. Schell J. *The Military Half: An Account of Destruction in Quang Ngai and Quang Tin.* New York, NY: Alfred A Knopf; 1968.

48. Hersh SM. *My Lai 4: A Report on the Massacre and its Aftermath.* New York, NY: Random House; 1970.

49. Vietnam Veterans Against the War. *The Winter Soldier Investigation: An Inquiry Into American War Crimes.* Boston, Mass: Beacon Press; 1972.

50. Hauser W. *America's Army in Crisis: A Study in Civil-Military Relations.* Baltimore, Md: Johns Hopkins University Press; 1973.

51. American Psychiatric Association. *Diagnostic and Statistical Manual of Mental Disorders II.* Washington, DC: American Psychiatric Association; 1968.

52. Datel WE. *A Summary of Source Data in Military Psychiatric Epidemiology.* Alexandria, Va: Defense Technical Information Center; 1976. Document No. AD A021265.

53. Nobel Foundation. Available at: http://www.nobelprize.org/nobel_prizes/peace/laureates/1973/index.html. Accessed 12 June 2013.

54. Starr JM. The peace and love generation: changing attitudes toward sex and violence among college youth. *J Social Issues.* 1974;30(2):73–106.

55. Seligman D. A special kind of rebellion. *Fortune.* January 1969: 66–69, 172–175.

56. Lang K. American military performance in Vietnam: background and analysis. *J Polit Mil Sociol.* 1980;8:269–286.

57. Camp NM, Stretch RH, Marshall WC. *Stress, Strain, and Vietnam: An Annotated Bibliography of Two Decades of Psychiatric and Social Sciences Literature Reflecting the Effect of the War on the American Soldier.* Westport, Conn: Greenwood Press; 1988.

58. Boettcher TD. *Vietnam: The Valor and the Sorrow—From the Home Front to the Front Lines in Words and Pictures.* Boston, Mass: Little, Brown; 1985.

59. Emerson G. *Winners and Losers: Battles, Retreats, Gains, Losses, and Ruins From the Vietnam War.* New York, NY: Random House; 1976.

60. Fitzgerald F. *Fire in the Lake: The Vietnamese and the Americans in Vietnam*. Boston, Mass: Little, Brown; 1972.

61. Gibson JW. *The Perfect War: Technowar in Vietnam*. Boston, Mass: Atlantic Monthly Press; 1986.

62. Horne AD, ed. *The Wounded Generation: America After Vietnam*. Englewood Cliffs, NJ: Prentice-Hall; 1981.

63. Kendrick A. *The Wound Within: America in the Vietnam Years, 1945–1974*. Boston, Mass: Little, Brown; 1974.

64. Kirk D. *Tell It to the Dead: Memories of a War*. Chicago, Ill: Nelson-Hall; 1975.

65. Lewy G. The American experience in Vietnam. In: Sarkesian SC, ed. *Combat Effectiveness: Cohesion, Stress, and the Volunteer Military*. Beverly Hills, Calif: Sage Publications; 1980: 94–106.

66. MacPherson M. *Long Time Passing: Vietnam and the Haunted Generation*. Garden City, NY: Doubleday; 1984.

67. Millett RA, ed. *A Short History of the Vietnam War*. Bloomington, Ind: Indiana University Press; 1978.

68. Peake LA. *The United States in the Vietnam War, 1954–1975: A Selected, Annotated Bibliography*. New York, NY: Garland Publishing; 1986.

69. Wheeler J. *Touched With Fire: The Future of the Vietnam Generation*. New York, NY: Franklin Watts; 1984.

70. Herring GC. *America's Longest War: The United States and Vietnam 1950–1975*. New York, NY: Knopf; 1986.

71. Duiker WJ. *Historical Dictionary of Vietnam*. Metuchen, NJ: Scarecrow Press; 1989.

72. Sheehan N. *A Bright and Shining Lie: John Paul Vann and America in Vietnam*. New York, NY: Random House; 1988.

73. Herring GC, ed. *The Pentagon Papers: Abridged Edition*. New York, NY: McGraw-Hill; 1993.

74. Heath GL, ed. *Mutiny Does Not Happen Lightly: The Literature of the American Resistance to the Vietnam War*. Metuchen, NJ: Scarecrow Press; 1976.

75. Stern L. America in anguish, 1965 to 1973. In: Millett AR, ed. *A Short History of the Vietnam War*. Bloomington, Ind: Indiana University Press; 1978: 3–12.

76. Gallup GH. *The Gallup Poll: Public Opinion, 1935–1971*. New York, NY: Random House; 1972.

77. Baskir LM, Strauss WA. *Chance and Circumstance: The Draft, the War, and the Vietnam Generation*. New York, NY: Alfred A. Knopf; 1978.

78. Hughes HS. Emotional disturbance and American social change, 1944–1969. *Am J Psychiatry*. 1969;126(1):21–28.

79. Yankelovich DA. *The Changing Values on Campus: Political and Personal Attitudes of Today's College Students*. New York, NY: Washington Square Press; 1972.

80. Yankelovich DA. *The New Morality: A Profile of American Youth in the 70's*. New York, NY: McGraw-Hill; 1974.

81. Taylor JE. *Freedom to Serve: Truman, Civil Rights, and Executive Order 9981*. New York, NY: Routledge; 2012.

82. Binkin M, Eitelberg MJ. *Blacks in the Military*. Washington, DC: Brookings Institution; 1982.

83. Mullen RW. *Blacks and Vietnam*. Washington, DC: University Press of America; 1981.

84. Terry W, ed. *Bloods: An Oral History of the Vietnam War by Black Veterans*. New York, NY: Random House; 1984.

85. Terry W. The angry blacks in the Army. In: Horowitz D and the editors of Ramparts. *Two, Three . . . Many Vietnams: A Radical Reader on the Wars in Southeast Asia and the Conflicts at Home*. San Francisco, Calif: Canfield Press; 1971: 222–231.

86. Figley CR, Leventman S. Introduction: estrangement and victimization. In: Figley CR, Leventman S, eds. *Strangers at Home: Vietnam Veterans Since the War*. New York, NY: Prager; 1980: *xxi-xxxi*.

87. Johnston J, Bachman JG. *Young Men Look at Military Service: A Preliminary Report*. Ann Arbor, Mich: University of Michigan, Survey Research Center, Institute for Social Research; 1970.

88. Bell DB. *Characteristics of Army Deserters in the DoD Special Discharge Review Program*. Arlington, Va: US Army Research Institute for the Behavioral and Social Sciences; 1979.

Report No. 1229. [Available at: Alexandria, Va: Defense Technical Information Center. Document No. AD A78601.]

89. Nicholson PT, Mirin SM, Schatzberg AF. Ineffective military personnel, II: An ethical dilemma for psychiatry. *Arch Gen Psychiatry.* 1974;30:406–410.

90. Moskos CC Jr. Surviving the war in Vietnam. In: Figley CR, Leventman S, eds. *Strangers at Home: Vietnam Veterans Since the War.* New York, NY: Praeger; 1980: 71–85.

91. Hayes JH. The dialectics of resistance: an analysis of the GI movement. *J Soc Issues.* 1975;31(4):125–139.

92. Brown CC, Savage C. *The Drug Controversy.* Baltimore, Md: National Educational Consultants; 1971.

93. O'Donnell JA, Voss HL, Clayton RR, Slatin GT, Room RGW. *Young Men and Drugs: A Nationwide Survey.* Rockville, Md: National Institute on Drug Abuse; 1976. Research Monograph 5.

94. Flanagan CH Jr. Review of psychiatric admissions for drug-related causes, Walter Reed General Hospital (unpublished). In: Baker SL Jr. Drug abuse in the United States Army. *Bull N Y Acad Med.* 1971;47:541–549.

95. Greden JF, Morgan DW, Frenkel SI. The changing drug scene: 1970–1972. *Am J Psychiatry.* 1974;131(1):77–81.

96. Black S, Owens KL, Wolff RP. Patterns of drug use: a study of 5,482 subjects. *Am J Psychiatry.* 1970;127(4):420–423.

97. Callan JP, Patterson CD. Patterns of drug abuse among military inductees. *Am J Psychiatry.* 1973;130(3):260–264.

98. Tennant FS Jr, Preble MR, Groesbeck CJ, Banks NI. Drug abuse among American soldiers in West Germany. *Mil Med.* 1972;137(10):381–383.

99. Sapol E, Roffman RA. Marijuana in Vietnam. *J Am Pharm Assoc.* 1969;9(12):615–619.

100. Stanton MD. Drugs, Vietnam, and the Vietnam veteran: an overview. *Am J Drug Alcohol Abuse.* 1976;3(4):557–570.

101. Frenkel SI, Morgan DW, Greden JF. Heroin use among soldiers in the United States and Vietnam: a comparison in retrospect. *Int J Addict.* 1977;12(8):1143–1154.

102. Frank IM, Hoedemaker FS. The civilian psychiatrist and the draft. *Am J Psychiatry.* 1970;127(4):497–502.

103. Liberman RP, Sonnenberg SM, Stern MS. Psychiatric evaluations for young men facing the draft: a report of 147 cases. *Am J Psychiatry.* 1971;128:147–152.

104. Roemer PA. The psychiatrist and the draft evader. *Am J Psychiatry.* 1971;127(9):1236–1237.

105. Ollendorff RH, Adams PL. Psychiatry and the draft. *Am J Orthopsychiatry.* 1971;41(1):85–90.

106. Moskowitz JA. On drafting the psychiatric "draft" letter. *Am J Psychiatry.* 1971;128(1):69–72.

107. Lifton RJ. Advocacy and corruption in the healing professions. *Conn Med.* 1975;39(3):803–813.

108. Spragg GS. Psychiatry in the Australian military forces. *Med J Aust.* 1972;1(15):745–751.

109. Boman B. The Vietnam veteran ten years on. *Aust N Z J Psychiatry.* 1982;16(3):107–127.

110. Brass A. Medicine over there. *JAMA.* 1970;213(9):1473–1475.

111. Maier T. The Army psychiatrist: an adjunct to the system of social control. *Am J Psychiatry.* 1970;126(7):1039–1040.

112. Barr NI, Zunin LM. Clarification of the psychiatrist's dilemma while in military service. *Am J Orthopsychiatry.* 1971;41(4):672–674.

113. Camp NM. The Vietnam War and the ethics of combat psychiatry. *Am J Psychiatry.* 1993;150(7):1000–1010.

114. APA members hit meeting disruptions in opinion poll results. *Psychiatr News.* 3 March 1971;6:1.

115. Psychologists, MH groups attack Vietnam War. *Psychiatr News.* 5 July 1972;7:1.

116. Johnson AW Jr. Combat psychiatry, II: The US Army in Vietnam. *Med Bull US Army Europe.* 1969;26(11):335–339.

117. Bloch HS. Dr Bloch replies (letter). *Am J Psychiatry.* 1970;126:1039–1040.

118. Colbach EM, Parrish MD. Army mental health activities in Vietnam: 1965–1970. *Bull Menninger Clin.* 1970;34(6):333–342.

119. Parrish MD. A veteran of three wars looks at psychiatry in the military. *Psychiatr Opinion.* 1972;9(6):6–11.

120. Gibbs JJ. Military psychiatry: reflections and projections. *Psychiatr Opinion*. 1973;10(1):20-23.

121. Bey DR, Chapman RE. Psychiatry—the right way, the wrong way, and the military way. *Bull Menninger Clin*. 1974;38:343–354.

122. US Army Chaplains Corps, The Cold War and the chaplaincy. In: *Origins of the American Military Chaplaincy, Chapter 7*. Available at: http://www.chapnet.army.mil/usachcs/origins/chapter_7.htm; accessed 25 June 2013.

123. Andrade D, Willbanks JH. CORDS/Phoenix: Counterinsurgency lessons from Vietnam for the future. *Mil Rev*. 2006;(Mar–Apr):9–23.

124. Van Creveld M. The helicopter and the computer. In: Van Creveld M. *Command in War*. Cambridge, Mass: Harvard University Press; 1985: 232–261.

CHAPTER 2

Overview of the Army's Accelerating Psychiatric and Behavioral Challenges: From Halcyon to Heroin

. . . Public, congressional, and even media support of an earlier day . . . dropped off precipitously once it was clear that the United States had opted out of the war. Societal problems of drug abuse, racial disharmony, and dissent, . . . reached epidemic proportions in the United States and, inevitably, spilled over to the forces in the field. Cumulatively, these differences constituted one of the most difficult challenges to leadership in the military history of the United States, and eventually their effects were felt throughout the forces in every theater.[1(p347)]

Lewis Sorley, PhD
Lieutenant Colonel, US Army (Retired)
Military historian and Vietnam veteran

Dust-off helicopter retrieving a casualty in the field. Despite Vietnam's challenging physical environment, sick and wounded soldiers were provided rapid access to sophisticated medical support, especially through the utilization of the new helicopter ambulance capability. This proved to be one of the chief stress-buffering influences on troops throughout the war. Photograph courtesy of Richard D Cameron, Major General, US Army (Retired).

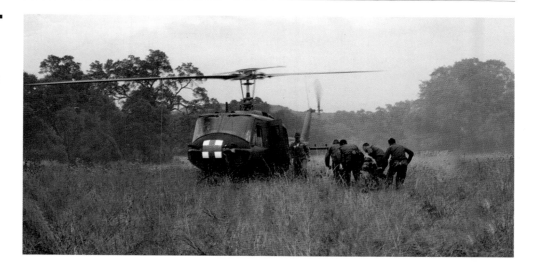

Whereas Army planners anticipated that once US forces were fully committed in Vietnam the war would be short and America and its allies would prevail, they also presumed, based on experience in the main force wars that preceded Vietnam—World War I, World War II, and Korea—there would be large numbers of soldiers disabled by combat exhaustion. As a consequence they incorporated in Vietnam the structure and doctrine of military and combat psychiatry that had been pragmatically established in the course of fighting those earlier wars to prevent and treat these types of casualties. In particular this meant that the allocation and the preparation of psychiatric assets throughout all 8 years of the war was weighted in favor of combat-committed soldiers[2,3] (the US Army Medical Department mission is "conserve the fighting strength"[4])—despite the fact that such troops would only represent roughly a quarter[5] to a third[6] of the Army personnel deployed in South Vietnam. This arrangement, nonetheless, seemed satisfactory for the first few years of the war as evidence indicated overall rates for psychiatric attrition and misconduct were exceptionally low for a combat theater.

However, as was described in Chapter 1, the ultimate reality in Vietnam proved to be far different than anticipated. The enemy reverted to mostly counterinsurgency/guerrilla tactics and was far more resilient and committed than expected. (Guerrilla warfare can be defined as irregular warfare in which a small group of combatants use mobile military tactics in the form of ambushes and raids to defeat a larger and less mobile formal army.) This led to a prolongation of the fighting along with rising costs and losses, which provoked the American public into increasingly passionate opposition to the war. In turn, as the war lengthened, the morale of the deployed force declined dramatically and troops—noncombat as well as combat—demonstrated in a wide variety of ways their reluctance to soldier and their antagonism to military authority, including accelerating rates for psychiatric conditions and behavioral problems.

In fact, among the wars in the 20th century, Vietnam became historically unique in having rising psychiatric hospitalization rates as the fighting waned and combat-generated physical casualties declined. Matters became substantially worse in 1970, when a heroin epidemic quickly spread among the lower-ranking soldiers—an unprecedented problem that seriously undermined soldier health, morale, and military preparedness. Military leaders as well as law enforcement, administrative, and medical/psychiatric elements were all severely tested before the last US military forces were withdrawn in March 1973.

This chapter provides an overview of the dominant patterns of psychiatric conditions and behavioral problems that arose within the Army in Vietnam and the consequent challenges faced by Army leaders and allied mental health personnel. Its approach is one of linking rising rates for traditional (psychiatric), as well as nontraditional, measures of soldier dysfunction, including misconduct, with the kaleidoscope of social, political, and military features that changed over time. In so doing it becomes evident that, although it prepared itself well for large numbers of combat stress reactions, the Army was not prepared for eventual morale

inversion and the associated upsurge in what might be referred to as "(combat theater) deployment stress reaction." (It is acknowledged that this distinction— ie, between combat stress-generated reactions [psychiatric and behavioral] and deployment stress reactions contradicts current trends in Army psychiatry. As codified in the 2009 US Army Field Manual 6-22.5, *Combat and Operational Stress Control Manual for Leaders and Soldiers*, acute dysfunctional combat stress reactions are lumped in with other stress-generated psychiatric and behavior problems under "Combat and Operational Stress Reaction" [COSR], a concept that includes noncombat personnel and does not even require that the affected individual is in a combat theater.[7] Adding further confusion, current doctrine also utilizes the term "COSR/combat misconduct stress behaviors" for soldiers who commit "serious" disciplinary infractions, whether the behavior is combat-related or not.[8])

Furthermore, with respect to providing humanitarian care, if not strictly that of serving force conservation, the data indicate that many who returned home from Vietnam subsequently experienced serious and sustained readjustment problems, including frank posttraumatic stress disorder (see Chapter 6, Exhibit 6-3, "The Post-Vietnam Era and Posttraumatic Stress Disorder"). Following their return to stateside life, many Vietnam veterans complained of emerging irritability and difficulty concentrating, recurrent nightmares of disturbing combat experiences, overreaction to environmental stimuli that reminded them of Vietnam, estrangement from others and serious relationship difficulties, and emotional numbing and disabling feelings of guilt and depression, which they often sought to tame with alcohol and drugs.[9–12] Although, as mentioned in the Preface, a comprehensive review of postdeployment adjustment and psychiatric morbidity is outside the scope of this work, it should be noted that some investigators have suggested that the prevalence of debilitating psychological and social problems among Vietnam veterans greatly exceeded that for earlier US wars; and that when postdeployment adjustment difficulties are included with psychological problems that arose in the theater, the psychosocial cost for the Vietnam War was unprecedented. This chapter will close with additional discussion of the postdeployment difficulties found among many Vietnam veterans.

US ARMY PSYCHIATRY IN VIETNAM: AN EXAMPLE OF "PREPARING TO FIGHT THE LAST WAR"?

Combat Stress Reactions and Conservation of the Fighting Force

Acute, disabling psychological symptoms among soldiers subjected to the extreme circumstances of combat have been variously labeled *shell-shock* (World War I), *combat neurosis* and *combat fatigue* (World War II), and *combat exhaustion* (Korean War and Vietnam War),[13,14] as well as newer names: *combat stress reaction* and *battle shock* (both of which Jones labeled "transient anxiety states"[15]). In the 20th century, these sorts of "bloodless casualties" were described beginning with the Russo-Japanese War of 1904–1905, but at that time they did not arise in numbers sufficient to constitute a military-medical problem.[2,3,16,17]

The introduction of weapons with greater lethal potential in World War I ushered in the era of the modern battlefield, and combat-generated psychiatric casualties were seen in much larger numbers[14]—numbers that could determine the outcome of a battle or a war. Furthermore, from the observations made through these later wars it became evident that not only could these reactions to combat present in a wide variety of psychological and behavioral forms, but they could also spread among soldiers by suggestion.[18] Although the term *combat exhaustion* was used in Vietnam—defined by the Army's Medical Field Service School in 1967 as "a transient emotional disease caused by the stress of combat [and by] fear [and] prolonged mental and physical exhaustion"[18(p10)]—this work will also use interchangeably the terms *combat reaction*, *combat stress reaction* (CSR), and *combat breakdown*.

The importance of combat stress reactions for military planners can be seen in these three examples:

1. In World War II, because of the mistaken belief that thorough induction screening could eliminate susceptible men and therefore prevent combat breakdown, 970,000 men (5.4%) of the almost 18 million men examined at induction stations were rejected for mental or emotional reasons.[3(p72)] Studies of a group of rejectees who were subsequently allowed to serve revealed that 79% served successfully.[14]

2. Also in World War II, psychiatric casualties were admitted to military hospitals at twice the rate in World War I, and psychiatric disabilities accounted for more World War II disability discharges (486,000) than any other medical reason—nearly three times the rate in World War I.[2]

3. To focus on just one campaign in World War II, but one that included an especially notable example of how psychiatric casualties can seriously undermine an army at war, forward deployment of psychiatrists in the early phases of the fighting in North Africa was not begun until late in the campaign and psychiatric casualties were therefore evacuated far from the fighting. Not only was the neuropsychiatric casualty rate unusually high (25%–35% of all nonfatal casualties), only 3% ever returned to combat duty.[19] At one point the rate of psychiatric evacuation from the area of fighting exceeded the rate of theater replacements.[20]

Psychiatric experiences during these wars also indicated that, sooner or later, the psychological stamina and resiliency of any soldier could be exceeded by the rigors, dangers, losses, or horrors (ie, the trauma) of the combat situation, and that such a "breakdown" was not primarily a measure of weakness of character or cowardice. For example, a study of 1,000 infantrymen fighting in the Mediterranean theater in World War II reported that the breaking point of the average rifleman was 88 days of company combat.[21] Furthermore, through projection it was estimated that, considering psychiatric attrition alone, a unit could become 90% depleted by combat day 210.[21]

These wars also taught military psychiatry that a vigorous, crisis-oriented, but conservative, forward treatment aimed at quickly restoring affected soldiers to duty function was mostly effective in reversing these combat reactions. By way of example, in August 1950 during the Korean War, before the forward placement of mental health personnel was instituted, the annualized rate for psychiatric admissions was 250 per 1,000 troops.[22(p25)] In 1951, following the implementation of the three-echelon system of psychiatric care, the rate dropped to 70 per 1,000 troops. In 1952, during the 6 months preceding the armistice, the rate fell to 21 per 1,000 troops.[22]

Finally, it also was made evident from past experience that if these combat stress casualties received premature evacuation, or even overly sympathetic treatment, not only was there needless elimination of capable soldiers from the fighting force, but levels of morbidity among these soldiers (ie, chronicity) greatly increased as well.[20]

Combat Stress Reaction and the Individual Soldier: Adapting the Combat Psychiatry Forward Treatment Doctrine in Vietnam

The following clinical material will illustrate the presentation and management of a soldier with acute combat exhaustion (or combat stress reaction) in Vietnam:

CASE 2-1: "Classic" Combat Exhaustion

Identifying information: Specialist 4th Class (SP4) Delta was a 20-year-old, single, white infantryman who had been assigned to one of the infantry divisions in Vietnam for 5 months and was transported from the field by helicopter to the 93rd Evacuation Hospital near Saigon along with other combat casualties.

History of present illness: (See clinical course)

Past history: Negative for psychopathology

Examination: Upon his arrival SP4 Delta was observed by the psychiatrists of the 935th Psychiatric Detachment, which was attached to the 93rd Evacuation Hospital, to be strapped to a litter, grunting incomprehensibly, and posturing. He was quite disorganized and could not communicate with his examiners. He was easily startled by noises and walked with a slow, shuffling gait, needing support and guidance. When he sat in a chair, he rocked with his eyes closed and occasionally mumbled "Mama." He spoke only if urged, and then in immature sentences. SP4 Delta reported unemotionally that many of his men had been killed while moving up a hill; no other information was obtainable. His physical examination was otherwise normal.

Clinical course: On the psychiatric unit, the patient was given a shower and reassurance and was "put to sleep" with Thorazine (dose not available). When he awoke 18 hours later he appeared alert, coherent, and rational. He was issued a fresh uniform and received instructions about the quasi-military ward routine. The staff told him that he was recovering from overexposure to combat, and that he could expect to be returned to his military unit soon. In the group therapy meeting, SP4 Delta emotionally described how he had been serving as a fire team leader when six of his friends were killed and mutilated by enemy fire, and that he had become agitated and began screaming while loading their bodies into a helicopter. He talked despondently of his revulsion at the killing and his regret that he had "gone to pieces" such that another squad leader had to take charge of his men. He said he felt torn because he always sought to be "good" and wanted to be a good soldier, but it just wasn't his "makeup" to kill. SP4 Delta said that he could not return to the field. The record noted that the psychiatric staff responded to his feelings "with reality-testing and ego support of his duty and mission." That night he was informed that he would be returning to his unit the following day, and he was again given Thorazine.

Discharge diagnosis: Combat exhaustion.

Disposition: SP4 Delta was returned to his unit and combat duty with a recommendation that he receive follow-up care at his battalion aid station.

Source: Adapted with permission from Camp NM. The Vietnam War and the ethics of combat psychiatry. *Am J Psychiatry.* 1993;150(7):1005.

Because SP4 Delta rapidly improved while in treatment and because he had no past psychiatric history, he was discharged back to his unit with a diagnosis of combat exhaustion—implying a temporary, stress-induced, nondisabling condition. Apart from prescribing chlorpromazine (Thorazine), a neuroleptic tranquilizer, rather than barbiturates and other sedatives of an earlier era, a patient like this one would have been managed similarly by military psychiatrists and allied medical personnel in late World War I, World War II, and the Korean War. This refers to a treatment regimen for psychologically overwhelmed combat soldiers that was pragmatically developed during those earlier conflicts and adapted by the 935th Psychiatric Detachment psychiatrists to the unique circumstances in Vietnam.[23]

Historically, this treatment regimen—referred to throughout this work as the combat psychiatric forward treatment doctrine, or the "doctrine"—included brief, simple, mostly restorative measures such as: safety; rest and physical replenishment; peer support; sedation, if necessary; and opportunities for emotional catharsis of the soldier's traumatic events. Such conservative treatment elements were to be applied as close to his unit as practical and accompanied by the expectation that he would quickly recover, rejoin his comrades, and resume his military duties.[24,25] Leading up to and throughout the Vietnam War, the Army confidently advocated this approach believing that it would serve both the needs of force conservation and those of the individual soldier.[26,27] (Pathogenesis, diagnosis, and treatment of combat stress disorders in Vietnam will be explored in Chapters 6 and 7.)

Available records from the 935th Psychiatric Detachment indicated that SP4 Delta was not rehospitalized at the 93rd Evacuation Hospital during the remaining 7 months of his assignment in Vietnam. However, because of the fluid nature of the military situation in Vietnam and frequent variations in the pattern of medical evacuations, it cannot be said with certainty that he was not subsequently treated somewhere else in the theater for a recurrence of his psychiatric symptoms. It is also not known if SP4 Delta was later killed or wounded, or suffered with delayed, postdeployment readjustment problems or psychiatric symptoms, including those that were later incorporated in the entity that was codified in 1980—posttraumatic stress disorder (PTSD).[28] However, in the absence of such information, by the standards passed down from earlier wars, his apparent recovery and return to duty after treatment at the 935th Psychiatric Detachment would have been a favorable outcome.

Army Psychiatry in Vietnam Was Organized to Treat Large Numbers of Combat Stress Casualties

Army medical and psychiatric planners anticipated sizeable numbers of combat exhaustion cases in Vietnam and therefore replicated the system of care that was pragmatically established in World War I by Major Thomas Salmon, chief psychiatrist of the American Expeditionary Forces, and validated in subsequent wars.[17] It was furthermore intended to conform to the Army's doctrinal three-tier (echelon) medical treatment system in Vietnam.[14,29] According to this system of psychiatric care (codified in US Army, Republic of Vietnam [USARV] Regulation 40-34, *Mental Health and Neuropsychiatry*[30]), soldiers with psychiatric symptoms who failed to respond to unit-based first aid, which consisted of efforts at increasing morale and confidence through counseling, reassurance, exhortation, and leadership, were to be provided graduated levels of psychiatric care as follows:

1st echelon psychiatric care: The soldier with more than temporary psychiatric symptoms and disability, including those with combat exhaustion, would enter the medical system through the battalion aid station (1st echelon treatment facility), where basic physical and emotional treatment would be provided by field medics working under the direct supervision of a general medical officer (battalion surgeon). In some instances the battalion aid station personnel would be augmented by an attached social work/psychology technician/specialist (91G military occupational specialty [MOS]), an enlisted corpsman with additional education and training who was under the technical, if not direct, supervision of the division psychiatrist. If these symptoms extended beyond 24 to 48 hours, the soldier would typically be evacuated further from the fighting to the division's medical clearing company for more specialized care.

2nd echelon psychiatric care: Throughout the war, combat divisions maintained a small clearing company treatment facility at a brigade's, or the division's, base camp. Here a broader range of support and treatment could be provided to combat stress casualties by the division psychiatrist, the division social work officer, and the enlisted social work/psychology technicians. If the soldier's symptoms failed to respond to treatment here within 3 to 5 days, he would be evacuated out of the operational area of the division to one of the Army-level hospitals in Vietnam.

3rd echelon psychiatric care: This refers to the more extensive psychiatric care provided at either of the two psychiatric specialty detachments in Vietnam. Each psychiatric treatment and rehabilitation center was attached to an evacuation hospital and was fully staffed with psychiatrists and other mental health professionals as well as enlisted personnel with specialized training. It was expected to provide up to 30 days inpatient treatment for soldiers from divisional as well as nondivisional units. (Apparently their high staffing allocations were primarily based on predictions that they would be required to treat up to 100 combat fatigue cases/24-hour period.[31]) The second priority for psychiatric specialty detachments was to provide outpatient treatment and mental health consultation services

(MHCS) for the nondivision, mostly noncombat, units in their coverage area.[29]

There were other evacuation hospitals (10 at most) and field hospitals (three at most) in Vietnam, each of which had an authorized psychiatrist position; however, these positions were often not filled because of lack of available personnel, they were generally not staffed with allied mental health personnel, and they did not have dedicated psychiatric wards. In instances when they did have a psychiatrist assigned, the inpatient treatment was limited to about 10 days and took place on a general medical ward. (Additional distinctions between the structure, staffing, and treatment capabilities of these echelons of psychiatric care will be provided in Chapter 7.)

As it turned out, the psychiatric assets deployed in Vietnam were not distributed in proportion to the professional challenges that arose. If 1969 is used as an example, on the surface numerical balance appears to be in effect. On April 30, Army strength peaked in Vietnam at 363,300,[32] with the seven full combat divisions accounting for approximately 126,000 of those (a figure derived from multiplying the number of divisions times an estimated 18,000 troops per division), that is, the full divisions accounted for one-third of the Army personnel in Vietnam. Furthermore, one-third (seven) of the 22 Army (clinical) psychiatrists in Vietnam were assigned as division psychiatrists (as indicated by the Walter Reed Army Institute of Research psychiatrist survey [to be discussed in Chapter 5]) with the remainder assigned to the two psychiatric specialty detachments or as solo psychiatrists at selected evacuation or field hospitals. However, four factors suggest that this allocation of psychiatric capability was out of balance:

1. Although the organizational structure dictated the prioritization of psychiatric attention in favor of staffing the combat divisions in anticipation of large numbers of combat stress casualties, they never materialized.

2. About half of the evacuation and field hospitals (excepting the two with psychiatric specialty detachments) did not have assigned psychiatrists, yet it was the job of these hospitals to support the approximately 237,000 nondivisional support and service support troops. Arranging for their psychiatric care would prove more awkward and unpredictable.[33] (Appendix 8, a summary of a presentation by Johnson to a 1967 expert panel discussion of Army psychiatry in Vietnam, addresses these difficulties.)

3. The Army's heavy reliance on heliborne medical evacuation meant that the overall echelon-based system of medical care in Vietnam was often not followed. Casualties of all types (including psychiatric patients from the field) frequently bypassed the 1st, and even 2nd, treatment echelon to be taken directly to field and evacuation hospitals (so-called overflying).[24]

4. Support troops, who constituted most of the nondivisional units, generally had greater rates of psychiatric disorders and behavior problems except during periods of high-combat activity.[15]

Furthermore, as the war progressed, this arrangement became increasingly out of balance. This is partly because as the war passed the midpoint there was a dramatic shift in the character of psychiatric and related problems. After 1969, when combat activities were being scaled back, troop demoralization, dissent, and drug use—disabling psychiatric and behavioral conditions in and of themselves—accelerated, apparently especially within the ranks of the nondivisional units—the noncombat, combat support and service support units (ie, the "rear").[5(p55)] However, no structural changes were made in the organization of mental health assets in Vietnam or modifications in the selection, preparation, or deployment of mental health personnel in order to offset this growing psychiatric challenge.

Army Psychiatrists Deploying to Vietnam Were Primarily Prepared to Treat Large Numbers of Combat Stress Casualties

Equally problematic, the training and indoctrination of physicians who would be assigned in Vietnam, including psychiatrists, mostly emphasized the psychological limits of soldiers in combat, the causes of breakdown (social, physical, and emotional) under sustained fire, and the prevention or management of large numbers of combat-generated psychiatric casualties. Other psychiatric or behavior problems associated with low morale and indiscipline—unrelated, or only indirectly related to combat exposure—were evidently presumed to be less pressing. This was the case in the Army's two psychiatric residency-training programs (Walter Reed General Hospital, Washington, DC, and Letterman General Hospital, San Francisco, California), where the principles of prevention and

TABLE 2-1. Expected Neuropsychiatric Casualties Among Troops as a Function of Combat Intensity and Cumulative Time in Combat*

Cumulative Combat Days	Wounded in Action (WIA) Per Thousand Troops Per Day (Combat Intensity)							
	0 WIA	5 WIA	10 WIA	20 WIA	30 WIA	40 WIA	50 WIA	60 WIA
1–5 days	0.3	1.0	1.6	2.9	4.2	5.5	6.8	8.1
6–10 days	1.7	2.4	3.0	4.3	5.6	6.9	8.2	9.5
11–20 days	3.9	4.6	5.2	6.5	7.8	9.1	10.4	11.7
21–40 days	6.4	7.1	7.7	9.0	10.3	11.6	12.9	14.2
41–80 days	8.6	9.3	9.9	11.2	12.5	13.8	15.1	16.4

*In means of estimates for infantry, armored, and airborne troop neuropsychiatric casualties.

Adapted from: Medical Field Service School. *Expected Neuropsychiatric Casualties Among Infantry, Armored, and Airborne Troops as a Function of Combat Intensity and Cumulative Time in Combat*. Fort Sam Houston, Tex: Department of Neuropsychiatry, Medical Field Service School; distributed July 1967. Training Document GR 51-400-104-105.

treatment of combat breakdown were central elements in the curricula (see Prologue).

Similarly, at Fort Sam Houston in San Antonio, Texas, newly commissioned, civilian-trained psychiatrists, including those who would be assigned in Vietnam, received their orientation to Army psychiatry at the Army's Medical Field Service School along with other new Medical Corps officers (physicians), and they were provided only a few hours of instruction in military psychiatry, most of which centered on combat-stress generated casualties. In July 1967, this training included the following three presentations:

1. A lecture with handout on the organization of psychiatric services in the combat division— especially the division psychiatrist's critical role in supporting the recovery and redeployment of the scores of men who were predicted to become overwhelmed with the stress of sustained combat operations in Vietnam:

> The organization of the psychiatric services of a division is based upon the requirements generated by expected combat experiences. The design and structure of these services are based largely upon the necessity of preventing, detecting, treating, and disposing of cases of combat exhaustion. Whether [the psychiatric services] deal with problems of mental illness or other problems of mental health in the [division] are of secondary importance.[34(p1)]

2. A lecture with handout addressing the etiology and presentation of combat exhaustion: It made reference to four severity levels and acknowledged the wide range of possible disabling symptoms. Theories as to pathogenesis centered on fear and exhaustion as primary and combat avoidance as secondary.[18]

3. Repeated warnings as to the likelihood of a flood of combat exhaustion psychiatric casualties in Vietnam ("Projecting psychiatric casualty rates an additional 4–6 months . . . most of the divisions in World War II would have been completely ineffective from the number of combat exhaustion cases alone"[18(p11)]). Table 2-1 is a combat stress casualty prediction schedule that was distributed to the Medical Field Service School participants illustrating the covariance of combat breakdown with combat intensity/duration derived from earlier military experience. The shaded box (6.5) has been selected here to serve as a conservative hypothetical example: If a combat division has 12,000 combat-committed soldiers engaged in a fight of moderate intensity (ie, 20 wounded-in-action/1,000 troops/day) over a moderate period of time (11–20 days), this schedule indicates that the division psychiatrist would be responsible for the care of *78 new combat exhaustion casualties per day* [emphasis added] (eg, 12 x 6.5). For simplicity's sake the physician participants were also given these rules of thumb: "One combat exhaustion case for every four wounded"[18(p11)] and "For every

four soldiers wounded in combat, there is a soldier that requires medical attention because of combat exhaustion."[34(p1)]

The Low Incidence of Classic Combat Stress Reaction Casualties in Vietnam

Over the course of the war senior military psychiatrists observed that the large number of combat exhaustion cases that were anticipated and planned for never materialized, at least not in their classical form.[17] Anecdotally the psychiatrists assigned to the Army combat divisions during the first few of years of the war reported a range from no combat exhaustion cases[35] to four to 12 per month,[36] with the higher numbers being associated with episodes of increased combat activity.[37,38]

Further substantiation of a low incidence for combat exhaustion appears to come from the observation that, although all hospitals were required to provide combat exhaustion casualty statistics to USARV medical command, the official summary of US Army medical experience in Vietnam (1965 through May 1970, two-thirds through the war) made no mention of combat exhaustion as a military medical problem.[27] Also, the official overview of the psychiatric problems in the Vietnam War, which was published after the war by Jones and Johnson when Johnson served as the Chief, Psychiatry and Neurology Consultant Branch, Office of The Surgeon General, US Army, did not report theater-wide incidence statistics for combat exhaustion; but the authors did attest to the fact that the incidence throughout the war was extremely low.[39]

An alternative means of measuring the clinical challenge represented by combat exhaustion cases in Vietnam was their percentage of all hospitalized psychiatric conditions. In the process of comparing US Army psychiatric hospitalization rates in Vietnam with those of the Army of the Republic of Vietnam during the first 6 months of 1966, early in the buildup phase, Peter G Bourne, Chief, Division of Neuropsychiatry, Walter Reed Army Institute of Research Medical Research Team in Vietnam (1965–1966) found only 6% of US Army psychiatric admissions were diagnosed as combat exhaustion.[40] Later, in a preliminary overview of US Army mental health activities in Vietnam, Matthew D Parrish, who was Chief, Psychiatry and Neurology Consultant Branch, Office of The Surgeon General, and Edward M Colbach, who was Assistant Psychiatric Consultant, reported only 7% of all psychiatric

admissions through the first two-thirds of the war were diagnosed as combat stress reaction.[41]

All this is not to say that the specialized treatment of combat stress reactions was not an important challenge in Vietnam; rather, that these casualties apparently never achieved the incidence rates that had been anticipated—or perhaps not in the more incapacitating forms anticipated. Still, it is regrettable that true combat reaction incidence figures are missing—data that could contribute to further understanding the various efforts of the US Army Medical Department to adapt the traditional psychiatric doctrine of forward treatment to Vietnam. This appears to be especially important considering: (*a*) the irregular, counterinsurgency/guerrilla warfare that was waged, and (*b*) the widespread use of newly developed psychopharmacologic medications for the treatment of combat stress reaction cases. (These themes will be developed further in Chapters 6 and 7.) In any event, in time psychiatric concerns for soldiers affected by combat stress in Vietnam became greatly overshadowed by the increases in other, unanticipated psychiatric conditions and behavior problems—essentially psychosocial disorders—that ultimately dismayed Army leaders and swamped mental health capabilities. As previously noted, the incidence of these problems was evidently greater among noncombat troops, thus the center of effort for mental health personnel shifted progressively to the understaffed nondivisional medical treatment facilities (the field and evacuation hospitals and the psychiatric specialty detachments).

A SYNOPSIS OF ARMY PSYCHIATRY'S TWO, SEQUENTIAL VIETNAM WARS

In presenting an overview of the clinical (and personal) challenges faced by Army psychiatrists assigned in Vietnam, this chapter draws upon selected references from the literature that provide markers bearing on the Army psychiatric experience there with respect to the ground war. These have been divided roughly along lines of the principle military deployment phases, that is, buildup (1965–1967), a transition phase (1968–1969), and drawdown (1970–1973), and placed against the war's shifting backdrops and contexts noted in Chapter 1.

The Buildup Phase (1965–1967)

By the end of 1965, the first year the US Army deployed in Vietnam, there were 116,800 Army troops; by the end of 1966 there were 239,400; and by the end of 1967 there were 319,500.[32] As noted in Chapter 1, during these years, opposition to the war was gradually building at home while draft call-ups quickly gathered momentum to meet the huge manpower needs in Southeast Asia. Because Reserve units and the National Guard were, for all practical purposes, exempted from deployment throughout the war, the ground forces were composed of a mix of career soldiers, draftees, and volunteers. The latter included many draft-motivated volunteers—soldiers who anticipated being drafted and who enlisted with a promise of a more advantageous training or assignment with regard to risk or privation. Thus, whereas officially only 39% of the Army's enlisted personnel in Vietnam were technically draftees,[42] regarding the matter of low morale and associated difficulties, the many "draft-motivated" volunteers should also be considered as conscripts.

Combat could be very intense during these initial years, and the cities and countryside were not secure; however, troops maintained high morale and a sense of purpose. According to General William C Westmoreland, the overall commander of US forces in Vietnam (Commander, US Military Assistance Command, Vietnam [MACV]), the troops operating in Vietnam during the buildup years were "the toughest, best trained, most dedicated American servicemen in history."[43(p34)] More specific to the Army in Vietnam, retired Brigadier General SLA Marshall, combat veteran of World War I and front-line observer in World War II and Korea, commented after his visit to Vietnam in 1966:

> My overall estimate was that the morale of the troops and the level of discipline of the Army were higher than I had ever known them in any of our wars. There was no lack of will to fight and the average soldier withstood the stress of engagement better than ever before.[43(p34)]

Nonetheless, the stress on the typical serviceman assigned in Vietnam was considerable. Navy Lieutenant Stephen Howard, who served as a Marine battalion surgeon, provided the following portrayal of the initial shock experienced by all newly arrived troops. According to Howard, alienation and depersonalization begin upon arrival in Vietnam.

> He is torn from everything that is familiar and comforting to him: his family and friends, his country, even the familiar routine of stateside barracks life; his normal hopes and troubles and ways of relating. He finds himself in a strange Asian country, knowing nothing of its language, history, or meanings, surrounded by desolation and threatened with death; *he is the alien* [emphasis added]. . . . He is a non person . . . a thing expected to function, while everything around him is strange and lacking in meaning. . . . And the excruciating boredom which he frequently must endure in the hiatus between military operations, along with the deprivation of privacy, only reinforces his experience of himself as a thing which is [expected to perform] in a prescribed way. . . .[44(p123)]

There are at least several additional stressors that should be added to Howard's synopsis. The first would be simply the presumed stress borne by the high numbers of very young, first-term, draftees and enlistees who entered Vietnam as their first assignment. Equally potent and linked would be the new replacement's difficulty in having to manage his shock alone as a consequence of the military's individual rotation policy. Of course, members of the receiving unit likewise incurred a stress in having to accommodate green troops who arrived singularly to replace seasoned troops.[45]

More specific to the fact of being assigned in an active theater of combat operations, innumerable accounts attest to how the type of warfare in Vietnam (ie, a counterinsurgency/guerrilla war) meant that no setting could be assumed safe from enemy-directed violence (eg, rocket and mortar attacks, ambush, terrorist activities, sniper fire). This meant that all troops were at least diffusely subjected to some degree of combat stress.[46–48] Of course the risk varied considerably by locale and role (especially, combat vs noncombat), and, as expected, great tensions arose between troops with higher combat exposure, as well as hardship in general, and those considered "rear echelon" (the despised "REMF"—"rear echelon mother f--ker"), although this was a relative measure.[5] For example, Major Douglas R Bey, a division psychiatrist with the 1st Infantry Division, underscored how deeply the combat troops resented the REMF who had it relatively safe and comfortable. "Grunts (infantry or ground soldiers) in the field often claimed that they had more in common with Charlie (the VC [Viet Cong] enemy) than they did with the REMFs."[49(p80)] Cincinnatus, a military historian, remarked that predictable resentment of the noncombat troops and those in the rear by those facing combat was a far greater irritant in Vietnam overall because of the "circular" nature of the tactics—soldiers perpetually returned to their secure base camp after going out to seek contact with the enemy, and there would encounter others who remained clean, comfortable, and, most of all, safe.[50] "Swarming base camps were filled with officers functioning in staff jobs or service support activities who were never in danger of being sent into combat despite the fact that they were serving in a 'war zone.'"[50(p149)] According to Cincinnatus, resentment of opportunism among those with rank or status advantage was corrosive to morale from early on:

> The war was torture for those who fought it, yet they saw others using that conflict for personal gain. They saw American contractors enriching themselves through multimillion-dollar building projects. Everyone seemed hell-bent . . . to manipulate currency, to deal in whiskey trades, to hoard a little gold or a few diamonds. They were often forced to live in flimsy tents and ramshackle quarters while their more fortunate noncombat brethren were housed in concrete-block, air-conditioned buildings. They swatted mosquitoes and despised the leeches they pulled from their crotches while others picked up fresh laundry from government-provided base facilities.[50(p151)]

Nonetheless, despite the rigors of the counterinsurgency warfare and the extremely inhospitable setting, morale and combat motivation remained high during the buildup years. The observations and interpretations by Moskos, a military sociologist, from his time in Vietnam as a war correspondent between 1965 and 1967 provided some explanation, at least for combat troops. He believed this arose from a linkage between the soldiers' individual self-concern (heightened because of the 1-year, individual rotation system) and devotion to the other soldiers in the immediate combat group (eg, instrumental interdependencies motivated by the functional goal of survival).[51] Moskos also noted their shared belief in an exaggerated masculine ethic as well as a latent ideology of devotion to US ideals that stemmed from their conviction regarding the supremacy of the US way of life. Furthermore, the soldiers he

studied were notably apolitical and antagonistic toward peace demonstrators ("privileged anarchists") at home.[51]

Comments by Bourne from his year in Vietnam are also illuminating. He reported that soldiers in these early years maintained a positive motivation in part through what he labeled "combat provincialism."

> They are not only unconcerned about the political and strategic aspects of the war; they are also disinterested in the outcome of any battle that is not in their own immediate vicinity . . . [The soldier] retains certain deep allegiances and beliefs in an . . . amorphous positive entity, 'Americanism,' which allow him to justify his being sent to Vietnam.[52(p44)]

Bourne especially credited the fixed, 1-year tour for soldiers for the high morale, but he also expressed concern for its consequent disturbance to the "solidarity of the small unit"—the traditional stress-protection system for combat soldiers.[53]

Buildup Phase Psychiatric Overview

Correlating with the observations of high esprit and commitment, troop attrition due to psychiatric or behavioral dysfunction was exceptionally low during those first few years. The Army psychiatric evacuation rates from Vietnam through mid-1968 averaged 1.97 per 1,000 troops per year (compared with a rate of 2.6 in the Korean War and 13.8 in Europe during World War II).[54(p59)] Similarly, the proportion of medical evacuations out of Vietnam for psychiatric diagnoses early in the war (3%–4%)[39] compared quite favorably with that for the Korean War (6%) and for World War II (23%).[14] Reporting from the Vietnam theater in January 1967, Johnson, the senior Army psychiatrist (the USARV Neuropsychiatry Consultant), observed:

> A cross section of psychiatric patients seen in Vietnam would include patients having symptoms of psychosis, psychoneurosis and character disorder in approximately the same proportion as a similar body of troops in the continental United States but with a relatively small increment of patients with more directly combat-induced symptoms.[55(p305)]

On a more granular basis, over the first 6 months of 1967 it was reported that among all medical causes, psychiatric cases accounted for only 6.7% of Army evacuees from Vietnam to Travis Air Force Base,

California (a rate that was almost one-third of that for the Navy/Marines or the Air Force). Furthermore, soldiers with character and behavior disorder diagnosis only accounted for 11.5% of Army psychiatric evacuees (US Navy/Marines = 53.5%; and US Air Force = 17.6%).[56(Figure 2)]

Rates for misconduct in the theater were also low (eg, the annual stockade confinement rate for 1966–1967 was 1.15/1,000 soldiers/year as compared to the expected overseas rate of 2.2).[57] According to Major General George S Prugh, former Staff Judge Advocate at the US Military Assistance Command in Vietnam,

> Criminal offenses in the Army were not a serious problem in the early years of U.S. involvement in Vietnam. At the beginning of 1965 the monthly Army court-martial rate in Vietnam was 1.17 per 1,000; at the end of 1965 it was 2.03 per 1,000. Yet the Army-wide court-martial rate for 1965 was even more; 3.55 per 1,000.[58(p98)]

Some senior Army psychiatrists attributed these favorable metrics to an array of operational and preventive factors that appeared to protect the soldiers from psychiatric and behavioral difficulties: (a) technological superiority; (b) the professionalism of the troops; (c) fixed, 1-year assignments; (d) high-quality leadership; and (e) adequate supplies, equipment, and support—especially medical support.[13,24,39] Others also credited the application of the aforementioned doctrine of combat psychiatry.[59,60]

Evidently also quite important in reducing the psychiatric attrition rate was the type of warfare waged in Vietnam. According to Colonel William J Tiffany, then Chief, Psychiatry and Neurology Consultant to The Surgeon General, US Army, and Lieutenant Colonel William S Allerton, his Assistant Chief:

> The fighting in Vietnam is in brief, intensive, and sporadic episodes, with periods of relative calm and safety interspersed. Troops are not pinned down by enemy fire for prolonged periods of days or weeks. The fact that no large artillery barrages exist may also be significant.[24(p813)]

However, quite presciently, these senior psychiatrists warned that the low psychiatric rates may be somewhat based on the deployment of "seasoned and motivated troops"; and that the greener or less motivated troops who follow may produce "a change," that is, deterioration.[24]

Alcohol use and abuse was predictably a common stress outlet for the soldiers of the buildup phase,[39] but military leaders and the psychiatric contingent expressed more concern for the use of illegal drugs by troops,[58,61,62] especially the locally grown marijuana that was readily available and highly potent. In their survey of drug use patterns of lower-ranking enlisted soldiers departing Vietnam in 1967, Roffman and Sapol reported that of the 32% who acknowledged ever smoking marijuana, 61% began in Vietnam and one-quarter were considered heavy users (greater than 20 times during their 1-year tour in Vietnam).[63] The authors also noted that the extent of marijuana use by soldiers in Vietnam was very similar to their civilian peers.[63] Furthermore, Bourne observed that marijuana use created almost no psychiatric problems in the theater.[52] Use of opiates was also mentioned, but it was not as pure as that which was sold after 1970 and was not used by soldiers in sufficient numbers to constitute a serious problem for command.[64] The senior psychiatric leaders in Vietnam were also not very concerned about effects of antiwar sentiment in the United States.[33]

One psychological phenomenon that did attract a fair amount of attention from military psychiatrists was the phasic nature of stressors, moods, and attitudes affecting soldiers as a consequence of the individual, 12-month tour of duty.[39,47,48] To paraphrase the observations by Army psychiatrists Gary L Tischler and Jerome J Dowling, (a) there is a period of initial emersion shock, fearfulness, and highest levels of psychiatric symptomatology; (b) followed by one of mastery and reduced preoccupation with home, but with some depression, resignation, and flight into a "hedonistic pseudocommunity" (peer-group sanctioned hypomanic pursuit of pleasure and materialism); (c) followed by growing combat apprehension and perhaps expressions of a "short-timer's syndrome." The latter refers to a low-grade form of disability often exhibited in soldiers within 4 to 6 weeks of their date of their expected return from overseas. Symptoms consisted of reduced combat tolerance and efficiency; preoccupation with fears about being killed; and sullen, irritable, or withdrawn behavior. This had also been noted among troops serving in the Korean War after individualized tour limitations were introduced there in mid-1951.[65(p73)]

The following is an account provided by Captain Harold SR Byrdy, who served during the first year of the war as division psychiatrist with the 1st Cavalry Division (August 1965–June 1966). It is especially illustrative of the cumulative stress experienced by many of the division's combat troops over time and their efforts to adapt.

During the course of the year there were vast changes in people and changes in the kinds of patients I saw. When the Cavalry troops first took over the safety of the perimeter of the base camp from the 1st Infantry Division in mid-September of 1965 they fired thousands of rounds throughout the first night. That was the main body getting used to being in Vietnam. I had the impression that we often saw a new trooper in his 2nd week in Vietnam. I speculated that it must take a while before the novelty of the place wore off, before he finally became familiar with the routine of his unit and learned its expectations of him and before compulsive mechanisms of adjustment were strained by the realization of a year of sad separation from home, tedious days of work and anxious nights.

The troops would make adjustments to being in the field. They would make some sort of adjustment to the mobility wherein they would sleep perhaps 3 or 4 hours a night and eat 1 or 2 meals a day. I don't think it was an exact plan of any sort, but they would attempt to develop this pattern. When they'd return to the base camp they would have to perhaps make a rapid adjustment from being in the field back to being in garrison where 'spit-shine' boots and polished brass then became the obsession. Often after the return to camp there would be some sort of explosion in the trooper who had done well out in the field. We believed that with time troops were less successful in protecting themselves against repeated loss. I think that during the Ia Drang campaign people tended to spring back to their usual selves with resiliency, but during the Bong Son campaign they wouldn't make it all the way back. Ambivalence would be more prominent. About that time I began seeing more depressed sergeants. A guilt for leading the troops was building up. Also we had several cases in which new sergeants without combat experience came to take over troops who were obviously battle seasoned. These men felt quite inadequate in a leadership role and realistically, they were.

The troops would steel themselves against repeated life-threatening situations and repeated loss of buddies. One fellow was a self-referral through his commanding officer; that is, he referred himself, then the CO [commanding officer] agreed. His complaint was simply that he just didn't feel right. With time due to loss of men through malaria, battle casualties and rotation he had seniority in his company. Having even lost friends among the newly rotated, he had no inclination to make friends and indeed had none. Denial to my mind was the most important mechanism for survival in the area, at all levels.[66(pp51–52)]

However, by the standards of military leaders, the short-timer's syndrome was not the only problem in Vietnam associated with the personnel turbulence brought about by the individualized, 1-year tours; apparently unit cohesion and combat effectiveness were also becoming seriously compromised.[5] (Short-timer's syndrome will be explored further in Chapters 3 and 8.)

Buildup Phase Psychiatrist Reports

The morale and confidence of the deployed Army psychiatrists during these early years also appears to have been high. This is suggested both in the large numbers who were motivated to publish professional accounts (Exhibit 2-1) and in the role satisfaction that these reports reveal. Taken together, these psychiatrists reflect optimism and they tout the effectiveness of the traditional doctrine of forward treatment in Vietnam, the extension of principles of social psychiatry to military leaders (command consultation), and the utilization of newly developed pharmacologic agents (neuroleptics, anxiolytics, and antidepressants) for the treatment of symptoms related to combat stress and other conditions. However, regarding the use of these medications, whereas a limited survey in 1967 confirmed a high level of this type of prescribing by Army physicians, including psychiatrists,[67] no associated clinical or research studies were undertaken to address risks and benefits under the unique circumstances of a combat zone. Buildup phase psychiatrist reports will be reviewed in more detail in subsequent chapters; however, simply scanning the titles provides an impression as to the predominant psychiatric challenges faced through these early years in the war.

With regard to the growing antiwar sentiment in the United States, Captain Arthur S Blank Jr and Captain H Spencer Bloch, two Army psychiatrists who served in the buildup phase and who published accounts, indicated that they did not believe the growing opposition to the war was significantly affecting their patients. Blank, who served during the first year of the war, was very specific: "Do the ambiguities of the war seem to be a problem for the soldiers? The answer is very simply, 'No.' I did not see a single patient in whom I felt that any kind of conflict about the war on any level was primary in precipitating his visits to me."[68(p58)]

Bloch served as the Chief of the Psychiatry and Neurology Inpatient Service of the 935th Psychiatric Detachment, a unit in which Blank had served approximately 2 years earlier. Even then, nothing in Bloch's review suggested either low morale among the troops they encountered or among the psychiatric staff of the 935th. He asserted that in his experience soldiers who struggled with concerns regarding the morality of the conflict typically were driven by pre-Vietnam psychological conflicts. In fact, he spoke favorably about the 935th Psychiatric Detachment's adaptation of the military's psychiatric treatment doctrine, including use of the new psychoactive medications, to the conditions of the irregular counterinsurgency/guerrilla warfare in Vietnam. He also made evident his team's alignment with military priorities in response to persisting conflicts that might arise within the soldier-patient.[23]

Nevertheless, the morale and attitude of deployed ground troops may have already started to slip by that point. Shortly after he returned to the United States from Vietnam, Lieutenant Colonel Jack R Anderson, who was the commanding officer of the 935th Psychiatric Detachment (September 1967–September 1968) when Bloch served, not only expressed concern for a rising incidence of soldiers with drug-induced psychoses and other forms of misconduct, he was also struck by the emergence of the "dedicated soldier turned 'dropper-outer.'"[54(pIII-56)] This refers to the drafted soldier with a stable background and a history of academic and military achievement who would "suddenly and steadfastly refuse to fight any more, and then steadfastly maintain this refusal, even after repeated courts-martial and stockade sentences."[54(pIII-56)]

Perhaps the morale of some of the deployed Army psychiatrists was starting to ebb as well. Captain John A Talbott, a drafted civilian-trained psychiatrist who reported that, pre-Vietnam service, he disagreed with the government and with the war,[69(pG-1)] nonetheless served in Vietnam during the same period as Bloch and Anderson. In an interview following his year there, he said: "[Unique for Vietnam] is the degree of complaining and dislike for this particular war. . . . Almost without

question, all nonpsychotic individuals who appeared at the mental health clinics complained of being in Vietnam and wanted to get out immediately."[70(pIII-58)] Talbott believed that although these were labeled psychiatric problems, they were primarily expressive of a "widespread negative sociologic phenomenon."[70(pIII-58)]

Buildup Phase Impressions

Measures of psychiatric and behavior difficulties among the deployed Army troops in Vietnam during these years was no greater than comparable stateside units. In addition, most military and psychiatric leaders were satisfied that adequate psychiatric resources had been deployed from the start in contrast to previous wars.[14,29,33]

However, as will be demonstrated in this volume, as the years passed, the positive morale in Vietnam did not hold, nor did the low psychiatric attrition rate. In fact, the contentious and protracted counterinsurgency war was already starting to have its corrosive effects on successive cohorts of replacement troops. Quoting a former infantryman:

[Soldiers] did not know the feeling of taking a place and keeping it. . . . No sense of order and momentum. No front, no rear, no trenches laid out in neat parallels, no Patton rushing for the Rhine, no beachheads to storm and win and hold for the duration. They did not have targets, they did not have a cause. . . . On a given day they did not know where they were in Quang Ngai or how being there might influence larger outcomes.[71(p270)]

The Transition From Buildup to Drawdown (1968-1969)

There were 354,300 US Army troops in Vietnam by the end of 1968. Army troop strength peaked at 363,300 by April 1969, and from there it gradually declined. At the end of 1969 there were still 331,100 Army troops in Vietnam.[32] However, as the war lengthened, the Army had been forced to rely increasingly on relatively inexperienced officers and noncommissioned officers, young draftees, and volunteers as more experienced troops rotated back after their year-long tours. According to Spector, a Marine field historian in Vietnam in 1968 and 1969, the negative consequences of not calling up the (experienced) reserves and the constant turnover of troops produced a very ineffective "Vietnam-only Army."[5] Years later, Sorley, a military historian, came

EXHIBIT 2-1. Selected Publications by Buildup Phase Army Psychiatrists (including research reports)

Years in Vietnam	No. Who Published Articles/ Total No. Deployed Army Psychiatrists (as a percentage)*	Publications
1965	1/7 (14.2%)	Huffman RE. Which soldiers break down: a survey of 610 psychiatric patients in Vietnam. *Bull Menninger Clin.* 1970;34:343–351. Bourne PG. Urinary 17-OHCS levels in two combat situations. In: Bourne PG, ed. *The Psychology and Physiology of Stress: With Reference to Special Studies of the Viet Nam War.* New York, NY: Academic Press; 1969: 95–116. Research report.
1966	6/16 (37.5%)	Conte LR. A neuropsychiatric team in Vietnam 1966–1967: an overview. In: Parker RS, ed. *The Emotional Stress of War, Violence, and Peace.* Pittsburgh, Penn: Stanwix House; 1972: 163–168. Johnson AW. Psychiatric treatment in the combat situation. *US Army Vietnam Med Bull.* 1967;January/February:38–45. Jones FD. Experiences of a division psychiatrist in Vietnam. *Mil Med.* 1967;132:1003–1008. Dowling JJ. Psychological aspects of the year in Vietnam. *US Army Vietnam Med Bull.* 1967;May/June:45–48. Tischler GL. Patterns of psychiatric attrition and of behavior in a combat zone. In: Bourne PG, ed. *The Psychology and Physiology of Stress: With Reference to Special Studies of the Viet Nam War.* New York: Academic Press; 1969: 19–44. Kenny WF. Psychiatric disorders among support personnel. *US Army Vietnam Med Bull.* 1967;January/February:34–37.
1967	12/22 (54.6%)	Roffman RA, Sapol E. Marijuana in Vietnam: a survey of use among Army enlisted men in two southern corps. *Int J Addict.* 1970;5:1–42. Research report. Anderson JR. Psychiatric support of the 3rd and 4th Corps tactical zone. *US Army Vietnam Med Bull.* 1968;January/February:37–39. Baker WL. Division psychiatry in the 9th Infantry Division. *US Army Vietnam Med Bull.* 1967;November/December:5–9. Bloch HS. Brief sleep treatment with chlorpromazine. *Comp Psychiatry.* 1970;11:346–355. Bostrom JA. Management of combat reactions. *US Army Vietnam Med Bull.* 1967;July/August:6–8. Casper E, Janacek J, Martinelli H. Marijuana in Vietnam. *US Army Vietnam Med Bull.* 1968;September/October:60–72. Evans ON. Army aviation psychiatry in Vietnam. *US Army Vietnam Med Bull.* 1968;May/June:54–58. Fidaleo RA Marijuana: social and clinical observations. *US Army Vietnam Med Bull.* 1968;March/April:58–59. Gordon EL. Division psychiatry: documents of a tour. *US Army Vietnam Med Bull.* 1968;November/December:62–69. Motis G. Psychiatry at the battle of Dak To. *US Army Vietnam Med Bull.* 1968;March/April:57. Pettera RL, Johnson BM, Zimmer R. Psychiatric management of combat reactions with emphasis on a reaction unique to Vietnam. *Mil Med.* 1969;134:673–678. Talbott JA. The Saigon warriors during Tet. *US Army Vietnam Med Bull.* 1968;March/April:60–61.

*These numbers do not count research reports, although they are listed in the Publications column.

to the same conclusion following his review of the American experience in Vietnam.[1]

Fatefully, in early 1968 the enemy's intensification of combat activities (the surprise, countrywide Tet offensives; the 77-day siege of the US Marine base at Khe Sanh; and the extended battle for Hue) following almost 3 years of bloody fighting convinced the American public that the costs incurred in Vietnam overshadowed the war's ostensible objectives.[1(p12),72(p546),73(pp68–69)] The resultant spike in public protest led President Johnson to announce the administration's intention to pursue peace with North Vietnam. Yet the fighting and dying continued during the tortuous peace negotiations, as did the assignment of replacement troops (albeit in decreasing numbers), and the progressively confrontational antiwar/antimilitary faction in the United States grew louder. The war took on characteristics of a tedious, agonizing stalemate, and the lack of tangible measures of progress contributed to the widespread feelings of futility and frustration about the war.

According to Spector:

[A]s the war ground on through its third and fourth year, the prestige of performing a mission well proved increasingly inadequate to men who more and more could see no larger purpose in that mission, and no end to the incessant patrols, sweeps, and ambushes which appeared to result only in more danger, discomfort, and casualties.[5(p61–62)]

Kirk, a journalist, reported from the field in 1969 that the attitudes of troops did not turn seriously negative until fall of 1968, when President Johnson stopped the bombing of North Vietnam and agreed to enter into peace talks.

The change in attitudes was so sudden . . . the overwhelming sentiment was that the war was a waste, that 'We aren't fighting it like we should. . . . We should go home and let the dinks fight their own war' . . . [soldiers] by and large applauded the [antiwar] demonstrators . . . the senselessness of the struggle.[74(pp61–62)]

Sterba, a correspondent, provided observations on the shifting demographics and particularly the attitudes of the soldiers who went to fight in Vietnam in 1969.

(On 8 June 1969, President Nixon, in concert with South Vietnam's President Thieu, had announced his intention to withdraw the first US troops [25,000] from South Vietnam during July and August.[1(p128),72(p684)]) Sterba demonstrated how the rapidly unfolding political events in the United States caused the romance and idealism of the early war to be replaced by a "hated, dreary struggle"[75(p447)] in which the soldier's overriding preoccupation was that of self-protection:

These were the grunts of the class of 1968—they had come out of that America some of their commanders had seen only from the windows of the Pentagon. They were the graduates of an American nightmare in 1968 that stemmed mostly from the war they had now come to fight—the year of riots and dissention, of assassinations and Chicago, the year America's ulcer burst.[75(p447)]

Transition Phase Psychiatric Overview

The pivotal year, 1968, started off well enough. A few of the psychiatrists in the field in Vietnam indicated that US forces had held up well despite the enemy's countrywide Tet surprise attacks.[76,77] Furthermore, Frank W Hays, a US Air Force psychiatrist who monitored medical evacuations from the theater to Travis Air Force Base in the United States, reported that the proportion of evacuation out of Vietnam for psychiatric conditions dropped to a low 2.7% of all medical evacuations during and immediately following the Tet fighting. "[T]his seems to indicate that the Army has set a new record in the management of psychiatric patients within a combat zone as well as in support areas."[60(p506)] Counterpoint came from Colonel Matthew D Parrish, the USARV Neuropsychiatric Consultant (1967–1968), whose summary of the medical problems and solutions associated with the enemy's Tet offensive observed that under these extreme conditions, by necessity psychiatric patients were evacuated instead of being sent to lower-echelon psychiatric care facilities; in fact, they were evacuated out of Vietnam at three times the usual rate. Parrish worried that, in having their treatment applied offshore and remote from the soldier's primary unit and comrades, these psychiatric conditions would become more intractable.[78]

But concern for soldier reactions to combat stress would soon fade in importance in Vietnam as the war started to have a more generally corrosive effect on the attitude and performance of successive cohorts

TABLE 2-2. Army Incidence Rate for Psychiatric Hospitalizations in Vietnam [and in Europe] in Cases/1,000 Troops/Year

	Total Psychiatric Conditions	Psychosis	Psychoneurosis	Character and Behavior Disorder	Other Psychiatric Conditions
1965	*10.8 [7.7]	1.6 [0.7]	2.3 [1.0]	3.1 [2.2]	3.8 [3.8]
1966	11.6 [7.3]	1.4 [0.8]	2.5 [1.0]	2.8 [2.2]	4.9 [3.3]
1967	9.8 [8.2]	1.7 [0.9]	1.3 [1.0]	2.9 [2.2]	3.9 [4.1]
1968	12.7 [7.9]	1.8 [0.9]	2.2 [1.2]	3.7 [1.8]	5.0 [4.0]
1969	15.1 [7.8]	3.4 [1.6]	1.9 [1.5]	4.2 [1.6]	5.6 [3.1]
1970 (Jan–Sep)	24.0 US [9.7]	3.8 [2.4]	3.3 [1.8]	8.4 [1.9]	8.5 [3.6]

Data source: Neel SH. *Medical Support of the US Army in Vietnam*, 1965–1970. Washington, DC: GPO; 1973; Table 5.
*Neel's rate for 1965 is discrepant with the 6.98 reported by Datel (Datel WE. *A Summary of Source Data in Military Psychiatric Epidemiology.* Alexandria, Va: Defense Technical Information Center; 1976. Document No. AD A021265).

of replacements. Budding demoralization and dissent during these pivotal years began to reveal itself especially in racial incidents and widening drug use (particularly marijuana, but also commercially marketed stimulants and barbiturates) by soldiers. Law enforcement figures demonstrated an increase of over 260% in the number of soldiers involved with possession or use of marijuana during 1968 as compared to the previous year.[5] Also, excessive combat aggression (atrocities) seemed to become more prevalent.[79–82] The official Army overview of medical support for the war showed that overall psychiatric attrition rates (soldiers hospitalized or confined to quarters for at least 24 hours) among all types rose steadily after 1968 through the third quarter of 1970 (from 13.3/1,000 for 1968, to 25.1/1,000),[27(Table 3,p36)] and overall psychiatric hospitalization rates doubled similarly during that period (Table 2-2). Although psychiatric hospitalization rates among Army troops stationed in Europe also increased during the same time frame, the increase was far more pronounced in the Vietnam theater.[27(Table 5,p46)]

As noted earlier, the official summary of Army medical activities in Vietnam (mid-1965 through mid-1970), authored by Major General Spurgeon Neel, made no mention of combat stress reactions as such. However, it did express concern that the overall psychiatric hospitalization rate was rising despite the falling wounded in action (WIA) rate—a contradiction of the covariance that was found in previous, high-intensity wars.[27(p47)] Neel attributed this increase to dissenting soldier subgroups who were motivated by racial, political, or drug culture priorities and to the

widening use of illegal drugs by soldiers in Vietnam. (This work was regrettably not published until 1973, after troops were withdrawn from Vietnam.)

Published more contemporarily (in 1970), Parrish and Colbach, both of whom had served in Vietnam, indicated that morale had been generally good in Vietnam; and they acknowledged their satisfaction that "The average soldier . . . has not seemed overly concerned with the justification for the war."[41(pp339–340)] Nonetheless, they did express "real concern"[41(p340)] for the doubling of the psychiatric casualty rate between 1968 and mid-1970 and speculated that this was fueled by increased racial tensions and a decrement in perception of military purpose within the soldier. They also correctly predicted that the intent to disengage from Vietnam would likely produce accelerating psychiatric problems among those newly assigned there.[41]

Regarding spreading drug use in Vietnam, M Duncan Stanton's survey of drug use patterns among soldiers entering or departing Vietnam in late 1969 revealed sizable increases in the use of most drugs compared to the 1967 survey by Roger A Roffman and Ely Sapol.[64] Stanton speculated, however, that marijuana and some other drugs might actually allow certain types of individuals to function under the stresses of a combat environment and separation from home.[64]

Problems for the US Marines fighting in Vietnam paralleled those of the Army. Lieutenant Commander John A Renner Jr, a Navy psychiatrist who served in the Vietnam theater in 1969, noted a similar rise in disciplinary problems, including racial disturbances, attacks on superiors, combat atrocities, drug abuse, and

EXHIBIT 2-2. Selected Publications by Transition Phase Army Psychiatrists (Including Research Reports)

Years in Vietnam	No. Who Published Articles/ Total No. Deployed Army Psychiatrists (as a percentage)*	Publications
1968	3/22 (13.6%)	Colbach EM, Crowe RR. Marijuana associated psychosis in Vietnam. *Mil Med.* 1970;135:571–573. Colbach EM, Willson SM. The binoctal craze. *US Army Vietnam Med Bull.* 1969;March/April:40–44. Forest DV, Bey DR, Bourne PG. The American soldier and Vietnamese women. *Sex Behav.* 1972;2:8–15. Postel WB. Marijuana use in Vietnam: a preliminary report. *US Army Vietnam Med Bull.* 1968;September/October:56–59.
1969	2/22 (9.1%)	Bey DR. Change in command in combat: a locus of stress. *Am J Psychiatry.* 1972;129:698–702. Bey DR, Smith WE. Organizational consultant in a combat unit. *Am J Psychiatry.* 1970;128:401–406. Bey DR, Zecchinelli VA. Marijuana as a coping device in Vietnam. *Mil Med.* 1971;136:448–450. Master FD. Some clinical observations of drug abuse among GIs in Vietnam. *J Kentucky Med Assn.* 1971;69:193–195. Stanton MD. Drug use in Vietnam. *Arch Gen Psychiatry.* 1972;26:279–286. Research report.

*These numbers do not count research reports, although they are listed in the Publications column.

the number of men diagnosed with character disorders (all of which he lumped under "hidden casualties").[83] He expressed concern that military psychiatrists were premature in touting the low rate for psychiatric difficulties in the war. Still, although he agreed there was a growing "morale problem," he believed that "the average soldier, despite complaints about his duties and possible reservations about involvement in Vietnam, seems to adapt to the situation."[83(p171)] (His work was not published until 1973, after the Marines left Vietnam.)

Transition Phase Psychiatrist Reports

Army psychiatrists serving in these years were mostly not motivated to publish accounts of their professional experience in Vietnam compared to those who served in the buildup phase (Exhibit 2-2). The titles of the articles that were published suggest increasing attention to challenges surrounding drug use and other morale issues and away from combat-related problems. Still, dissent within the ranks appears not to be a subject of major concern among these psychiatrists.

Especially notable were the postdeployment observations of Captain John Imahara, an Army psychiatrist. His tour (September 1968–September 1969) was unique in that, although assigned to the 935th Psychiatric Detachment, he volunteered to provide specialized services for the confinees of the USARV Installation Stockade ("Long Binh Jail") following the August 1968 riot (". . . the 'worst prison riot in the modern history of the US Army'"[84(pIII-57)]). Imahara recalled the innumerable soldiers who were in the stockade who might have otherwise warranted psychiatric attention. Singled out among this group of disruptive, deviant, and sometimes violent soldiers were the "restive 'soul brothers' whose . . . certain gestures, ornaments, and modes of behavior were known to intimidate white soldiers."[84(pIII-57)] According to Imahara, their intense hostility expressed a belief that the military was an oppressive institution, and that whites were the oppressors. Imahara also acknowledged the widening drug use in Vietnam and its potential to fuel violent incidents.

[E]xplosive situations arising from the combination of drugs, available weapons, and stress, necessitated confinement of the passive resistive marihuana smoker, the paranoid methamphetamine injector, the hyperactive amphetamine user, the AWOL [absent without leave] emaciated opium injector, and the moody individual who takes barbiturates.[84(pIII-57)]

A contrasting picture came from Bey. He spent his year in Vietnam (1969–1970) as division psychiatrist with the 1st Infantry Division and authored or coauthored 11 timely articles reporting on his experiences in the war along with associated matters such as psychiatric problems within other cultures in Vietnam, adjustment issues for returning veterans, and problems facing waiting wives. Bey's efforts constituted a rich and optimistic exposition of the means and achievements of a division psychiatrist and his staff. He especially commended his enlisted mental health technicians for their work with the widely dispersed commanders, physicians, and soldier-patients of the division.[85] Regarding his sustained confidence, it appears that Bey was unique among the Army psychiatrists assigned in Vietnam during this phase. Despite having received his psychiatric training in a civilian setting, evidently his additional background in organizational consultation, his family heritage of military service, and a predeployment military assignment equipped him for the challenges he faced in Vietnam and allied him with the military organization. Bey's more positive take on his year in Vietnam,[86] despite serving there a year after Imahara, may also reflect that morale and associated psychiatric and behavior problems were less prevalent among combat units than in noncombat units.

Transition Phase Impressions

America's war in Vietnam had become prolonged, stalemated, and costly during this transition phase. Waging war during the highly contentious, off-and-on peace negotiations with the enemy and the ever-widening antiwar sentiment at home was wearing away the initial sense of national purpose and resolve among those who were nonetheless sent to fight as replacements. In retrospect, the gradually rising rates for psychiatric conditions and behavior problems during these pivotal years, including drug abuse and racial conflicts, signaled brewing discontent and dissent among the deployed troops. Still, falling morale and its psychological and behavioral repercussions do not generally appear to be of major concern among the Army psychiatrists in Vietnam through these years.

The Drawdown Phase (1970–1973)

There were 249,600 US Army troops in Vietnam by the end of 1970 and 119,700 by the end of 1971.[32] Six months later, in July 1972, Army strength had dropped to 31,800 support troops.[32] During these final years, although more troops were leaving than were being sent as replacements, hostilities and dangers continued, even if attenuated. Unrelenting public opposition to the war may have accelerated the American pullout, but the process severely demoralized those who were sent there during the drawdown years. Many soldiers interpreted antiwar sentiment as criticism of them personally—not the war more generally. In addition to accelerating rates for psychiatric conditions and behavior problems, two new and very alarming behavior problems emerged in 1970, primarily among lower-ranking enlisted troops: (1) widespread heroin use and (2) soldier assaults on military leaders with explosives ("fragging")—symptoms unmistakably indicating that the US Army in Vietnam was becoming seriously compromised. Despite the reduction in combat activity, Army leaders and the medical/psychiatric contingent in Vietnam became increasingly consumed with problems associated with the wholesale alienation and dysfunction of soldiers.[87] Furthermore, by now the deployed psychiatrists were surrounded by a professional literature that was mostly critical of the military psychiatric structures and priorities there.[88]

Shelby Stanton, distinguished military historian and the author of *Vietnam Order of Battle*, provided this description of the problems in maintaining military order and discipline among US military units as the end of the war approached:

Lowered troop morale and discipline were manifested in increased crime, racial clashes, mutinous disregard of orders, anti-war protests, and monetary corruption in black market currency exchanges, as well as drug use. The Army had become extremely permissive as it tried to cope with changing societal attitudes, and standards of soldiering eroded proportionally. In Vietnam serious disciplinary problems resulted in disintegrating unit cohesion and operational slippage. In the field, friendly fire accidents became more prevalent as more short rounds and misplaced fire were caused by carelessness. There was an excessive number of "accidental" shootings and promiscuous throwing of grenades, some of which were deliberate

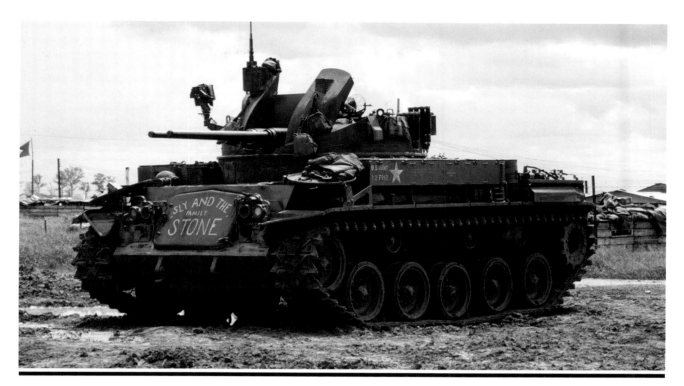

FIGURE 2-1. M42 Duster self-propelled antiaircraft gun "Sly and the Family Stone" This particular M42 Duster was given the name of a popular rock band by its crew. This choice likely alludes to the group's iconic hit song from the 1969 counterculture Woodstock festival, "I Want to Take You Higher," which is also suggestive of the growing popularity of the drug culture. More-broadly it connotes the counterculture attitude shared by young adults of that time, which was captured in the phrase popularized by hippie guru, Timothy Leary, "Turn on, tune in, drop out". This name is in striking contrast to those commonly applied to planes and tanks in earlier wars that were intended to be ferocious and intimidating; and it seems to reflect a generation of troops fightingin Vietnam—resonant with their civilian counterparts—who were ambivalent regarding the military mission and values. Photograph courtesy of Richard D Cameron, Major General, US Army (Retired).

fraggings aimed at unpopular officers, sergeants, and fellow enlisted men. Redeploying units gave vent to years of frustration as their speeding [A]rmy vehicles tore down the frequently ambushed highways, shooting and hurling rocks, cans and insults at the Vietnamese alongside the roads.

Widespread breakdowns in troop discipline forced the military police into a front-line role serving as assault troops against other soldiers. These actions were typified by two instances. Composite military police Whisky Mountain Task Force was engaged in a rather spectacular standoff on 25 September 1971. Fourteen soldiers of the 35th Engineer Group had barricaded themselves in a bunker and were holding out with automatic weapons and machine guns. A homemade explosive device was exploded in the rear of the bunker, and all 14 surrendered and

were treated for wounds. Chinook helicopters had them in Long Binh Stockade the next day. A month later, on 27 October 1971, another military police strike force air-assaulted the Praline Mountain signal site near Dalat. Two fragmentation grenades had been used in an attempt to kill the company commander two nights in a row. Initial escorts had proved insufficient protection, and military police had to garrison the mountaintop for a week until order was restored.[87(pp357–358)]

Validation for these observations came from an exceptionally comprehensive historical series by The Boston Publishing Company. It provided vivid accounts of the various expressions of contempt for the war and the South Vietnamese shared by US military forces in the war's last years. In particular, they noted that, "The daily round of random death and incapacitation from

EXHIBIT 2-3. A Specimen of Leadership in Late Vietnam

The 1st Battalion, 5th Cavalry, 1st Cavalry Division (Airmobile), and its commander in early 1971, Lt. Col. Richard Kattar, was one example of a unit that remained effective and disciplined.

When Kattar took command . . . his men received a jolt. "He energized the battalion," said Captain Eugene J. White, Jr., Company A commander. "He pulled me out of the field and brought me back to the base and said, 'My name's Kattar. Here's what you can expect from me, and here's what I expect from you.' That's the first time a battalion commander had talked to me like that." . . . Company B commander Captain Hugh Foster at first was skeptical. Kattar came on too strong for Foster. "But he was supportive and he gave his people credit for common sense," said Foster. Many of the troops at the time grumbled about going into the field. But Kattar told operations officer Lieutenant John D. Stube, "We cannot have that attitude. People will be sloppy, make mistakes, and get killed."

Kattar immediately improved firebase security. He ordered more patrolling and required his men to change the positions of the 105MM howitzers after dark. He had them loaded with fléchette rounds (an antipersonnel round containing short, nail-like projectiles) for direct fire against any attackers. Units returning from patrol were given additional tasks to keep them busy on the base; the prior habit of "flopping out" had raised the level of boredom.

In his second tour after serving as an advisor in 1963–1964, Kattar believed that the soldiers "deserved to be inspired to believe in a cause," and their own survival was an excellent cause. Kattar visited each company separately and gave the men a version of the following speech:

No one in his right mind wants to be shot at, indeed killed. Unless you're a crackpot, and I'm certainly not a crackpot. But I am a professional soldier. I've been here before, I've been shot at before, and I have lived as you live, on the trail with my whole life on my back. I am not here to demonstrate courage under fire. Because I'm scared to death every time somebody shoots at me. The only thing I'm delighted with is that the army took the time to train me well enough so I react properly under fire. Because that's all it is—a reaction. No one really thinks about what the hell they're doing.

Now I have a beautiful wife, three lovely children and a great life ahead of me. I want to get this done and get back to that. The things I can guarantee you are that I will die for you, if it's necessary, and that I will never experiment with you, and that if you listen to what I tell you and do as I say and am prepared to do with you, then your opportunity to fight and win will be the greatest, will be maximized. Because it makes no sense to me at all for someone to draw the conclusion that they're giving themselves an opportunity to get back home by walking around the jungle in a stupor, either because of dope or preoccupation of mind. . . . When you walk through that jungle, you'll walk through there sharp and intent upon insuring that if that sonofabitch raises his goddam ugly head to blow you away, you're going to blow him away first. And then we're going home.

mines and booby traps, combined with short-timer's fever and skepticism about the worth of 'search and clear' missions steadily lowered American morale."[89(p97)] The pervasive demoralization in the theater and the brittle nature of race relations, especially within noncombat units, became associated with a weakening of the military legal system. According to these authors, combat refusals, drug problems, and racial strife often proved impossible to resolve in the last years in Vietnam. Although punishments tended to be increasingly lenient, commanders openly acknowledged that, rather than hunt the enemy or carry out a tactical mission, they considered their primary responsibility to be to return their men safely home. "It sometimes seemed to be little more than a ragtag band of men wearing bandannas, peace symbols, and floppy bush hats, with little or no

fight left in it"[43(p16)] (Figure 2-1).

Similarly Balkind's historical review of the severe breakdown in morale and effectiveness of the US military in Southeast Asia during the drawdown phase of the war provided thoroughly referenced data indicating an unprecedented increase in rates of combat refusals, combat atrocities, heroin use, assassinations (or threats) of military leaders, racial conflicts, AWOL, and desertion, and the emergence of the soldier antiwar movement.[65] Balkind also underscored the corrosive effects on morale and cohesion consequent to emergent careerism among military leaders ("ticket punching"), a criticism similarly brought to bear by Gabriel and Savage[90] and by Cincinnatus.[50]

Firsthand observations came from Kirk, a journalist:

EXHIBIT 2-3. A Specimen of Leadership in Late Vietnam, continued

Kattar forbade the wearing of bandannas and required his men to wear steel helmets. He also put a stop to one of the characteristic "grunt" symbols of the war—the wearing of "Pancho Villa" bandoliers of M60 ammunition crossed over the shoulders [because dirt got in the ammo links]. . . . Kattar required company commanders to attach [the heavy] "secure" scrambler devices to the standard PCR-77 radio for communications security. . . .

Under the prevailing circumstances of 1971, Kattar's insistence on tight discipline and "by-the-book" procedures might have made him a candidate for "fragging" by disgruntled troops. But most of the men responded to his leadership. "He took care of the soldiers," said Captain Foster. Operating from Firebases Apache and Mace, the 1st Battalion's mission was to pursue the 33d NVA Regiment. "Kattar always came out into the field," Foster said. "He talked with the soldiers. He went out on sweeps with the company. He showed that he shared the risks."

The 1st Battalion also had had its share of the problems of the times—combat refusals, drug problems, racial strife—which the weakened "system" proved incapable of resolving. Punishments for offenses that once were considered to be serious had become lenient. A squad leader who had refused Foster's order to stake out an ambush was court-martialed and found guilty, fined only $100, and was not demoted. Another soldier, a machine gunner, threatened to kill a squad leader if he forced his men to advance down a certain trail. Sent to the rear for prosecution, the man returned shortly without having been court-martialed. The legal authorities said that since he had not fired his weapon, he had committed no offense. . . .

As the battalion came off the helicopter pad at Bien Hoa to stand down prior to leaving Vietnam, the troops were enthusiastic, shouting "All the way!" and "Airborne!" as they left the war behind them. . . . A writer from the division historical office . . . asked operations officer Lt. Stube how the battalion commander had managed to get these troops to act as they did. "He is the finest leader I have ever known," Stube answered. "He motivated soldiers and officers to do the right thing."

Reproduced with permission from Fulghum D, Maitland T, & the editors of Boston Publishing Co. *The Vietnam Experience: South Vietnam on Trial.* Boston, Mass: Boston Publishing Co; 1984: 22–24.

[I]t is, in reality, a desultory kind of struggle, punctuated by occasional explosions and tragedy, for the last Americans in combat in Vietnam. It is a limbo between victory and defeat, a period of lull before the North Vietnamese again seriously challenge allied control over the coastal plain, as they did for the last time in the Tet, May and September offensives of 1968. For the average "grunt," or infantryman, the war is not so much a test of strength under pressure, as it often was a few years ago, as a daily hassle to avoid patrols, avoid the enemy, avoid contact—to keep out of trouble and not be the last American killed in Vietnam.[74(p65)]

More ominous was the investigative report by Linden, another journalist, from his visit in 1971. Linden covered much of the same ground as those mentioned above, but in addition he provided case examples and other observations. These included corroboration from Captain Robert Landeen, an Army psychiatrist assigned to the 101st Airborne Division. Linden dynamically depicted the circumstances and meanings that combined to produce a "class war" between leaders and subordinates in Vietnam—often with fragging as its final result. He described the mounting tensions that commonly arose when bitter, dispirited enlisted soldiers, black activism, and heroin combined within small, isolated units, especially noncombat units; and how common it was for fraggings and threats of violence to be used as means of controlling officers and noncommissioned officers (NCOs). "[Fragging in Vietnam became] prevalent, passionless, and apparently unprovoked, representing the grisly game of psychological warfare that [soldiers] use."[91(p12)]

Not surprisingly, the Army's pernicious morale and discipline problems were mirrored on a comparable scale among the Marines fighting in Vietnam. The official review of US Marine activities late in the war acknowledged rampant combat atrocities, "friendly fire" accidents, combat refusals, racial strife, drug abuse, "fraggings," and dissent.[92] William Corson, a retired Marine lieutenant colonel (and an expert on revolution and counterinsurgency warfare and veteran of World War II, Korea, and Vietnam), blamed the military's problems in late Vietnam on both America's failure in Vietnam and an "erosion of moral principle within the military."[93(p100)] He referred to the rise in "fragging" incidents as a new service-wide form of psychological warfare and an aspect of institutionalized mutinous behaviors (along with sabotage, evasion of leadership responsibilities, and internecine conflict). According to Corson, "[a]s with fragging, the potential for a mutinous refusal to carry out an order is so widespread [in Vietnam] that routine actions are being avoided by those in charge."[93(p99)]

The subject of the role and effectiveness of military leaders, including in Vietnam, is beyond the scope of this work, but history has amply illustrated the inexorable tie between high caliber of leadership (eg, intelligence, skills, tact, knowledge, personality, maturity, ethics, and devotion to the mission and to the welfare of the troops) and high morale within military units. Observers and commentators have acknowledged a critical downturn in Army leadership as the war in Vietnam lengthened, American opposition to the war grew more forceful, and troop morale slumped ever lower. Many officers and senior enlisted personnel also lost their commitment to the war and thus had little with which to inspire their troops. (See Appendix 6, "Administrative Elimination Under Provisions of AR 635-212.")

However, even though the yearly rotation of these senior grades in and out of Vietnam was especially responsible for deficiencies in leadership, there were other policies that also contributed to the problem.[1,5] For instance, within Vietnam officers commonly served only 6 months as commanders, while being utilized in the remaining 6 months of their tour in a staff position. For the enlisted soldier this meant that, at any given point, his unit officers had either been in a command less than 3 months and, in many respects, were still learning their jobs and the personnel, or they had less than 3 months before rotating out and were perhaps experiencing their own short-timer's syndrome of emotional withdrawal.

One postwar critic utilized the term "institutional inexperience" to refer to the tentative, clumsy, and indecisive style of American operations in Vietnam consequent to the short command tours for officers.[5] Illustrating the problem, John Paul Vann, who served as an Army officer in Vietnam and later became the II Corps senior advisor, provided the oft-quoted and cynical line, "The United States has not been in Vietnam for ten years . . . but for one year ten times."[43(p47)] Others noted the emergent careerism that had replaced commitment to military objectives in Vietnam (so-called "ticket punching," ie, an officer's belief that service in Vietnam would advance his career through collecting

experiences and awards that would push him ahead of his contemporaries).[90] Exhibit 2-3, "A Specimen of Leadership in Late Vietnam," presents the description of one exceptional battalion commander who opposed this trend and remained disciplined and effective during the drawdown phase in Vietnam, evidently with salutary consequences.[43]

It seems remarkable in retrospect that the enemy did not find ways to exploit these serious fault lines in the morale and discipline of the American forces late in the war. However, according to Sorley, the military historian, "Perhaps, even in the midst of the undeniably widespread problems of drugs, race, and indiscipline, there were enough good soldiers left to do what had to be done."[1(p295)] He posited that the Army's problems in Vietnam, although substantial, had been exaggerated by those who were opposed to the war. Still, it was a precarious situation as exemplified by the incident on 28 March 1971, when elements of the 196th Light Infantry Brigade at Fire Support Base Mary Ann suffered severe casualties (33 American soldiers killed and 78 wounded) when they were infiltrated by enemy sappers.[87] By Sorley's report, this arose because the unit was "riddled with drugs and incompetence."[1(p295)]

Drawdown Phase Psychiatric Overview

The drawdown years saw a dramatic increase in the traditional indices of psychiatric attrition. As noted in the Preface to this book, through the early years of the war, the Army psychiatric hospitalization rate had hovered between 12 and 16.5 per 1,000 soldiers per year,[14,39,94] which was very favorable compared to rates for the preceding wars. However, the rate in Vietnam started to rise in 1968, doubled by April 1970, and doubled again by July 1971 (reaching an annualized rate of 40/1,000/year).[39] From there it rapidly dropped until the remaining combat troops were pulled out in mid-1972. New policies that permitted troops detected as narcotic-positive by urine testing to be medically evacuated out of Vietnam were largely responsible for this reversal (marijuana use was not detectable at that time).[95] Figure 2-2 illustrates the independence of the accelerating psychiatric hospitalization rate from the variable of combat intensity in Vietnam (as measured by the Army battle death rate) after 1968.

The rising out-of-country psychiatric evacuation rate is especially striking. This remained at the favorable rate of below four to five per 1,000 troops per year through 1970. By July 1971 it had risen to 42.3, and by the following year, July 1972, the rate had climbed to

FIGURE 2-2. US and Army Vietnam rates per 1,000 troops for battle deaths,[1] psychiatric hospitalization,[2] and psychosis[3]

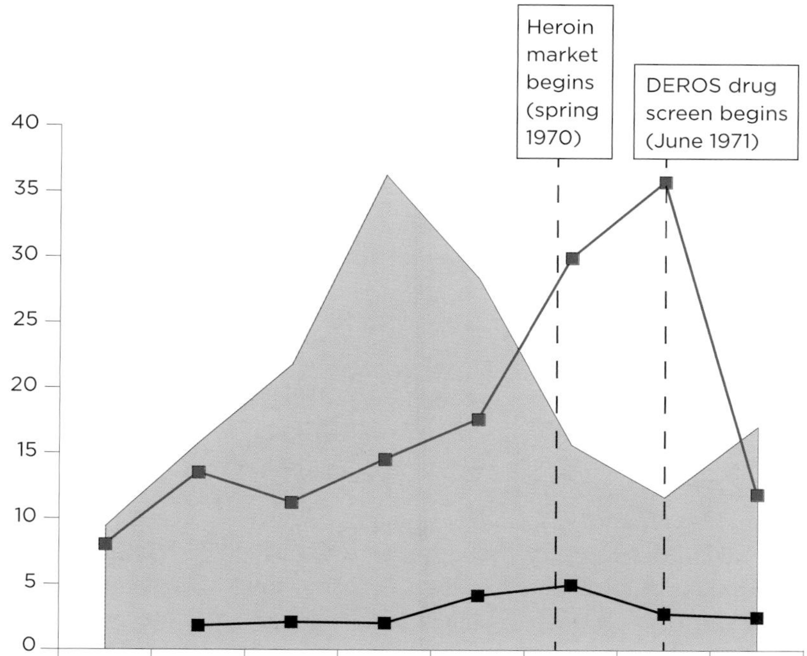

	1965	1966	1967	1968	1969	1970	1971	1972
Army battle death rate	9.42	15.6	21.6	36.3	28.4	15.7	11.7	17.1
Army psychiatric hospitalization rate	6.98	11.8	9.8	12.7	15.4	25.2	31.3	10.4
Army psychosis rate		1.58	1.83	1.78	3.63	4.35	2.43	2.2

Within figure: "Heroin market begins (spring 1970)" and "DEROS drug screen begins (June 1971)"

[1] US Army Adjutant General, Casualty Services Division (DAAG-PEC). Active duty Army personnel battle casualties and nonbattle deaths Vietnam, 1961–1979, Office of the Adjutant General counts. February 3, 1981.

[2] Datel WE. *A Summary of Source Data in Military Psychiatric Epidemiology.* Alexandria, Va: Defense Documentation Center, 1976. Document ADA 021-265.

[3] Jones FD, Johnson AW Jr. Medical and psychiatric treatment policy and practice in Vietnam. *J Social Issues*; 1975;31(4):49-65.

DEROS: date of expected return overseas

129.8.[39(Figure 2)] In other words, at that point in the war, *one out of every eight soldiers* was medically evacuated from Vietnam for psychiatric reasons (primarily for drug dependency, especially heroin).

A corollary measure of the rapidly deteriorating mental health of soldiers assigned in Vietnam was the skyrocketing percentage of neuropsychiatric cases among medical evacuations for all causes from Vietnam. It had remained below 5% through the first two-thirds of the war but rose to 30% in late 1971 (at which point more soldiers were being evacuated from Vietnam for drug use than for war wounds[96]). By late 1972, the percentage of neuropsychiatric evacuations was at 61% of evacuations,[39] a rate almost triple that during World

War II (23%[29]). However, taken alone this metric could overstate the case for spiraling neuropsychiatric rates because the WIA rate was simultaneously declining.

It is of special note that the doubling rate for psychosis in 1969 and 1970 in Vietnam (see Figure 2-1) from its historically predictable 2 per 1,000 troops per year presented a paradox for Army psychiatry. Because it coincided with an Army-wide rise in the psychosis rate, it was initially explained by Jones and Johnson as secondary to the influence of illegal drugs in confusing the diagnosis.[39] Jones subsequently noted that in 1971 the psychosis rate reverted back to its historical levels but only in the Vietnam theater after the Army allowed drug-dependent soldiers to utilize medical evacuation

TABLE 2-3. Rates for Fragging Incidents and Narcotic Overdose Deaths in Vietnam (All Branches/1,000 US Troops/Year)

	1969	1970	1971	1972
Fragging rates[1]	0.5	1.12	2.4	2.3
Narcotic overdose death[2] rates[†]	0	0.34*	0.3	No data

*The 1970 narcotic overdose death rate is annualized from the 49 deaths confirmed between August and December. Ninety-five percent pure heroin only became widely marketed in South Vietnam in spring of 1970, and the first heroin overdose death proven by autopsy was in August 1970.[3]
†These figures are discrepant from those provided by Baker, a senior Army psychiatrist, who suggested an even higher rate in 1970 (75 confirmed or suspected incidents between August 1 and October 18, which provides an annualized rate of 1.05). Baker also said there were 11 confirmed by autopsy in 1969, and 14 in 1970 before August[4]; however, these must involve other drugs such as barbiturates because heroin was not yet available.

Data sources: (1) Gabriel RA, Savage PL. *Crisis in Command: Mismanagement in the Army*. New York, NY: Hill and Wang; 1978; (2) US Department of Defense. *Drug Abuse in the Military—A Status Report (Part II)*. Washington, DC: Office of Information for the Armed Forces; August 1972. DoD Information Guidance Series No 5A-18: 1-3; (3) Colonel Clotilde Bowen, USARV Psychiatric Consultant. End of Tour Report, 8 June 1971; (4) Baker SL Jr. Drug abuse in the United States Army. *Bull N Y Acad Med*. 1971;47(6):541–549.

channels.[21] He speculated that the rising rates may have also reflected the tendency for Army psychiatrists and other physicians in Vietnam to mislabel soldiers "who did not belong overseas" as psychotic (eg, insinuating the physicians' intent to manipulate the system).[21]

In themselves, these traditional measures of psychiatric attrition are startling. However, they must be viewed in conjunction with the equally alarming rise in behavioral problems during the drawdown years in Vietnam: (*a*) judicial and nonjudicial (Article 15) disciplinary actions,[58] (*b*) noncombat fatalities,[97] (*c*) combat refusals,[89] (*d*) corruption and profiteering,[5,65] (*e*) racial incidents,[5,65] (*f*) convictions for the specific crime of "fragging,"[98,99] (*g*) suicides,[100] and, especially, (*h*) use of illegal drugs. Table 2-3 presents grim, "tip-of-the-iceberg" statistics for the most dramatic of these: fragging incidents and narcotic overdose deaths. Army mental health personnel were often called upon to intervene with these types of problems and sought to apply traditional means and models but with uncertain results.

Drawdown Phase Psychiatrist Reports

As it turned out, as soldier morale, psychological fitness, and military readiness were declining in Vietnam, greater numbers of Army psychiatrists with little or no military experience were sent as replacements. Similarly, those serving in Vietnam as the senior Army psychiatrist (the USARV Neuropsychiatry Consultant) had progressively less Army psychiatry experience as the war extended.[101] The psychiatrists deployed during the drawdown phase of the war were

generally not motivated to publish accounts of their experience. Perhaps somewhat contributory was the fact that publication of the *USARV Medical Bulletin* was discontinued in 1970. The few who published wrote exclusively about the heroin epidemic and implied a relative failure of traditional psychiatric approaches to solve this problem and ones stemming from soldier demoralization and dissent (Exhibit 2-4).

Two publications from this period warrant special attention. In a lay publication, Major Richard Ratner, an Army psychiatrist, described his service with the 935th Psychiatric Medical Detachment ("Drugs and Despair in Vietnam") 2 years after Bloch left Vietnam. Ratner's recollections centered on the challenge of the drug epidemic, and he summarized the patterns of use, clinical presentations, and treatment results (poor) for over 1,000 drug-dependent soldiers who were voluntary residents in the Army Amnesty Center on Long Binh Post near Saigon between January 1971 and July 1971. In the process he conveyed a dark picture of military life in Vietnam at that time. He considered that his caseload was only a fraction of the estimated 30% of the young, lower-ranking soldiers who use heroin regularly, and that they in turn only partially reflected the pervasive demoralization within the larger military force in Vietnam. Although alluding to likely predeployment factors in the drug-dependent soldiers he saw, Ratner credited more their universal despair, which he believed was due to a combination of societal factors (eg, America's motivation for waging war in Southeast Asia represented a displacement of its "racial hostilities") and an "inhumane" Army. Ratner acknowledged the sense

EXHIBIT 2-4. Selected Publications by Drawdown-Phase Army Psychiatrists (Including Research Reports)

Years in Vietnam	No. Who Published Articles/ Total No. Deployed Army Psychiatrists (as a percentage)*	Publications
1970	2/20 (10%)	Char J. Drug abuse in Vietnam. *Am J Psychiatry*. 1972;129:463–465. Ratner RA. Drugs and despair in Vietnam. *U Chicago Magazine*. 1972;64:15–23.
1971	1/13 (7.7%)	Joseph BS. Lessons on heroin abuse from treating users in Vietnam. *Hosp Community Psychiatry*. 1974;25:742–744. Holloway HC. Epidemiology of heroin dependency among soldiers in Vietnam. *Mil Med*. 1974;139:108–113. Research report.
1972	0/1 (0.0%)	Holloway HC, Sodetz FJ, Elsmore TF, and the members of Work Unit 102. Heroin dependence and withdrawal in the military heroin user in the US Army, Vietnam. In: *Annual Progress Report, 1973*. Washington, DC: Walter Reed Army Institute of Research; 1973: 1244–1246. Research report.

*These numbers do not count research reports, although they are listed in the Publications column.

of clinical impotence he and his colleagues experienced ("there seems to be no place for a psychiatrist to begin"); he also seemed to share the cynicism of his soldier-patients.[102]

Equally troubling is the account by Lieutenant Commander Howard W Fisher, a Navy psychiatrist who served with the 1st Marine Division during the same year as Ratner only further north near Da Nang ("Vietnam Psychiatry: Portrait of Anarchy"[103]). According to Fisher, of 1,000 consecutive Marine referrals, 960 warranted personality disorder diagnoses ("usually antisocial"), with 590 of these presumed to be involved with illegal drugs. Although he differed from Ratner in attributing more of their dysfunction to predeployment defects of character, Fisher also faulted the officers and NCOs who encouraged their misconduct and rebellion. He felt this occurred because of vacillations in enforcing regulations, and he argued that these problems were exacerbated by expectations that psychiatry would either provide these Marines medical evacuation out of Vietnam or recommend administrative separation from the service in lieu of punishment.

Finally, the 1982 Walter Reed Army Institute of Research survey (mentioned in the Prologue) of Army psychiatrists who were veterans of the Vietnam War confirmed that, in large part, those who served in the second half of the war felt overwhelmed when trying to treat soldiers affected by a raging drug epidemic, incendiary racial animosities, and outbreaks of violence. Compared to their counterparts in the first half of the war, these late war psychiatrists tended to be more vocal, more divided according to training differences (military vs civilian), and, in some cases, quite defensive. They also were more likely to be critical of their preparation and utilization by the Army.[101,104]

Drawdown Phase Impressions

During these final 3 years, as the US military was carefully reducing its presence in South Vietnam and turning the fighting over to the Army of the Republic of Vietnam (ARVN), deployed troops increasingly expressed their opposition to serving through antimilitary behaviors and psychosocial disability. Collectively this represented a rampant social/military breakdown within the deployed force—an "inverted" morale. Replacement Army psychiatrists and allied mental health personnel in Vietnam found themselves in a radically different war—with a radically different Army—than was faced by those who served in previous wars or even those who preceded them in Vietnam. The record from this phase suggested that the psychiatric contingent, like the military leaders, failed to anticipate these emergent psychiatric and conduct disorders. Furthermore, psychiatrists with appreciably less military experience, including those in leadership positions, were sent to the theater as the problems there were multiplying. Ultimately the morale of the later Army psychiatrists paralleled the flagging morale of the deployed soldiers.

A Case Example of "Deployment Stress Reaction"

The following case material (disguised) was extracted from the report of an Army Sanity Board hearing for Private (PVT) Echo, which was held at the 98th Psychiatric Detachment in Da Nang, Republic of South Vietnam, in early 1971. In many important respects PVT Echo personified the avalanche of soldiers seen by the psychiatric component during the final third of the war, especially including the fact that he had a good pre-Vietnam service history and little or no active exposure to combat risk at the time of the incident. Perhaps he should be labeled a "(combat theater) deployment stress reaction" as defined earlier.

CASE 2-2: Sanity Evaluation of a Private Who Threatened His Platoon Leader and First Sergeant

Identifying information: PVT Echo was a 19-year-old, single, black E-2 with 17 months of Army service and 4 months duty in Vietnam. He was facing a general court-martial after he had pointed a gun at Lieutenant (LT) K, threatened to kill him and the First Sergeant (1st SGT), and demanded the LT's shirt, which he put on.

History of present illness: Although rated as a light weapons infantryman, at the time of the incident PVT Echo was permanently assigned as a jeep driver for Headquarters Company of one of the battalions of his division—an assignment with little, if any, direct exposure to hostile enemy forces. On the day prior to the incident PVT Echo had received an upsetting letter from his mother in which she admonished him for getting into trouble with military authorities (some months earlier he had been convicted in a court-martial for threatening a superior officer and demoted). Also on that day, PVT Echo injured his leg and had been excused from duty. On the morning of the incident, he had become very distressed when he learned that another soldier had been assigned to drive his jeep, and he believed he would be financially responsible if something were to happen to it. After smoldering with anger throughout most of the day,

PVT Echo got his M16A1 rifle and went to his platoon leader, LT K, with the intention of demanding he get his vehicle back. PVT Echo could not explain to the Sanity Board why he had threatened LT K and the 1st SGT; only that he "lost control" and wasn't himself. He argued that there should not be an attempted murder charge against him because he was certain that he could have killed them had he wanted to. His explanation as to why he put on LT K's shirt was that he had been "pushed around enough" as a private; and that Army rank and regulations "Don't mean nothing."

Past history: PVT Echo was raised in the rural South as the fourth of five children. His family's standard of living was near the poverty level. His father worked at various semiskilled jobs and was described as "mean" during the week and docile on the weekend when he would be drinking. PVT Echo's parents often fought, and he was closer to his mother than to his father. His description of his psychosocial development was not notably abnormal. He was a popular youth and a valued member of various athletic teams. He did not have a history of violent behavior. He completed high school by receiving special help because of his status as an athlete. Following his graduation he enlisted in the Army to gain some measure of independence from home. He admitted to recreational drug use in the United States after entering the Army and acknowledged he smoked marijuana and heroin "with the brothers" on occasion in Vietnam, but he denied using drugs or alcohol on the day of the incident in question. He had no civilian history of arrests or convictions, and the character of his military service before being sent to Vietnam was excellent. He had received numerous awards while in the Army including several for marksmanship.

Examination: The report of examination indicated that PVT Echo was a large, muscular, black male with a neat, military appearance. He was alert, pleasant, and cooperative. His mood was lowered and consistent with his circumstance. His thinking was completely rational and centered on the sequence of events that landed him in the stockade and caused him to worry about his fate. He expressed dismay that he would be punished when he had not, in fact, hurt anyone. His cognitive capacities appeared intact and his intellect appeared to be in the range "dull normal." This impression was confirmed with formal psychological testing.

Clinical course: Not applicable.

Diagnosis: The board arrived at an impression of acute situational maladjustment, without current impairment for further military duty.

Disposition: Regarding the court-martial allegations, the board judged him to have been capable of distinguishing right from wrong (as evidenced by a statement by one witness who reported PVT Echo saying he was "going to make the [news]papers and go out in a big splash and take some people with him"), but to have diminution in his ability "to adhere to the right secondary to his distress over his mother's letter, his leg injury the day before, and his misunderstanding that he would be held accountable for damages to his vehicle if he was ordered to let someone else drive it" [plus the combination of a socioeconomic background that made it difficult to solve problems by use of intellect and reasoning or to delay impulse gratification, and the limitations imposed by a dull-normal intellect]. The board also recommended clemency.

Source: Medical Board report prepared by the Mental Hygiene Consultation Clinic, 98th Psychiatric Detachment.

The medical board concluded that PVT Echo had an episode of serious, even dangerous, breakdown of mental functions, but their diagnosis—acute situational maladjustment—indicated they believed that this was temporary and uncharacteristic for him. They also did not believe he suffered with a more sustained psychiatric condition or that this incident was caused principally by compromised brain function secondary to substance abuse or mental deficiency. Still, there are two, potentially etiologic, features of the case that warrant amplification:

1. *Mental impairment secondary to drug and alcohol use.* Considering PVT Echo's drug use history, his denial of use on the day of the incident may be questionable (the Sanity Board had no medical information to rule in or out the presence of intoxicating substances during the incident). In a study of men convicted and sentenced for using explosives in attacks on superiors in Vietnam, investigators found that 87.5% acknowledged being intoxicated at the time of the incident.[105]

2. *Mental impairment secondary to low intellect.* Early in the war, the Department of Defense lowered its educational and physical requirements for induction for selected individuals to increase the eligible pool of potential recruits ("Project 100,000," which came to be known as "McNamara's 100,000").[42,106] In one study in Vietnam, soldiers who had entered the Army through this program were represented among mental health referrals at ten times the rate as those who were not.[107] Because the program ultimately mandated that Project participants could not be identified, PVT Echo's military record would not have contained information as to whether he was a Project 100,000 participant or not; however, his low IQ (intelligence quotient) scores, which were ascertained during the Sanity Board proceedings, suggested that he was.

In limiting the scope of their opinion to PVT Echo's individual mental and physical state regarding the charges, the Sanity Board psychiatrists acted true to the Army's charge to them. However, should there also have been some recognition of the social pathology associated with PVT Echo's incident, that is, that he also represented a "deployment stress reaction"? His presentation strongly mirrored the extraordinarily demoralizing influences apparently borne by all young, first-term, enlisted soldiers to some degree late in the war: racial tensions, class tensions, tensions with military authority, a sense of purposelessness, and, especially, a sense of persecution by those in the United States at that time consequent to the repudiation of the war and those serving in Vietnam. Even the factors of drug/alcohol use and limited intelligence—both of which would represent PVT Echo's features as an individual—don't diminish the prospect that he was also expressive of a larger social pathology, or more specifically, of disintegrating morale and military order, that is, a breakdown of commitment and cohesion. Such a perspective would be consistent with the tenants of social/community psychiatry as adapted to military populations. However, despite concerted efforts on the part of several prominent Army psychiatrists,[20,24] the social/community psychiatry perspective among Army psychiatrists in Vietnam at that time was mostly recessive.

VIETNAM VETERANS AND READJUSTMENT PROBLEMS

Estimates as to the prevalence of sustained postwar adjustment and psychiatric problems among Vietnam veterans seem to vary as widely as the political reactions to the war itself.[3,108–113] Furthermore, comparisons of the psychosocial effect of combat service in Vietnam with earlier US wars is especially challenging because measures are inconsistent.[114] Somewhat reassuring, a 1980 Harris Poll of Vietnam veterans commissioned by the then-Veterans' Administration found 91% reporting they were glad they had served their country, 74% said they enjoyed their time in the service, and nearly two-thirds said they would go to Vietnam again, even knowing how the war would end.[1]

Nonetheless, there was rising professional concern for the psychological injury of veterans secondary to service in Vietnam, and in the decade that followed the war, the *International Classification of Disease,* 9th edition, *Clinical Modification* (ICD-9-CM),[115] and the *Diagnostic and Statistical Manual of Mental Disorders,* 3rd edition (DSM-III),[28] both contained the new category "Post-Traumatic Stress Disorder or PTSD," which had been originally called "post-Vietnam syndrome."[14] The inclusion of PTSD in DSM-III reflected the political efforts of the Vietnam veterans who were seeking greater recognition, as well as Americans with residual antiwar sentiment and psychiatrists who believed that DSM-II had neglected the ordeal of combat veterans.[116] However, many took this new diagnosis to mean that the *acute* effects of overwhelming combat stress were indistinguishable from those associated with civilian catastrophes—an arguable equivalency. Others confused PTSD with the reversible, if temporarily disabling, combat stress reactions. For example, the glossary to DSM-III (published separately) commented that combat fatigue is "an obsolete term for posttraumatic stress disorder." Another example can be found in Kentsmith's review of principles of battlefield psychiatry.[117] This misunderstanding can also be found in mainstream psychiatric textbooks published decades later. For example, the 2001 edition of the American Psychiatric Association's *Introductory Textbook of Psychiatry* (3rd edition) included the comment, "[Before the term posttraumatic stress disorder was introduced], the disorder was recognized as shell shock or war neurosis because it was seen most commonly in wartime situations."[118(p236)]

The most commonly referenced findings regarding PTSD prevalence and incidence following the Vietnam War come from the government-sponsored National Vietnam Veterans Readjustment Study (NVVRS). At the time of the study (mid-1980s), approximately 30% of male and 27% of female study participants had evidenced PTSD at some point since serving in Vietnam, and for many PTSD had become persistent and incapacitating (15% and 9% of study participants, respectively).[119] However, some challenge to the validity of the PTSD diagnostic construct has arisen from the observation that among the over 30% of Vietnam veterans complaining of these symptoms, only 15% had been assigned to combat units in Vietnam, and the incidence of reported PTSD is higher among those who served later in the war despite the fact that the combat intensity, as measured by killed-in-action and wounded-in-action rates, was falling.[120] Others, like Nadelson, the former Chief of Psychiatry at the Boston Veterans Administration Hospital, feel that the character of some postwar psychiatric conditions cannot be approached with a checklist of symptoms as does the DSM for posttraumatic stress disorder ("Labeling [a veteran's preoccupation] with visions of exploding bodies, of carnage, and of devastation. . . , 'posttraumatic stress disorder,' virtually trivializes a consuming experience."[121(p103)]

Noticeably, over the years there has been a gradual divergence from the original PTSD model's emphasis that the "trauma" is singularly explanatory, and disputes have arisen as to the relative weight to give various etiologic influences (eg, predisposition and personality, traumatic extent of combat theater circumstance, and, particularly, social dynamics[111,122–128])—differences in perspective that have complicated the diagnosis and treatment of PTSD and related adjustment difficulties. Regarding the latter, a more recent review of the myriad studies of the postwar adjustment of Vietnam veterans by Wessely and Jones, British investigators, concluded that the origins of posttraumatic stress disorder appear to be less often from the purportedly traumatic Vietnam combat experiences, and more from opposition to the war.[129,130] The logical extension is that, at least among some veterans, continuing adjustment difficulties and chronic psychiatric conditions in part serve to (unwittingly) obtain, through the "sick role,"[131] an honorable adaptation to impossibly contradictory public (moral) pressures that surrounded the war (eg, "Foolish for going, wrong for participating, and inadequate for losing"[132]). According to Blank, a psychiatrist who served with the Army in Vietnam and subsequently served for many years as National Director for the Department of Veterans Affairs (DVA) Readjustment Counseling Centers,

[S]ince 1973 I have treated, evaluated, supervised the treatment of, or discussed the cases of approximately 1,400 veterans of Viet Nam with PTSD and have yet to hear a single case where the veteran's symptoms were not accompanied by either: (1) significant doubts or conflicts about the worthiness of the war, or (2) considerable anger about perceived lack of support for the war by the government or the nation. Furthermore, *although researchers have been barred from exploring the relationship between the occurrence of PTSD and the overwhelmingly conflicted nature of the war* [emphasis added], it is the observation of almost all clinicians who have treated substantial numbers of Viet Nam veterans with PTSD that the clinical condition is almost always accompanied by a deeply flawed sense of purpose concerning what happened in Viet Nam.[133]

Following the cessation of hostilities in Southeast Asia, the ethical challenges to military psychiatry voiced during the war[88] shifted to speculations on the harmful long-term consequences of field psychiatric practices in Vietnam (the aforementioned doctrine). The criticism was that these forward treatment methods may have expeditiously served the military priority of force conservation, but in the process they ignored the needs of the soldier and unnecessarily fostered the development of PTSD.[122,134–136] Offsetting opinion came from Blank, who noted that acute combat stress reactions usually do not meet the criteria for PTSD and do not generally evolve into diagnosable PTSD later.[137] It also came from Franklin Del Jones, a senior Army psychiatrist who also served in Vietnam and who argued vigorously that postwar sympathies for maligned Vietnam veterans may have led psychiatrists without military experience to misunderstand the unique aspects of a soldier's state when his psychological defenses become overwhelmed in combat. As a consequence, they failed to appreciate the fluid and reversible nature of the resultant acute stress disorder and the increased risk for psychiatric morbidity (including PTSD) if

treatments do not promote symptom suppression and rapid return to military function and comrades.[138]

SUMMARY AND CONCLUSIONS

This chapter provided an overview of the emergent patterns for psychiatric conditions and behavior problems that challenged Army medical and psychiatric resources over the 8 years that ground troops fought in Vietnam. It also correlated them with the military, social, and political events that increasingly roiled America throughout the period. Salient observations include:

- **Army psychiatrists in Vietnam apparently did not encounter the large numbers of combat exhaustion cases that were predicted, at least not in the forms seen in earlier wars.** The organization of Army psychiatric services in Vietnam was weighted in favor of the combat divisions in anticipation of large numbers of combat exhaustion cases (combat stress reactions). Preparation included the promulgation of the combat psychiatry doctrine that was developed in World War I and World War II and validated in Korea (ie, a vigorous, crisis-oriented, forward treatment aimed at quickly restoring the soldier's duty function). Unfortunately, incidence rates for combat stress reaction cases for Vietnam were never released by the Army. The preliminary official overview of US Army mental health activities in Vietnam (through years 1–5 of 8) did indicate that only 7% of all psychiatric admissions were diagnosed as combat exhaustion, and anecdotal reports from some of the psychiatrists who served during the buildup phase of the war appeared to corroborate a very low CSR rate.

- **The overall low levels for psychiatric conditions and behavioral problems were limited to the buildup years.** In that during the first half of the war psychiatric attrition rates for all types of conditions, including behavior problems, remained uncharacteristically low for a combat theater, the allocation of mental health resources that favored the combat divisions in Vietnam did not present a problem. Unfortunately the situation reversed itself in the second half of the war but without modifications in the selection, preparation, or deployment of mental health personnel.

• Anecdotal and published reports indicate that the newly developed psychotropic medications were commonly prescribed in Vietnam, but their use and effects were not systematically documented or studied. Neuroleptic (antipsychotic), anxiolytic (antianxiety), and tricyclic (antidepressant) medications were available for the first time during the Vietnam War, and anecdotal reports, at least from the first half of the war, indicate they were commonly prescribed by military physicians throughout the theater for a full range of combat and noncombat stress-related symptoms. A limited survey in 1967 confirmed a high prescribing level of these medications and enthusiasm for their salutary effects, but there were no associated clinical or research studies.

• Over time medical/psychiatric capabilities became overwhelmed by the numbers of soldiers with psychiatric conditions and behavior problems— expressions of "(combat theater) deployment stress reaction." Rates for psychiatric hospitalization and evacuations, as well as those for behavior problems, began to increase throughout the theater beginning in 1968 following the enemy Tet offensives and associated political turbulence at home, and they rapidly accelerated once the American troop withdrawals had begun in 1969. By then Americans had become intolerant of the war and impatient for peace. Prolongation of the fighting over the next 3 years aggravated the smoldering societal crisis at home, which was expressed in increasingly radical, sometimes violent, American politics and an expanding drug culture. These attitudes quickly spread among the US forces in Vietnam through the 1-year rotation schedule and rapid troop transport. The growing collection of psychiatric disorders and behavior problems seen by the mental health personnel in Vietnam had little or no apparent connection to combat risk or the falling combat casualty rates, and ultimately they reached unsustainable proportions and likely threatened military preparedness. Because most of the affected soldiers had demonstrated an adequate predeployment military service record, in failing to adapt to the changing circumstance in Vietnam and becoming symptomatic they warranted a generic descriptor such as "(combat theater) deployment

stress reaction" in addition to their primary psychiatric diagnosis.

• Command was equally burdened by the effects of widespread dissent and indiscipline—expressions of "inverted morale." From 1970 through 1972, when the last Army combat units in Vietnam finally redeployed, an unprecedented proportion of troops—especially lower-ranking, enlisted replacement troops—exhibited wholesale demoralization, a reluctance to soldier, antagonism to military authority, and a propensity to disable (or demobilize) themselves through racial conflicts, drug use, and other forms of misconduct. Like Army psychiatry, Army leaders in Vietnam faced an avalanche of dysfunctional soldiers and a degradation of military order and discipline—a situation that thankfully went unchallenged by the enemy—for which the traditional models of military leadership proved marginally effective. From the standpoint of these soldiers collectively, this mostly passive-obstructionistic movement was expressive of antimilitary authority and warranted the descriptor "inverted morale."

• Heroin use eclipsed other medical and psychiatric problems in the late war. The popular and casual use of heroin by soldiers in the last few years of the war represented a new form of soldier dissent as well as disability. Enabled by an extremely accommodating indigenous heroin market, this became an especially disruptive problem for the Army and one for which military psychiatry had no answers. By late 1971 more soldiers were being evacuated from Vietnam for drug use than for war wounds; in the month of July 1972, one out of every eight soldiers in Vietnam was medically evacuated back to the United States for psychiatric reasons, primarily for drug dependency, especially heroin.

• Attacks on military leaders also accelerated in the last years of the war. Associated with the rapid rise in dissent and misconduct in the last few years of the war were vicious assaults on military leaders, especially attacks using explosives ("fragging"). Whereas assassination of unpopular officers and noncommissioned officers had been seen in earlier wars to a limited degree while in combat, the

Vietnam theater is distinct in that not only was the prevalence of such incidents exceptionally high, but the attacks apparently occurred more often in rear areas and among support troops. More broadly, threats of enlisted member attacks were utilized to intimidate and control military leaders, that is, they were expressions of class warfare.

- **Army psychiatry expertise and morale in the theater declined as problems accelerated.** The record of psychiatric effort through the course of the war in Vietnam is unquestionably laudatory. Still, as the problems mounted, the collective expertise among replacement Army psychiatrists declined substantially; the evidence suggests that the mental health component ultimately became overwhelmed, depleted, and demoralized. Furthermore, a large proportion of the psychiatrists who served during the drawdown phase and who responded to the Walter Reed Army Institute of Research survey complained, often bitterly, of inadequate predeployment preparation and poor professional support in the theater.

- **The evidence of large numbers of Vietnam returnees with sustained adjustment difficulties, including psychiatric conditions, provoked postwar questions regarding the adequacy and appropriateness of in-theater military mental healthcare as well as that provided by the government for veterans.**

The chapters that follow will amplify these themes and explore more fully the Army's mental health problems in Vietnam and the professional (and personal) challenges faced by successive cohorts of Army psychiatrists assigned there over 8 years of war.

REFERENCES

1. Sorley L. *A Better War: The Unexamined Victories and Final Tragedy of America's Last Years in Vietnam.* New York, NY: Harcourt Books; 1999.

2. Ingraham L, Manning F. American military psychiatry. In: Gabriel RA, ed. *Military Psychiatry: A Comparative Perspective.* Westport, Conn: Greenwood Press; 1986: 25–65.

3. Gabriel RA. *No More Heroes: Madness & Psychiatry in War.* New York, NY: Hill and Wang; 1987.

4. Office of the Adjutant General. *Coat-of-Arms for Medical Field Service School.* Washington, DC: War Department; 1921: 424.5 Coats of Arms. Memorandum.

5. Spector RH. *After Tet: The Bloodiest Year in Vietnam.* New York, NY: The Free Press; 1993.

6. McGrath JJ. *The Other End of the Spear: The Tooth-to-Tail Ratio (T3R) in Modern Military Operations.* Fort Leavenworth, Kan: Combat Studies Institute Press; 2007.

7. US Department of the Army. *Combat and Operational Stress Control Manual for Leaders and Soldiers.* Washington, DC: Headquarters, Department of the Army; 18 March 2009: Chapter 1. Army Field Manual 6-22.5.

8. Brusher EA. Combat and operational stress control. In: Ritchie EC, ed. *Combat and Operational Behavioral Health.* In: Lenhart MK, ed. *The Textbooks of Military Medicine.* Washington, DC: Department of the Army, Office of The Surgeon General, Borden Institute; 2011: 59–74.

9. Hendin H, Haas AP. *Wounds of War: The Psychological Aftermath of Combat in Vietnam.* New York, NY: Basic Books; 1984.

10. Sonnenberg SM, Blank AS Jr, Talbott JA. The *Trauma of War: Stress and Recovery in Viet Nam Veterans.* Washington, DC: American Psychiatric Press; 1985.

11. Friedman MJ. Post-Vietnam syndrome: recognition and management. *Psychosomatics.* 1981;22(11):931–943.

12. Figley CR, ed. *Stress Disorders Among Vietnam Veterans: Theory, Research, and Treatment.* New York, NY: Brunner/Mazel; 1978.

13. Glass AJ. Introduction. In: Bourne PG, ed. *The Psychology and Physiology of Stress: With Reference to Special Studies of the Viet Nam War.* New York, NY: Academic Press; 1969: xiii–xxx.

14. Baker SL Jr. Traumatic war disorders. In: Kaplan HI, Freedman AM, Sadock BJ, eds. *Comprehensive Textbook of Psychiatry.* 3rd ed. Baltimore, Md: Williams & Wilkins; 1980: 1829–1842.

15. Jones FD. Reactions to stress: combat versus combat support troops. Presentation to World Psychiatric Association, 29 August 1977, Honolulu, Hawaii.

16. Keegan J. *The Face of Battle: A Study of Agincourt, Waterloo and the Somme.* New York, NY: Penguin Books; 1978.

17. Glass AJ. Military psychiatry and changing systems of mental health care. *J Psychiat Res.* 1971;8(3):499–512.

18. Cooke ET. *Another Look at Combat Exhaustion.* Fort Sam Houston, Tex: Department of Neuropsychiatry, Medical Field Service School; distributed July 1967. Training Document GR 51-400-320, 055.

19. Drayer CS, Glass AJ. Introduction. In: Mullens WS, Glass AJ, eds. *Neuropsychiatry in World War II.* vol 2. *Overseas Theaters.* Washington, DC: Medical Department, United States Army; 1973: 1–23.

20. Hausman W, Rioch DMcK. Military psychiatry. A prototype of social and preventive psychiatry in the United States. *Arch Gen Psych.* 1967;16(6):727–739.

21. Jones FD. Psychiatric lessons of war. In: Jones FD, Sparacino LR, Wilcox VL, Rothberg JM, Stokes JW, eds. *War Psychiatry.* In: Zajtchuk R, Bellamy RF, eds. *Textbooks of Military Medicine.* Washington, DC: Department of the Army, Office of The Surgeon General, Borden Institute; 1995: 3–33.

22. Peterson DB. The psychiatric operation, Army Forces, Far East, 1950–1953, with statistical analysis. *Am J Psychiatry.* 1955;112(1):23–28.

23. Bloch HS. Army clinical psychiatry in the combat zone: 1967–1968. *Am J Psychiatry.* 1969;126(3):289–298.

24. Tiffany WJ Jr, Allerton WS. Army psychiatry in the mid-'60s. *Am J Psychiatry.* 1967;123(7):810–821.

25. Jones FD. Traditional warfare combat stress casualties. In: Jones FD, Sparacino LR, Wilcox VL, Rothberg JM, Stokes JW, eds. *War Psychiatry.* In: Zajtchuk R, Bellamy RF, eds. *Textbooks of Military Medicine.* Washington, DC: Department of the Army, Office of The Surgeon General, Borden Institute; 1995: 37–61.

26. US Department of the Army. *Military Psychiatry.* Washington, DC: HQDA; August 1957. Technical Manual 8-244.

27. Neel SH. *Medical Support of the US Army in Vietnam, 1965–1970.* Washington, DC: GPO; 1973.

28. American Psychiatric Association. *Diagnostic and Statistical Manual of Mental Disorders.* 3rd ed (DSM-III). Washington, DC: APA; 1980.

29. Allerton WS. Army psychiatry in Vietnam. In: Bourne PG, ed. *The Psychology and Physiology of Stress: With Reference to Special Studies of the Viet Nam War.* New York, NY: Academic Press; 1969: 1–17.

30. US Department of the Army. *Mental Health and Neuropsychiatry.* March 1966. US Army Republic of Vietnam Regulation 40-34. [This material is available as Appendix 2 to this volume.]

31. Conte LR. A neuropsychiatric team in Vietnam 1966–1967: an overview. In: Parker RS, ed. *The Emotional Stress of War, Violence, and Peace.* Pittsburgh, Penn: Stanwix House; 1972: 163–168.

32. Department of Defense, Office of the Assistant Secretary of Defense (Comptroller). Directorate for Information Operations. US Military Personnel in South Vietnam 1960–1972; 15 March 1974.

33. Johnson AW Jr. In: Johnson AW Jr, Bowman JA, Byrdy HS, Blank AS Jr. Panel discussion: Army psychiatry in Vietnam. In: Jones FD, ed. *Proceedings: Social and Preventive Psychiatry Course, 1967.* Washington, DC: GPO; 1968: 41–76. [Available at: Alexandria, Va: Defense Technical Information Center; 1980. Document No. AD 950058. An abbreviated version of this material is presented as Appendix 7 to this volume.]

34. Organization of Psychiatric Services at Division Level. Fort Sam Houston, Tex: Department of Neuropsychiatry, Medical Field Service School; distributed July 1967. Training Document GR 51-400-960, 015.

35. Jones FD. Experiences of a division psychiatrist in Vietnam. *Mil Med.* 1967:132(12):1003–1008.

36. Baker WL. Division psychiatry in the 9th Infantry Division. *US Army Vietnam Med Bull.* 1967;November/December:5–9.

37. Motis G. Psychiatry at the battle of Dak To. *US Army Vietnam Med Bull.* 1967;November/December:57.

38. Byrdy HSR. Division psychiatry in Vietnam (unpublished), 1967. [An abbreviated version of this descriptive material is available as Appendix 8 to this volume.]

39. Jones FD, Johnson AW Jr. Medical and psychiatric treatment policy and practice in Vietnam. *J Soc Issues.* 1975;31(4):49–65.

40. Bourne PG. A comparative study of American and Vietnamese neuropsychiatric casualties. In: Bourne PG. *Men, Stress, and Vietnam.* Boston, Mass: Little, Brown; 1970: 63–81.

41. Colbach EM, Parrish MD. Army mental health activities in Vietnam: 1965–1970. *Bull Menninger Clin.* 1970;34(6):333–342.

42. Dougan C, Lipsman S, Doyle E, and the editors of Boston Publishing Co. *The Vietnam Experience: A Nation Divided.* Boston, Mass: Boston Publishing Co; 1984.

43. Fulghum D, Maitland T, and the editors of Boston Publishing Co. *The Vietnam Experience: South Vietnam on Trial, Mid-1970 to 1972.* Boston, Mass: Boston Publishing Co.; 1984.

44. Howard S. The Vietnam warrior: his experience, and implications for psychotherapy. *Am J Psychother.* 1976;30(1):121–135.

45. Bey DR. Group dynamics and the "F.N.G." in Vietnam: a potential focus of stress. *Int J Group Psychother.* 1972;22(1):22–30.

46. Bloch HS. The psychological adjustment of normal people during a year's tour in Vietnam. *Psychiatric Q.* 1970;44(4):613–626.

47. Tischler GL. Patterns of psychiatric attrition and of behavior in a combat zone. In: Bourne PG, ed. *The Psychology and Physiology of Stress: With Reference to Special Studies of the Viet Nam War.* New York, NY: Academic Press; 1969: 19–44.

48. Dowling JJ. Psychological aspects of the year in Vietnam. *US Army Vietnam Medical Bull.* 1967;May/June:45–48.

49. Bey D. *Wizard 6: A Combat Psychiatrist in Vietnam.* College Station, Tex: Texas A & M University Military History Series, 104; 2006.

50. Cincinnatus. *Self-Destruction: The Disintegration and Decay of the United States Army During the Vietnam Era.* New York, NY: Norton; 1981.

51. Moskos CC Jr. *The American Enlisted Man: The Rank and File in Today's Military.* New York, NY: Russell Sage Foundation; 1970.

52. Bourne PG. *Men, Stress, and Vietnam.* Boston, Mass: Little, Brown; 1970.

53. Marlowe DH. The human dimension of battle and combat breakdown. In: Gabriel RA, ed. *Military Psychiatry: A Comparative Perspective.* Westport, Conn: Greenwood Press; 1986: 7–24.

54. Allerton WS. In: Allerton WS, Forrest DV, Anderson J, et al. Psychiatric casualties in Vietnam. In: Sherman LJ, Caffey EM Jr. *The Vietnam Veteran in Contemporary Society: Collected Materials Pertaining to the Young Veterans.* Washington, DC: Veterans Administration; 1972: III: 54–59.

55. Johnson AW Jr. Psychiatric treatment in the combat situation. *US Army Vietnam Med Bull.* 1967;January/February:38–45.

56. Hays FW. Military aeromedical evacuation and psychiatric patients during the Viet Nam War. *Am J Psychiatry.* 1969;126:658–666.

57. Johnson AW Jr. Combat psychiatry, I: A historical review. *Med Bull US Army Europe.* 1969;26(10):305–308.

58. Prugh GS. *Law at War: Vietnam 1964–1973.* Washington, DC: GPO; 1975.

59. Bourne PG. Military psychiatry and the Viet Nam experience. *Am J Psychiatry.* 1970;127(4):481–488.

60. Hays FW. Psychiatric aeromedical evacuation patients during the Tet and Tet II offensives, 1968. *Am J Psychiatry.* 1970;127(4):503–508.

61. Fidaleo RA. Marijuana: social and clinical observations. *US Army Vietnam Med Bull.* 1968;March/April:58–59.

62. Talbott JA. Pot reactions. *US Army Vietnam Med Bull.* 1968;January/February:40–41.

63. Roffman RA, Sapol E. Marijuana in Vietnam: a survey of use among Army enlisted men in two southern corps. *Int J Addict.* 1970;5(1):1–42.

64. Stanton MD. Drug use in Vietnam. A survey among Army personnel in the two northern corps. *Arch Gen Psychiatry*. 1972;26(3):279–286.

65. Balkind JJ. *Morale Deterioration in the United States Military During the Vietnam Period* [dissertation]. Ann Arbor, Mich: University Microfilms International; 1978: 235. [Available at: *Dissertations Abstracts International*, 39 (1-A), 438. Order No. 78-11, 333.]

66. Byrdy HSR. In: Johnson AW Jr, Bowman JA, Byrdy HSR, Blank AS Jr. Panel discussion: Army psychiatry in Vietnam. In: Jones FD, ed. *Proceedings: Social and Preventive Psychiatry Course, 1967*. Washington, DC: GPO; 1968: 41–76. [Available at: Alexandria, Va: Defense Technical Information Center. Document No. ADA 950058.]

67. Datel WE, Johnson AW Jr. *Psychotropic Prescription Medication in Vietnam*. Alexandria, Va: Defense Technical Information Center; 1981. Document No. AD A097610. [Or search http://www.dtic.mil/cgi-bin/GetTRD oc?AD=ADA097610&Location=U2&doc=Get TRDoc.pdf.]

68. Blank AS. In: Johnson AW Jr, Bowman JA, Byrdy HSR, Blank AS Jr. Panel discussion: Army psychiatry in Vietnam. In: Jones FD, ed. *Proceedings: Social and Preventive Psychiatry Course, 1967*. Washington, DC: GPO; 1968: 41–76. [Available at: Alexandria, Va: Defense Technical Information Center. Document No. ADA 950058.]

69. Steinbach A. Psychiatry plus conscience. *Baltimore Sun*. 8 December 1985.

70. Talbott JA. In: Allerton WS, Forrest DV, Anderson J, et al. Psychiatric casualties in Vietnam. In: Sherman LJ, Caffey EM Jr. *The Vietnam Veteran in Contemporary Society: Collected Materials Pertaining to the Young Veterans*. Washington, DC: Veterans Administration; 1972: III: 54–59.

71. O'Brien T. *Going After Cacciato*. New York, NY: Delacorte; 1978.

72. Karnow S. *Vietnam: A History*. New York, NY: Viking; 1983.

73. Dougan C, Weiss S, and the editors of Boston Publishing Co. *The Vietnam Experience: Nineteen Sixty-Eight*. Boston, Mass: Boston Publishing Co; 1983.

74. Kirk D. *Tell It to the Dead: Memories of a War*. Chicago, Ill: Nelson-Hall; 1975.

75. Sterba JP. Cover your ass. In: Falk RA, Kolko G, Lifton RJ, eds. *Crimes of War*. New York, NY: Random House; 1971: 445–458.

76. Talbott JA. The Saigon warriors during Tet. *US Army Vietnam Med Bull*. 1968;March/April:60–61.

77. Edmendson SW, Platner DJ. Psychiatric referrals from Khe Sanh during siege. *US Army Vietnam Med Bull*. 1968;July/August:25–30.

78. Parrish MD. The megahospital during the Tet offensive. *US Army Vietnam Med Bull*. 1968;May/June:81–82.

79. Yager J. Personal violence in infantry combat. *Arch Gen Psychiatry*. 1975;32(2):257–261.

80. Schell J. *The Military Half: An Account of Destruction in Quang Ngai and Quang Tin*. New York, NY: Alfred A. Knopf; 1968.

81. Norden E. American atrocities in Vietnam. In: Falk RA, Kolko G, Lifton RJ, eds. *Crimes of War*. New York, NY: Random House; 1971: 265–284.

82. Vietnam Veterans Against the War. *The Winter Soldier Investigation: An Inquiry Into American War Crimes*. Boston, Mass: Beacon Press; 1972.

83. Renner JA Jr. The changing patterns of psychiatric problems in Vietnam. *Compr Psychiatry*. 1973;14(2):169–181.

84. Imahara JK. In: Allerton WS, Forrest DV, Anderson J, et al. Psychiatric casualties in Vietnam. In: Sherman LJ, Caffey EM Jr. *The Vietnam Veteran in Contemporary Society: Collected Materials Pertaining to the Young Veterans*. Washington, DC: Veterans Administration; 1972: III: 54–59.

85. Bey DR, Smith WE. Mental health technicians in Vietnam. *Bull Menninger Clin*. 1970;34(6):363–371.

86. Bey DR. Division psychiatry in Viet Nam. *Am J Psychiatry*. 1970;127(2):228–232.

87. Stanton SL. *The Rise and Fall of an American Army: US Ground Forces in Vietnam, 1965–1973*. Novato, Calif: Presidio Press; 1985.

88. Camp NM. The Vietnam War and the ethics of combat psychiatry. *Am J Psychiatry*. 1993;150(7):1000–1010.

89. Lipsman S, Doyle E, and the editors of Boston Publishing Co. *The Vietnam Experience: Fighting For Time.* Boston, Mass: Boston Publishing Co; 1983.

90. Gabriel RA, Savage PL. *Crisis in Command: Mismanagement in the Army.* New York, NY: Hill and Wang; 1978.

91. Linden E. The demoralization of an army: fragging and other withdrawal symptoms. *Saturday Review,* 8 January 1972:12–17, 55.

92. Cosmas GA, Murray TP. *US Marines in Vietnam: Vietnamization and Redeployment, 1970–1971.* Washington, DC: GPO; 1986: 343–369. Available at: http://ehistory.osu.edu/vietnam/books/vietnamization/index.cfm. Accessed 13 June 2012.

93. Corson WR. The military establishment. In: *Consequences of Failure.* New York, NY: Norton; 1974: 74–105.

94. Datel WE. *A Summary of Source Data in Military Psychiatric Epidemiology.* Alexandria, Va: Defense Technical Information Center; 1976. Document No. AD A021265.

95. Jones FD. Disorders of frustration and loneliness. In: Jones FD, Sparacino LR, Wilcox VL, Rothberg JM, Stokes JW, eds. *War Psychiatry.* In: Zajtchuk R, Bellamy RF, eds. *Textbooks of Military Medicine.* Washington, DC: Department of the Army, Office of The Surgeon General, Borden Institute; 1995: 63–83.

96. Stanton MD. Drugs, Vietnam, and the Vietnam veteran: an overview. *Am J Drug Alcohol Abuse.* 1976;3(4):557–570.

97. US Army Adjutant General, Casualty Services Division (DAAG-PEC). *Active Duty Army Personnel Battle Casualties and Nonbattle Deaths Vietnam, 1961–1979,* Office of the Adjutant General counts. 3 February 1981.

98. Bond TC. The why of fragging. *Am J Psychiatry.* 1976;133(11):1328–1331.

99. Gabriel RA, Savage PL. Cohesion and disintegration in the American Army: an alternative perspective. *Armed Forces Soc.* 1976;2(3):340–376.

100. Adams DP, Barton C, Mitchell GL, Moore AL, Einagel V. Hearts and minds: suicide among United States combat troops in Vietnam, 1957–1973. *Soc Sci Med.* 1998;47(11):1687–1694.

101. Camp NM, Carney CM. US Army psychiatry in Vietnam: preliminary findings of a survey, I: Background and method. *Bull Menninger Clin.* 1987;51(1):6–18.

102. Ratner RA. Drugs and despair in Vietnam. *U Chicago Magazine.* 1972;64:15–23.

103. Fisher HW. Vietnam psychiatry. Portrait of anarchy. *Minn Med.* 1972;55(12):1165–1167.

104. Camp NM, Carney CM. US Army psychiatry in Vietnam: preliminary findings of a survey, II: Results and discussion. *Bull Menninger Clin.* 1987;51(1):19–37.

105. Gillooly DH, Bond TC. Assaults with explosive devices on superiors: a synopsis of reports from confined offenders at the US Disciplinary Barracks. *Mil Med.* 1976;141(10):700–702.

106. Starr P. *The Discarded Army: Veterans After Vietnam.* New York, NY: Charter House; 1973.

107. Crowe RR, Colbach EM. A psychiatric experience with Project 100,000. *Mil Med.* 1971;136(3):271–273.

108. Pols H, Oak S. War & military mental health: the US response in the 20th century. *Am J Public Health.* 2007;97(12):2132–2142.

109. Stretch RH. Posttraumatic stress disorder among US Army Reserve Vietnam and Vietnam-era veterans. *J Consult Clin Psychol.* 1985;53(6):935–936.

110. Centers for Disease Control Vietnam Experience Study. Health status of Vietnam veterans, I: Psychosocial characteristics. *JAMA.* 1988;259(18):2701–2707.

111. Marlowe DH. *Psychological and Psychosocial Consequences of Combat and Deployment, With Special Emphasis on the Gulf War.* Santa Monica, Calif: National Defense Research Institute/RAND; 2001.

112. Dean ET Jr. *Shook Over Hell: Post-Traumatic Stress, Vietnam, and the Civil War.* Cambridge, Mass: Harvard University Press; 1997.

113. Kaylor JA, King DW, King LA. Psychological effects of military service in Vietnam: a meta-analysis. *Psychol Bull.* 1987;102(2):257–271.

114. Magruder KM, Yeager DE. The prevalence of PTSD across war eras and the effect of deployment on PTSD: a systematic review and meta-analysis. *Psych Annals.* 2009;39:778–788.

115. Centers for Disease Control. International Classification of Disease-9th ed-Clinical Modification. Available at: http://www.cdc.gov/nchs/icd/icd9.htm. Accessed 13 June 2012.

116. Shephard B. *A War of Nerves*. Cambridge, Mass: Harvard University Press; 2000.

117. Kentsmith DK. Principles of battlefield psychiatry. *Mil Med*. 1986;151:89–96.

118. Andreasen NC, Black DW. *Introductory Textbook of Psychiatry*. 3rd ed. Washington DC: APA; 2001.

119. Kulka RA, Schlenger WE, Fairbank JA, et al. *Trauma and the Vietnam War Generation: Report of Findings From the National Vietnam Veterans Readjustment Study*. New York, NY: Brunner/Mazel; 1990.

120. McNally RJ. Can we solve the mysteries of the National Vietnam Veterans Readjustment Study? *J Anxiety Disord*. 2007;21:192–200.

121. Nadelson T. *Trained to Kill: Soldiers at War*. Baltimore, Md: The Johns Hopkins University Press; 2005.

122. Boman B. The Vietnam veteran ten years on. *Aust N Z J Psychiatry*. 1982;16(3):107–127.

123. Holloway HC, Ursano RJ. Viet Nam veterans on active duty: adjustment in a supportive atmosphere. In: Sonnenberg SM, Blank AS Jr, Talbott JA, eds. *The Trauma of War: Stress and Recovery in Viet Nam Veterans*. Washington, DC: American Psychiatric Press; 1980: 321–338.

124. Fleming RH. Post Vietnam syndrome: neurosis or sociosis? *Psychiatry*. 1985;48(2):122–139.

125. Frueh BC, Grubaugh AL, Elhai JD, Buckley TC. US Department of Veterans Affairs disability policies for posttraumatic stress disorder: administrative trends and implications for treatment, rehabilitation, and research. *Am J Public Health*. 2007;97(12):2143–2145.

126. McFarlane AC. The duration of deployment and sensitization to stress. *Psych Annals*. 2009;39:81–88.

127. Wilson D, Barglow P. Posttraumatic stress disorder. *Psych Times*. 2009 (July):30.

128. Kutchins H, Kirk SA. *Making Us Crazy: DSM: The Psychiatric Bible and the Creation of Mental Disorders*. New York, NY: Free Press; 1997.

129. Jones E, Wessely S. *Shell Shock to PTSD: Military Psychiatry From 1900 to the Gulf War*. New York, NY: Psychology Press; 2005.

130. Wessely S, Jones E. Psychiatry and the "lessons of Vietnam": what were they, and are they still relevant? *War Soc*. 2004;22:89–103.

131. Parsons T. *The Social System*. New York, NY: Free Press; 1951.

132. Jay JA. After Vietnam: in pursuit of scapegoats: the veteran as pariah. *Harper's Magazine*. 1978, July:14–15, 18–23.

133. Blank AS, Jr. Personal communication. 4 May 2008.

134. Abse DW. Brief historical overview of the concept of war neurosis and of associated treatment methods. In: Schwartz HJ, ed. *Psychotherapy of the Combat Veteran*. New York, NY: Spectrum Publications; 1984: 1–22.

135. Perlman MS. Basic problems of military psychiatry: delayed reaction in Vietnam veterans. *Int J Offender Ther Comp Criminol*. 1975;19:129–138.

136. Scurfield RM. Post-traumatic stress disorder in Vietnam veterans. In: Wilson JP, Raphael B, eds. *International Handbook of Traumatic Stress Syndromes*. New York, NY: Plenum Press; 1993: 285–296.

137. Blank AS Jr. The longitudinal course of posttraumatic stress disorder. In: Davidson JRT, Foa EB, eds. *Posttraumatic Stress Disorder: DSM–IV and Beyond*. Washington, DC: APA; 1993: 3–22.

138. Jones FD. Chronic post-traumatic stress disorders. In: Jones FD, Sparacino LR, Wilcox VL, Rothberg JM, Stokes JW, eds. *War Psychiatry*. In: Zajtchuk R, Bellamy RF, eds. *Textbooks of Military Medicine*. Washington, DC: Department of the Army, Office of The Surgeon General, Borden Institute; 1995: 409–430.

CHAPTER 3

Organization of Army Psychiatry, I: Psychiatric Services in the Combat Divisions

The peak incidence of our combat exhaustion cases occurred during [the battle of the Ia Drang Valley]. . . . [K]nowing what was going on [from the commanding general's briefing] was vital so that one could realistically perceive the difficulties that the troopers were confronting and give the individual trooper some feeling that his story was falling on knowledgeable ears. Perhaps this was just to alleviate my own anxiety, but I think this is a real thing, that as the troopers pass back [through the evacuation chain] nobody sits down and listens; and one of the major needs of distressed people of this sort is for someone to sit and listen. Often this was one of the prime functions of the corpsmen in dealing with the combat exhaustion patient.[1(p48)]

Captain Harold SR Byrdy, Medical Corps, US Army
Division psychiatrist with the 1st Cavalry Division (Airmobile)
August 1965 to June 1966

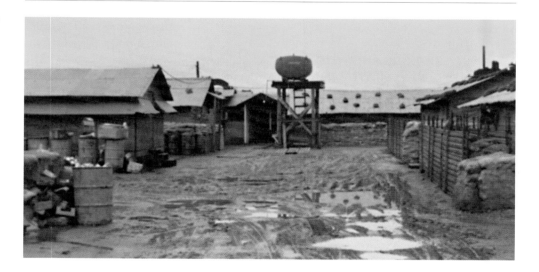

The 326th Medical Battalion, 101st Airborne Division, Phu Bai, 1971. The building beyond the orange water tank housed the division's mental hygiene clinic, medical dispensary, and small inpatient unit for medical and psychiatric conditions. On the right are the officers' quarters, while on the left is a "club" where personnel could get beer and soft drinks. Photo courtesy of Phillip W. Cushman.

US Army psychiatrists were deployed in Vietnam to provide specialized clinical services and leadership for allied medical and mental health personnel to aid in the conservation of the force in support of the military mission and to provide humanitarian care for the sick and wounded. The first Army psychiatrist in South Vietnam was Major Estes Copen. He was assigned to the 8th Field Hospital in Nha Trang for 5 months in 1962 to provide specialized care for the approximately 8,000 assigned US personnel.[2,3] In the decade that followed, an estimated 135 to 140 psychiatrists served with the US Army in South Vietnam, typically for 1-year assignments. The last Army psychiatrist in Vietnam, Major Dennis Grant, left Vietnam in March 1973.

One hundred forty psychiatrists is considerably fewer than the more than 2,400 who served with the Army in World War II, and, more generally, the scope of America's war effort in World War II dwarfs that of the Vietnam War. Still, the war in Vietnam brought new, and in many regards unanswered, challenges for Army psychiatry as it undertook to support the US military's efforts to defeat an enemy that employed a guerrilla/counterinsurgency strategy and capitalized on roiling social and political events at home.

This chapter begins a more detailed account of US Army psychiatry in the war with a description of the organization of Army psychiatric services in Vietnam. It also draws upon published and otherwise available written accounts by the division psychiatrists and allied mental health personnel to construct a composite picture of the psychiatric care that was provided within the combat units. Reports from the psychiatrists and allied mental health professionals assigned to the hospitals and psychiatric specialty detachments will be presented in Chapter 4, as will information regarding the professional activities of the nine psychiatrists who served as the senior Army psychiatrist in the theater (the Neuropsychiatry Consultant to the Commanding General, US Army Republic of Vietnam [CG/USARV] Surgeon).

THE ORGANIZATION OF ARMY PSYCHIATRY IN VIETNAM

Medical Command Authority and the US Army Republic of Vietnam Surgeon

Throughout the ground war years—1965 to 1973—the US Army Republic of Vietnam (USARV) Surgeon was responsible for command and control of Army-level medical resources in Vietnam (Figure 3-1): Army hospitals and all other medical units that were not components (ie, "organic") of combat divisions or independent brigades. The USARV Surgeon was also responsible for advising the USARV commander on matters pertaining to the health of the command; providing technical supervision for all medical activities in the theater, including those that were organic to combat units; and assuring the availability of adequate medical support, that is, personnel, supply, and maintenance.[4]

The Mission, Structure, and Deployment of Army Psychiatry in Vietnam

The Army Regulation (AR) governing the provision of psychiatric care when America entered the Vietnam War, AR 40-216, *Medical Service: Neuropsychiatry* (dated 18 June 1959), directed neuropsychiatry to "aid command to conserve the manpower of the Army and maintain it at the highest possible peak of efficiency through the application of sound psychiatric principles."[5(§I,¶2,p1)] This mission statement directed Army psychiatrists and allied mental health personnel to prioritize military and combat objectives, an emphasis that coincided with the overall mission of the Army Medical Department. The regulation stipulated that the responsibilities of psychiatrists should include "professional services in the prevention, diagnosis, and treatment of emotional and personality disorders, mental illness, and neurological diseases and in the evaluation and disposition of such involved military personnel."[5(§I,¶3,pp1–2)] Further specifications directed Army psychiatrists to provide state-of-the-art, specialized psychiatric care for soldier-patients; clinical/psychiatric authority and leadership for other deployed military health professionals and paraprofessionals (enlisted specialists); and consultation to commanders regarding factors affecting the morale and mental health of their troops.[5]

In March 1966, Headquarters (HQ)/USARV published Regulation No. 40-34, *Medical Services: Mental Health and Neuropsychiatry*,[6,7] which provided more specifics pertaining to the Vietnam theater (USARV Regulation 40-34 is reproduced in Appendix 2). This regulation tasked both commanders and the deployed medical/mental health elements for "the maintenance of high standards of mental health and for the management of psychiatric and neurologic problems in this command."[6(§I,¶1,p1)] The regulation was clear that: (*a*) prevention is as critical as treatment; (*b*) outpatient management is emphasized over inpatient; (*c*) hospitalization is to be avoided when possible, especially in the case of soldiers who primarily need "custodial care" (ie, supervision while awaiting administrative or judicial processing); and (*d*) Army psychiatrists should serve as consultants to unit commanders.

From the outset of hostilities in Vietnam, US Army planners committed ample mental health assets to avoid a problematic shortage situation similar to that which had arisen in the startup phases of previous campaigns.[8(pp819–821)] In fact, during the first year of the buildup period, the ratio of deployed Army psychiatrists to troops was higher than in any previous engagement.[9] The mental health component in Vietnam consisted of psychiatrists, allied mental health professionals (social workers, psychologists, psychiatric nurses),

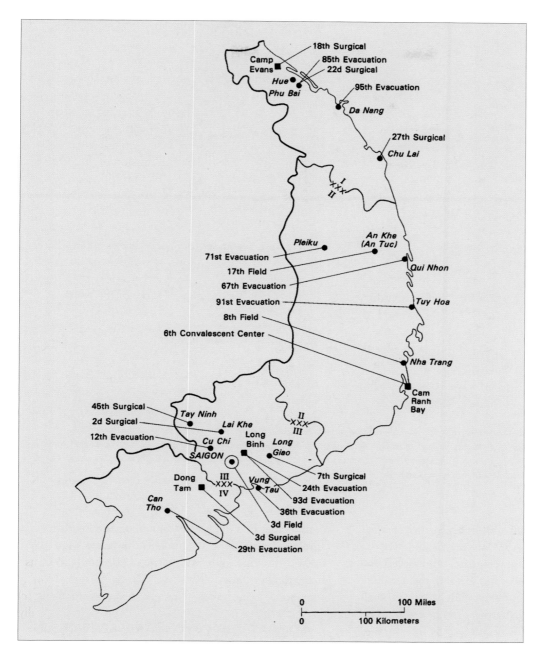

FIGURE 3-1. A map of South Vietnam dated 31 December 1968 shows the locations of US Army hospitals. Source: Ognibene AJ. Full-scale operations. In: Ognibene AJ, Barrett O'N Jr, eds. *General Medicine and Infectious Diseases.* Vol 2. In: Medical Department, United States Army. *Internal Medicine in Vietnam.* Washington, DC: Department of the Army, Office of The Surgeon General, and Center of Military History; 1982: 51.

and paraprofessionals (enlisted specialists, which included many who had college or even graduate-level degrees) who were provided behavioral science training by the Army.[10] They were referred to variously as "neuropsychiatric specialists," "social work/psychology specialists," and "psychology technicians," but most often they were simply referred to as "psych techs." As will be described, the complement of mental health assets was deployed in the theater congruent with the Army's three-echelon doctrine for the system of medical care mentioned in Chapter 2.

Army psychiatrists assigned in Vietnam served either close to the combat troops and the fighting when assigned as division psychiatrists, or in rear echelons when assigned to an evacuation or field hospital or to one of the two neuropsychiatry specialty detachments, so-called KO teams, the 98th and the 935th.[3,7,11,12] (The initial "K" indicated that these were medical specialty detachments, which were typically attached to selected evacuation hospitals; the choice of the second letter was arbitrary.) In addition, in each year of the war a psychiatrist served as staff officer for the Army

TABLE 3-1. US Army Psychiatry Assignment Types in Vietnam

Organization Level	Psychiatrist Position
Division level medical resources	1) As division psychiatrist
Army level medical resources in Vietnam	2) As solo psychiatrist with an evacuation or field hospital
	3) As staff with a psychiatric specialty detachment (935th or 98th)
Headquarters, United States Army, Republic of Vietnam (USARV)	4) As Neuropsychiatry Consultant to the CG/USARV Surgeon

CG/USARV: Commanding General, US Army, Republic of Vietnam

TABLE 3-2. Full US Army Divisions Deployed in Vietnam

Initially Deployed (main body)[1]	Combat Division	Withdrawal (main body)[2]	Approximate number of years in Vietnam*
September 1965	1st Cavalry Division (Airmobile)	April 1971	5.5
October 1965	1st Infantry Division	April 1970	4.5
March 1966	25th Infantry Division	December 1970	4.75
October 1966	4th Infantry Division	December 1970	4.25
December 1966	9th Infantry Division	August 1969	2.75
September 1967	23d Infantry Division (American) *Formed in Vietnam*	November 1971	4.25
November 1967	101st Airborne Division (Airmobile)	January 1972	4.25
	TOTAL "DIVISION YEARS"		30.25

* Represents the time span between when the main body of the division arrived and when it withdrew, rounded to nearest quarter year.
Data sources: (1) Maitland T, McInerney P, and the editors of Boston Publishing Co. *The Vietnam Experience: A Contagion of War*. Boston, Mass: Boston Publishing Co; 1983: 10–11. (2) Fulghum D, Maitland T, and the editors of Boston Publishing Co. *The Vietnam Experience: South Vietnam on Trial: Mid-1970 to 1972*. Boston, Mass: Boston Publishing Co; 1984: 23.

commanding general and his staff as "Neuropsychiatry Consultant" to the CG/USARV Surgeon (Table 3-1).

The numbers of Army psychiatrists who served in clinical psychiatry positions in the Vietnam theater (ie, the division psychiatrists combined with hospital and psychiatric detachment psychiatrists) can be estimated to be six in 1965, 15 in 1966, 22 in each of the years 1967 to 1969, 20 in 1970, 14 in 1971, and two in 1972 and 1973. These numbers are extrapolations from Tiffany and Allerton,[9(p813)] Allerton,[3(p9)] and information collected in 1982 from participants in the Walter Reed Army Institute of Research (WRAIR) Vietnam psychiatrists survey mentioned in the Preface and the Prologue. It should be noted that there were more established positions than there were psychiatrists to fill them. The USARV Psychiatric Consultant was responsible for deciding which positions got filled depending on anticipated need and psychiatrist availability. In some years, psychiatrists were also assigned as division, brigade, or battalion surgeon, commander of a medical battalion, or as a flight surgeon, and in these assignments they often were called upon to provide some psychiatric care in addition to their primary duties.

COMBAT UNIT PSYCHIATRIC SERVICES IN VIETNAM: THE DIVISION MEDICAL BATTALION AND THE DIVISION PSYCHIATRIST

Organization of Psychiatric Care in the Combat Units

At the conclusion of the buildup of ground troops in Vietnam there were seven full Army divisions and two Marine divisions operating in the theater. Table 3-2 lists Army divisions arranged in the order of arrival of the main body of each division. Also provided are their withdrawal dates and the approximate number of years they were in Vietnam.

EXHIBIT 3-1. Ratio of Combat Troops to Noncombat/Support Troops in Vietnam

There has been controversy regarding the so-called tooth-to-tail ratio during the war in Vietnam, with accusations that it was unreasonably lopsided in the direction of noncombat troops. For example, military psychiatry historian Franklin Del Jones indicated that each combat soldier in Vietnam was supported by about eight noncombat troops.[1] This was refuted in a more recent review by military historian JJ McGrath. He calculated a far lower ratio in Vietnam (one combat to two noncombat), one that was very similar to that in the Korean War.[2] According to McGrath, whereas since the World War I era the US Army's functional tooth-to-tail ratio has risen in favor of noncombat elements, this primarily occurred during the period between the two world wars because of improvements in mass motorization and mechanization. Since the onset of World War II, combat elements have averaged 32.5%. They have ranged between 40% and 25%, with recent trends hovering toward the lower end.

In Vietnam the typical Army combat division was a "light" infantry division consisting of about 17,000 soldiers. In the light configuration, much of the heavy equipment was deleted in favor of additional infantry companies and battalions. Based on the Table of Organization and Equipment for these divisions, the combat components comprised roughly 58% of troops, logistics were 11%, and headquarters/administration were 31%.[2(Figure 21)] Among the latter were the so-called life support functions or MWR (morale, welfare, and recreation) and base camp support.

McGrath also notes that if April 1968 is used as a measuring point, when Army troop strength was at its peak, although the seven deployed combat divisions represented only 22% of the deployed force, the numbers of soldiers comprising the other, nondivisional combat troops raised the level of combat troops to 35%.[2(Figure 22)] In other words, by these calculations, the ratio of combat troops to noncombat troops was 1:2. (See also Chapter 1 for estimates by Spector.)

1.   Jones FD. Psychiatric lessons of war. In: Jones FD, Sparacino LR, Wilcox VL, Rothberg JM, Stokes JW, eds. *War Psychiatry*. In: Zajtchuk R, Bellamy RF, eds. *Textbooks of Military Medicine*. Washington, DC: Department of the Army, Office of The Surgeon General, Borden Institute; 1995: 1–33.
2.   McGrath JJ. *The Other End of the Spear: The Tooth-to-Tail Ratio (T3R) in Modern Military Operations*. Fort Leavenworth, Kan: Combat Studies Institute Press; 2007.

For the full combat divisions, 1st and 2nd echelon medical support came from medical assets within their organizational structure, that is, division level resources. A typical combat division in Vietnam was composed of 15,000 to 18,000 soldiers (and by one estimate roughly 60% of those served in combat assignments while the remainder filled noncombat positions[13]). (See Exhibit 3-1.)

The division's schedule of organization called for a medical battalion of four companies, each with three platoons. The three-echelon medical care system implemented at the outset of the war meant that 1st echelon care would consist of treatments provided by unit medics and battalion aid station medical personnel under the direction of the battalion surgeon, and more extensive 2nd echelon medical care, which provided fixed beds, would be administered by medical personnel at the brigade or division headquarters/division clearing station (Figure 3-2). Soldiers who failed to respond within 3 to 5 days would ordinarily be sent to Army-level hospitals beyond the division (but within Vietnam) for more prolonged, that is, 3rd echelon care. Requirements for additional care beyond the 3rd

echelon meant evacuation out of the Vietnam theater.

Beginning in World War I, combat-generated psychiatric problems proved capable of reaching a magnitude that could significantly undermine the integrity and capability of the force and affect the outcome of the battle. As a consequence, in World War I and again in the later stages of World War II and in Korea, the US Army came to recognize the importance of military/combat psychiatry and assigned a psychiatrist to each combat division to provide specialized care for troops and guidance regarding troop morale and mental health.[14] During the war in Vietnam, each combat division had included in its organizational structure (its Table of Organization and Equipment— the TO&E) a position for a division psychiatrist who was assigned to the division's Headquarters and Headquarters Company.

The division psychiatrist was assisted by the division social work officer and six to 10 enlisted social work/psychology technicians (the "psych techs").[3] Whereas 1st echelon, nonspecialized, mental healthcare was to be provided by battalion surgeons and field medics, the division psychiatrist and his staff were

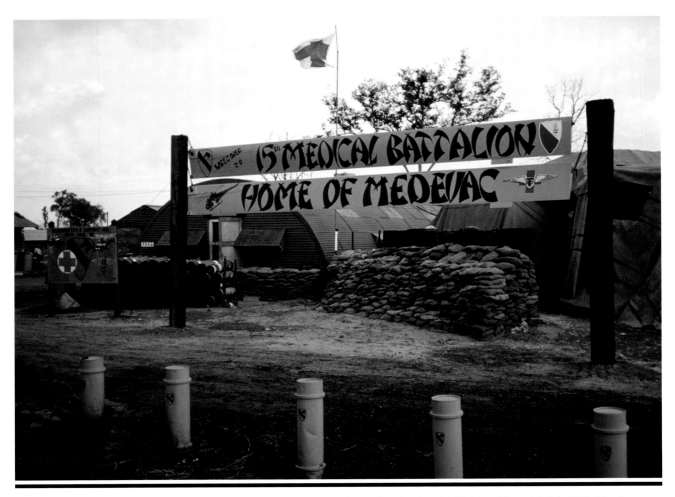

FIGURE 3-2. Headquarters and Headquarters Company, 15th Medical Battalion, 1st Cavalry Division, Phouc Vinh in 1970. The Army medical care doctrine at the outset in Vietnam called for a three tier, or echelon, system of treatment. Within the divisions, 1st echelon care was to consist of treatment provided by a unit's medics and battalion aid station medical personnel under the direction of the battalion surgeon; more extensive, 2nd echelon medical care, including that requiring fixed beds, was to be administered by medical personnel at the brigade or division headquarters/division clearing station level, such as at the 15th Medical Battalion. Only soldiers who failed to recover within roughly 3 to 5 days were to be evacuated out of the division to Army-level hospitals within Vietnam for more prolonged, that is, 3rd echelon care. However, because of the widening use of helicopters in Vietnam for medical evacuation, the lower echelons of medical care were often bypassed (so-called overflying). Photograph courtesy of Richard D Cameron, Major General, US Army (Retired).

expected to operate a small treatment facility and provide more extensive and specialized 2nd echelon mental healthcare. This took place in conjunction with the clearing company medical facility (clearing station), which was located with the division's medical battalion at a brigade, or the division's, base camp (Figure 3-3). Also, because a key objective in providing psychiatric care for a combat division is to place mental health assets as far forward as possible, it was common for one or two enlisted social work/psychology technicians to be attached to the division's forward operating brigades

to provide timely, specialized support of the battalion surgeons and other 1st echelon medical personnel.[7]

By policy, authority to evacuate psychiatric patients out of the division to the Army-level hospitals in Vietnam (ie, 3rd echelon care facilities) was restricted to the division psychiatrists who were to distinguish which casualties required additional specialized care. Finally, being assigned with a line unit (ie, in a nonmedical unit versus in a hospital or psychiatric specialty detachment) meant that division psychiatrists had a broader scope of duties than those assigned to the hospitals or psychiatric

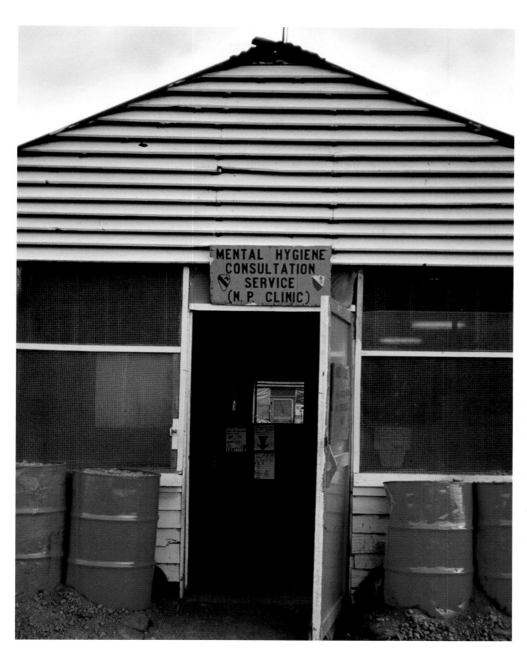

FIGURE 3-3. The central psychiatric treatment facility of the 1st Cavalry Division base camp at Phuoc Vinh in 1970. During the war each of the seven full combat divisions in Vietnam included a position for a division psychiatrist who was assigned to the division's Headquarters and Headquarters Company. He was assisted by the division social work officer and six to 10 enlisted social work/psychology technicians. They operated a small treatment facility such as this one where they offered more extensive, specialized mental health-care for troops than was available in the field. Some of the enlisted technicians were also attached to forward units to provide acute treatment of psychiatric casualties and consultation to unit cadre and other medical personnel. Photograph courtesy of Richard D Cameron, Major General, US Army (Retired).

detachments. In addition to their clinical responsibilities, they also were expected to be readily accessible to provide professional consultation to unit commanders and the division surgeon.[15] (See Chapter 7 for more specifics regarding the management and treatment capabilities for combat divisions.)

In Vietnam, because of the great distances that typically separated elements of the divisions, these duty requirements were often quite challenging because of transportation and communication impediments. This was partially remedied by having the enlisted psychiatric technicians attached to forward operating brigades as noted. Still, the scattered nature of the brigades often complicated the division psychiatrist's supervision of these techs as well as consultations with the various battalion surgeons and unit commanders. Furthermore, the fluid nature of the tactical situation and new heliborne medical ambulance capability often led to deviations from the triple echelon care and evacuation plan, and this invariably affected the system of treatment of psychiatric casualties as well.[9]

In fact, because of the common practice of helicopters evacuating casualties directly to division clearing stations,[16] as well as to surgical, field, and evacuation hospitals (so-called overflying), after he left the theater in 1969, Major General Spurgeon Neel, former Military Assistance Command, Vietnam (MACV) Surgeon, recommended that the battalion surgeon positions no longer be filled.[4] (The 1st Infantry Division's Regulation 40-13, *Medical Service: Division Mental Hygiene Program*, dated 25 October 1967, which explained the policies, procedures, and functions of the division's Mental Hygiene Program, can be found in Gordon.[17])

Four independent brigades were also deployed in Vietnam: (1) 11th Armored Cavalry Regiment; (2) 1st Brigade, 5th Infantry Division (Mechanized); (3) 199th Infantry Brigade (Light); and (4) 173rd Airborne Brigade. Each was about one-third the size of a division and was composed of approximately 30 company-size units (about 5,000 soldiers). They did not typically have a dedicated psychiatrist position. In some situations these brigades were attached to a combat division and utilized the division psychiatrist's staff; otherwise they arranged for specialized mental healthcare to be provided by the nearest evacuation or field hospital or one of the two psychiatric detachments.

Even the full divisions in Vietnam may not have had a psychiatrist assigned for periods of time because of personnel shortages. In these instances, specialized psychiatric care and consultation also had to be obtained from a hospital-based psychiatrist, but there were predictable disadvantages to such an arrangement.

Accounts by Division Psychiatrists and Allied Mental Health Personnel

Establishing a reasonably accurate history of the medical care and support provided combat units during a war should be a priority. However, as has been stated, this did not happen in the aftermath of Vietnam regarding the psychiatric components of the combat units and the care they provided. Whereas psychiatrists were directed by HQ/USARV Regulation 40-34, *Mental Health and Neuropsychiatry*,[6] to be responsible for "keeping accurate records of all outpatients and inpatients, and for coordinating with registrars so that accurate morbidity figures are obtained and forwarded [to higher command]"[6] (see Appendix IV in Appendix 2, Army Regulation 40-34), evidently there was no sustained effort at a central level to analyze and retain this data from the combat (division) psychiatrists

distinct from medical data from other sources. As a consequence, overall epidemiologic documentation for the combat units is missing.

Notably, Major General Neel's official summary of Army medical care in Vietnam through the first two-thirds of the war did not specifically mention combat stress reaction casualties. He also did not break out the yearly psychiatric rates among the major diagnostic subgroupings for combat units (refer back to Chapter 2, Table 2-2, Army Incidence Rate for Psychiatric Hospitalizations in Vietnam and [in Europe] in Cases/1,000 Troops/Year).[4] Colbach and Parrish's overview of the first two-thirds of the war did indicate that combat stress reaction cases accounted for 7% of psychiatric hospitalizations,[12] but the fuller review of psychiatric care in Vietnam by Jones and Johnson did not include measures for combat stress reaction cases. Whereas they differentiated the psychosis rate from other causes for hospitalization, and generally distinguished inpatient rates and outpatient rates, there are no breakouts for the combat units.[7]

In search of an alternative means for understanding the fuller story, the available accounts of individual division psychiatrists and their mental health colleagues are reviewed below. These are arranged in a rough chronological order to provide some impression of the changing nature of the war and associated psychiatric challenges. (All quotation marks identify the terms used by the reporting individual.) Selected aspects will be presented in more detail in subsequent chapters. Additionally, a few psychiatrists assigned with the divisions reported on circumscribed problems, and these will be noted in subsequent chapters as well. Finally, as will be made evident, attempting to reconstruct the history of psychiatry in the combat divisions by this means is incomplete because the majority of the deployed mental health professionals did not produce records, or, if they did, most served in the first half of the war.

25th Infantry Division

Background. At the opening of the Vietnam War, the 25th Infantry Division was the only trained counterguerrilla unit in the US Army. The division's 3rd Brigade deployed to the central highlands at Pleiku, 28 December 1965. The rest of the division completed its deployment by March 1966. The soldiers of the 25th Infantry Division fought in some of the toughest battles of the war. During the Tet offensives in 1968 and 1969, they were instrumental in defending the besieged city of Saigon. In 1970 the division became heavily involved

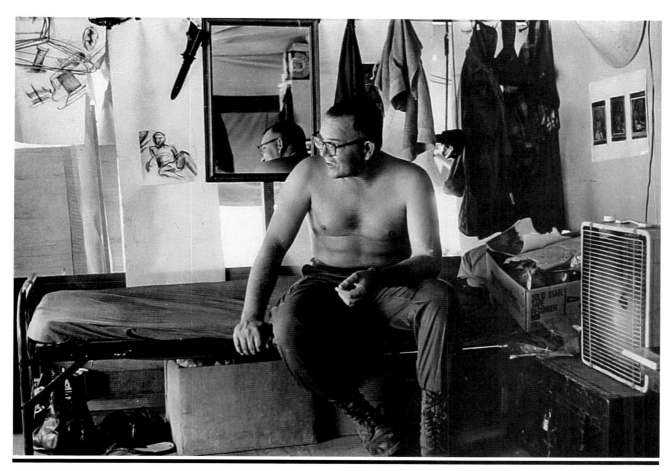

FIGURE 3-4. Major Franklin Del Jones, Medical Corps, Division Psychiatrist with 25th Infantry Division. Jones, an Army-trained psychiatrist, accompanied the division when it deployed to Vietnam in February 1966. In September he was transferred to the 3rd Field Hospital in Saigon where he completed his yearlong assignment in Vietnam. Jones is credited with publishing the first overview of the psychiatric problems arising in a combat division in Vietnam. Also, the postwar summary of the Army's psychiatric problems in the Vietnam War he published (with Johnson) provided the only theater-wide statistics released by the Army that spanned all 8 years of the war. Photograph courtesy of June Jones.

in the "Vietnamization" program and participated in Allied thrusts deep into enemy sanctuaries in Cambodia. By the end of that year, elements of the 25th Infantry Division began redeployment back to the United States. Overall, between battle deaths and deaths from other causes, the division lost 4,540 men in Vietnam.[18]

Major Franklin Del Jones, Medical Corps. An Army-trained psychiatrist, Jones (Figure 3-4) was the first division psychiatrist to serve with the 25th Infantry Division in Vietnam (March 1966–September 1966) and the only one to publish an account. Jones traveled with the division when it deployed to Vietnam in early 1966.[19] According to his published account, the division set up its base camp near Cu Chi, about 20 miles northwest of Saigon and 10 miles from the Cambodian

border, among abandoned peanut fields, rice paddies, and graveyards. This initially required heavy contact with the Viet Cong guerrillas. Dense vegetation, orchards, and rubber plantations were within the enemy's rifle range, but sniping and mortaring on the base camp ceased after the establishment of an effective perimeter of concertina wire, mines, and bunkers.

The heat and the dust in the dry months, and the heat, humidity, and mud in the rainy months, were debilitating. Establishment of reliable generators allowed for an array of electrical conveniences and diversions (fans, refrigerators, televisions and radios, and movies—but not air conditioning). Jones recalled that there was remarkable logistical support in that "almost no material deprivation was suffered by the men,"[19(p1004)] and he felt this contributed to the maintenance of high morale within the division. On the other hand, he complained about his dependency on the goodwill of medical battalion for staff and equipment. Whereas he was authorized a .45 caliber pistol, a compass, and psychological testing equipment, what he really needed were "a jeep, a typewriter, a . . . tent to house [my mental health clinic], a desk, and a locking file cabinet."[19(p1008)]

According to Jones, "Casualties of all kinds were relatively few, and psychiatric casualties were quite infrequent."[19(p1005)] He ultimately averaged 75 referrals per month; of those, approximately four per month (5.3%) required hospitalization. Most of the referrals were from support units and presented problems similar to those seen among garrisoned troops, for example, regarding disciplinary action or for alcohol-related incidents. Approximately two-thirds of referrals were diagnosed as character and behavior disorders (ie, personality disorders[20]). The other third were for psychiatric "clearance" in conjunction with legal or administrative difficulties and generally received a diagnosis of "no disease found." The few individuals who became psychotic were quickly evacuated out of the division.

Alcohol abuse incidents became a special problem category. Jones reported that beer was easier to obtain than soft drinks, and that incidents of soldiers going "berserk" became enough of a problem that command developed a coordinated response plan to disarm drunken soldiers who were brandishing weapons and threatening others. He also noted that there was no available treatment for chronic alcoholism, and that these individuals typically received administrative processing out of the Army.

The other major group of soldiers that required attention from Jones and his staff were variations of "combat avoidance" (including "helmet headaches" in soldiers seeking to avoid patrol duty, or sleepwalking in those who did not want to be quartered near the perimeter). Jones indicated that he never saw a case of combat fatigue, but he did see a few combat-generated "fright reactions [which were] occasioned by imminent danger or witnessing the death of a friend."[19(p1005)] He diagnosed these as situational reactions but nonetheless lumped them with the character and behavior disorders. In particular, there were no related psychiatric cases in the aftermath of a mortar attack on the base in July that left two dead and 100 wounded.

Jones speculated that the lack of psychiatric sequelae was the consequence of the command/psychiatric policy of opposing "environmental change." This refers to a policy against reassigning away from danger soldiers who had some potential for becoming anxious after such an attack.

Jones mentioned the emergence of "short timer's" syndrome ("mild anxiety and some phobic feelings") seen among combat soldiers approaching their date of expected return from overseas (DEROS). He noted that commanders who routinely reduced combat exposure of such troops as a prophylactic measure found these symptoms arose even sooner among the other troops (Jones opposed commanders allowing the soldier's 11th month to be his last in the field).

Finally, Jones reflected on the overall low psychiatric attrition rate he and other psychiatrists encountered at that early stage of the war. Although he credited the same features noted by other psychiatric observers detailed in Chapter 2, he also favored "the fact that we began to win the war in an observable fashion in 1966."[19(p1007)]

1st Cavalry Division (Airmobile)

Background. The 1st Cavalry Division was the first full combat division to be deployed in Vietnam. In August 1965, its initial elements arrived in An Khe, which was located between Qui Nhon on the coast and Pleiku in the central highlands. The division was fully deployed by September 1965. Among its more prominent combat operations were participation in the Battle of Ia Drang Valley in 1965; the battle to recapture Quang Tri and Hue; relief of the Marine units besieged at Khe Sanh; clearing operations in the A Shau Valley in 1968; and participation in the Cambodian incursion in 1970. The bulk of the division was withdrawn in April 1971, but its 3rd Brigade was one of the final two major US ground combat units in Vietnam, departing in June 1972. Overall, between battle deaths and deaths from other causes, the 1st Cavalry Division lost 5,439 men in Vietnam.[18]

Captain Harold SR Byrdy, Medical Corps. Byrdy had been draft-deferred under the Army's "Berry Plan" (permitting the completion of civilian medical specialty training) and was commissioned as an Army Medical Corps officer shortly before being deployed to Vietnam as the 1st Cavalry Division's first division psychiatrist in Vietnam. (In the previous segment, Jones was identified as an Army-trained psychiatrist; Byrdy is

TABLE 3-3. Diagnostic Distribution of Referrals to the
1st Cavalry Division Mental Health Service, August 1965–
June 1966 (N = 503)

Diagnosis	% of cases
Psychotic reactions	2.4%
Psychoneurosis	13.9%
Personality disorders	40.4%
Psychophysiologic reactions	4.8%
Combat exhaustion	4.4%
Acute (alcoholic) brain syndrome	4.4%
Adult situational reaction	3.6%
Miscellaneous	26.2%
	100%

Data source: extracted from Byrdy HRS. Division Psychiatry in Vietnam.
[Appendix 8 to this volume]. Table 2.

identified as a civilian-trained psychiatrist. The salience
of this pre-Vietnam training distinction is considered in
this chapter and the next. It is described more fully in
Chapter 5, and it is utilized throughout the remaining
chapters as a key background variable that may explain
differences in the deployed psychiatrists' appraisal of the
challenges they faced in Vietnam and their professional
decisions.) Byrdy arrived in the summer of 1965 with
the division's advance party immediately after attending
the 5-week Medical Field Service School training at
Fort Sam Houston, Texas. During his 10 months with
the 1st Cavalry (also referred to as the 1st Cav), Byrdy
was assisted by the division social work officer, but
they were short five of their allotted eight enlisted social
work/psychology technicians.

Descriptive aspects of Byrdy's experience in the 1st
Cavalry are found in his unpublished manuscript[21] (see
Appendix 8, "Division Psychiatry in Vietnam") and his
participation in a 1967 panel discussion.[1] According
to Byrdy, despite the trying conditions associated with
conducting military operations while establishing the
division in Vietnam, the troops maintained high morale
by drawing upon the 1st Cav's airmobile status as a
new, albeit experimental, means of conducting warfare.
However, transportation and communication obstacles
faced by Byrdy and his team were substantial.

The division psychiatrist must try to compromise
between his potential skills and his ability to be
realistically effective. Telephone calls . . . would often
take up to 45 minutes for a completion through the
switches. I could borrow a vehicle at times from the
surgeon or from the medical battalion. At other times
I hitch-hiked. It is at this grass-roots level that the

best preventive measures are probably carried out for
units in the division area. For units in the field outside
of the base camp, travel, when indicated, was a major
operation of scheduling. The net result was that we
responded to crises rather than "heading them off at
the pass."[1(p50)]

Byrdy also referred to interpersonal impediments in
providing primary prevention/command consultation to
the various units of the 1st Cavalry.

I did not feel in the least that it was professionally
desirable that we sell ourselves to the division. By
that I mean that, though I did go and talk with unit
commanders, I felt it an awful thing to sort of ferret
out problems as though we were drumming up
business. I thought this was a rather uncomfortable
role for me. . . . Indeed, there were elements in
the division that strongly felt that, because of the
nature of the combat (we were in the Airmobile
Division and moved around quite rapidly), there
would be no psychiatric casualties . . . I was assured
at the very beginning by some people that really I
was just unnecessary baggage because I would have
no work.[1(p47)]

During the division's initial 9½ months in Vietnam,
he and his staff had 503 referrals, or 53 per month.
These were seen in 1,065 outpatient visits, which
averaged two visits per patient and three patient visits
per day. Table 3-3 presents the distribution of referrals
by diagnostic groupings.

According to Byrdy, the combat troops bore the
greatest stress, and most of the referrals were from
the enlisted ranks, E-2 through E-6. The majority of
soldiers who were diagnosed as personality disorders
were passive-aggressive. Byrdy hospitalized 116
referrals (23%), averaging one admission every 3
days (maximum bed capacity was six, and maximum
stay was about 3 days). Of these, 30 (26%) were
evacuated out of the division for additional treatment
(representing 6% of referrals and an estimated evacuation rate for the 1st Cavalry Division of 2.2/1,000
troops/year). This number included all 12 soldiers
diagnosed as psychotic. Byrdy indicated that he often
prescribed Thorazine and Librium; but, apart from the
latter, he opposed the use of psychoactive medications
for outpatient maintenance because of their potential
for impairing reactions in combat.

Thirty-two soldiers (6.4% of referrals) received an initial diagnosis of combat exhaustion, that is, soldiers presenting disorganizing anxiety related to an active combat situation.[1] Most of these arose in conjunction with the division's two sustained combat operations: the Battle at the Ia Drang Valley near Pleiku (October 1965–November 1965) and the Bong Son campaign (February 1966–March 1966). However, 10 of the 32 failed to respond to brief, simple treatments—the Army's combat psychiatry forward treatment doctrine, which was augmented with "tranquilization"—and consequently received various amended diagnoses (including two as "alcohol agitations"[sic]). The incidence rate for the remaining 22, which by implication Byrdy considered to be the true combat exhaustion cases, was 1.6 per 1,000 troops per year (vs his rate for all psychiatric referrals, 22/1,000 troops/year).[21]

Finally, Byrdy provided this account of an attempt to forestall the development of the short-timer's syndrome by one unit,

> [An] outgoing commander had instituted a program in which the "short-timers" in the unit would have a terminal, non-combatant status. I don't remember what the time duration was—perhaps 15, perhaps 30, days prior to rotation. The result was chaos in the unit with bitterness and breakdown in morale among the whole unit so that he had to rescind this time concession. I also feel that it was significant that the commander was getting to be a "short-timer."[1(p52)]

Captain John A Bostrom, Medical Corps. Some appreciation for psychiatric activities in the 1st Cavalry Division later in the buildup phase can be derived from two publications by Bostrom, the division psychiatrist (February 1967–February 1968). He also was trained in psychiatry in a civilian program and joined the 1st Cavalry Division in February 1967, some 9 months following Byrdy's departure. Bostrom's publications were limited in scope compared to those by Byrdy and Jones. In his first, he proposed a taxonomy of the combat stress-generated cases derived from his experiences with cases who were referred to the mental hygiene clinic over a 3-month span:

> **Type I–Normal Combat Syndrome** (two cases): included soldiers who were frightened or experiencing "realistic anxiety," but not to the extent that combat effectiveness was impaired.

Bostrom noted that most cases of this type were not referred to the mental hygiene clinic because they were effectively treated in the battalion aid stations.

> **Type II–Pre-Combat Syndrome** (11 cases): included soldiers who were experiencing significant anxiety, psychosomatic complaints, and sleeplessness, and which degraded combat performance.

> **Type III–Combat Exhaustion** (four cases): included soldiers who were experiencing a state of psychosis or near-psychosis, and resulting in a complete loss of combat effectiveness.[22(pp6–8)]

With regard to treatment of combat exhaustion cases, Bostrom, like Byrdy, utilized a blend of rest, physical replenishment, and empathy combined with emphatic expectation of return to combat duty. Some also received psychotropic medication. In the more severe cases he prescribed sufficient Thorazine to induce arousable sleep for about 24 hours—so-called *dauerschlaf*.[22] This refers to a sleep therapy regimen that was also used by Bloch at the 935th Psychiatric Detachment, and later by Major Douglas R Bey with the 1st Infantry Division. (*Dauerschlaf* will be described in Chapter 4 and Chapter 7.) Bostrom's other publication provided case examples of two hypothetical referrals—one a soldier with psychosomatic back pain and the other a "troublemaker"—to demonstrate the unit consultation approach utilized by his enlisted social work/psychology technicians with good effect.[23]

Additional information regarding the psychiatric challenges in the 1st Cavalry Division was provided by two Army psychiatrists: (1) Jerome J Dowling (June 1966–March 1967) described commonly seen soldier stress and adjustment patterns through the course of the 1-year tour early in the war (see Chapter 8) and (2) Frank Ramos (October 1970–May 1971) described the division's heroin detoxification/rehabilitation program late in the war (see Chapter 9).

9th Infantry Division

Background. The 9th Infantry Division was reactivated on 1 February 1966 and arrived in Vietnam in December 1966. Upon deployment the division was assigned to the III Corps Tactical Zone of Vietnam where it commenced operations in the Dinh Tuong and Long An provinces in Operation Palm Beach. Division headquarters, which initially housed the division's 3rd

Brigade, was at Camp Bearcat some 20 miles northeast of Saigon. The permanent base, Camp Dong Tam, was established in the Viet Cong-infested Mekong Delta near My Tho in January 1967.

In March the 2nd Brigade moved into Camp Dong Tam, and the 3rd Brigade relocated northward to Tan An. To improve division mobility in the inundated Mekong Delta, in June two battalions from the 2nd Brigade joined a US Navy Task Force afloat to establish the Mobile Riverine Force (with South Vietnamese Marines and units of the ARVN [Army of the Republic of Vietnam] 7th Division). In February 1968, the division's armor reconnaissance squadron relocated to the far north to Wunder Beach in I Corps Tactical Zone, 15 miles south of the demilitarized zone. This reassignment distinguished the 9th Infantry Division as the most widespread division in Vietnam. The 1st and 2nd Brigades, along with division headquarters, departed Vietnam in July and August 1969, leaving the 3rd Brigade at Tan An to operate as an autonomous combat unit. The 3rd Brigade withdrew a year later, September 1970. Overall, between battle deaths and deaths from other causes, the 9th Infantry Division lost 2,625 men in Vietnam.[18]

Captain William L Baker, Medical Corps. Baker was trained in psychiatry in a civilian program and was assigned as the division psychiatrist to the 9th Infantry Division between January 1967 and September 1967. He joined the division 1 month after the division arrived in Vietnam and in the midst of some of the heaviest fighting in the war. He published information regarding his tour with the 9th Infantry Division in the *US Army Vietnam Medical Bulletin*.[24] Baker's initial cases were not primarily combat-generated but were a heterogenic group of other psychological disorders such as situational, reactive, or chronic characterological problems.

After the fifth month and as combat activities became more regular, a few cases of combat stress reaction began to appear, which he labeled classic combat fatigue. Baker reported that most of these were managed at the 1st echelon care level by the battalion surgeons using rest and sedation (no details as to medications prescribed). Over time, the incidence of combat soldiers undergoing more severe regression ("brief periods of psychotic symptoms") went from rare to four to 12 per month. These received 2nd echelon care by Baker and his staff at the division base camp. Ultimately more challenging were "modified combat stress reactions," which became more frequent as the

division passed its 10th month in Vietnam. These were soldiers with good performance records, including in combat, who variously developed disabling anxiety, functional gastrointestinal disturbances, recurrent traumatic dreams, or "short-timer's syndrome."

Baker's impression was that the rapid rise in all these reactions represented a time-stress continuum in response to combat exposure. However, soldier stress was apparently compounded by the loss of unit bonding from: (*a*) combat losses, and (*b*) a command decision to transfer large numbers of soldiers to different units to reduce the impact of impending rotations back to the United States. Most of the combat stress reaction cases Baker saw responded to supportive psychotherapy, 2 to 3 days of rest, recreation, and pharmacologic support (Combid Spansules, Compazine, Probanthine, and Donnatal for the gastrointestinal symptoms; and nighttime Seconal for sedation). Baker also thought the treatment results were better when these soldiers were not hospitalized but were instead kept at the base camp and followed by his staff as outpatients. Still, some had persisting symptoms and required reassignment to noncombat duties (so they would not be a "liability in the field"). "True psychosis" (ie, schizophrenia or manic-depression) accounted for about 1% of Baker's caseload, and with these he saw no correlation with external stressors.[24]

Lieutenant Colonel Robert L Pettera, Medical Corps. Two publications by Pettera, a military-trained psychiatrist who succeeded Baker, provided some further appreciation for psychiatric challenges that faced the 9th Infantry Division as the war intensified. In one, Pettera (with Basil M Johnson and Richard Zimmer, his colleagues) distinguished three varieties of combat stress-generated casualties seen:

1. A "nebulous, ill-defined transient anxiety reaction with little or no specific etiology"—which responded easily to supportive therapy;
2. Acute incapacitating "combat fatigue"—of which there were few, apparently because of the lack of sustained (ie, fatiguing) combat activities; and
3. "Vietnam combat reaction"—a disabling psychophysiological condition with anorexia, nausea, and vomiting; severe anxiety with tremulousness; insomnia and traumatic nightmares; and survivor guilt with incomplete grieving (this condition was commonly found among seasoned combat soldiers who were approaching the end of their tour).[25(pp673–674)]

Captain Edward L Gordon, Medical Corps.
Although not constituting an overview, some perspective on the psychiatric activities in the 1st Infantry Division during the buildup phase in Vietnam came from Gordon, the division psychiatrist (June 1967–June 1968), who published in the *US Army Vietnam Medical Bulletin* several of his interim reports to Colonel Matthew D Parrish, the senior theater Army psychiatrist (Neuropsychiatry Consultant to the CG/USARV) at the time. Among Gordon's reports was the 1st Infantry Division's Regulation No. 40-13, which detailed the division's mental hygiene program. Gordon also indicated that among the more than 1,000 soldier-patients seen in 1967 (Camp: estimated to be over a 6–7 month span) by him, his social work officer, or the enlisted social work/psychology techs, 6.8% required evacuation out of the division for additional care, and, of those, about one-third were further evacuated out of Vietnam (none of whom were combat exhaustion cases).[17]

Additional information from the same time frame comes from an article by Specialist 6th Class Dennis L Menard, one of Gordon's enlisted social work/psychology technicians. Menard observed that unusually high psychiatric referral rates usually came from units in the combat arms battalions. Believing that many of these referrals likely also represented dysfunctional units, the mental health service began a field consultation program in July 1967. Two social work/psychology technicians were assigned to the medical companies located at each of three brigade base camps—Di An, Lai Khe, and Quan Loi—and functioned under the technical supervision of the division psychiatrist. Through increased contacts with the unit cadres of problem units, early detection and effective intervention was improved at both the level of the individual soldier and with the unit's leaders.[30] (Menard also provided information on troop living conditions in the field [Chapter 1, Exhibit 1-2] and consultation to a combat battalion by a social work specialist [Chapter 10, Exhibit 10-1].)

Major Douglas R Bey, Medical Corps. A much fuller description of the psychiatric experiences during the transition phase of the war comes from civilian-trained Bey, the division psychiatrist for the 1st Infantry Division (April 1969–April 1970) who arrived in Vietnam a year after Gordon's departure. Bey (Figure 3-5), whose promilitary training and pre-Vietnam service background was mentioned in Chapter 2, was uniquely prepared to serve as a division psychiatrist. He

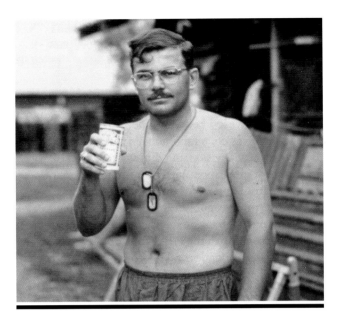

FIGURE 3-5. Major Douglas R. Bey, Medical Corps, Division Psychiatrist with the 1st Infantry Division. Bey, a civilian-trained psychiatrist, served with the 1st Infantry Division between April 1969 and April 1970. His many publications are noteworthy in themselves, but they are also unique because he was the only division psychiatrist assigned in Vietnam after 1968 to describe his professional experiences in detail. Photograph courtesy of Douglas R Bey.

provided a rich legacy regarding his tour in the form of a series of publications, an unpublished professional treatise, and a personal account published 35 years after he left Vietnam.[31] His observations and impressions were especially valuable because he was the only psychiatrist deployed in Vietnam after 1968 to write about his experiences.

In his principle publication, he described the "tertiary preventive" care (ie, direct care) provided by him, his social work officer, and eight enlisted social work/psychology technicians. This involved the diagnosis and treatment of 180 to 200 new patients (plus 200 follow-up visits) per month who were either referred by battalion surgeons, chaplains, units, and the judge advocate's office, or were walk-ins. ("We are geared toward rapid evaluation and treatment near the soldier's unit—[a treatment] aimed at restoring him to duty as soon as possible."[15(p229)]) By routine, an enlisted technician took a detailed history of each new case before the soldier was interviewed by Bey or the social work officer. The soldier's unit was also contacted to provide further historical and observational data[15] (initial interviews of officers and senior sergeants were conducted by Bey or the social work officer[32]).

Bey also described various practical frustrations borne by all division psychiatrists in Vietnam.

> [The division psychiatrist] is not officially provided with the wherewithal to carry out this mission. [W]hile consultation and prevention are urged, [he] is not provided . . . a jeep or other consistent means of land transportation. He is not provided with a typist, yet is expected to prepare reports. His staff [that is, social work officer and enlisted social work/psychology technicians] are under the command of the medical battalion who decide if and when they will be available for work with the psychiatrist.[32(pIII-17)]

According to Bey, he found his first medical battalion commander to be a significant obstacle: "So you're the new [division psychiatrist]. I'm not sure I believe in psychiatry." Bey and his team had to resort to "midnight requisitions" (unofficial appropriation of materials) and procurement of personnel through means such as bartering in order to acquire a jeep, build their offices, and arrange to have a clerk typist assigned. As it turned out, subsequent medical battalion commanders were much more supportive of the mental health team's mission as were the company commander and the executive officer of Headquarters and A Company ("[who] helped us to avoid pitfalls and bottlenecks and enabled us to devote ourselves to our work"[32]). Overall, Bey indicated that he and his staff maintained high morale despite their manifold challenges "because we could see that we were providing a useful service to our comrades and because we made the effort to do out best under difficult circumstances."[32(pIV-1)]

The following was Bey's description of the widely dispersed 1st Infantry Division's medical battalion and requirements of the mental health component:

> Headquarters and A Company were located at support command headquarters in Di An which was the location of our psychiatric headquarters. The patients requiring hospitalization in the Division were treated at the A Company clearing station for the most part. The psychiatrist, social work officer, a clerk typist and three or four social work psychology technicians were stationed at this base camp. B Company was originally in Di An,

TABLE 3-4. Estimated Diagnostic Distribution Among Referrals to the 1st Infantry Division Mental Health Service, April 1969–April 1970 (N = Average 180/mo)

Diagnosis	% of cases
Psychotic reactions (including drug induced)	5%
Psychoneurosis	10%
Character-behavior reactions	40%
Acute situational reaction (including combat exhaustion cases and "short-timer's syndrome")	20%
No psychiatric diagnosis	25%
	100%

Data source: Bey DR. Division psychiatry in Viet Nam. *Am J Psychiatry*. 1970;127(2):228–232.

but later moved to Dau Tieng with two social work psychology techs assigned to it. D and C Companies were located in Lai Khe and had two technicians assigned to each company. In addition, we provided supervision and back-up for a corpsman in Phu Lai who was interested in the mental health field, so that in fact we had mental health services available in that base camp as well.[32(ppV-2–3)]

> . . . . The Division's psychiatrist and/or social work officer traveled regularly by jeep or helicopter to Lai Khe to supervise the technicians, to see patients directly and to consult with units. Dau Tieng was visited infrequently because of difficulties arranging helicopter transportation there. Land transportation was not possible because the roads were unsafe. Thus the technicians at [B] Company at Dau Tieng functioned with less direct supervision but did an excellent job. Communication by radio and landline was available but often difficult to most base camps. . . . [F]or example, after spending an hour getting the Di An operator to connect with Lai Khe and Lai Khe to connect with Dau Tieng and Dau Tieng to connect with the battalion radio frequency and the battalion to switch to get the company, one would hear a distant voice of the company commander who would then be cut off and the whole process would need to be repeated.[32(pV-7)]

Table 3-4 presents Bey's case distribution during his year. As indicated, combat exhaustion cases were subsumed in the category of acute situational reaction, and there was no indication as to numbers of these cases who required treatment for combat stress reaction at either the 1st echelon of care (ie, at the battalion aid station, perhaps including treatment by a social work/psychology technician) or at the 2nd echelon of care (ie, the division clearing station). According to Bey, "[W]e did have a number of cases that were situational reactions precipitated by combat stress most of which were treated by their unit corpsman, the battalion surgeons, or our nearest social work/psychology technician."[32(pIX-2)] Thus despite the exacerbating "frustrations of the hot, hostile environment," the evidence suggests a low combat stress reaction incidence for the 1st Infantry Division for this later year in the war, and this is consistent with the more defensive military posture adopted by American forces.[33] However, Bey's case examples did include a "combat exhaustion" case as well as a case of a soldier who developed dissociation and mutism in the aftermath of his first fire fight.

Otherwise, the types of problems Bey described among his relatively high rate of referrals (approximately 127/1,000/year) appeared to be more consistent with troops in a demobilizing mode as opposed to those with a high combat intensity/stress quotient. Bey estimated that 25% of soldiers in Vietnam during his year used marijuana, primarily those in lower ranks. These included troops in the field who wished to reduce their fear and anxiety. However, although Bey did not provide statistics, incidents of misuse of alcohol (especially those contributing to acts of violence), acute alcohol-induced organic brain syndromes with paranoia and hallucinosis, as well as the more insidious problem of alcoholism ("the alcoholic sergeant") were far more problematic for the division. Bey reported they had few referrals for suicidal behavior, and only one of those, a sergeant with a serious alcohol addiction, subsequently killed himself. Cases of barbiturate intoxication and addiction were occasionally treated, but evidence of narcotic use was rare. Bey underscored the need to distinguish functional psychotic disorders from organic/metabolic or toxic-delirious brain syndromes. As examples he recalled a patient with a combination of drug or alcohol intoxication and a skull fracture with subdural hematoma; a patient with severe hypoglycemia secondary to a pancreatic tumor; and patients with cerebral malaria or heat stroke.

Bey hospitalized 10% of referrals for up to 2 to 3 days at the division clearing station. Treatment strategies included the use of Thorazine for both nonpsychotic

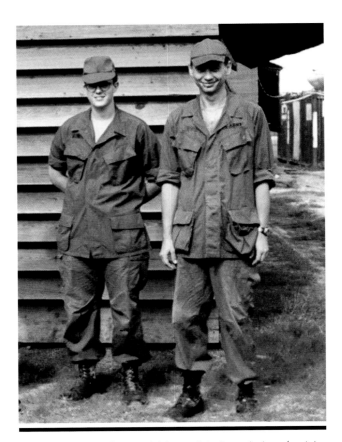

FIGURE 3-6. 1st Infantry Division enlisted psychology/social work technicians Vincent Zecchinelli (left) and Louis Stralka. Zecchinelli and Stralka served in the 1st Infantry Division in 1969–1970 with the Division Psychiatrist, Major Doug Bey, and the Division Social Work Officer, Captain Ray Troop. Overall, enlisted "psych techs" proved invaluable in Vietnam as they provided roughly 80% of the treatment of psychiatric patients. Photograph courtesy of Douglas R Bey.

combat exhaustion and as sleep therapy (*dauerschlaf*) for more disorganized psychiatric states. Regarding final dispositions, 85% of all referrals were returned to duty, 14% were psychiatrically "cleared" for administrative separation from the Army (meaning no psychiatric diagnosis), and less than 1.0% were evacuated out of the division to one of the psychiatric specialty detachments for further treatment or evacuation out of Vietnam.

In other publications, Bey provided examples of command consultation regarding specific unit stresses affecting 1st Infantry Division troops, especially change of command[34] and the introduction of a new unit member[35] (see Chapter 6 and Chapter 8). He also wrote about soldier-on-soldier violence[36] (see Chapter 8), and soldier use and misuse of marijuana[37] (both with Vincent A Zecchinelli, Figure 3-6) (see Chapter 9).

Bey collaborated with Specialist 5th Class William E Smith, an enlisted social work/psychology technician, on a pair of publications illustrating the mental hygiene unit's vigorous primary and secondary psychiatric prevention activities within the 1st Infantry Division.[10,38] They described how they targeted especially stressed units by monitoring selected parameters (eg, sick call and mental hygiene referrals and rates for nonjudicial punishments and courts-martial, Inspector General complaints, accidents, venereal disease, and malaria) and employed a formal organizational case study and unit intervention method adapted from the civilian social psychiatry model. In so doing they demonstrated the enlisted social work/psychology technician's potential for providing both case-centered clinical approaches and organization-centered consultative ones for the often geographically separated units of the 1st Infantry Division. Attention was given to the process of educating unit commanders and others about special combat group stress points as well as stressors affecting individual soldiers (such as "short-timer's syndrome," having less education, being foreign born, or having a language handicap).

It is noteworthy that Bey did not describe a drop in troop morale or increased dissention in the 1st Infantry Division during his year, despite their occurrence more generally throughout the theater. Perhaps this is explainable on the basis that there was some measure of lag in the spread of the antimilitary sentiments to the combat divisions that was noted to be more prevalent in noncombat units. Yet scattered throughout his publications there are suggestions that morale was beginning to seriously sag and antimilitary sentiment was on the rise. For example, Bey and Smith provide the example of a black enlisted soldier who was described by his commander as "uncooperative, hostile, provocative, disrespectful, and incapable of soldiering."[10(p367)] He became the center of a fruitful unit consultation in which they brokered an expanded tolerance by the unit cadre for "expressions of 'Black pride' and 'brotherhood.'"[10(p368)] They similarly eased the tensions (and reduced referrals) through consultation to a commander who punished the "heads" (presumably habitual marijuana-using soldiers) in his unit unnecessarily —his "ten least wanted men."[38(p404)] Over the course of the consultation process, a more flexible attitude emerged that served

to acknowledge "the stress they were all under and the command's recognition of the men's positive efforts under trying conditions"[38(p405)]; and "[t]he men's provocative behavior diminished."[38(p405)] Also, in Bey's paper regarding the stresses associated with a change in command, he referred to an incident when a claymore mine was placed in a new commander's quarters with a note warning him "not to try any chicken shit with this unit."[34(p700)]

23rd Infantry Division/American

Background. The 23rd Infantry Division (American) was reactivated in Vietnam in September 1967 through the consolidation of three independent units— the 11th, 196th, and 198th Light Infantry Brigades— which had deployed in Vietnam to participate in Task Force Oregon. In spite of a large number of successful operations in and around Quang Ngai and Quang Tin provinces, the American Division's history ultimately came to be severely marred by the massacre of the villagers of My Lai on 16 March 1968 by one of the companies of the 11th Light Infantry Brigade (C Company, 1st Battalion, 20th Infantry), led by 2nd Lieutenant William Calley[39] (mentioned in Chapters 1 and 6). Further embarrassing the division, another company, part of the 196th Light Infantry Brigade, suffered severe casualties when it failed to rebuff an enemy attack on Fire Support Base Mary Ann in March 1971 (as described in Chapter 2).[33,40]

The 198th and 11th Brigades were withdrawn from Vietnam in November 1971, and the division was inactivated. The 196th Brigade remained until June 1972, the last major combat unit to be withdrawn. The last battalion in Vietnam, its 3rd Battalion, 21st Infantry, left on 23 August 1972. Overall, between battle deaths and deaths from other causes, the 23rd Infantry Division lost 4,041 men in Vietnam.[18]

None of the psychiatrists who served with the 23rd Infantry Division (American) rendered an overview. However, some perspective on the psychiatric activities in its 11th Infantry Brigade in early 1968 came from a publication by Specialist 5th Class Paul A Bender, an enlisted social work specialist. More broadly illuminating was a 1970 directive issued by Captain Larry E Alessi, Medical Corps, the division psychiatrist, 2 years following Bender's tour.

11th Light Infantry Brigade and Specialist 5th Class Paul A Bender. The 11th Infantry Brigade (Light) was deployed in early 1968, and Bender and three other mental health technicians were assigned to its base camp at Duc Pho on the northern coast of South Vietnam. They were under the technical supervision of the American Division psychiatrist who was based elsewhere with the division's other two brigades and divisional support units. The following is Bender's description of the impediments to communication and transportation he faced in providing clinical services for the troops of the 11th Light Infantry Brigade.[41]

> Part of my [medical battalion] is located at Duc Pho, the 11th Brigade's base camp. One company is attached to a task force about forty miles north of Duc Pho. The other three line companies operate out of a fire base approximately fifteen miles from this task force and the final element is located about ten miles from the fire base. I am located with the latter element in an aid station within helicopter range of all the others. The medical aid men in these respective line platoons send in any psychiatric casualties with field medical tags describing the man's behavior and need for treatment. At this point, I interview the individual at the aid station. If necessary, I transport him [by helicopter] to the Americal Division Psychiatrist, Major Edmund Casper, for evaluation and necessary treatment, which includes advice as to how to handle the patient in my follow-up.[41(p63)]

By necessity, the wide dispersion of these units meant that most soldiers had to be evaluated and counseled in one session and sent back to duty. According to Bender, it also meant that information as to a soldier's progress might come through his executive officer or first sergeant. Also, because the social work/psychology technician was in the medical platoon, he could easily get a report from the unit's medical aid man. Bender divided his caseload into: (1) passive-aggressive disciplinary problems; (2) anxious patients with secondary somatic symptomatology; (3) cases with functional somatic symptoms as primary symptoms; and (4) combat exhaustion cases, which he indicated were his most acute cases. His report especially illustrated the enlisted social work/psychology technician's critical place in the echelon system of medical care as the mental health representative for his battalion. As such he served both as a link between the primary care medical system and the division psychiatrist, and between the medical and psychiatric system and the soldier's unit. More

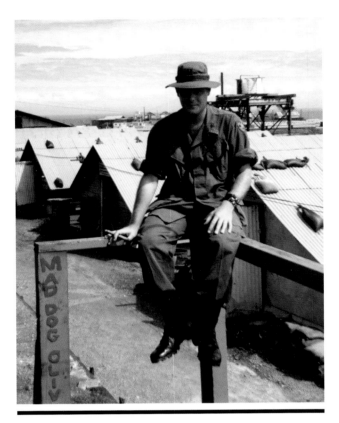

FIGURE 3-7. Captain Larry E Alessi, Medical Corps, Division Psychiatrist with the 23rd Infantry Division (Americal). Alessi, a civilian-trained psychiatrist, served with the 23rd Infantry Division from August 1970 to August 1971. His letter of instruction to the division's battalion surgeons, which provided advice regarding the treatment and referral of psychiatric and behavior problems, is especially notable because it is all that survives pertaining to the management of these problems during the drawdown phase of the war. Photograph courtesy of Larry E Alessi.

detail on Bender's approach can be found in Exhibit 3-2, "Problems Associated With One-Session Counseling," and in Chapter 7, Exhibit 7-3, "Counseling the Soldier With Combat Stress Symptoms in Vietnam."

Captain Larry E Alessi, Medical Corps. Alessi (Figure 3-7), a civilian-trained psychiatrist, served as the division psychiatrist for the 23rd Infantry Division (Americal) from August 1970 to August 1971. His November 1970 directive, "Principles of Military Combat Psychiatry," which was distributed to the division's brigade and battalion surgeons, provides a unique window into the psychiatric services available to the division during the drawdown phase of the war (provided as Appendix 9, "Principles of Military

Combat Psychiatry"). Alessi's communiqué sought to discourage the primary care physicians from making a "large number of inappropriate referrals"[42(p1)] to his mental hygiene team. Instead he urged them to screen "every soldier with an emotional or drug problem"[42(p1)] and manage the ones they could using him as consultant.[42] On the surface this appears to be an unremarkable directive. However, a closer look at it reveals that a very unusual pattern had developed by the fall of 1970:

- Army commanders, as well as the mental health component, were becoming overtaxed by the burgeoning emotional, behavioral, morale, and discipline problems;
- Rising levels of drug dependency, especially heroin addiction, had become an especially prevalent type of behavior problem among the troops of the 23rd Infantry Division (Alessi advised battalion surgeons to manage these soldiers using their unit's rehabilitation program—with some cases also benefitting from treatment with the neuroleptic tranquilizer Mellaril);
- Psychophysiologic symptoms had become the most common combat-generated psychiatric reaction (he advised them to manage these soldiers in a fashion consistent with the military psychiatry treatment doctrine— with some cases also benefitting from treatment with Mellaril); and
- There were growing numbers of anxious combat soldiers with "non-psychiatric emotional problems," that is, fear of the field and refusal to go to the field, who should be regarded as having normal aversion (and managed with reassurance, peer support, and firm opposition to claims of psychiatric impairment—again, with some cases also benefitting from treatment with Mellaril).[42]

Further perspective on psychiatric challenges in the 23rd Infantry Division (American) can be derived from results of the 1968 marijuana use surveys of the division's soldiers conducted by Edmund Casper, the division psychiatrist, and James Janacek, an Army psychiatrist with the 98th Psychiatric Detachment (with the assistance of Hugh Martinelli Jr, an enlisted specialist) (see Chapter 9).

101st Airborne Division

In July 1965, the 1st Brigade and support troops of the 101st Airborne Division arrived in Vietnam and saw much action before the remainder of the division arrived in November 1967. For most of the war the 101st was deployed in the northern I Corps region operating against ARVN infiltration routes through Laos and the A Shau Valley. Elements of the 101st participated in 15 campaigns including the Battle of Hamburger Hill in 1969 and the 23-day defense of Firebase Ripcord in 1970. The 101st withdrew from Vietnam in January 1972. It was the last US Army division to leave the combat zone. Overall, between battle deaths and deaths from other causes, the 101st Airborne Division lost 3,902 men in Vietnam.[18]

No available accounts of the provision of psychiatric care for the 101st Airborne Division exist. However, there is a report of a drug use survey conducted in the fall of 1970 by Major Jerome Char, the division psychiatrist, in which 41% of departing lower-ranking enlisted soldiers admitted to using drugs while in Vietnam, with roughly one-third of those acknowledging use of heroin or other "hard" drugs (see Chapter 9).[43] To get some further appreciation for the enormous morale and psychiatric challenges faced in the 101st Airborne Division during the drawdown phase, Char's study can be joined with Linden's disturbing report from late 1971 that described the unraveling military discipline in Vietnam ("Fragging and Other Withdrawal Symptoms"[44])—a journalist's report that especially centered on the 101st Airborne Division and included a series of quotes from Captain Robert Landeen, Medical Corps (1971–1972), a civilian-trained Army psychiatrist who followed Char. Linden's account highlighted rampant heroin use by soldiers, incendiary racial tensions, and leader assassinations ("fragging") and threats; Landeen provided commentary on their psychosocial causes, but without reference to clinical challenges. According to Landeen, there were two enlisted factions who were most likely to resort to fraggings (what Linden referred to as a "lethal fad")—(1) heroin users and dealers, and (2) black radicals. He felt this was partly explainable because the typical soldier of 1971 came from a lower socioeconomic strata and was more inclined to act out his frustrations, was opposed to serving in Vietnam, believed his work was purposeless, and felt "helpless and paranoid" because of the Army's vacillating discipline (too much flexibility, followed by overly harsh punishments). On the other

EXHIBIT 3-2. Problems Associated With One-Session Counseling

Providing psychological counseling for soldiers in a combat zone presents additional challenges because of the preeminence of the combat mission and because of practical impediments to accessing treatment. In early 1968, a piece appeared in the USARV Medical Bulletin that described firsthand experience in attempting to surmount these challenges in Vietnam. This unique article was written by Specialist 5th Class Paul A Bender, an enlisted social work/psychology technician, who was assigned to the 11th Infantry Brigade (Light). Like many of the social work/psychology technicians operating in Vietnam, Bender functioned semiautonomously while under the technical supervision of Major Edmund Casper, the division psychiatrist for the Americal Division, who was based elsewhere with the division's other two brigades and divisional support units. The information provided by Bender is especially salient in that it is estimated that 80% of the direct psychiatric care in Vietnam was provided by "psych techs." In his report Bender emphasizes that by necessity, the typical counseling patient from a combat unit is seen, evaluated, and counseled in only one session and sent back to duty. That makes helping him achieve insight into his problem much more difficult. However, underscoring a basic paradox in doing counseling in a combat zone, Bender also surmises that even if repeated visits were possible, it might actually oppose therapeutic progress (because, under the special stresses of the combat zone, the soldier-patient has the potential for so-called secondary gain in illness). Furthermore, such a situation might also contribute to reducing his unit's combat effectiveness. The following are excerpted from Bender:

Initiating Short-Term Counseling

Rapport is relatively easy to develop between the individual and the technician since both persons are enlisted men from the same organization and experiencing many of the same problems in relation to the Army. The individual realizes that the technician can empathize with the situation. In essence he 'knows what is happening.' [Also] the technician should spend maximum time in the battalion area so that he is thought of as being part of the unit and not an outsider.[1(p68)]

Defining the Problem

I first try to have the patient identify his primary problem while exploring his feelings and attitudes toward this problem. We explore ways of handling the specific enigma [that] is causing the trouble within the patient. If he is able to understand why he has reacted to a situation and what the consequences of this reaction are, he can usually change his maladaptive way of contending with environmental pressures.[1(p63–64)]

Undoubtedly, the most often heard complaint from soldiers is that of being 'harassed' too much by his superiors in the unit. . . . I would rather think of it as self-devaluation on the part of the man concerned. When an individual is forced to perform a function [that] he considers below his self-concept, anxiety is produced. His self ideal is now incongruous with his real position, and [he] cannot accept it since he does not conceive of himself as one controlled to the extent that he is. When discipline reaches the point where he cannot act out without serious repercussions, the individual becomes angry and resentful. He can't rid himself of these feelings by directing them toward the source of his conflicts, and he becomes stymied. We now find the person in a perplexing dilemma with no solution to his problem and a great deal of anxiety.[1(p68–69)]

Maladaptive Defenses, Resistance to Treatment, and Counseling Approaches

The individual's preconceived solution to his problem resisted the effects of counseling. Most often he attributed his conflict to outside sources and concluded that if the technician could change these environmental conditions his problem would he solved. . . . A job or area transfer is easier to accept than a basic personality defect.[1(p66)]

The technician [must] impress upon the patient that this conflict was not just a product of his environment but was also a result of his own perceptions, attitudes, and the manner in which he coped with conflicts.[1(p66)]

Most individuals do not realize that their conflicts can be resolved through change in their behavior and that this behavior or their coping techniques are the elements to be examined rather than merely an isolated incident when they were challenged. In other words, it's not just the 'what,' but also the 'why,' that must be explained.[1(p68)]

[But] the technician has to maintain an atmosphere of reality. The patient will tend to pursue a solution colored with fantasy, but all illusions must be destroyed, no false hopes extended, and only pragmatic avenues followed.[1(p68)]

Once the individual accepts this, the actual therapy can ensue. In essence, the technician takes away the individual's definition of the problem and presents an entirely different aspect to him which typically is not easily accepted.[1(p66)]

EXHIBIT 3-2. Problems Associated With One-Session Counseling, continued

If [the patient] resists understanding, the technician must then define for him just what the conflict is and what his own behavior is doing for him. The technician finally has him explore various ways to adapt to this problem, and then it is up to the individual to take the initiative in adjusting his actions.[1(p66–67)]

In dealing with psychosomatic symptoms I found it useful to treat them as being far less serious than the person had supposed they were. . . . Also, if the patient realizes that his own behavior is causing the ailment, additional impetus may be provided to resolve his conflicts.[1(p68)]

If an individual complains of difficulties in peer relationships, we may explore his own attitudes toward people in general and discover a basic mistrust or dislike of them. We then attempt to get him to realize that feelings are transmitted to those he now associates with and are reciprocated. The individual usually then realizes how he must change his own attitudes to foster more amiable relations with his peers.[1(p64)]

[Overall] this is a very difficult situation to resolve, and therapy must allow for much ventilation and empathy. The underlying purpose is to direct the patient toward accepting this period of his life as one which he must adjust to and even get some daily benefits out of so as to make life as pleasant as possible.[1(p69)]

Psychological Stress on the Counselor

[I]t would he easier to sympathize with the patient, leave him in a relaxed mood, and have him return to duty temporarily relieved and convinced his behavior is not the cause of his problems. To project his difficulties onto the external environment is more palatable to the individual and provides an amiable atmosphere for interview. All these effects must be avoided. The conflict or problem has to be identified by both the patient and the technician before an attempt is made to work through it. This is going to involve resistance, denial, but hopefully insight in the end.[1(p67)]

Many times when a patient leaves the interview, I wonder if I have helped him to understand himself since most of the time his problems persist, and the new knowledge gained must still be put into practice in his relationships. However, I am beginning to respect the will and resourcefulness of each person in solving his interpersonal problems when he really has to. I also respect his ability to accept parts of his behavior which, up to this time, he has been unable to understand.[1(p69)]

Follow-Up

One of the drawbacks to the psychiatric patient's returning to duty is the stigma attached to the concept of mental illness. This stigma must be minimized as much as possible. It can best be accomplished by the technician [because] he, more than anyone else at the clinic, is in familiar communication with the unit. He must deemphasize the notion that the patient is dangerous, aggressive, or hostile and emphasize the best way to handle him. The soldier must be seen as a behavior problem expected to feel and respond like his peers and not as a psychotic patient.[1(p67)]

In Vietnam continuous direct contact is not feasible, the resulting indications of a [soldier's] progress are gained through his unit executive officer or First Sergeant. The best source though, is the patient's medical aid man. Since the technician was in the medical platoon, he can easily get a report from the medical aid man.[1(p66)]

1. Bender PA. Social work specialists at the line battalion. *US Army Vietnam Med Bull.* 1968;May/June:60–69.

hand, Landeen believed that many of the officers and noncommissioned officers who were fragged contributed to this outcome by excessive rigidity, pettiness, hypocrisy, or zeal for the war. (More on Linden's report can be found in Chapters 2, 8, and 9.)

Discussion of Reports by Division Psychiatrists and Allied Personnel

The foregoing review of the available written accounts of the Army's division psychiatrists and allied

mental health personnel deployed in Vietnam permitted some appreciation of the exceptional efforts expended by the psychiatric assets that were organic to the combat divisions. Unfortunately, at best these reports represent only a small portion of the Army's 30.25 division-years in Vietnam (from Table 3-2). Furthermore, they were mostly limited to the first half of the war. Explanations for the sparse number of reports would certainly include that to study, document, and write up observations for publication would rely on the personal initiative of the deployed mental health practitioners—activities that might compete for resources with mission-required ones. However, the fact that the extant reports from Vietnam were limited to the earlier years of the war could also be explained by a lowered morale among the mental health representatives in the divisions over time as suggested in Chapter 2. Further discussion of these reports by stages of the war follows.

Early Buildup Phase Reports (1965–1966)

Reports by Jones (25th Infantry Division [ID]) and Byrdy (1st Cav) can be compared as they both deployed early in the buildup phase (1965–1966), and both provided details regarding the considerable practical difficulties they faced as their respective divisions established themselves in Vietnam. In general, their professional activities were more reflective of the psychosocial stress associated with deployment and the newness of each division to their specific combat environment than combat stress per se. Both Jones and Byrdy indicated that requisite troop morale in their respective divisions was sustained, and apparently this contributed to the overall low levels of psychiatric symptoms and referrals. Jones reported only mild combat stress symptoms among the soldiers of the 25th Infantry Division, whereas Byrdy diagnosed at least 22 1st Cavalry soldiers as "combat exhaustion" and 10 others with combat stress reactions in conjunction with other diagnoses; nonetheless, combat stress reactions were not predominant among psychiatric referrals to either psychiatrist.

Distinct differences existed as well. Jones had 50% more referrals per month than Byrdy, yet he only "hospitalized" 5.3% compared to Byrdy's 23%. Also, Jones only evacuated a few psychotic soldiers out of the division for additional treatment. Byrdy evacuated 6% of all referrals, the majority of whom were not designated as psychotic. Finally, although presumably Jones and Byrdy had the same medications available, Byrdy mentioned prescribing Thorazine and Librium, but Jones made no mention of using medications. Aside from the prospect that Byrdy's division had some greater combat intensity levels than Jones's, another possible explanation for these differences may come from distinctions in pre-Vietnam military psychiatry training and experience. Jones's extensive military background may have influenced him to see symptomatic soldiers as struggling to adapt to the unique rigors of a combat deployment (ie, less pathological), which in turn may

have led him to be more restrictive with regard to medications and hospitalization. Byrdy, on the other hand, with his civilian-based professional background, may have been somewhat more inclined to see soldier symptoms as representing fixed deficits needing more extensive treatment. (Important differences in clinical perspective stemming from military vs civilian medical orientation will be amplified below as well as discussed in Chapter 5 and Chapter 11.) Perhaps also influential was that Byrdy reported being understaffed in social work/psychology technicians. This would have limited the extent to which he could extend his psychiatric expertise closer to the fighting units and thus could have contributed to some greater morbidity among combat stress affected soldiers.

Peak Combat Activity Phase Reports (1967–1968)

Reports by four division psychiatrists—Bostrom (1st Cav), Motis (4th ID), Baker (9th ID), and Pettera (9th ID)—from the next 2 years, 1967 and 1968, centered on a rising incidence of combat stress reactions, which seemed to trump concern for other psychiatric problems. This coincided with the theater-wide increase in combat activity, as well as combat intensity, in those years. Nonetheless, the relatively low numbers of combat stress reaction cases these psychiatrists reported is still consistent with a generally low combat stress reaction incidence rate throughout the war.

It is interesting to note the variability in the diagnostic criteria utilized by these psychiatrists for combat-generated casualties. Bostrom's taxonomy was consistent with the one Byrdy (1st Cav) utilized in the first year of the war, which coincided with the historically based spectrum of psychiatric and behavior symptoms: demonstrable apprehension but with retained combat performance; followed by moderate dysfunction; followed by severe disorganization/ dysfunction (see Table 6-1). The last stage, severe disorganization/dysfunction, Bostrom referred to as combat exhaustion, and Pettera as combat fatigue (these terms were used interchangeably in the literature). In contrast, Baker's "classic combat fatigue" cases were the less severe cases—those that were reversible at the 1st echelon care level; and he distinguished them from the more severe cases (no label) who required treatment by him and his staff at the 2nd echelon care level, the division clearing company. Baker also described the "modified combat stress reaction," a class of soldier-patient with over 10 months of credible combat experience in Vietnam who became combat-ineffective associated with an array of psychological and psychosomatic disturbances. Pettera, who followed Baker at the 9th ID, repeated this observation but renamed them "Vietnam combat reaction." Together these two psychiatrists seemed to have identified the "old sergeant syndrome," which was first described in World War II. This referred to the capable and responsible combat soldier who underwent a loss of his psychological resiliency after enduring months of sustained combat. This in turn caused him considerable depression and guilt at abdicating his responsibilities with his combat unit.[45] But inasmuch as the cases reported by Baker and Pettera were nearing the end of their year in Vietnam (as opposed to the soldiers who faced indeterminate combat exposure in World War II), they also resembled the short-timer's syndrome, which arose for the first time in Korea after tour limits were instituted and again in Vietnam.

Still, labeling differences aside, these four psychiatrists reported the consistent application of the established military treatment doctrine for combat stress affected soldiers, which was augmented by judicious use of Thorazine (according to Motis, "to aid in rest and restraint")—apparently with favorable results. They also valued the decentralized use of enlisted social work/psychology technicians as psychiatrist extenders. In fact there appears to have been an overwhelming consensus that these enlisted specialists proved critical to the smooth operation and effectiveness of the mental health contingent in the combat units. (In this regard, the publication by Bey, the 1st ID psychiatrist, and Smith, his social work/psychology technician, provided an especially rich review of background, training, deployment, utilization, and supervision of these paraprofessionals in Vietnam. The authors noted how the technicians' medical/psychiatric responsibilities and activities often exceeded those performed in stateside settings because of the extremes of the combat situation. They also provided case examples illustrating both case-oriented clinical approaches and organization-oriented consultative ones.[10]) With regard to attrition secondary to combat stress reactions, both Pettera and Motis suggested that approximately 15% of referred soldiers could not be recovered for further combat duty but were able to assume other military duties in the division.

On the other hand, there was a fair amount of divergence among these division psychiatrists regarding the pathogenic variables assumed to be responsible for the more acute combat-generated psychiatric disabilities (eg, specific combat events, features of the unit, personality elements, or other distinctions). The only division psychiatrist to provide a specific case example was Motis, and that soldier was felt to be especially susceptible because of personality deficits.[46]

Finally, none of these four division psychiatrists provided figures for overall psychiatric evacuations out of their divisions. However, Gordon, who served as division psychiatrist with the 1st ID contemporaneously with them, did note that 6.8% of his over 1,000 referrals required evacuation beyond the division (presumably to the 935th Psychiatric Detachment), and that some were combat exhaustion cases. This figure is very close to the 6% reported by Byrdy with the 1st Cav among his over 500 referrals in 1965 to 1966 during the early buildup phase, and collectively they suggest very low rates for psychiatric attrition from combat divisions in an active theater of war.

Transition Phase Reports (1969 to Early 1970)

The inauguration of Richard Nixon as President of the United States in 1969 brought a change of command in Vietnam and a new strategy. The new strategy sought to insure area security while the primary combat roles were gradually shifted to South Vietnamese military forces. As a consequence the second half of the war took on a distinctly different character than that of the first half, with American combat operations steadily declining along with troop strength.

Regrettably, the reports from the 1st Infantry Division by Bey and his colleagues were the only descriptions from the combat divisions for this pivotal phase in the war. On the other hand, they do serve as an elaborate record because Bey was committed to providing and documenting a model of psychiatric care for a deployed combat division that included a full range of primary, secondary, and tertiary prevention activities. Highlights include that:

- Whereas USARV Regulation 40-34, *Mental Health and Neuropsychiatry*, stipulated that support (both material and personnel) would be made available for those who provided psychiatric services, it was not automatically supplied by the division (a complaint shared earlier by Jones and Gordon); consequently it was necessary for Bey to employ improvisation and ingenuity in recruiting command support.

- The proportion of psychiatric cases with combat stress symptoms evidently had dropped from that of the preceding 2 years (an assumption based on the observation that they were statistically subsumed within the broader category of acute situational reactions), and "drug-induced" problems apparently became more prevalent.

- Bey's mental health team devoted a great deal of attention to ameliorating stress-inducing group and interpersonal factors. Still, despite these preventive activities, his unit averaged 180 referrals per month. This is almost 3½ times the 53 per month reported by the shorthanded Byrdy and almost 2½ times Jones's 75 per month—the only other division psychiatrists who provided these rates. Furthermore, Bey's significantly higher referral rate 3 years after Jones and Byrdy cannot be explained by rising combat intensity. Thus the elevated rate and other indicators of rising stress and dysfunction levels, like his reference to racial tensions and problematic "heads" (the marijuana-using subculture), suggest that Bey and his staff were seeing the beginnings of the serious erosion of mental health and military order and discipline that was spreading throughout the theater.

- Like Bostrom earlier with the 1st Cavalry Division, Bey advocated the use of phenothiazines both for nonpsychotic combat exhaustion and for sleep therapy (*dauerschlaf*) for more disorganized psychiatric casualties.

- Bey's reported psychiatric attrition rate (actually, proportion of referrals hospitalized or evacuated to a psychiatric specialty detachment) is intermediate between rates reported by Jones (25th ID) and Byrdy (1st Cav) (Table 3-5). Even though Jones and Byrdy served during the early buildup years, their experiences may be reasonably compared with Bey's because during Bey's year the overall combat stress levels in Vietnam (at least as measured by battle death rate) dropped to the levels seen when Jones and Byrdy were there. As mentioned earlier, a possible explanation for higher hospitalization and evacuation rates is the psychiatrist's lack of military training or experience. Unfortunately, these are the only division psychiatrists who provided this data, so this hypothesis cannot be further tested. Gordon, who preceded Bey with the 1st ID, reported eva-

cuating 6.8% of referrals out of the division, but his training and military experience background is not known. Again, the importance of the distinction between civilian and military training will be further developed in Chapter 5 and Chapter 11.

Drawdown Phase Reports (Late 1970 to 1972)

Following Bey, professional observations from the mental health component assigned to the combat units in Vietnam become scant. The evidence provided by Alessi (23rd Infantry Division, 1970–1971), followed a year later by Landeen (101st Airborne Division, 1971–1972), suggested morale and discipline had dropped to a new and dangerous low, and psychiatric and psychosocial problems continued to rise, especially in novel forms (eg, soldier dissent, open racial conflicts, widespread heroin use, and attacks on superiors).

US Marine Corps/Navy Experience in Vietnam

From March 1965, when the 9th Marine Expeditionary Brigade landed on the northern coast of the Republic of South Vietnam, until April 1971, when the last elements of the 1st Marine Division departed Vietnam, approximately 360,000 Marines fought in Vietnam,[47] mostly as members of the 1st and the 3rd Marine Divisions. Navy Lieutenant Ted D Kilpatrick, the division psychologist of the 3rd Marine Division, reported on the diagnostic, dispositional, and selective demographic data regarding 823 psychiatric admissions (14% of all medical admissions) to the 10-patient psychiatric ward of a division field hospital during 9 months of 1967.

Overall, approximately two-thirds of the casualties came directly from field units actively fighting well-trained North Vietnamese troops along the demilitarized zone. Kilpatrick and Harry A Grater, his coauthor, blamed the especially high out-of-country psychiatric evacuation rate (42% of referrals) on the high admission rate, inadequate staffing, the absence of 3rd echelon treatment facilities in-country, and the limited number of support billets that would allow patients to be reassigned to noncombat duty. Whereas some cases received 3rd echelon treatment offshore on either the USS *Sanctuary* or the USS *Repose* (the Navy's two hospital ships), most were evacuated out of the combat zone.

The diagnosis of combat fatigue was reserved for the few Marines who conformed to the "classic" combat fatigue diagnostic criteria *and* had "experienced

TABLE 3-5. A Comparison of Division Psychiatrists' Pre-Vietnam Military Training and Experience, the Percentages of Referrals in Vietnam They Hospitalized, and the Percentages They Evacuated out of the Division

	Jones (25th ID) February 1966–September 1966	Bey (1st ID) April 1969–April 1970	Byrdy (1st Cav) August 1965–June 1966
Army Psychiatric Residency Training	Yes	No	No
Pre-Vietnam Army Assignment	Yes	Yes	No
% of Referrals Hospitalized in the Division	5.3%	10%	23%
% of Referrals Ultimately Evacuated out of the Division	"a few" ("psychotics")	1%	6%

ID: Infantry Division
Cav: Cavalry

intolerable stress over a prolonged period of time." On the other hand, the diagnosis of "combat reaction" (which they regarded as a version of "situational maladjustment" as defined in the *Diagnostic and Statistical Manual of Mental Disorders*, 1st edition [1952][48(p802)]) was applied to all other acute psychiatric casualties referred from units actively engaged in combat (16.7% of referrals). The majority of these were returned to duty. Other categories of cases seen were: personality disorders (29.6%), most as passive-aggressive personality type; neurotic disorders (28.6%), most as anxiety reaction type; and "no diagnosis" (19.7%). It was the authors' impression that the threat of combat was the basic precipitating factor for most of the psychiatric casualties, but in 75% of the cases, personality defects were contributory. They also noted that 10% of admissions had a previous psychiatric contact in Vietnam.[48]

Further perspective on psychiatric challenges for the Marines in Vietnam include the reports in this volume by Navy medical personnel Robert E Strange and Ransom J Arthur, who recounted their psychiatric experience aboard the USS *Repose* during the ship's first year stationed off the northern coast of South Vietnam (1966) (Chapter 4); Stephen W Edmendson and Donald J Platner, who reviewed the psychiatric evacuations from Khe Sanh during the siege (1968) (Chapter 6); Stephen Howard (1968) and Herman P Langner (1967–1968), who both reported on the rise in excessive combat aggression and atrocities (Chapter 6); John A Renner Jr, regarding the epidemiology of psychiatric and related difficulties among Marine and Navy personnel hospitalized aboard the hospital ship USS *Repose* (1969) (Chapter 6); and Howard W Fisher, who described the exceedingly high rate of personality disorders among his

referrals from the 1st Marine Division (March 1970–February 1971) (Chapter 2).

SUMMARY AND CONCLUSIONS

This chapter utilized the available reports provided by the Army mental health professionals and paraprofessionals who were assigned to combat units in Vietnam in order to construct a composite picture of the psychiatric problems they encountered, the conditions under which they worked, and their professional responses and results. When combined with the next chapter, which pertains to psychiatric care provided in the Army hospitals in Vietnam, a richly descriptive and informative story emerges depicting a mental health contingent that was trained, organized, and supplied to support the deployment of many thousands of troops into the combat theater and, in particular, to aid the recovery of large numbers of soldiers who were expected to be disabled by combat stress. Furthermore, the documentation indicates they met these challenges with commitment and effectiveness.

The chapter's review began with an overview of the organization of psychiatric care implemented in South Vietnam in support of US Army forces—a system based on forward treatment of affected soldiers that replicated one utilized with good effect in World War I, in the later stages of World War II, and in the Korean War. The system in Vietnam was a component of the larger Army medical system, and its ultimate authority in Vietnam was the CG/USARV Surgeon. It centered on the (combat) division psychiatrists who were assisted by allied mental health personnel, that is, social work officers and enlisted mental health specialists, as well as general medical assets, all of whom were assigned to the divisions. Beyond the divisions, specialized psychiatric care was provided by the mental health personnel assigned to the two psychiatric detachments (KO teams), and at times by the psychiatrists assigned to Army-level evacuation and field hospitals in Vietnam. The mental health assets at these hospitals and detachments also provided mental health care on a regional basis for the large numbers of nondivision personnel deployed throughout the theater, but often this system was thinly allocated. By the time the Army was fully deployed in Vietnam (1967) there were 23 psychiatrists rotating into and out of Vietnam each year, which included the seven division psychiatrists, and it is estimated that a total of 135 to 140 psychiatrist positions were assigned there over the course of the war. The Army Neuropsychiatry Consultant to the CG/USARV Surgeon provided the psychiatric leadership for this system. This was the senior Army psychiatrist in South Vietnam who served as staff officer and advisor for the Army commander in Vietnam and directed the coordination of Army psychiatric facilities and program planning throughout the country.

This chapter also reconstructed as much of the history of Army psychiatry in Vietnam as possible through the available reports provided by psychiatrists and other mental health personnel assigned to the combat divisions. In addition to their descriptive value, these reports suggested the following trends:

- **Clinical challenges associated with combat stress reaction casualties were significantly lower than that seen in earlier wars.** This held true despite the increased combat intensity in Vietnam through years 2 through 4, as well as episodic spikes in combat activity associated with specific campaigns.
- **Division psychiatrists appeared confident in the effectiveness of the military doctrine of forward treatment, especially for soldiers with combat stress reactions.**
- **Troop morale appeared sustained in the early years, numbers of referrals were at manageable levels, and psychiatric conditions and behavior problems were generally more challenging than those stemming from direct combat exposure.**
- **For soldiers in combat roles, the chronic strain associated with fighting an elusive guerrilla/**counterinsurgency force appeared to produce more low-grade forms of combat stress reaction, especially psychosomatic symptoms and behavior problems.** This is in contrast to the more extensive breakdown in psychological functioning seen in earlier wars under conditions of continuous operations and high intensity combat.
- **Division psychiatrists utilized extensively, and highly valued, the capabilities of the psych techs (enlisted corpsmen with additional social work/ psychology training), including those who were dispersed among the division's scattered brigades and battalions and functioned semiautonomously and effectively as psychiatrist extenders.** The success of this arrangement confirmed the benefits of decentralized care.
- **Division psychiatrists also utilized extensively, and highly valued (and encouraged other medical personnel to as well), the new anxiolytic and neuroleptic medications to accelerate the recovery of function of soldiers with disabling psychological and psychosomatic symptoms.**
- **Division psychiatrists, with one exception, rarely devoted mental health resources to command-centered social/community psychiatry prevention programs.** Notably, the exception occurred after the US strategy shifted to a defensive one and combat intensity dropped.
- **Very little record exists of the activities of the division psychiatrists during the last 2 years of the war, mid-1970 through 1972.** This is regrettable because other data indicated that these were the most difficult years for Army psychiatry from the standpoint of low morale and a substantial rise in psychiatric conditions and behavior problems, especially soldier dissent, racial conflicts, widespread heroin use, and attacks on superiors.

The portrayal of the organization and experience of Army mental health assets resumes in the next chapter. It will review reports from psychiatrists who served in evacuation and field hospitals and in the two psychiatric specialty detachments (KO). It also presents available information describing the professional activities of the senior Army psychiatrists in Vietnam (Neuropsychiatry Consultant to the CG/USARV Surgeon).

REFERENCES

1. Byrdy HSR. In: Johnson AW Jr, Bowman JA, Byrdy HSR, Blank AS Jr. Panel discussion: Army psychiatry in Vietnam. In: Jones FD, ed. *Proceedings: Social and Preventive Psychiatry Course, 1967.* Washington, DC: GPO; 1968: 41–76. [Available at: Alexandria, Va: Defense Technical Information Center. Document No. ADA 950058.]

2. Copen EG. Discussed in: Jones FD, Johnson AW. Medical and psychiatric treatment policy and practice in Vietnam. *J Soc Issues.* 1975;31(4):49–65.

3. Allerton WS. Army psychiatry in Vietnam. In: Bourne PG, ed. *The Psychology and Physiology of Stress: With Reference to Special Studies of the Viet Nam War.* New York, NY: Academic Press; 1969: 1–17.

4. Neel SH. *Medical Support of the US Army in Vietnam, 1965–1970.* Washington, DC: GPO; 1973.

5. US Department of the Army. *Medical Service: Neuropsychiatry.* Washington, DC: DA; June 1959. Army Regulation 40-216.

6. Headquarters US Army Republic of Vietnam. *Medical Services: Mental Health and Neuropsychiatry.* 30 March 1966. USARV Regulation 40-34. [This material is presented as Appendix 2 to this volume.]

7. Jones FD, Johnson AW Jr. Medical and psychiatric treatment policy and practice in Vietnam. *J Soc Issues.* 1975;31(4):49–65.

8. Peterson DB. Discussion. In: Tiffany WJ Jr, Allerton WS. Army psychiatry in the mid-'60s. *Am J Psychiatry.* 1967;123(7):810–821.

9. Tiffany WJ Jr, Allerton WS. Army psychiatry in the mid-'60s. *Am J Psychiatry.* 1967;123(7):810–821.

10. Bey DR, Smith WE. Mental health technicians in Vietnam. *Bull Menninger Clin.* 1970;34(6):363–371.

11. Johnson AW Jr. Combat psychiatry, II: The US Army in Vietnam. *Med Bull US Army Europe.* 1969;26(11):335–339.

12. Colbach EM, Parrish MD. Army mental health activities in Vietnam: 1965–1970. *Bull Menninger Clin.* 1970;34(6):333–342.

13. McGrath JJ. *The Other End of the Spear: The Tooth-to-Tail Ratio (T3R) in Modern Military Operations.* Fort Leavenworth, Kan: Combat Studies Institute Press; 2007.

14. Hausman W, Rioch DMcK. Military psychiatry. A prototype of social and preventive psychiatry in the United States. *Arch Gen Psych.* 1967;16(6):727–739.

15. Bey DR. Division psychiatry in Viet Nam. *Am J Psychiatry.* 1970;127(2):228–232.

16. Motis G, Neal RD. Freud in the boonies, II: The 4th Infantry Division psychiatric field program at work in a sustained combat situation. *US Army Vietnam Med Bull.* 1968;January/February:27–30.

17. Gordon EL. Division psychiatry: documents of a tour. *US Army Vietnam Med Bull.* 1968;November/December:62–69.

18. National Archives and Records Administration, Archival Databases, Vietnam Conflict Extracts Data File. Available at: http://aad.archives.gov. Accessed 20 June 2013.

19. Jones FD. Experiences of a division psychiatrist in Vietnam. *Mil Med.* 1967:132(12):1003–1008.

20. American Psychiatric Association. *Diagnostic and Statistical Manual of Mental Disorders.* 2nd ed. (DSM-II). Washington, DC: APA; 1968.

21. Byrdy HSR. Division psychiatry in Vietnam (unpublished); 1967. [Full text available as Appendix 8 to this volume.]

22. Bostrom JA. Management of combat reactions. *US Army Vietnam Med Bull.* 1967;July/August:6–8.

23. Bostrom JA. Psychiatric consultation in the First Cav. *US Army Vietnam Med Bull.* 1968;January/February:24–25.

24. Baker WL. Division psychiatry in the 9th Infantry Division. *US Army Vietnam Med Bull.* 1967;November/December:5–9.

25. Pettera RL, Johnson BM, Zimmer R. Psychiatric management of combat reactions with emphasis on a reaction unique to Vietnam. *Mil Med.* 1969;134(9):673–678.

26. Pettera RL. What is this thing called "field consultation" in psychiatry. *US Army Vietnam Med Bull.* 1968;January/February:31–36.

27. Stern DB. The social work/psychology specialist with the Mobile Riverine Force. *US Army Vietnam Med Bull.* 1968;May/June:70–74.

28. Motis G. Freud in the boonies: a preliminary report on the psychiatric field program in the 4th Infantry Division. *US Army Vietnam Med Bull.* 1967;September/October:5–8.

29. Motis G. Psychiatry at the battle of Dak To. *US Army Vietnam Med Bull.* 1967;November/December:57.

30. Menard DL. The social work specialist in a combat division. *US Army Vietnam Med Bull.* 1968;March/April:48–57.

31. Bey D. *Wizard 6: A Combat Psychiatrist in Vietnam.* College Station, Tex: Texas A & M University Military History Series, 104; 2006.

32. Bey DR. *Division Psychiatry in Vietnam* (unpublished).

33. Stanton SL. *The Rise and Fall of an American Army: US Ground Forces in Vietnam, 1965–1973.* Novato, Calif: Presidio Press; 1985.

34. Bey DR. Change of command in combat: a locus of stress. *Am J Psychiatry.* 1972;129(6):698–702.

35. Bey DR. Group dynamics and the 'F.N.G.' in Vietnam: a potential focus of stress. *Int J Group Psychother.* 1972;22(1):22–30.

36. Bey DR, Zecchinelli VA. G.I.'s against themselves. Factors resulting in explosive violence in Vietnam. *Psychiatry.* 1974;37(3):221–228.

37. Bey DR, Zecchinelli VA. Marijuana as a coping device in Vietnam. *Mil Med.* 1971;136(5):448–450.

38. Bey DR Jr, Smith WE. Organizational consultation in a combat unit. *Am J Psychiatry.* 1971;128(4):401–406.

39. Dougan C, Weiss S, and the editors of Boston Publishing Co. *The Vietnam Experience: Nineteen Sixty-Eight.* Boston, Mass: Boston Publishing Co; 1983.

40. Sorley L. *A Better War: The Unexamined Victories and Final Tragedy of America's Last Years in Vietnam.* New York, NY: Harcourt Books; 1999.

41. Bender PA. The social work specialist at the line battalion. *US Army Vietnam Med Bull.* 1968;May/June:60–69.

42. Alessi LE. 23d Infantry Division Mental Hygiene Consultation Service: Principles of Military Combat Psychiatry. November 1970 (unpublished). [Full text available as Appendix 9 to this volume.]

43. Char J. Drug abuse in Vietnam. *Am J Psychiatry.* 1972;129(4):463–465.

44. Linden E. The demoralization of an army: fragging and other withdrawal symptoms. *Saturday Review,* 8 January 1972:12–17, 55.

45. Johnson AW Jr. Psychiatric treatment in the combat situation. *US Army Vietnam Med Bull.* 1967;January/February:38–45.

46. Motis G, West HE. The case of the dumbstruck soldier. *US Army Vietnam Med Bull.* 1968;March/April:70–73.

47. US Military Personnel in South Vietnam 1960–1972. Department of Defense, Office of the Assistant Secretary of Defense (Comptroller), Directorate for Information Operations,15 March 1974: 60.

48. Kilpatrick TD, Grater HA Jr. Field report on Marine psychiatric casualties in Vietnam. *Mil Med.* 1971;136(10):801–809.

CHAPTER 4

Organization of Army Psychiatry, II: Hospital-Based Services and the Theater Psychiatric Leadership

A frequent source of contention between [division] psychiatrists and the KO team involves patients who are seen as psychotic . . . in the division setting, but who present essentially characterologic problems [on] our ward. Problems potentially get worse because of the . . . fact that character disorders are not removed through medical channels in the Army. . . . [W]e are [thus] left with a man who we feel is character disordered and cannot evacuate [from Vietnam] through medical channels with good conscience, but on the other hand [he is] a man whom [you] feel is psychotic and cannot be returned to duty with good conscience. . . . So, what to do??[1(pp1–2)]

Captain H Spencer Bloch, Director, Inpatient Psychiatry Service
935th Psychiatric Detachment (KO)
August 1967 to August 1968

At the peak of the buildup phase there were 10 Army-level evacuation hospitals in Vietnam, such as the 95th Evacuation Hospital pictured here (1970), and five field hospitals, each of which had a psychiatrist position. There were also two psychiatric treatment centers, the Neuropsychiatric Medical Specialty Detachments (KO), which were staffed by psychiatrists, allied mental health professionals, and enlisted technicians. Photograph courtesy of Norman M Camp, Colonel, US Army (Retired).

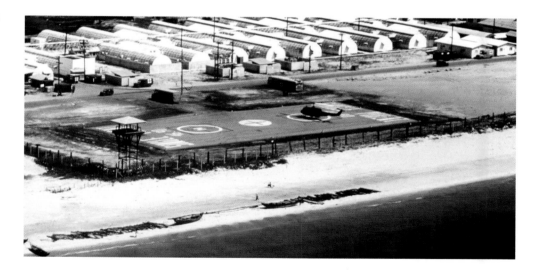

This chapter extends the description of Army psychiatry in Vietnam begun in Chapter 3 by reviewing the published accounts by hospital psychiatrists and those assigned to the Neuropsychiatric Medical Specialty Detachments ("KO teams"). It concludes with a review of the available record of the professional activities and recollections of the senior psychiatrists deployed in Vietnam as Neuropsychiatry Consultant to the Commanding General, US Army Republic of Vietnam Surgeon.

ARMY-LEVEL PSYCHIATRIC SERVICES IN VIETNAM: EVACUATION AND FIELD HOSPITALS AND THE TWO NEUROPSYCHIATRIC MEDICAL SPECIALTY DETACHMENTS (KO)

Army-level hospital care was abundantly provided for Army personnel in South Vietnam through a collection of semipermanent, air-conditioned, 200- to 400-bed, medical treatment facilities and their associated dispensaries. These hospitals had sophisticated equipment, surgical suites, and intensive care wards and were located throughout the country in secure base camps. Because the ecology of the battlefield meant that there was no front line, and because of the advent of the heliborne medical evacuation capability, there was little reason to have hospitals physically follow the combat units in the war. These hospitals and their various medical specialty detachments were rapidly introduced in Vietnam as the war progressed, commensurate with the escalating troop strength. By the end of 1968, there were 23 Army hospitals in South Vietnam with a bed capacity of 5,283 (11 evacuation hospitals, five field hospitals, and seven surgical hospitals, augmented by the 6th Convalescent Center at Cam Ranh Bay).[2] At various times, Army patients, including psychiatric patients, were hospitalized and treated at the 483rd US Air Force Hospital, which was also located in the Cam Ranh Bay area. Psychiatrists were assigned to the Army hospitals in either of two arrangements: (1) as a solo psychiatrist assigned directly to an evacuation hospital or a field hospital, or (2) as a member of the one of two neuropsychiatric specialty detachments: the 935th (KO) or the 98th (KO).

Data collected in the Walter Reed Army Institute of Research survey of Vietnam veteran psychiatrists indicated there were at least eight Army field or evacuation hospitals with solo psychiatrists assigned at one time or another:

- 3rd Field Hospital (Saigon)
- 17th Field Hospital (Saigon)
- 8th Field Hospital (Nha Trang)
- 36th Evacuation Hospital (Vung Tau)
- 67th Evacuation Hospital, which sometimes had two psychiatrists (Qui Nhon and later, Pleiku)
- 85th Evacuation Hospital (Qui Nhon and later, Phu Bai)
- 71st Evacuation Hospital (Pleiku)
- 95th Evacuation Hospital (Da Nang)

In 1970–1971, at least one Army psychiatrist was assigned to the 3rd Surgical Hospital (Binh Thuy), and another was attached to the 483rd US Air Force Hospital (Cam Ranh Bay).

Also, the two psychiatric detachments were located as follows:

- The 935th Psychiatric Detachment was attached to the 93rd Evacuation Hospital on Long Binh post near Saigon from December 1965 until near the end of the war. In April 1971, its inpatient unit became attached to the 24th Evacuation Hospital, also on Long Binh post.
- The 98th Psychiatric Detachment was attached to 8th Field Hospital at Nha Trang from May 1966 through mid-1970 (Figure 4-1), when it moved further north on the coast to the Da Nang area where it became attached to the 95th Evacuation Hospital. It remained there until it was inactivated near the end of the war.

EVACUATION AND FIELD HOSPITALS STAFFED WITH SOLO PSYCHIATRISTS

Structure of Psychiatric Services in the Evacuation and Field Hospitals

The evacuation and field hospitals without attached neuropsychiatric specialty detachments were allocated only one psychiatrist position and none for social work officers, psychologists, psychiatric nurses, or mental health paraprofessionals (enlisted specialists).[3] Psychiatrists were assigned to these hospitals depending on anticipated need and psychiatrist availability. There they functioned solely in a clinical capacity, providing mostly inpatient care and consultation for the soldiers who were referred from the various nondivisional units in their area. The fact that they had no specialized staff meant they could not typically provide a dedicated psychiatric inpatient ward. However, local deviations did occur in some instances when hospital commanders were faced with unmanageable clinical demand.[3]

Soldiers who failed to respond within approximately 10 days to simple inpatient treatments at these hospitals were evacuated to one of the two psychiatric detachments in Vietnam. Staffing limitations also reduced the capacity of these psychiatrists to provide outpatient services and mental health consultation to the command cadre of nearby units. Command consultation

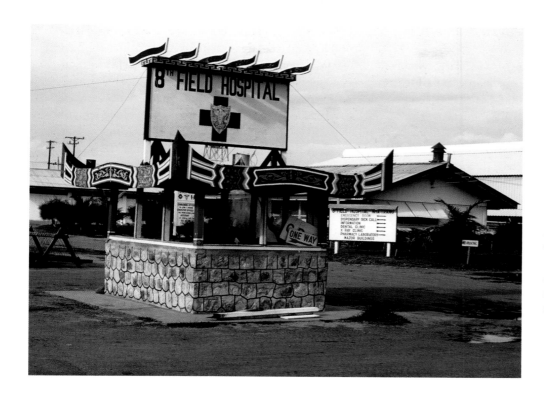

FIGURE 4-1. Entrance to the 8th Field Hospital, Nha Trang, midway along the coast of South Vietnam, 1969. The 98th Psychiatric Detachment was attached to the 8th Field Hospital from May 1966, when it was first deployed in Vietnam, through early 1970 when it moved farther north to the Da Nang area and became attached to the 95th Evacuation Hospital. Photograph courtesy of Richard D Cameron, Major General, US Army (Retired).

was additionally constrained by the fact that the hospital psychiatrists were not organizationally connected to these units as they were in the combat divisions. As a result of these shortcomings, some areas, especially those containing large numbers of nondivisional units, experienced chronic difficulties in the management and outpatient treatment of soldiers with psychiatric and behavior problems (this was especially true for the Qui Nhon and Cam Ranh Bay areas—See Johnson's panel remarks in Appendix 7).

Accounts by Psychiatrists Assigned as Solo Specialists to Field and Evacuation Hospitals

Among the estimated three dozen psychiatrists who served as solo specialists with the Army field and evacuation hospitals during the ground war, only a few provided an overview of their experience. These are summarized below, and selected aspects will be reviewed in more detail in subsequent chapters. Also, a few Army psychiatrists published reports of circumscribed problems treated at these facilities, and they will be mentioned in subsequent chapters as well. Reports by psychiatrists who were assigned to the two psychiatric detachments are summarized in the next section.

During the advisor phase, Army-trained Major Estes Copen was assigned in South Vietnam to provide psychiatric care for US military personnel (October 1962 and February 1963). Although Copen did not provide an account of his professional activities, the following quote survived:

> Support troops, although exposed to little physical danger or hardship, nevertheless were stressed by separation from family, boredom, and job frustration. These men were frequently seen because of excessive drinking, psychosomatic complaints, and behavioral problems. [These] individuals . . . were contrasted with advisors to combat units in which there was constant physical danger and far less comfortable environmental surroundings. These stresses resulted in casualties referred to as combat fatigue, although this entity tended frequently to be disguised in the form of antisocial behavior or vague physical symptoms.[4]

There is no record of Copen's treatment of these casualties, but he did indicate that those with significant emotional or behavioral problems were transferred out of South Vietnam to avoid "unpleasant relationships with the host government."[4]

8th Field Hospital (Nha Trang) / 3rd Field Hospital (Saigon)

Captain Robert E Huffman, Medical Corps. Huffman was the first Army psychiatric specialist assigned in Vietnam (May 1965–May 1966) following the commitment of American ground troops. He published an account of his professional activities in Vietnam—initially with the 8th Field Hospital at Nha Trang, midway up the coast (before the 98th Psychiatric Detachment arrived), and then with the 3rd Field Hospital in Saigon.[5] Huffman had not received formal training in psychiatry, but he had received 14 weeks of on-the-job training at an Army hospital in the United States. Nonetheless, he expressed dismay at discovering that he was the only physician representing Army psychiatry through the first 4 months of his assignment in the theater. Until August, when additional Army psychiatrists began to arrive in Vietnam, he was responsible for all cases from units in the northern half of South Vietnam, whereas Army troops in the southern half were treated at the Navy hospital in Saigon.

Among his cases at the 8th Field Hospital and subsequently at the 3rd Field Hospital (N = 573 American military personnel), 74% were referred by battalion surgeons and dispensary physicians, with the remainder in trouble and sent by their commanders to insure that there was no psychiatric condition that would preclude administrative or judicial proceedings. Demographic data indicated that 97% of referrals were from enlisted ranks and 11% were draftees; 62% had not completed high school; 15.6% had previous psychiatric consultation; and 28% reported previous legal difficulties. Huffman also provided the following clinical observations:

- for 8%, "the stress of combat was related to the onset of emotional difficulties";
- 18.5% were diagnosed as having severe problems with alcohol intoxication;
- fewer than 1% had drug-induced reactions; and
- 6.1% had suicide attempts or gestures (one was completed).

3rd Field Hospital (Saigon)

Captain Arthur S Blank Jr, Medical Corps. Blank was a civilian-trained psychiatrist who served with the 1st Infantry Division and later with the 935th Psychiatric Detachment before being assigned to the 3rd Field Hospital (April 1966–September 1966).

A record of Blank's experiences with the 3rd Field Hospital can be found in his remarks in a 1967 panel discussion (Appendix 10).[6] The 3rd Field Hospital shared responsibility with the 17th Field Hospital for the medical care of the US military personnel in the Saigon area. These two facilities, along with the 93rd Evacuation Hospital (with its 935th Psychiatric Detachment), which was located 20 miles away on the American post at Long Binh, also provided direct care for combat units operating in the Mekong Delta (support and combat).

Although Blank's referrals came from a wide variety of primary care sources, that is, from battalion surgeons in the field, dispensaries in Saigon, doctors assigned to ships off the coast, and flight surgeons in aviation battalions in the Delta, the evacuation system at that time was in a state of flux, and soldier-patients were just as likely to be taken to the 17th Field Hospital Saigon or the 93rd Evacuation Hospital/935th Psychiatric Detachment. During his first 3 months with the 3rd Field Hospital, Saigon was unusually tense because of the clashes between the Buddhists and the Catholics as well as episodic Viet Cong terrorist activity in the form of grenades thrown in jeeps, sniping, burning of vehicles, and mortar attacks on US facilities. However, only one individual was admitted to either hospital in Saigon with an apparent psychiatric reaction to these events. Blank was left with the impression that the terrorist behavior did not generate significant psychiatric problems among the assigned American military population.

According to Blank, his workload at the 3rd Field Hospital was manageable, but matters of administration and communication took an inordinate amount of time. During his 6 months there he saw approximately 300 outpatients and treated 61 inpatients (length of stay averaged under 5 days; daily census averaged two patients). Blank provided only a little clinical information regarding his inpatients. Demographically, only two (3%) were combat soldiers (whereas 20% of all psychiatric referrals were from combat units, indicating that noncombat troops from combat units were overrepresented). Also, 25 (41%) inpatients had psychiatric histories before Vietnam, and 12 (20%) were initially admitted by other physicians for psychosomatic problems. This last observation led him to speculate there may be substantial numbers of covert psychiatric casualties in Vietnam who are in the care of nonpsychiatrists. Also, he reported there was one completed suicide of a chronically depressed alcoholic sergeant.

Blank noted that his referrals had a minor peak at around 4 weeks after a soldier's arrival in Vietnam, with a much larger peak at about 5 months in-country. The predominant diagnosis overall was transient situational reaction. Approximately one-fourth of his referrals (70–80) were categorized as passive-dependent personalities who developed an anxiety syndrome within 4 to 6 weeks of arrival in Vietnam as a consequence of difficulties separating from mothers or wives and the extraordinary hours that most personnel worked (12–16 hours/day, 7 days/week). With the help of psychotherapy and Librium these individuals were able to maintain their duty performance levels.

Another 50 (17%) referrals were from commanders seeking psychiatric clearance for administrative separation from the service. These were overtly hostile soldiers who had repeated incidents of either verbal abuse or physical assault on superiors, usually while armed and often with some degree of intoxication. These soldiers were mostly untreatable. Although tending to have had an absent or inadequate father in their development, because they were careerists and had good military records before Vietnam, Blank was puzzled. "There was something about being in Vietnam, something about the situation, something about the war, something about the invitation to violence, which had changed their attitudes with respect to the military."[6]

However, Blank refuted an explanation centered on demoralization secondary to antiwar sentiment. (To illustrate the extreme challenge of these types of soldiers, in the panel proceedings Jones added: "Reference is made to an incident in which one of Blank's patients brought a grenade into his office and exploded it after warning him to leave. Although Blank was uninjured, the patient sustained frontal lobe brain damage."[6 (p58)]) Also see Chapter 8 for results of Jones' review of diagnostic and demographic data for 120 consecutive enlisted referrals at the 3rd Field Hospital during the 6 months following Blank.

Captain John A. Talbott, Medical Corps. A limited follow-on to Blank's experience with the 3rd Field Hospital came from Captain Talbott, a civilian-trained psychiatrist, who served there (February 1968–May 1968) almost 2 years later. Talbott reported observations and psychiatric incidence figures surrounding the intense fighting waged in and around Saigon in conjunction with the enemy's 1968 surprise Tet offensives (January

31st through the end of February 1968). He recalled the common characterization of the "Saigon Warrior" ("an overweight, contented man working decent hours at a regular jobs, surrounded by bars, bar-girls, restaurants, taxis, and all the trappings of civilization") and noted that, "in one night [it all] changed from the Paris of the East to the Algiers, from war stories to war experiences, and from luxury to horror. Street-fighting, dive-bombing, snipers, and nightly mortars and rockets replaced the entertainment."[7(p60)]

Among his first 100 patients, 18 manifested anxiety related to the fighting, and another six he labeled combat reactions (a "transient disorganized" syndrome). Among the latter, he indicated that the incidence rate for these was 6 times that of the preceding 6 months. Of the remaining cases, 44 were diagnosed as character and behavior disorders, with 26 of those subcategorized as alcoholics. Still, the number of individuals psychologically affected by the fighting was smaller than predicted, which led Talbott to conclude that the personnel who lived and worked in the relative luxury of Saigon were at no greater risk for combat reactions than would have been predicted for a similar sized infantry unit.[7]

17th Field Hospital (Saigon)

Captain William F Kenny, Medical Corps. Blank's psychiatric counterpart in Saigon, Kenny, a civilian-trained psychiatrist, came to Vietnam in May 1966 and was assigned to the 17th Field Hospital. Kenny's account of the psychiatric challenges he faced over his 8 months there was limited to the types of psychiatric disorders that presented among Saigon's urban (support) personnel, and he did not refer to the combat troops in the area. In fact, he categorically stated that he saw almost no cases where precipitating factors included the strain of combat.

According to Kenny, his daily inpatient caseload averaged two or three (with an average stay of 3–4 days), which was similar to that of Blank's at the 3rd Field Hospital. If a patient's condition did not respond to acute care, he was evacuated to the nearby 93rd Evacuation Hospital/935th Psychiatric Detachment on Long Binh post. Kenny's outpatient visits averaged 110 to 120 per month, or roughly four each day (40% for evaluation and 60% for treatment). They often presented as acute, transient, anxiety states—including under the influence of alcohol—but many were diagnosed as depressions, chronic anxiety states, emotionally unstable personalities, or psychopathic personalities. Their difficulties stemmed from heightened dependency needs, underlying separation anxiety, and primitive defense mechanisms.

Psychotherapeutic strategies involved encouraging them to verbalize their angry feelings toward the authorities whom they perceived were responsible for their situation, setting firm limits, and the therapist offering himself as a figure for positive identification—as well as use of a mild tranquilizer (no specifics). Kenny also conducted a study of 64 soldiers (nonpatient) seeking official permission to marry Vietnamese women and found them to be mostly immature, dependent men who had fears of being dominated by women and a consequent preference for a presumably submissive Vietnamese wife.[8]

67th Evacuation Hospital (Qui Nhon)
Captain Gary L Tischler, Medical Corps.
Contemporaneously with Blank and Kenny in Saigon, Tischler (Figure 4-2), an Army psychiatrist who was also civilian-trained, was assigned to the 67th Evacuation Hospital at Qui Nhon (March 1966–March 1967), which was located on the coast of South Vietnam, midway between Saigon to the south and Da Nang to the north. In contrast to the large urban population surrounding the Saigon hospitals, the catchment area for the 67th Evacuation Hospital consisted of a sprawling collection of nondivisional, mostly support, units. In a brief publication, Tischler noted that most of the patients he saw fell into three types: (1) those affected by combat stress; (2) those with dependent, symbiotic personalities who were disabled by the requirement for functioning overseas; and (3) those with preservice patterns of conflict with societal norms.[9]

Much more extensive was Tischler's description of the dominant patterns of stress and adaptation affecting all those deployed in that area of the combat zone in 1966 and 1967, primarily as seen through the perspectives of the patients he treated.[10] What impressed him most were the phases of adaptation (or in some instances, maladaptation) of the typical soldier as he struggled with the environmental hazards and privations attendant to the individualized 1-year tour in Vietnam. The peak psychiatric casualty rate was in the first 90 days, which gradually diminished over the next 6 months, followed by a rapid drop over the last 90 days. Although Tischler did not provide an overview of the psychiatric activities at the 67th Evacuation Hospital,

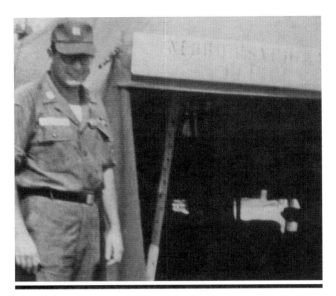

FIGURE 4-2. Captain Gary L Tischler, Medical Corps, psychiatrist with the 67th Evacuation Hospital in Qui Nhon. Early in the war, between March 1966 and March 1967, Tischler was assigned to the 67th Evacuation Hospital, which had recently deployed in Vietnam to Qui Nhon, located on the coast of South Vietnam between Nha Trang to the south and Da Nang to the north. The primary mission for the 67th Evacuation Hospital was to provide medical care for a large collection of nondivisional, mostly support, units in the area. Tischler, who was civilian-trained, was the only psychiatrist who served solo in an Army hospital that was not located in Saigon who published an account of his professional experiences. Photograph courtesy of Gary L Tischler.

in reviewing the demographic features of 200 enlisted referrals and their diagnostic breakdown, he did permit a view of the psychiatric challenge there (Table 4-1).

Whereas Tischler alluded to soldiers affected by combat stress ("[a] number of men were referred after being overwhelmed in an encounter of high hazard potency"), short-timer's syndrome, and combat aversion, it is not evident where these cases fit in his diagnostic groupings. They may have been included under the transient situational disorder category; however, their numbers may have been very low anyway because most of the troops treated at the 67th Evacuation Hospital were support troops. Like the reports from hospital psychiatrists from early in the buildup phase (Blank and Kenny), Tischler did not explicitly mention illegal drugs. On the other hand, also like them, he indicated that alcoholic intoxication was frequently found to be associated with suicidal and assaultive behavior.

TABLE 4-1. Estimated Diagnostic Distribution Among Enlisted Referrals to the 67th Evacuation Hospital, March 1966–March 1967 (N = 200)

Diagnosis	% of referrals
Psychotic reactions	3%
Psychoneurosis	10%
Transient situational disorders	18%
Character-behavior reactions	58.5%
Other, including neurological disorders	10.5%
	100%

Data source: Tischler GL. Patterns of psychiatric attrition and of behavior in a combat zone. In: Bourne PG, ed. *The Psychology and Physiology of Stress: With Reference to Special Studies of the Viet Nam War.* New York, NY: Academic Press; 1969: 26 (Table 1).

Additional perspectives on psychiatric challenges at the 67th Evacuation Hospital came from Colbrach (Figure 4-3), who summarized findings from his study (with Crowe) described in Chapter 8 that demonstrated an increased incidence of psychiatric problems among soldiers inducted into the Army under a program of relaxed educational and physical requirements ("Project 100,000"); a clinical report by Colbach (with Crowe) described in Chapter 9 regarding marijuana psychosis cases and increasing use of barbiturates by troops in the region; and Master's report on the growing polydrug use problems seen the following year, Chapter 9.

Discussion of Documentation by Those Who Served as Solo Psychiatrists With Field and Evacuation Hospitals

These accounts permit some appreciation for the psychiatric challenges early in the war and the commendable service these psychiatrists provided; however, it is unfortunate that only five individuals provided a record of their experiences while assigned to Army field or evacuation hospitals as solo psychiatrists. Furthermore, generalizability is not possible because, except for Talbott's circumscribed observations from early in 1968, the other reports are limited to the initial 2 years of the war (1965 and 1966). As noted previously, combat intensity and associated stress increased after that point, and deployment stress levels accelerated after 1968. The value of these reports is also somewhat limited because, with the exception of Tischler's from the 67th Evacuation Hospital, they

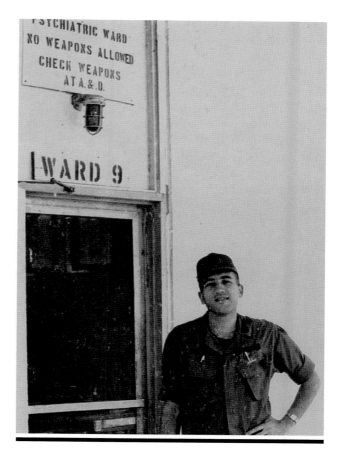

FIGURE 4-3. Captain Edward M Colbach, Medical Corps, psychiatrist with the 67th Evacuation Hospital in Qui Nhon. Colbach was a civilian-trained psychiatrist who was assigned to the 67th Evacuation Hospital at Qui Nhon between November 1968 and October 1969, the peak year for Army troop strength in Vietnam. He is notable for his publications (with Crowe) describing clinical experiences with marijuana psychosis cases and reviewing the psychiatric problems presenting among soldiers inducted into the Army under a program of relaxed educational and physical requirements. Also, Colbach's post-war overview (with Parrish) of the Army's psychiatric experience in Vietnam through 1970 permitted a fuller appreciation of the dominant forms of morale and psychiatric problems seen by the midpoint of the war. Photograph courtesy of Edward M Colbach.

center on experiences at the 17th Field Hospital and the 3rd Field Hospital, both of which were in Saigon. The 25,000 to 30,000, mostly noncombat, personnel operating in Saigon served in a crowded and hectic Vietnamese urban environment and were occasionally subjected to guerrilla attacks by the enemy—a distinctly different combat ecology than was faced by soldiers operating in the rest of South Vietnam.

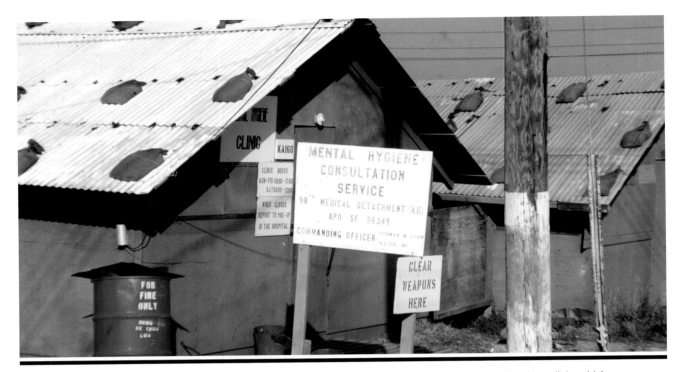

FIGURE 4-4. The 98th Neuropsychiatric Medical Specialty Detachment (KO) headquarters and mental hygiene clinic, which was attached to the 95th Evacuation Hospital outside of Da Nang, in the fall of 1970. Earlier in the year the 98th "KO Team" had relocated there from Nha Trang, farther south along the coast, where it had initially been attached to the 8th Field Hospital. The 98th (KO) was one of two definitive psychiatric treatment facilities in Vietnam. Its principal mission was to provide specialized hospital-level care (up to 30 days) for troops evacuated by Army psychiatrists operating in the northern half of South Vietnam and to stage out-of-country evacuations for patients needing additional care. It also provided outpatient services for the large number of nondivisional units in the area and scattered along the northern coast of South Vietnam. Photograph courtesy of Norman M Camp, Colonel, US Army (Retired).

Each of the psychiatrists in this set included rather different types of information with little apparent synchronization regarding diagnostic criteria and groupings or measures of psychiatric attrition (rates or proportions of those hospitalized, returned to duty, or evacuated to the psychiatric specialty detachments). Still, the data suggest that the incidence of inpatient-level psychiatric problems was relatively low, and that, despite having few or no specialized staff available, these hospital-based psychiatrists were able to reasonably manage a steady stream of referrals representing a mix of problems more centered on combat theater stress than combat stress. (See Johnson's panel remarks in Appendix 7 for contrary evidence with respect to the Qui Nhon support area/67th Evacuation Hospital.) In fact, there is little mention of combat stress casualties per se among this group except for Tischler's passing reference to combat stress as etiologically significant in some cases, and Talbott's observations and demographic data pertaining to the psychiatric casualties generated

among noncombat personnel in Saigon because of the Tet fighting in 1968. In contrast, Blank, who served at the 3rd Field Hospital during the first year of the war, noted that over a 6-month span, only two soldiers were transferred to him from the combat divisions.

Although Huffman mentioned drug abuse very early in the war (<1% of referrals), he is the only one; however, all five psychiatrists reported substantial alcohol-related problems. Notably, none suggested they maintained any consultative dialogue with unit commanders. This is not surprising given the limitations of psychiatric staffing in these hospitals and the fact that the hospitals were organizationally distinct from the surrounding units. However, because all of these psychiatrists received their psychiatric training in civilian programs, they may also have favored a model of individual pathogenesis as opposed to one embracing the interplay of the soldier's psychological dynamics with the small group dynamics within his unit.

THE TWO NEUROPSYCHIATRIC MEDICAL SPECIALTY DETACHMENTS (KO TEAMS)

Structure of Psychiatric Care in the Neuropsychiatric Medical Specialty Detachments: The 935th (KO) and the 98th (KO) Teams

The Neuropsychiatric Medical Specialty Detachments, the so-called KO teams, primarily treated soldiers who failed to respond sufficiently to short-term hospital treatment by the division psychiatrists or the solo psychiatrists at the evacuation or field hospitals (Figure 4-4). The mission for the KO detachments was to establish 3rd echelon psychiatric treatment and evacuation centers that would provide the full range of inpatient care for up to 30 days.[11] Cases requiring additional specialized care were evacuated out of Vietnam to Army treatment facilities in Japan, Hawaii, and the continental US.[12] If the KO detachment staff members concluded a soldier-patient was unlikely to recover within 30 days or be able to return to duty within Vietnam, they could evacuate him as soon as it could be arranged.[11]

KO teams also provided outpatient psychiatric care, referred to as mental health consultation services (MHCS), for the nondivisional units in their coverage area and hospitalized their soldiers when necessary. Overall, referrals from nondivisional units were either command-directed or were from the primary care physicians assigned to the various hospital-based dispensaries who provided 1st echelon medical and mental healthcare.

Because the 935th and the 98th Psychiatric Detachments were terminal psychiatric treatment facilities in the in-country evacuation chain, an important service they provided was a second level of psychiatric review regarding the medical necessity for evacuation out of Vietnam (US Army Republic of Vietnam Regulation No. 40-34[13]). As far back as the British experience in World War I, psychiatric observers noted a dramatic increase in psychiatric morbidity associated simply with removal from the combat theater.[12] Army medical planners for Vietnam also imposed this system of reassessment to minimize unnecessary manpower losses (including through what later became referred to as evacuation syndromes, ie, soldiers who may exaggerate their symptoms to be removed from the theater[14]). According to SL Baker Jr, a senior Army psychiatrist, in anticipation of such a possibility, "clear and firm policies [restricting] medical

evacuation were issued early by the [military medical] authorities there."[15(p1831)] However, as this chapter's introductory quotation indicated, this arrangement was not always popular.

Army TO&E 8-500D provided for the psychiatric detachment to be organized with the following professional staff: three psychiatrists, one neurologist, two social workers, one clinical psychologist, and one psychiatric nurse. The unit also was staffed with 12 to 15 enlisted corpsmen ("techs") who had additional military mental health training, for example, those with military occupational specialty (MOS) codes: 91-F (neuropsychiatric specialists), 91-G (social work specialists), and 91-H (clinical psychology specialists).[16] The psychiatric detachments were also allocated an electroencephalograph machine, and, because the psychiatric detachments were designated to be semi-mobile, three vehicles (two jeeps and a 2½-ton truck) and other specialized equipment, such as tents, which would permit rapid relocation to areas with greater need. However, like the Army hospitals in Vietnam, both of the psychiatric detachments operated as fixed facilities throughout the war. The one exception was the relocation of the 98th Psychiatric Detachment from the 8th Field Hospital in Nha Trang to the 95th Evacuation Hospital in Da Nang in early 1970. Finally, the inpatient wards were typically run as open units, and physical restraints were used on a brief and selective basis; the staff did not have the capability for providing electric convulsive therapy.

Reports by Psychiatrists and Allied Mental Health Personnel Assigned to Neuropsychiatric Medical Specialty Detachments (KO)

Below are summaries of the overviews provided by deployed Army psychiatrists that permit some appreciation of the professional challenges faced in the KO teams. Selected aspects will also be noted in subsequent chapters. A few psychiatrists published reports of circumscribed problems seen in these facilities, and these will be mentioned in subsequent chapters as well.

935th Neuropsychiatric Medical Specialty Detachment (KO) During the Early Buildup Phase (1965–1966)

The first KO team deployed in Vietnam was the 935th. It was formed at Valley Forge General Hospital in Pennsylvania in preparation for overseas movement. The staff and their equipment traveled to Vietnam by ship and arrived on 23 December 1965, and it became attached to the 93rd Evacuation Hospital on the Long Binh post 20 miles outside of Saigon.

Major John A Bowman, Medical Corps. Bowman was the first commander of the 935th Psychiatric Detachment (December 1965–October 1966). He had trained in psychiatry in an Army program, and his overview of the experiences of the 935th can be found in a transcript of a panel discussion held in 1967,[17] his unpublished manuscript,[18] and his "Unit History of the 935th Medical Detachment (KO), 20 September 1965 to 1 September 1966,"[16] also unpublished. Bowman's account, which mostly spanned his first 6 months in Vietnam, described how the 935th provided specialized psychiatric inpatient care for soldiers from Army combat and noncombat units throughout the country, 24 hours per day outpatient care, consultation services for noncombat units on a regional basis, and psychological services and consultation to the stockade. At that early point in the war, the combat units for whom the KO team provided 2nd and 3rd echelon psychiatric care included the 25th Infantry Division, the 1st Infantry Division, the 1st Cavalry Division (Airmobile), and the 173d Airborne Brigade of the 101st Airborne Division. According to Bowman, these were primarily Regular Army professional soldiers who were well motivated and skillfully led. Overall troop morale was reportedly high, despite the fact that combat units regularly conducted search and destroy missions, and no area was considered safe from ambush, terrorist activities, or sniper fire.

> However, the practical impediments the 935th KO team had to surmount were substantial: [Y]ou really don't have enough supplies to get along. For instance, we didn't have any electricity so we couldn't run a ward very well at night; we had no generators. . . . We had no lanterns. When we put in our request for supplies, we found out how snarled things really could be.[17(p61)]

The 935th KO team averaged about 300 referrals per month and carried a daily inpatient census of 10 to 12. Bowman and his staff rarely saw uncomplicated combat exhaustion cases because most such cases were effectively treated at the level of 1st echelon care, that is, by field medics and battalion aid station personnel within the combat units. Bowman's staff used two criteria in the diagnosis of combat exhaustion: (1)

history of exposure to actual combat, and (2) evidence of fatigue, whether produced by physical causes such as exertion, heat, dehydration, diarrhea, and loss of sleep, or by psychological causes such as anxiety and insomnia.

Overall Bowman and the KO team encountered a very low rate of combat exhaustion and an increase in character and behavioral disorders as time progressed. Fewer than 5% of referrals were for psychosis, usually paranoid schizophrenia or manic depression, and fewer than 2% were for combat exhaustion. The remainder consisted of stress reactions, including those secondary to separation from home, which were commonly expressed through psychosomatic symptoms or manifestations of anxiety, depression, agitation, or behavior problems, especially aggressive behavior problems. Regarding the behavior problems, Bowman stated, "In almost every case the soldier was defined as somebody that his unit could no longer tolerate."[17(p65)]

Bowman indicated that because their ward (census of 10–12 patients) was visibly open to the other wings housing convalescing medical and surgical patients, peer pressure served to reduce patient acting out. His inpatient staff included a nurse and 12 corpsmen. They utilized brief psychotherapy, "sedation when appropriate,"[17(p6)] and a therapeutic ward milieu whose emphasis was rapid recovery of function and return to duty in Vietnam. New admissions were given clean clothing, a shower, a warm meal, and told they were expected to assist the staff in maintaining an orderly ward. They were to keep their area clean, help police up the ward, and participate in outside details (fill sand bags, help build bunkers, etc). A patient NCOIC (noncommissioned officer-in-charge) was appointed to manage a "buddy" system wherein soldier-patients helped each other as well as exerted controls on each other's behavior. According to Bowman:

> Treatment of soldiers admitted to the inpatient ward reflected proven principles of preventive psychiatry. An atmosphere of expectancy of return to duty was maintained for all soldiers, and at the same time each man was expected to display the same military bearing, behavior, and courtesies as he would in his own unit. At all times the soldier was reminded that he was a part of the US Army in a combat situation and was expected to behave accordingly.[16(p2)]

He also emphasized that despite the remoteness of tactical units, the 935th KO Detachment placed a priority on maintaining the soldier-patient's military identity through having his unit make regular visits to him, bring him his mail, and pay him on the ward; and that thanks to helicopter mobility, line commanders were fully cooperative, even though a unit might be 250 miles away. About 90% of all hospitalized soldiers were returned to duty, a high rate that Bowman in part credited to the military-centered clinical perspective held by the psychiatrists of the 935th. ("Unless, upon evaluation the soldier proved to be frankly psychotic, the presenting symptom was rarely considered sufficient reason to evacuate the soldier from Viet Nam. . . . In most cases the soldiers gave up their symptoms . . . and returned to duty asymptomatic or with less severity of symptoms."[16(p2)]) (See Appendix 11, "Recent Experiences in Combat Psychiatry in Viet Nam," for a further discussion.)

Bowman was especially appreciative of the support provided by the enlisted specialists assigned to his team:

> These men always worked an 8-hour shift, sometimes . . . they worked 12 hours. After their work was over they had all kinds of details. There was guard duty, latrine duty, KP ["kitchen patrol"], vehicle maintenance, maintenance on their weapons, etc. So, these men were really soldiers, and they were well trained. . . . I just can't say too much about the school at Ft. Sam [Fort Sam Houston, Texas] and the kind of men that they sent us. They really made the KO team function.[17(p62)]

The 935th KO During the Peak Combat Activity Phase (1967–1968)

Chapter 3 reviewed the observations from four division psychiatrists (Bostrom, Baker, Pettera, and Motis) who served during 1967–1968—a period in which the troop buildup reached its peak and American troops engaged in some of the most intense fighting of the war. Collectively their reports provided some appreciation of the growing numbers of combat stress casualties seen at the level of 1st and 2nd echelon care in the combat divisions. Fortunately three Army psychiatrists assigned to the 935th (KO) also served in that time frame and provided further documentation of the professional challenges associated with these events. Their reports are summarized below. By that point the other psychiatric detachment, the 98th KO, had arrived

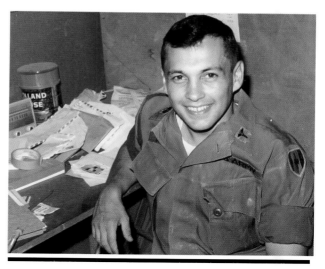

FIGURE 4-5. Captain H Spencer Bloch, Medical Corps, Director, Inpatient Psychiatry Service, 935th Neuropsychiatric Medical Specialty Detachment (KO). Bloch, a civilian-trained psychiatrist, served in Vietnam between August 1967 and July 1968 with the 935th KO team, which was attached to the 93rd Evacuation Hospital on Long Binh post near Saigon. Through his publications and notes he retained from his tour he played a critical role in documenting the more serious psychiatric challenges faced by the Army in Vietnam during the period of highest combat intensity. Photograph courtesy of H Spencer Bloch.

and assumed responsibility for psychiatric referrals in the northern half of the country (I and II Corps); thus the 935th was only responsible for units in the southern half (III and IV Corps).

Captain H Spencer Bloch, Medical Corps. Bloch (Figure 4-5), a civilian-trained Army psychiatrist, served as Director, Inpatient Psychiatry Service at the 935th Psychiatric Detachment between August 1967 and July 1968. He arrived a year after Bowman left. Two publications by Bloch permit a rich review of the psychiatric experience at the 935th during his year.[19,20] The outpatient service of the 935th provided care principally for nondivisional units and saw roughly 750 psychiatric patient visits per month. The inpatient service averaged 60 new cases per month, with a mean daily census of 12. Inpatients typically came in the form of admissions from the outpatient psychiatric service and refractory cases from the combat divisions and brigades and the other evacuation and field hospitals. Direct admissions also came from combat units in the area when it was necessitated by the tactical situation. Table 4-2 presents Bloch's diagnosis and disposition

TABLE 4-2. Diagnostic Groupings Among 600 Consecutive Admissions to the 935th Medical Detachment (KO) Inpatient Service Between 21 August 1967 and 27 July 1968*

Diagnosis	% of admissions (n)	Average hospital stay (days)	% returned to duty in Vietnam
Psychosis†	44.0% (264)	14	56%
Acute situational reaction	17.5% (105)	8	90%
Psychoneurosis	12.3% (74)	6	85%
Character-behavior reaction	11.2% (67)	8	90%
Alcohol and drug problems	6.8% (41)	2	98%
Combat exhaustion	5.7% (34)	3	100%
Observation/no NP disease (includes neurology patients)	2.5% (15)	N/A	80%

*59 patients (10%) were admitted a second time, and nine were admitted a third time. It is unclear whether these nine were included in the 59.
†32 psychosis patients were admitted a second time, and six were admitted a third time. It is unclear whether those admitted a third time were included in the 32.
N/A: not applicable
NP: neuropsychiatric
Data source: Bloch HS. Army clinical psychiatry in the combat zone 1967–1968. *Am J Psychiatry*. 1969;126(3):289–298,

breakdown among 600 consecutive admissions to the 935th Detachment/93rd Evacuation Hospital.

Although Bowman did not provide a comparable set of inpatient statistics from 2 years earlier, Bloch's 5.7% for combat exhaustion cases among his inpatients compared with Bowman's 2% is consistent with the sharp rise in combat intensity between 1966 and 1968.

Bloch and his staff sought to provide "psychiatrically sophisticated" treatment that took into account the context of this new type of war—a low-intensity conflict dominated by counterinsurgency/guerrilla tactics. The design of their inpatient service combined the traditional principles of the combat psychiatry doctrine ("immediacy, proximity, and expectancy") with concepts of milieu therapy to create a therapeutic community for all patients—not just those affected by combat stress (Exhibit 4-1, "The Therapeutic Milieu in the 935th (KO) Neuropsychiatric Specialty Detachment"). The ward routine included group therapy, work details, recreation programs, and a patient government—all within a quasimilitary atmosphere intended to reestablish the soldier-patient's military group identity and underscore the preeminence of the military mission ("conserve the fighting strength"[19(p292)]). The premium was placed on environmental manipulation and interpersonal techniques, versus intrapsychic approaches.

Professional military psychiatrists are essentially interpersonal psychiatrists, whose approach is oriented toward interventions in the interpersonal dimensions of the patients' problems. Their experience has proven that they can most efficiently utilize their time and skill by intervening in this manner rather than concentrating on underlying internal emotional conflicts, which are often thought to take much longer periods of time to resolve. [Thus] in helping a man back to a more functional state and maintaining him there, military psychiatrists work in two directions: aiding the man in developing behavior that is more tolerable to others, and getting his unit to become more accepting of idiosyncratic behavior that does not impede its mission.[19(p292)]

For selected inpatients the 935th KO provided psychoactive medications (especially Thorazine and Librium), as well as individual psychotherapy. In particular, Bloch and his colleagues, like division psychiatrists Bostrom and Bey, advocated a sleep therapy protocol (*dauerschlaf*) as the initial intervention for disorganized, agitated, or violent soldiers, regardless of the provisional diagnosis on admission.[20]

Finally, Bloch compared their results with those from the year before as follows: In the first 6 months of 1968, their military-centered milieu treatment program discharged 78% of patients back to duty in Vietnam. During the same time period the year before, when their predecessors operated what Bloch characterized as a diagnosis and disposition center, only 53% were

EXHIBIT 4-1. The Therapeutic Milieu in the 935th (KO) Neuropsychiatric Specialty Detachment

. . . [I]n establishing the treatment program it was decided to apply the three principles of combat psychiatry to all hospitalized patients. That is, the ideas of immediacy, proximity, and expectation were combined with concepts of milieu therapy to establish the ward as a therapeutic community aimed at the restitution of all men to duty.

The hospital in which this ward was located was composed of a series of one-story quonset buildings, each constructed in the form of a cross with four 16-bed wings diverging from a central area. The psychiatric ward comprised one wing in one of these buildings; the other three wings . . . were for preoperative and convalescent surgical patients. . . . The ward was completely open, without seclusion rooms, although all kinds of patients were treated there—psychotic and nonpsychotic, violent and withdrawn, officers and enlisted men, civilians, occasionally foreigners, and (rarely) women.

With such a diversity of patient type and lack of facilities for seclusion and isolation, expectation became vitally important in the ethos of treatment. A very high level expectation was maintained: patients were there to get well and to conduct themselves appropriately. Restraints and medications were available when patients' behavior was out of control or not controllable by other means, but actually restraints were required infrequently and rarely for more than a few hours at a time.

Regarding the milieu treatment program, all of the ward patients, even the sickest, got up together in the morning. They dressed in fatigue pants, T-shirts, and combat boots. . . . They ate together in the mess hall and then went to group therapy for one and a quarter hours, five mornings each week. Group therapy was run by the corpsmen and supervised by psychiatrists; it was oriented around the immediate difficulties that precipitated each patient's hospitalization. Following the group therapy session the patients cleaned up the ward together while the psychiatrist who had observed the meeting conducted a teaching session for the corpsmen who had led it. Then the patients went on a two-hour work detail together, . . . ate together, rested briefly, and then had a two-hour recreation period. Following this they showered, washed their clothes, and relaxed in a lounge playing cards, pool, or talking until dinner. Afterwards they held a patient government meeting on the ward.

They themselves decided about each patient's privilege status. A three-class system was utilized: Class I patients could not leave the ward without a corpsman; Class II patients could go off the ward with Class III patients; Class III patients could leave the ward unaccompanied when no group activity was scheduled. After the patient government meetings, the men watched television or wrote letters until bedtime.

The program was highly structured and geared toward much group activity as well as toward individual patient responsibility. Our rationale was that these men had run into some difficulty in interpersonal relationships in their units that caused them to be extruded from those groups. The therapeutic endeavor of this program was to facilitate the men's reintegration into their own groups (units) through integration into the group of ward patients. . . . [Although] we can consider intrapsychic psychopathology—that is, symptoms of emotional conflict and unrest within the individual . . . [since the aim of military psychiatry] . . . is to conserve the fighting strength . . . [we] want the man only to be able to function optimally, or as close to it as possible, in his or some other unit.

Reproduced with permission from Bloch HS. Army clinical psychiatry in the combat zone: 1967-1968. *Am J Psychiatry*. 1969;126:291–292.

discharged back to duty in Vietnam—a spread that suggests strikingly different clinical philosophies with significant outcome consequences. (See also in Appendix 12, Bloch's paper, "Interesting Reaction Types Encountered in a War Zone.")

Captain John A Talbott, Medical Corps. Before his assignment to the 3rd Field Hospital (mentioned earlier), Talbott served with the 935th Psychiatric Detachment (May 1967–February 1968). While there he participated in an ambitious community psychiatry program intended to extend primary and secondary prevention care to the troops in the catchment area, primarily those in units that were located on the sprawling post at Long Binh. The program, which utilized six mental health

professionals (psychiatry, psychology, and social work) and 10 enlisted social work/psychology technicians, offered outreach services and consultation for the Army stockade, 10 primary care medical dispensaries, the post chaplains, and units showing elevated rates for sick call or psychiatric referral. The program especially sought to identify military units that were experiencing internal difficulties to understand group factors contributing to individual psychopathology and to reduce the incidence of both individual and unit problems through active consultation/liaison with unit cadres. Although no outcome measures were presented by Talbott, he indicated that when commanders were open to consultation, the program was generally successful in increasing early psychiatric referrals of appropriate cases and reducing inappropriate referrals.[21]

Lieutenant Colonel Jack R Anderson, Medical Corps. Anderson, an Army-trained psychiatrist, served as the commanding officer of the 935th Psychiatric Detachment (September 1967–September 1968) at the same time Bloch and Talbott were assigned. Prior to obtaining his medical training, Anderson was an Army medical administrator in Europe in World War II and a clinical psychology officer stateside during the Korean War. His assignment in Vietnam immediately followed the completion of his psychiatry training at Letterman Army Hospital. Although his comments were general in nature, some appreciation of Anderson's experience in Vietnam could be gleaned from an interview soon after he returned to the United States. He spoke of becoming concerned with the "new breed" of delinquent and noneffective soldiers; soldiers exhibiting a schizophreniform toxic drug reaction (presumed secondary to marijuana use); and rising numbers of previously performing soldiers who became "dropper-outers."[9] In these observations, he appeared to have noticed early expressions of the demoralization and dissent that were gradually building in the theater.

Also, in a brief article published in the *USARV Medical Bulletin*,[22] Anderson expressed his opposition to assigning psychiatrists to the combat divisions in Vietnam and in effect offered a distinctly contrasting perspective to that prevailing in Army psychiatry. He believed the social psychiatry/unit consultation model had proved marginally successful within the combat divisions. His opinion derived from observations that there had been a low incidence of combat-generated psychiatric casualties, battalion surgeons had used phenothiazines effectively to treat these conditions, and helicopters had rapidly evacuated those who didn't respond to nearby hospitals. In Anderson's estimation the division-based social workers, social work/psychology technicians, and battalion surgeons appeared to be fully capable of handling the psychiatric problems in the divisions; consequently the division psychiatrists in the southern half of Vietnam would be more efficiently utilized if they were reassigned to the 935th Psychiatric Detachment.[22]

Additional perspectives on psychiatric challenges at the 935th Medical Detachment/93rd Evacuation Hospital in 1967 to 1968 came from Bloch regarding the soldier's adjustment during a year's tour in Vietnam (further discussed in Chapter 8); and Fidaleo on

marijuana use patterns and problems, Talbott on "pot (marijuana) reactions," and Talbott and Teague on marijuana-induced psychosis cases (in Chapter 9). The following year (September 1968–September 1969), Imahara described the increasing morale and behavior problems seen among the confinees of the US Army Republic of Vietnam Stockade (in Chapter 2); and Forrest described indicators of growing soldier polydrug use (in Chapter 9), as well as provided observations on the commercial sexual relationships between soldiers and Vietnamese women and the challenges faced by those who wished to marry (Chapter 8). From the drawdown years, Ives (August 1970–August 1971) described the heroin treatment provided for Army troops at the 483rd US Air Force Hospital at Cam Ranh Bay (Chapter 9), and Ratner (August 1970–August 1971) provided observations on the characteristics of heroin-using soldiers admitted to the Long Binh Post Amnesty Center (Chapter 2 and Chapter 9).

98th Neuropsychiatric Medical Specialty Detachment (KO)

In May 1966, 5 months after the 935th Psychiatric Detachment (KO) came ashore in Vietnam, its counterpart, the 98th Psychiatric Detachment (KO), arrived. It also traveled by troop ship, and it became located in Nha Trang in the central coastal region of South Vietnam. Initially the 98th was not attached to a hospital as the 935th was attached to the 93rd Evacuation Hospital. The 98th operated out of a medical clearing company, including its inpatient unit, a couple of miles from the 8th Field Hospital. This turned out not to be administratively and logistically practical so it was subsequently attached to the hospital and its inpatient ward relocated there; however the clinic/mental health consultation services (MHCS) activity stayed in the troop area some distance from the hospital. As already mentioned, once operational the 98th concentrated on serving Army units in the northern half of South Vietnam (I and II Corps) while the 935th continued to serve the units in the southern provinces. Three years later, in early 1970, the 98th relocated farther up the coast to the Da Nang area and became attached to the 95th Evacuation Hospital where it remained. Although there were an estimated two dozen psychiatrists assigned to the 98th KO team over its 6 years in Vietnam, except for its first year, little documentation of its activities is available.

Captain Louis R Conte, Medical Corps. Conte, a civilian-trained psychiatrist, was the first commander of the 98th Psychiatric Detachment (May 1966–May 1967). His overview of the activities of the 98th Detachment[23] suggested important differences from that of its sister detachment to the south, the 935th. First, evidently the caseload of the 98th was about a third lighter. Conte acknowledged the relatively low overall psychiatric casualty rate, made little mention of combat exhaustion cases specifically ("a relative minority of the problems that presented related directly to combat experience"[23(p167)]), and compared the outpatient caseload of the 98th Detachment, which averaged between three and four patients per day, to that found on a stateside post. Their outpatient catchment area was estimated by Conte to be 25,000 troops. Apparently most outpatients initially received an intense, multiday evaluation, often involving psychological testing, but ongoing outpatient treatment was rare because of transportation impediments. The 98th returned to duty 80% to 90% of the 1,000 or so outpatients they were referred ("[M]ost of the diagnoses were in the character and behavior disorder category"[23(p167)]). Their consultation service primarily provided secondary prevention (assessment of referrals, which, in some instances led to interaction with units), but team members also regularly visited the "community caretakers" (dispensary physicians, chaplains, Red Cross personnel, etc). Additionally, a psychiatrist, social worker, and technicians flew weekly to Cam Ranh Bay to conduct a satellite clinic for the many nondivisional Army units located there.

The 98th KO team averaged about one new inpatient admission per day, and, like the 935th, their bed capacity was 12. Most strikingly, they diagnosed 40%–50% of hospitalized patients with schizophrenia—an extremely high proportion—and they returned only 40% of inpatients to duty—an unusually low percentage. By Conte's account,

> [A]bout 50% of the patients we received were essentially untreatable from the perspective of rehabilitation for duty within 30 days. The ward then, for them at least, became little more than a way station preliminary to evacuation [out of Vietnam].[23(p165)]

Their inpatient therapeutic program included work therapy, recreational therapy, group therapy,

a patient government, and one unique feature: the detachment psychologist was regularly embedded into the ward milieu as a therapeutic participant-observer. Nonetheless, Conte reported considerable frustration associated with the "rapid influx of patients,"[23(p165)] burgeoning treatment requirements, and "much, much, paperwork."[23(p165)] Whereas his intention was that the ward "should be a place of humanness, giving, and feeding,"[23(p165)] the turnover pressure resulted in the ward becoming "more military and bureaucratically depersonalized,"[23(p165)] and the psychiatrist "felt more and more like a custodian administrator and less like a healer."[23(p165)] Finally, Conte was frank in acknowledging that he and his colleagues at the 98th "struggled to cope with our ambivalence toward the war, with anxieties and depression upon separation from our families . . . and with the exquisite frustrations from the primitive circumstances in which we lived."[23(p167)]

Captain Joel H Kaplan, Medical Corps. Kaplan was a civilian-trained psychiatrist who served as the commander of the 98th Psychiatric Detachment (November 1968–1969) while it was still located in Nha Trang and attached to the 8th Field Hospital. Some appreciation for the deteriorating clinical circumstances faced by him and his staff were provided through his publication regarding the drug problems in the northern half of Vietnam during his year[24] and his 1970 testimony before the Senate Subcommittee to Investigate Juvenile Delinquency.[25] According to Kaplan, 70% of psychiatric outpatients and 50% of psychiatric inpatients were drug abusers (defined as "using drugs heavily day in and day out"), with both combat and noncombat troops equally represented. To try to meet the demand, the 98th initiated a nightly group therapy program, but successes were mostly limited to soldiers close to the end of their tours. Kaplan acknowledged that there was no easy answer to the growing "subculture of drugs" in Vietnam, and he implored Congress to take action to address this serious and unacknowledged problem.[25]

Major Norman M Camp, Medical Corps. Camp [the author] was an Army-trained psychiatrist who served his tour in Vietnam (October 1970–October 1971) as the commander of the 98th Psychiatric Detachment, 4½ years after it arrived in Vietnam and a year following its relocation to Da Nang (Figure 4-6). This volume's Prologue presented Camp's account of the drawdown's bottoming morale in Vietnam and the rampant psychiatric and behavior consequences that greatly challenged the 98th KO team. These included

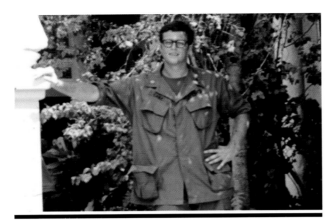

FIGURE 4-6. The author, Major Norman M Camp, Medical Corps, was an Army-trained psychiatrist who served in Vietnam between October 1970 and October 1971 as the commander of the 98th Neuropsychiatric Medical Specialty Detachment (KO), which was outside of Da Nang on the coast of the South China Sea. This photograph was taken in fall of 1970 while he was touring a Catholic-sponsored leper colony outside of Qui Nhon. Photograph courtesy of Norman M Camp, Colonel, US Army (Retired).

the rapidly spreading heroin epidemic and antimilitary behaviors, particularly soldiers threatening to assassinate their leaders.

Major Nathan Cohen, Medical Corps. Cohen was a civilian-trained psychiatrist who served with Camp as the Deputy Commander of the 98th Psychiatric Detachment (August 1970–1971). A record of Cohen's experience, which serves to corroborate Camp's observations, comes by way of a speech he made to the I Corps Medical Society (Da Nang, January 1971). In his remarks Cohen acknowledged the "raging (heroin) epidemic"; however, he was also frankly critical of the disjointed countermeasures by the Army in Vietnam, especially the poorly conceptualized and implemented Drug Amnesty Program and command's expectation that the solution should primarily be a medical and psychiatric one. According to Cohen, the majority of drug users in Vietnam had stable use patterns as long as their supply remained uninterrupted, and their day-to-day functioning was unimpaired, even if, to varying degrees, some were addicted. More critically, these soldiers did not agree with the Army that they had a problem. They blamed their drug use on being assigned in Vietnam and being "hassled by the lifers," or they maintained that the drug was controlling them.

Cohen also observed that the majority of heroin users who were referred to the 95th Evacuation Hospital/98th Psychiatric Detachment were not physically dependent (as tested with a narcotic antagonist). They exaggerated their symptoms so as to be hospitalized to evade duty responsibilities and disciplinary action ("ersatz R & R [ie, rest and recuperation]"). Compared to nonreferred users, those who were seen at the 98th KO either had character and behavior disorders or they were individuals with adolescent turmoil who were seriously maladapted to their circumstance in Vietnam. Cohen categorically refuted the general impression that they were psychiatrically ill and argued that this problem would not yield to the methods of clinical medicine or psychiatry. He recommended a broad-based, command-centered approach—with medical support—that assumed drug abuse was an expression of a much wider morale problem. Such an approach would emphasize "limit setting and the instilling of realistic models for dealing with the inherently frustrating nature [of serving in Vietnam]."[26(p9)]

Further perspectives on psychiatric challenges at the 98th Psychiatric Detachment are found in the Prologue and in the summary of social work officer Meshad's narrative describing his ethical struggle in 1969–1970 (in Chapter 11).

Discussion of the Documentation by Psychiatrists Who Served With the Neuropsychiatric Medical Specialty Detachments

Just as the earlier effort to reconstruct the history of Army psychiatry in Vietnam from the reports of the division psychiatrists and those assigned as solo psychiatrists to the evacuation and field hospitals was limited by the many gaps in information, the record provided by those who served with the specialized psychiatric detachments is similarly incomplete. Not only were the available reports inconsistent in the types of information provided, they also tended to be skewed toward the first half of the war and the southern psychiatric detachment, the 935th. Otherwise, with the exception of Ratner's portrayal of the clinical ordeal associated with the heroin epidemic at the Army Amnesty Center on Long Binh Post in 1971, there was little to represent the 935th between 1969 and 1972 when the last combat units left Vietnam. With regard to the 98th, Conte's description of circumstances there during its first year in Vietnam stands alone until the late war years when Kaplan's depiction of the clinical challenges associated with the growing marijuana problem, this author's postwar account (Prologue), and the talk by Cohen convey a picture of a hectic, dysfunctional drawdown Army.

The available information did indicate that the deployed mental health personnel assigned to the two KO teams worked very hard under very challenging circumstances, both physically and clinically, and provided commendable service. In fact, Bloch's description of his inpatient service at the 935th during the most intense period of combat activity served as a model treatment program given the circumstances. Similarly, Talbott's description of the consultation-liaison program spawned by the 935th that same year set an example for the provision of preventive services for a large collection of nondivisional support and service-support units in a combat zone. (Notably, his program is the only reference to command consultation activities provided by the psychiatric personnel assigned to the psychiatric detachments.)

With regard to clinical outcomes, Conte indicated that the 98th Detachment's inpatient service only returned 40% of patients to duty during its first year deployed (1966–1967). This was dramatically discrepant from Bowman's report that the 935th Detachment returned to duty 90% of hospitalized patients during roughly the same year of the war. Similarly remarkable, Conte reported that 40% to 50% of their patients were hospitalized for schizophrenia compared to the 5% reported by the 935th for "psychosis" (obviously not identical). It seems reasonable to speculate that the much higher rates for schizophrenia diagnosis by the 98th Detachment, as well as their much higher rates for evacuation out of Vietnam, in large part resulted from Conte's team's acknowledged civilian-centered clinical perspective ("healer"), in contrast to the military mission-centered one espoused by Bowman and the 935th—an emphasis derived from Bowman's strong military training and experience background (like the earlier comparison of division psychiatrists Jones, Bey, and Byrdy). However, Bloch's 78% return-to-duty rate a couple of years later was also much higher than Conte's, yet like Conte, Bloch was new to Army service and had no predeployment military experience. When asked about this, Bloch acknowledged that he was undoubtedly influenced by his father, who had combat experience in World War II, and by Anderson, his commanding officer at the 935th, who was trained in psychiatry by the Army and who had an extensive pre-Vietnam military background.[27] Chapters 5 and 11 will provide a fuller discussion of such potentially

divergent clinical philosophies that may stem from such background differences.

US Marine Corps/Navy Experience Offshore in Vietnam

The Navy did not establish 3rd echelon care hospitals in South Vietnam. Marines and Navy personnel who required treatment beyond that provided in the medical units ashore or the field hospitals were evacuated to either of the Navy's two hospital ships, the USS *Sanctuary* and the USS *Repose*, or out of the combat zone (to Okinawa, the Philippines, Japan, or the United States). Two Navy psychiatrists, Robert E Strange and Ransom J Arthur, published a report summarizing their experience aboard the USS *Repose* treating 143 psychiatric cases admitted between February 1966 and August 1966. Notably, at that early point in the war they highlighted the overall low psychiatric attrition rate in Vietnam for which they credited the "high sense of purpose and commitment on the part of the individuals facing combat." Their daily census averaged 12 to 15 patients. Intakes averaged 1.7 cases per day. The length of stay averaged 13.5 days, and they returned to duty approximately 50% of cases. (Subsequently, Strange said that 62% were returned to duty and 38% were evacuated out of the theater.[28]) In contrast with reports from the Army psychiatrists, their report presented additional demographic information as well as that pertaining to extent of combat exposure as a potential risk factor. They were also more explicit regarding use of pharmacotherapy and differences in return-to-duty rates comparing psychotic, psychoneurotic, and character and behavior disorders (Table 4-3).[29]

THE ARMY'S SENIOR THEATER PSYCHIATRIST: THE NEUROPSYCHIATRY CONSULTANT TO THE COMMANDING GENERAL/US ARMY, REPUBLIC OF VIETNAM SURGEON

The Position of US Army, Republic of Vietnam Neuropsychiatry Consultant

The position of USARV Neuropsychiatry Consultant, typically referred to simply as the Psychiatry Consultant, completes the description of the Army psychiatrist assignments in Vietnam. This individual was the senior Army psychiatrist in Vietnam and served on the staff of the Commanding General, US

FIGURE 4-7. Colonel Matthew D Parrish, Medical Corps, being awarded the Legion of Merit in Vietnam. Parrish served in Vietnam between July 1967 and July 1968 as the third Neuropsychiatry Consultant to the Commanding General, US Army Republic of Vietnam Surgeon. In this position he monitored psychiatric casualties and treatment capabilities throughout the theater, directed the coordination of psychiatric facilities and program planning, and advised the Army commander regarding psychiatric matters. Photograph courtesy of Marilyn Parrish.

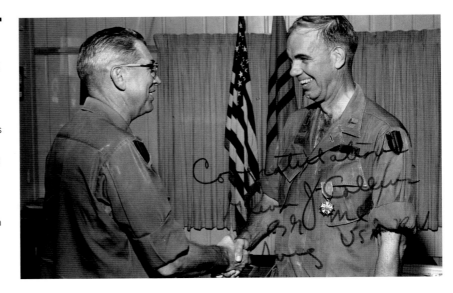

Army, Republic of Vietnam (CG/USARV) Surgeon. The Psychiatry Consultant's principle tasks were to monitor psychiatric casualties and treatment capabilities throughout the theater, direct the coordination of psychiatric facilities and program planning, and advise the Army commander regarding psychiatric matters. Although based at US Army Headquarters on the post at Long Binh, they traveled extensively throughout Vietnam, visited psychiatrists and programs, provided clinical leadership, and consulted with senior military leaders about issues affecting mental health and fitness.

The psychiatry consultant was also required to coordinate mental health operations with the US Air Force and Navy medical systems, which had their own psychiatric elements. At times there was a similar necessity to coordinate with counterparts within the Korean Army and the few psychiatrists serving with the Army of the Republic of Vietnam. Ultimately, nine Army psychiatrists served in this position between November 1965 and November 1972. Regrettably, none of the psychiatry consultants published accounts of their tour in Vietnam. However, some perspective can be gleaned from information from four of them provided through other means.

The US Army Republic of Vietnam Neuropsychiatry Consultants

Lieutenant Colonel John Gordon, Medical Corps

Gordon was the first USARV Psychiatry Consultant (November 1965–September 1966). He was a graduate of an Army psychiatry-training program and had over

12 years of experience as an Army psychiatrist before assuming this position in Vietnam.

Lieutenant Colonel Arnold W Johnson Jr, Medical Corps

Johnson was a Korean War veteran and received his psychiatric training in an Army residency program. He served as the second Psychiatry Consultant (July 1966–July 1967). In a 1967 panel discussion, Johnson provided an extensive overview of the psychiatric challenges faced by the Army early in the war, especially those consequent to the inevitable confusion attendant to the rapid influx of troops under combat conditions and the practical problems involving housing, communications, and especially transportation.[3]

With regard to combat troops, Army units were often widely scattered, ground transportation was risky, and the medical evacuation helicopters were not assigned directly to the combat units but operated on a regional basis. This meant the pattern of medical evacuation frequently deviated from the Army's echelon structure in which medical treatments were to be provided closest to the soldier's parent unit. The often-improvised area coverage of medical and psychiatric care that arose as a consequence did not seem to present major problems regarding combat-generated psychiatric problems because they were relatively infrequent. Most of those that did occur did not require evacuation as they were effectively handled at the 1st echelon care level by enlisted corpsmen in tandem with the battalion surgeons (at times assisted by enlisted social work/psychology technicians).

TABLE 4-3. Major Diagnostic Groupings for 143 Navy and Marine Admissions to the Psychiatric Service of the USS *Repose* Between February 1966 and August 1966*

Diagnosis	Character and Behavior Disorder (67%)	Psychoneurotic Disorder (20%)	Psychotic Disorder (13%)
Age in years	21.4	25	22.6
Rank	Majority were E-2	E-4 and above	Mostly E-3 and E-4
Military experience	Short, with disciplinary problems	> 3 years	No information provided
Married	35%	52%	23%
History of agitation, violence	45%	18%	18%
Combat exposure	63%	79%	32%
Combat judged to be a major precipitant	49%	47%	16%
Those treated with drugs	54%	82%	90%
Those returned to full duty	52%	75%	none

*By selected demographics, extent of exposure to combat, etiologic importance of combat stress, percentage treated with pharmacotherapy, and percentage returned to full duty.
Data source: Strange RE, Arthur RJ. Hospital ship psychiatry in a war zone. *Am J Psychiatry*. 1967;124(3):281–286.

According to Johnson, the Army mental health asset allocation in Vietnam favored the combat divisions despite the fact that the noncombat personnel outnumbered combat troops by 3-4:1. This disadvantaged the very large concentrations of support troops, especially in the Cam Ranh Bay and Qui Nhon areas, because of the formidable distances separating them from the psychiatric specialty teams. These challenges notwithstanding, Johnson spoke of his own job satisfaction, which was consistent with the overall "excellent level of morale and motivation" he noted throughout the theater and the unexpectedly low levels of psychiatric attrition, including from combat stress.

Colonel Matthew D Parrish, Medical Corps

Parrish (Figure 4-7) was the third USARV Psychiatry Consultant (July 1967–July 1968). He had served over 20 years as an Army officer before his assignment in Vietnam, including a tour in World War II as a bombardier and one in Korea during the war as an Army psychiatrist. He received his psychiatric training at Walter Reed General Hospital in the early 1950s. In his correspondence with the author 17 years after he returned from Vietnam, Parrish provided glimpses into his experience as the senior Army psychiatrist in Vietnam, as well as in the aftermath (see Appendix 13, "Parrish's Postwar Recollections"). Parrish indicated that he was somewhat dismayed that no history of psychiatry in Vietnam had been forthcoming from the Army and that there was no repository of the monthly reports he and the other psychiatry consultants in the Vietnam theater of operations were required to send to the Army Surgeon General's Office. On the positive side, he recalled that the psychiatrists who were assigned during his year—a year that included some of the most intense fighting of the war—were in ample numbers and adequately trained.

Parrish also approved of the regular use of neuroleptic tranquilizers in the theater and believed that there were no significant adverse consequences. On the other hand, he expressed regret that prescribing such drugs was part of a trend toward training psychiatrists to diagnose and medicate patients as opposed to clinical approaches that would provide (in Vietnam) more psychological support for the soldier's recovery, including reintegrating him into his military unit ("enmembering"). Parrish reflected a measure of cynicism in his thoughts on how the war was waged. In particular he worried that it became unwinnable because of a failure of the administration and the military to stay in touch with human dimensions as opposed to conducting the war as a "management war" (ie, overvaluing quantifiable elements). In this regard, he suspected there was "upper echelon" resistance to the analysis of psychiatric statistics coming out of Vietnam because it might be interpreted critically. As an example, he noted that the results of a 1967 soldier drug use survey, the first theater-wide study of marijuana use, was suppressed by the USARV Surgeon's office because of its negative findings.

Lieutenant Colonel George Mitchell, Medical Corps

Mitchell served as the fourth USARV Psychiatry Consultant (July 1968–July 1969). He was a graduate of an Army psychiatry-training program and had over 8 years of experience as an Army psychiatrist before assuming his position in Vietnam.

Colonel Thomas "Brick" Murray, Medical Corps

Murray (Figure 4-8) served as the fifth USARV Psychiatry Consultant (1969–1970). In 1960 he completed his training in psychiatry at Letterman General (Army) Hospital. This was followed by assignments at the US Military Academy at West Point, at Madigan General Hospital, and at Walter Reed General Hospital (Chief of Psychiatry), before he was assigned to Vietnam. Although Murray did not provide a summary of his tour of duty in Vietnam, Bey included the following description from contacts with him while serving as division psychiatrist with the 1st Infantry Division:

Col. [Colonel] Murray reviewed the psychiatric statistics from the various units in Vietnam and passed on information of epidemiological significance both to the psychiatrists in Vietnam as well as to BG [Brigadier General] Thomas who was the USARV Surgeon. Col. Murray held a conference on alcohol and drug abuse in Vietnam in conjunction with the Judge Advocate's Office and the CID [Criminal Investigative Division]. At this meeting the medical and legal branches had an opportunity to exchange information and to share their experiences in attempting to reduce the casualties resulting from drug abuse. Col. Murray regularly visited all of the psychiatric services in Vietnam. He provided direct professional supervision to us and shared his extensive knowledge of military psychiatry. . . . Col. Murray also set an example to his supervisees to keep on the go and to fly and consult and supervise their [social work/psychology] technicians and to visit units in their divisional areas. Col. Murray was well schooled as a military psychiatrist and felt at home consulting with outlying units. Through his rank and military experience he could consult with the generals and brigade commanders in the combat division in a way that was most helpful to the division psychiatrist's efforts to establish an effective unit consultation program. Through his continual contact with the psychiatrists in Vietnam and their

units, Col. Murray obtained much information which could not be learned from the monthly statistical reports sent to his office. Col. Murray was well liked by officers and men in the First Infantry Division and was a frequent and welcome guest in our Division. He did a great deal to support and ease our efforts within the Division.[30(Chap5,pp3–4)]

Colonel Clotilde D Bowen, Medical Corps

Bowen holds the distinction of being the first black female physician to serve in the US Army. Initially trained as a specialist in pulmonary medicine, she completed her civilian psychiatry training in the early 1960s and ultimately became the sixth USARV Psychiatry Consultant (July 1970–July 1971). She recalled receiving her orders to serve in that position, "[with] surprise and dismay," as she had only 3½ years of experience as an Army psychiatrist—considerably fewer than her predecessors. In her position as Psychiatry Consultant in Vietnam, Bowen not only monitored the work of the deployed mental health personnel in Vietnam as had earlier consultants, but in addition she was required to plan and coordinate the Army's hastily developing drug and race relations programs, submit reports about the morale and mental health of troops there, and brief congressmen, visiting foreign dignitaries and ranking officers, and representatives of the news media "who wanted to know what was really happening as we were losing the war."[31(B-11)]

Bowen's official End of Tour Report (see Appendix 14) was appropriately constrained, but it nonetheless provided a striking contrast to Johnson's optimistic overview from 4 years earlier. In particular Bowen provided a window into the enormous difficulties borne by the Army leadership in Vietnam during the last years of the war in trying to keep up with rapidly deteriorating soldier morale, discipline, and mental health while maintaining a capable fighting force. By her account Bowen did a commendable job in orchestrating the mental health assets amidst the drawdown's shortages of trained personnel, turbulence of military personnel more generally, and the rising incidence of psychiatric and behavior problems. Her report appeared to substantiate command's mixed results in counteracting these unprecedented problems:

- Bowen noted that the first autopsy confirmation of a heroin overdose death among Army troops occurred in August 1970—which suggested the

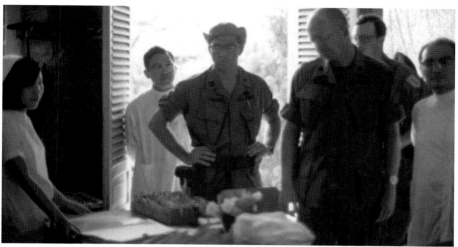

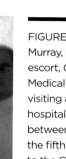
FIGURE 4-8. Colonel Thomas "Brick" Murray, Medical Corps, and his escort, Captain Ross Guarino, Medical Corps, 1st Infantry Division, visiting a Vietnamese psychiatric hospital. Murray served in Vietnam between July 1969 and July 1970 as the fifth Neuropsychiatry Consultant to the Commanding General, US Army Republic of Vietnam Surgeon. Photograph courtesy of Douglas R Bey.

soldier heroin problem had reached a new and disturbing level.

- She alluded to the "crash" project to publish a medical technical guidance manual about drug abuse in Vietnam (with Major Eric Nelson, Medical Corps, commanding officer of the 935th Psychiatric Detachment) for distribution to newly arriving physicians (implemented in January 1971)—which suggested how unprepared the Army in Vietnam was for the heroin problem.

- She described the shift of heroin detoxification centers from medical and psychiatric authority to command/disciplinary authority—which suggested the relative failure of the medical approach in reducing soldier heroin use.

- She mentioned persistent problems with the medical/psychiatric reporting system, especially for alcoholism, drug abuse, and psychosomatic conditions—which appeared to reflect disagreement as to whether soldier drug abuse should be regarded as a discipline problem, a medical condition, or a psychiatric disorder. It also indicated that the traditional measures of psychiatric morbidity had become distorted.

- She referred to the elimination of the Army Regulation 635-212 requirement that psychiatrists evaluate every soldier for whom a commander recommended administrative separation from the Army (implemented in October 1970)—which suggested an overwhelming rise in command referrals to psychiatry for soldiers with disciplinary problems or unsatisfactory performance.

- She advocated that nondivisional units have

unprecedented access to the mental health assets of the combat divisions—which suggested the disproportionate prevalence of problems regarding racial incidents, drug abuse, and soldier dissent within support units.

- She advocated an unprecedented elevation of the (staff) status of the division psychiatrists to be the equivalent with the division surgeons—which suggested a growing tendency for division commanders and division surgeons to disregard the expertise of their division psychiatrists, especially regarding racial incidents, soldier dissent, and drug abuse.

Major Francis J Mulvihill Jr, Medical Corps

Mulvihill was a recent graduate from a civilian psychiatry-training program and had no experience as an Army psychiatrist before his assignment in Vietnam. In Vietnam he served as a solo psychiatrist at the 67th Evacuation Hospital for 8 months before being reassigned to USARV HQ to serve as interim USARV Psychiatry Consultant (June 1971–September 1971).

Colonel Niklaus J A Keller, Medical Corps

Keller not only served as the eighth USARV Psychiatry Consultant (August 1971–April 1972), but he was also Chief of Professional Services for the CG/USARV Surgeon. He received partial training in psychiatry in a civilian program before he entered the Army in 1950. This was followed by 4 years of training in a combined neurology/psychiatry program at Walter Reed General Hospital. During most of the intervening years between his training at Walter Reed and his assignment in Vietnam, he served as a neurologist or in medical administration, including in Korea in 1964.

Major Ralph Green, Medical Corps

Upon completion of his Army psychiatry-training program in the Fall of 1971, Green was assigned to Vietnam to the Cam Ranh Bay Detoxification Center. Six months later he was reassigned to be the ninth USARV Psychiatry Consultant (May 1972–November 1972).

Discussion of the Documentation of the Activities of the Psychiatrists Assigned as USARV Psychiatry Consultant

Each of the available portraits of the senior Army psychiatrists in Vietnam is descriptively interesting. Johnson appeared to reflect confidence that Army psychiatry was doing its part in medically supporting the escalating war effort; and Murray (through Bey's description) appeared to be the model of the effective psychiatric advisor for command and mentor for the deployed mental health component. In contrast, Parrish (who preceded Murray but whose comments must be considered to be influenced by the negative postwar zeitgeist in America) and Bowen (who found herself in the middle of the war's most difficult drawdown problems) suggested a far more negative view. However, because these four individuals represented fewer than half of those who held the critical position of Neuropsychiatry Consultant to the USARV CG/Surgeon, and inasmuch, perhaps with the exception of Johnson's panel presentation, none of these accounts were drafted by the principals as reports summarizing their experiences, one again is left to speculate on all that is missing. This is even more disturbing when Parrish noted that the consultants were required to forward a monthly psychiatric report to the office of the Army Surgeon General in Washington, which were evidently discarded or destroyed.

SUMMARY AND CONCLUSIONS

This chapter, combined with the preceding one, featured the available records provided by 24 Army psychiatrists and paraprofessionals who fought the war in the psychological trenches in Vietnam in order to construct a composite picture of the psychiatric problems they encountered, the conditions under which they worked, and their professional responses and results. Taken together, these two chapters tell a story of a mental health contingent that was trained, organized, and supplied in a fashion to support the deployment of many thousands of troops into the combat theater and, in particular, to aid the recovery of large numbers of soldiers who were predicted to be disabled by combat stress. The extant documentation indicated they met these challenges with commitment and effectiveness.

This chapter presented more specifically summaries of the publications by some of those assigned as solo psychiatrists with the field and evacuation hospitals and some of those who served in the neuropsychiatric medical specialty detachments. It also reviewed the available information pertaining to the work of four (of nine) psychiatrists who were the Neuropsychiatry Consultants to the CG/USARV Surgeon. In addition to their descriptive value, these reports suggested the following trends:

- **The solo psychiatrists assigned to the field and evacuation hospitals treated a steady stream of referrals representing a mix of problems more centered on combat theater stress than combat stress.** Each psychiatrist provided basic inpatient care for a large catchment area of support troops, and the psychiatric conditions requiring such treatment were mixed in nature and mostly manageable despite the lack of additional specialized staff. Although only one (of five overviews) mentioned drug abuse as etiologically significant, this was clearly a consequence of the group serving during the first couple of years of the war. On the other hand, all of them reported substantial alcohol problems. Finally, none of them indicated they provided consultation to unit commanders or other Army agencies.
- **The psychiatrists assigned to the 935th and the 98th Neuropsychiatric Medical Specialty Detachments (KO)—the definitive psychiatric treatment facilities in Vietnam—verified that, as designed, they had a more challenging caseload than the other hospital psychiatrists.** Their cases included some soldiers with combat-stress generated psychopathology (fresh casualties, as well as treatment-resistant ones from the division psychiatrists), but most cases had conditions not primarily connected with combat. Inpatient programs provided an array of treatment elements including milieu therapy, psychotropic

medications, and, especially, the therapeutic relationships provided by the enlisted specialists. Inpatient treatment outcomes varied widely between these two specialized units; the percent of hospitalized soldiers recovered for duty in the theater ranged from 40% to 90%, with the higher recovery rates coinciding with the implementation of the combat psychiatry treatment doctrine. Very little was said regarding the treatment of outpatients, and only one report described a program of command and agency consultation.

- **The record from the psychiatrists assigned as USARV psychiatry consultant is both quantitatively and qualitatively sparse.** Although the available information regarding those who served as psychiatry consultant in years 2, 3, 5, and 6 of the war was mostly indirect, the composite strongly indicated how personally, professionally, practically, and ethically challenging this important leadership job became as the war lengthened.

- **Except for fragments derived from unconventional sources, the individual professional accounts mostly stopped after 1968 to 1969—the midway point in the war.** As a result, the collection of records provided by the psychiatrists assigned with the hospitals, those who served in the psychiatric medical specialty detachments, and those who served as USARV Psychiatry Consultant fell short of representing the psychiatric services provided throughout the war. As the surviving record, this is especially unsatisfactory because theater-wide indices of psychiatric and behavior dysfunction among the troops began to rise in 1968, a trend that accelerated sharply through 1969–1972 and was unrelated to the dropping levels of combat activity.

The chapters that follow will consider these resources in more depth, examine additional information from other sources, and present findings from the Walter Reed Army Institute of Research survey of Army psychiatrist veterans of Vietnam in an attempt to fill in some of the blanks left by this review.

REFERENCES

1. Bloch HS. *The Problem of Character Disorder vs. Psychosis*. Unpublished manuscript.

2. Neel SH. *Medical Support of the US Army in Vietnam, 1965–1970*. Washington, DC: GPO; 1973.

3. Johnson AW Jr. In: Johnson AW Jr, Bowman JA, Byrdy HS, Blank AS Jr. Panel discussion: Army psychiatry in Vietnam. In: Jones FD, ed. *Proceedings: Social and Preventive Psychiatry Course, 1967*. Washington, DC: GPO; 1968: 41–76. [Available as Appendix 7 to this volume.]

4. Quoted by Jones. In: Jones FD. Reactions to stress: combat versus combat support troops. Presentation to World Psychiatric Association, Honolulu, Hawaii, 29 August 1977.

5. Huffman RE. Which soldiers break down. A survey of 610 psychiatric patients in Vietnam. *Bull Menninger Clinic*. 1970;34(6):343–351.

6. Blank AS Jr. In: Johnson AW Jr, Bowman JA, Byrdy HS, Blank AS Jr. Panel discussion: Army psychiatry in Vietnam. In: Jones FD, ed. *Proceedings: Social and Preventive Psychiatry Course, 1967*. Washington, DC: GPO; 1968: 41–76. [Available as Appendix 10 to this volume.]

7. Talbott JA. The Saigon warriors during Tet. *US Army Vietnam Med Bull*. 1968;March/April:60–61.

8. Kenny WF. Psychiatric disorders among support personnel. *US Army Vietnam Med Bull*. 1967;January/February:34–37.

9. Allerton WS, Forrest DV, Anderson JR, et al. Psychiatric casualties in Vietnam. In: Sherman LJ, Caffey EM Jr. *The Vietnam Veteran in Contemporary Society: Collected Materials Pertaining to the Young Veterans*. Washington, DC: Veterans Administration; 1972: III: 54–59.

10. Tischler GL. Patterns of psychiatric attrition and of behavior in a combat zone. In: Bourne PG, ed. *The Psychology and Physiology of Stress: With Reference to Special Studies of the Viet Nam War*. New York, NY: Academic Press; 1969: 19–44.

11. Allerton WS. Army psychiatry in Vietnam. In: Bourne PG, ed. *The Psychology and Physiology of Stress: With Reference to Special Studies of*

the Viet Nam War. New York, NY: Academic Press; 1969: 1–17.

12. Rock NL, Stokes JW, Koshes RJ, Fagan J, Cline WR, Jones FD. US Army combat psychiatry. In: Jones FD, Sparacino LR, Wilcox VL, Rothberg JM, Stokes JW, eds. *War Psychiatry*. In: Zajtchuk R, Bellamy RF, eds. *Textbooks of Military Medicine*. Washington, DC: Department of the Army, Office of The Surgeon General, Borden Institute; 1995: 149–175.

13. US Department of the Army. *Mental Health and Neuropsychiatry*. March 1966. US Army Republic of Vietnam Regulation 40-34. [Available as Appendix 2 to this volume.]

14. Johnson AW Jr. Psychiatric treatment in the combat situation. *US Army Vietnam Med Bull*. 1967;January/February:38–45.

15. Baker SL Jr. Traumatic war disorders. In: Kaplan HI, Freedman AM, Sadock BJ, eds. *Comprehensive Textbook of Psychiatry*. 3rd ed. Baltimore, Md: Williams & Wilkins; 1980: 1829–1842.

16. Bowman JA. Unit History of the 935th Medical Detachment (KO), 20 September 1965 to 1 September 1966 (unpublished); undated.

17. Bowman JA. In: Johnson AW Jr, Bowman JA, Byrdy HS, Blank AS Jr. Panel discussion: Army psychiatry in Vietnam. In: Jones FD, ed. *Proceedings: Social and Preventive Psychiatry Course, 1967*. Washington, DC: GPO; 1968: 41–76. [Available at: Alexandria, Va: Defense Technical Information Center. Document No. AD A950058.]

18. Bowman JA. Recent experiences in combat psychiatry in Viet Nam (unpublished); 1967. [Available as Appendix 11 to this volume.]

19. Bloch HS. Army clinical psychiatry in the combat zone: 1967–1968. *Am J Psychiatry*. 1969;126(3):289–298.

20. Bloch HS. Brief sleep treatment with chlorpromazine. *Compr Psychiatry*. 1970;11(4):346–355.

21. Talbott JA. Community psychiatry in the Army. History, practice, and applications to civilian psychiatry. *JAMA*. 1969;210(7):1233–1237.

22. Anderson JR. Psychiatric support of III and IV Corps tactical zones. *US Army Vietnam Med Bull*. 1968;January/February:37–39.

23. Conte LR. A neuropsychiatric team in Vietnam 1966–1967: An overview. In: Parker RS, ed. *The Emotional Stress of War, Violence, and Peace*. Pittsburgh, Penn: Stanwix House; 1972: 163–168.

24. Kaplan JH. Marijuana and drug abuse in Vietnam. *Ann N Y Acad Sci*. 1971;191:261–269.

25. GIs called 'pot users' in Vietnam. *US Medicine*. 1 April 1970:7.

26. Cohen N. Drug use in Army personnel in Vietnam: A psychiatrist's view. Address to I Corps Medical Society, Camp Baxter, Republic of Vietnam, 2 January 1971 (unpublished).

27. Bloch, HS. Personal communication with the author. 19 February 2010.

28. Strange RE. Effects of combat stress on hospital ship psychiatric evacuees. In: Bourne PG, ed. *The Psychology and Physiology of Stress: With Reference to Special Studies of the Viet Nam War*. New York, NY: Academic Press; 1969: 75–93.

29. Strange RE, Arthur RJ. Hospital ship psychiatry in a war zone. *Am J Psychiatry*. 1967;124(3):281–286.

30. Bey DR. *Division Psychiatry in Vietnam* (unpublished); undated.

31. Bowen C. A different war, another time. *Denver Post*, 21 November 2001.

CHAPTER 5

The Walter Reed Army Institute of Research Survey of Army Psychiatrists Who Served in Vietnam

Conversion [r]eactions and [m]alingering . . . are not of major importance to the civilian psychiatrist whose patients exchange money, inconvenience, time, and in some cases an initial loss of self-esteem for the hope that the physician will relieve his discomfort. In the military, where cost is not a factor (and in fact illness could provide compensation), where time out of the field is a convenience (the longer the better), and where any medical procedure is preferable to the dangers and stress of combat, these topics become extremely important in the medical officer's daily workload.[1(ChapIX,pp5–6)]

Major Douglas R Bey
Medical Corps, Division Psychiatrist
1st Infantry Division (April 1969–April 1970)

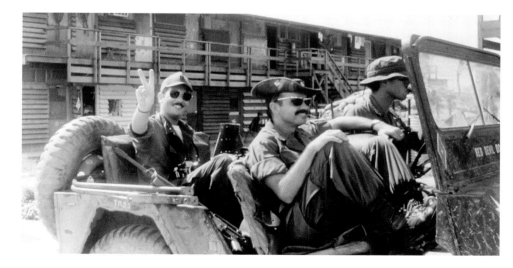

Major Nathan Cohen, Medical Corps, 98th Psychiatric Detachment (back seat), prepares to travel with an armed convoy 80 km north from Da Nang to Quang Tri near the demilitarized zone in Spring 1971 to provide care for troops of the 1st Brigade, 5th Infantry Division (Mech). Cohen was drafted into the service immediately following his civilian psychiatry training and, like the majority of psychiatrists who served there after 1968, Vietnam was his first post-residency assignment. Photograph courtesy of Norman M Camp, Colonel, US Army (Retired).

Construction of an official and, one might argue, essential history of Army psychiatric care in the Vietnam theater by the Army Medical Department was never accomplished, even if it was evidently intended.[2] Some documentation exists in conventional published sources; however, critical shortcomings persist, especially because of the drop-off in professional publications by assigned Army psychiatrists and other mental health professionals after the war passed its midpoint. Furthermore, the opportunity to develop a comprehensive history has been missed due to the passage of time and the loss of primary documents and personnel. The review of individual reports by Army psychiatrists who served in Vietnam and their mental health colleagues (Chapters 3 and 4) is very illuminating; however, large gaps remain. In an attempt to establish a more complete picture of the psychiatric challenge, practices, and results in Vietnam, albeit a decade after American ground troops were finally withdrawn, Walter Reed Army Institute of Research (WRAIR) conducted a survey in 1982 of all locatable psychiatrists who had served with the Army there. This chapter will describe that survey as well as present selected results. Additional findings will also be presented throughout this work.

THE WALTER REED ARMY INSTITUTE OF RESEARCH STUDY DESIGN, RESPONSE, AND MODE OF ANALYSIS

Study Rationale and Objectives

While assigned to WRAIR in the early 1980s, this author conducted a comprehensive review of the available psychiatric and behavioral science literature surrounding military psychiatry in the Vietnam war[3] and found it to be regrettably spotty and even misleading in places—especially in its limited perspective regarding the psychosocial and psychiatric deterioration of the deployed force in the second half of the war. Equally problematic, primary documents from the war such as clinical records or prevalence data could not be located by the Army at that time and evidently did not still exist.[4] Eight of the nine (one was deceased) psychiatrists who served as senior Army psychiatrist in Vietnam (US Army Neuropsychiatry Consultant to the Commanding General/US Army Republic of Vietnam [CG/USARV] Surgeon) were contacted personally and all acknowledged that they did not retain records from their tour; several commented that it was against Army policy to return to the United States with professional documents.

In 1982 the author developed and distributed a survey instrument to all who served as Army psychiatrists in Vietnam inquiring about their preparation, training, and assignments in Vietnam; their professional activities while in the theater; and their reactions regarding their tour. It was hoped that this alternative approach of systematically collecting the recollections of these trained professional observers could complement the fragmented record from the war and allow for a more comprehensive portrait of the dominant patterns of perceived psychiatric need, practices, and results.[5,6]

Survey Questionnaire

The questionnaire consisted of fill-in items and forced-choice questions regarding 10 aspects of Vietnam service. The fill-in questions addressed three areas:

1. professional background and preparation, such as the length and type of formal psychiatric training (ie, civilian or military), extent of pre-Vietnam military experience, and information on Vietnam assignments (ie, units, duties, and dates);

2. estimates of time commitments to military and professional duties in various types of assignments as well as estimates of the percentages of their clinical time devoted to categories of patients across a spectrum of diagnostic groups; and

3. recollections of the indications for prescribing psychotropic medications in the treatment of combat stress reactions as well as for psychiatric symptoms presenting among combat-exposed troops in general.

The forced-choice questions were grouped in seven additional areas for which the participants were asked to indicate extent of their agreement/disagreement along a 5-point scale regarding:

1. the perceived efficacy of various types of therapy for treating combat reactions;

2. circumstantial factors perceived as contributing to the pathogenesis of combat breakdown at both the level of the individual soldier and the level of the group;

3. estimates of troop morale and impressions of situational factors perceived as lowering morale;

4. perceptions of professional requirements regarding the treatment and management of behavioral problems;

5. estimates as to the utility of primary prevention activities, that is, command (program) consultation;

6. perceptions regarding the dominant patterns of substance abuse among troops; and

7. recollections regarding participants' operational frustrations and ethical dilemmas while assigned in Vietnam.

Interested readers can review the original questionnaire through the Defense Technical Information Center (http://handle.dtic.mil/100.2/ADA556223).

Survey Population

The first step—that of determining how many psychiatric positions there were in Vietnam and identifying who served in those positions—proved much more difficult than anticipated. Official Army sources yielded only 51 names, yet it could be estimated that the number of Army psychiatric positions over the 7 years of combat activity was in the range of 135 to 140 (taking into account that psychiatrist tours, as with all Army personnel deployed in the war, were limited to 1 year).[7] The sole remaining course was to build a personnel list from unofficial sources. This led to extensive correspondence with those already identified, inquiring as to whether they could help identify colleagues who also served there. Gradually, and with many false starts, the list of Vietnam Army psychiatrists grew to reach 123. Of the 123, three were not located and five were deceased, reducing the study's population to 115 (113 men, two women).

Survey Response

The response from the study population to the survey was robust in that 85 (74%) provided useable responses. Seventy-four psychiatrists completed the entire questionnaire and 11 completed an abbreviated version (sections 1–2 of the fill-in parts and sections 5 and 7 of the forced choice parts). Regarding response distribution, neither the stage of the war served, nor the setting of the psychiatrists' primary training (civilian or military), apparently introduced a skew in the willingness to participate in the survey. Respondents were evenly distributed over the years of deployment in Vietnam (60%–80% of psychiatrists who served during the advisor and build-up periods of the war [1962–1967], as well as the transition [1968–1969] and the withdrawal [1970–1972] stages). Also, it had been previously determined that the original target population of 115 consisted of 30% with military psychiatric training and 70% with training in civilian programs; a military-to-civilian training ratio of 1:2 was found for the 85 study participants.

Data Analysis

The retrospective and inferential nature of the study meant that it would primarily serve various descriptive or hypothesis-generating purposes as opposed to hypothesis testing. Thus an analytic approach to the data was utilized that primarily centered on descriptive categorization or simple inferential statistical analyses. In several instances, small sample sizes precluded more complex statistical approaches. However, on occasion, such approaches were utilized. Specifically, multi-item batteries were submitted to data reduction procedures, that is, factor analysis, for the purpose of trying to summarize the information contained in those

batteries. By so doing, regression analyses based on the composites derived from various subsets of items were not only likely to be more robust, but the overall analysis could also proceed more efficiently than would be the case if the analyses focused only on the individual items.

Because the survey questionnaire was designed to allow participants to skip sections that did not apply to their experience in Vietnam, numbers of respondents in various sections of the analysis are often less than 85. In this work the most definitive results are presented. Selected findings from the survey have been published in a preliminary form.[5,6]

Study Limitations

This research was not intended to replace studies that should have been conducted during and immediately after the war. As an alternative approach, the findings from this structured "debriefing" are subjective, requiring retrospection many years after the war ended. Nonetheless, the study's qualitative and quantitative results strongly indicated that, in most instances, the psychiatrists' recollections of their Vietnam experiences remained vivid, even if in some instances their interpretations of the meaning of those events have changed. Thus it is informed recollection. The "felt experience" of the war to the psychiatrists who were charged with "picking up the pieces," as it were, is critically important to understanding the psychological costs of the conflict as perceived by those most qualified to understand them. In other words, other than from first-person accounts of the war, which are by definition limited in their generalizability, the expert opinion distilled from the WRAIR psychiatrist survey is as close as a reader can get to obtaining a real "feel" for the emotional and behavioral effects of the war on those who fought it.

WALTER REED ARMY INSTITUTE OF RESEARCH SURVEY RESULTS: PRINCIPAL DISTINCTIONS AMONG ARMY PSYCHIATRISTS IN VIETNAM

Before addressing the WRAIR survey participants' recollections of the psychiatric challenge in Vietnam, it is important to acknowledge certain potentially confounding variables centered on the psychiatrists themselves. Whereas it may be convenient to think of Army psychiatrists as a single group, that is, interchangeable physicians with specialized training, three key differences have the potential to affect their experience in Vietnam as well as their perception of it: (1) phase of the war served in Vietnam, which takes into account associated changing social and military contexts; (2) military familiarity, which refers primarily to whether the psychiatrist received his or her psychiatric training in a military program versus in a civilian program, but in some analyses includes those with civilian training who had some stateside military experience before serving in Vietnam; and (3) combat unit assignment in Vietnam vs assignment to a hospital or psychiatric detachment there.

Phase of the War Served in Vietnam and Changing Social and Military Contexts

The survey psychiatrists' recollections could have been influenced by the half of the war in which they served. The preceding chapters have illustrated that later cohorts of replacement psychiatrists assigned in Vietnam faced an accelerating array of more complex, and in many ways unique and unanticipated, problems in Vietnam—while surrounded by a fractious American society and a hostile professional climate. Also suggested is that some of the deployed mental health personnel, primarily those serving in the later years, may have shared to some degree the demoralization and antimilitary passions of the soldiers whom they treated or may have even become uncertain of their own goals, procedures, and the Army's forward treatment doctrine for management of troops under those circumstances. A critical question then follows: were the clinical perceptions and decisions of these later Army psychiatrists affected by doubt and demoralization? As the nation turned progressively against the war, did later psychiatrists lean more in the direction of a protective, sympathetic overdiagnosis (ie, from the military's point of view) and overevacuation of soldiers[8]—even though in past wars such a clinical posture threatened force conservation and military success, as well as contributed to sustained disability among individual soldiers? Ethical and moral reactions to a war and its politics can measurably influence military psychiatrists regarding the diagnosis and management of their cases.[9]

Because of the small numbers of survey participants, the three phases of the war mentioned earlier were collapsed into two. Using a somewhat arbitrarily chosen dividing line, Army psychiatrists were categorized by their service during either of the two halves of the war, with "early" or "late" referring to whether they arrived in Vietnam before or after May 1968—before and after the pivotal 1968 enemy Tet offensives. Forty survey psychiatrists (47%) served in Vietnam in the first half of the war ("early" psychiatrists), and 45 (53%) were assigned in the second half ("late" psychiatrists). Some of the WRAIR survey data will be explored dichotomously from the standpoint of the effect of this variable.

Military Familiarity: Pre-Vietnam Training and Military Psychiatry "Orientation"

As suggested in the preceding chapters, there are several important experiences in the Army psychiatrist's pre-Vietnam professional background that had the potential to influence their reactions to the war and their professional perspective. These include: (*a*) setting of psychiatry residency training (ie, civilian or military); (*b*) extent and nature of the orientation and training provided by the Army; and (*c*) having a military assignment in the United States before deployment in Vietnam.

Military vs Civilian Psychiatry Training

In World War I, World War II, and the Korean War the mounting need for psychiatric manpower fell largely upon civilians. In the most dramatic example, on VE (Victory in Europe) Day in 1945, a total of 2,402 Army officers were in psychiatry positions. Yet, before the World War II mobilization began, there were fewer than 20 Army medical officers with training in psychiatry.[10] As was noted earlier, matters were distinctly more favorable for Vietnam in that roughly 30% of Army psychiatrists assigned in Vietnam were graduates of Army psychiatry training programs.[6]

As will be discussed here, before Vietnam the Army learned to be cautious with regard to the civilian-trained psychiatrist because of the critical leadership role demanded of every military psychiatrist in the treatment and restoration of the soldiers who succumb to battle stress (ie, because the requisite medical priority was that of force conservation). The history of military psychiatry repeatedly highlights a fundamental difference in clinical perspective that distinguishes psychiatrists with military professional training from those with civilian professional training. In particular it underscores the necessity that the "military inexperienced" civilian-trained psychiatrist accept the modified treatment goals that underlie the military doctrine of forward treatment for psychiatric and behavior disorders, especially combat stress reactions.[11] As articulated by Albert J Glass, a senior Army psychiatrist, and his colleagues:

> [The effective military psychiatrist] renders decisions and recommendations which are meaningful and relevant from a military standpoint. . . . The psychiatrist, new to the service, cannot hope to achieve such military sophistication by limiting his professional activities to a traditional office or hospital practice. [H]e must acquaint himself with the military environment, its rules, regulations, culture, mores and operational procedures.[12(p674)]

In a military setting, especially a combat situation, the civilian-trained psychiatrist is required to transcend his customary prioritization of the individual in the service of supporting the needs of "the group" (referring not only to the soldier's combat group and its combat mission, but also, by implication, American national interests more broadly). In practical terms, for the soldier who develops psychiatric or behavioral symptoms while in combat or anticipating combat, the clinical emphasis should be on his recovering sufficiently to return to combat duty or to function within the military structure—even if he has some residual symptoms or is reluctant.[13] Johnson, a senior Army psychiatrist, summarized the requisite attitude of the effective military psychiatrist as it relates to the rationale for the doctrine of forward treatment:

> If prompt treatment can be given in the individual's combat unit . . . this tends to catch the patient while the reaction is still in conflict between the interest in his group and his self-preservative interest. Appropriate handling at this level tends to preserve the group identification and submerge the self-preservative feelings which promote the symptoms. . . . An attitude of expectancy on the part of the physician and the other treatment personnel can be adequately implemented only if these personnel identify with the needs of the combat group [while also acknowledging] the discomfort of the person who presents with symptoms. . . . The criterion for return to duty is not comfort or complete absence of symptoms but rather ability to perform.[14(p307)]

Harris comments similarly from the Korean War, but he is more direct in distinguishing the problematic civilian perspective:

> The psychiatrist gets his expectations from his orientation—from others and his own experience he rather quickly learns what the score is. I doubt if many patients could ever be returned to duty if the division psychiatrist did not "expect" it. It is . . . a problem of the psychiatrist's own orientation and the means he finds for 'handling' (in contrast to what is usually called [in civilian practice] treating) patients.[15(p399)]

An example of the effects of this distinction from Vietnam can apparently be seen early in the war when comparing the reported experiences of Conte (a civilian-trained psychiatrist who indicated that the 98th KO treatment center returned only 40% of hospitalized soldiers back to duty in Vietnam) with Bowman (an Army-trained psychiatrist whose 935th KO treatment center returned 90% of hospitalized soldiers back to duty during the same timeframe), as discussed in Chapter 4. (Also see Exhibit 5-1, "Potential Identity Problems Facing the Drafted, Civilian-Trained Psychiatrist.")

Preassignment Military Orientation

To address these problems, early in World War II the Army created a 4-week School of Military Neuropsychiatry designed to systematically "indoctrinate" newly inducted psychiatrists. Until an acute shortage of trained psychiatrists later in the war forced conversion of these programs to provide basic psychiatric training for general physicians, over 400 civilian psychiatrists underwent this training.[16] A similar program was instituted for psychiatrists who were new to the Korean combat theater.[17]

The case of Vietnam revealed a much more limited preassignment training and indoctrination.[13] It had apparently been assumed from the beginning that Vietnam-bound psychiatrists would receive sufficient expertise from the generic, 5-week medical officer's basic training required of all physicians new to the Army (Medical Field Service School, Fort Sam Houston, San Antonio, Texas).[7,18,19] In that program, successive cohorts of Army Medical Corps officers received familiarization in the Army's medical mission and its associated structures and procedures as well as specific preparation for various combat environments, especially Vietnam (at least through July 1967). For example, they participated in exercises in traumatic wound debridement using goats wounded with an M16A1 rifle, and

EXHIBIT 5-1. Potential Identity Problems Facing the Drafted, Civilian-Trained Psychiatrist

Many "noncareer" [military] psychiatrists, finding themselves in an alien, time-limited situation (usually two years), prefer to maintain a degree of social and occupational isolation as a means of defending against the realization that they are, in fact, a part of the military system. Having deferred the issue of military service through the three years of residency training, many are reluctant to subordinate their personal and therapeutic efforts to an organization whose values they may not share. Under these circumstances, there is a tendency for [some] psychiatrists, and noncareer physicians in general, to huddle together in shared paranoia and distrust of the "line" military. Thus isolated, there is ample opportunity to construct a skewed image of those outside the hospital as belligerent, insensitive, and ill-informed, particularly when it comes to mental health matters. There is a tendency to cling to familiar therapeutic modalities (eg, office-based psychotherapy) despite indications that the overall mental health of the [military] community might be better served by efforts toward primary prevention. Where persons are referred for administrative, rather than therapeutic, purposes, a great deal of energy [should instead be] directed toward expediting the evaluation procedure and, on occasion, manipulating the bureaucracy in the patient's behalf (most commonly in the area of assignment change and discharge requests).

Understandably, those who practice in [the former] manner soon begin to doubt the magnitude of their therapeutic impact. As in the case of the young draftee, the psychiatrist's self-esteem is closely tied to a positive work identity. As one feels less "therapeutic" and more like a "tool" of the organization, there develops a propensity to identify with the "oppressed" patient. The result may be tacit support for continued "acting out" on the part of the patient, or the psychiatrist may expedite his premature discharge without examining the implications for future (civilian) adjustment. In either case, the patient may suffer. Many of those referred for psychiatric evaluation have already been subject to minor disciplinary action. Further belligerence not uncommonly precipitates courts-martial proceedings or administrative discharge. Where such a discharge is accompanied by a character and behavior disorder diagnosis, the psychosocial consequences can be quite severe. . . .

For [other] psychiatrists, the anxiety of being controlled by a powerful, sometimes unpredictable, system fosters identification with the perceived aggressor. Command values are quickly introjected, resulting in moralistic, as opposed to psychiatric, judgments. Adaptive failure is viewed solely as the result of a serviceman's psychopathologic disorganization, with little or no consideration for the environmental context. Concurrently, there is a tendency to think in administrative, rather than therapeutic, terms. This is not to deny that there are those cases where all concerned would be well served by prompt separation from military service. Rather, it is to point out that in a military setting, the doctor/patient relationship is subject to a number of dynamic pressures that may [be] characteristic of psychiatry in an institutional setting.

Reproduced with permission from Mirin SM. Ineffective military personnel I: A psychosocial perspective. *Arch Gen Psychiatry*. 1974;30:401.

they belly-crawled beneath live machine gun fire in a simulated night combat situation.

All attendees at this training received a few general hours of instruction on selected aspects of military psychiatry, which included key differences between the military and civilian practice of psychiatry. Beyond that, however, the new Army psychiatrists who would be assigned in Vietnam were relegated to on-the-job training there. However, in Vietnam their situations varied widely regarding the extent of their initial on-site supervision through overlap with the psychiatrists who preceded them. Overall it was quite limited if at all (per information collected separately from participants in the WRAIR Vietnam psychiatrists survey). Finally,

throughout the war there was no effort made to debrief the Army psychiatrists returning from Vietnam so as to distill the collective wisdom for dissemination to the psychiatrists who were replacing them in Vietnam or to the Army residency training programs in the United States.

Practical Alternatives to Military Psychiatry Training

Because of the haste to mobilize the forces during World War I and World War II, civilian-trained psychiatrists (most) typically had no prior military experience before they assumed their new positions as military psychiatrists. Army residency training programs

EXHIBIT 5-2. The Jones-Dr A Correspondence

The following profiles and correspondence serve to illustrate the growing differences between the military trained and civilian trained psychiatrists who served with the Army in Southeast Asia during the war—differences that had the potential to affect clinical decisions in the theater and may have shaped American psychiatry and military psychiatry after the war. This subject will be amplified in Chapter 11. The identity of one of the correspondents has been disguised. His specific name is not as important as his view on military psychiatry.

Upon completion of his medical and psychiatric specialty training, Dr A was drafted into the Army. His first assignment was to Vietnam (early in the war) where he served with a psychiatric detachment near Saigon, followed by service with the 3d Field Hospital in Saigon. For his service in Vietnam he was awarded the Bronze Star Medal. His professional publications substantiate his valuable clinical contributions there. Upon his return to the United States and discharge from the Army, Dr A became politically active in the antiwar movement, including serving on the national steering committee of the Vietnam Veterans Against the War. In the intervening years following the end of the war, he achieved considerable professional distinction through his vigorous work on behalf of the psychiatric needs of the seriously mentally ill. In the late 1970s, he was instrumental in the development of the 3rd edition of the *Diagnostic and Statistical Manual of Mental Disorders* (DSM-III), the new psychiatric nomenclature that revolutionized the field of psychiatry. By the mid-1980s, Dr A had become the president of a major national professional organization, the editor of a prominent professional journal, and chairman of a Department of Psychiatry at a medical school. In a newspaper interview at the time of his appointment as department chair, he remarked that when he was drafted into the Army, he was so opposed to the war that he was tempted to move to Canada to avoid serving; yet the experience there was pivotal for him. In particular he was impressed there by the larger picture as opposed to dealing with the individual patient—the need to comprehend the overriding effects of the social and societal situation. Simultaneously in a journal column, he spoke of Vietnam as a national tragedy that represented America's political and economic decline.

Dr A's mostly civilian personal/professional trajectory and orientation can be contrasted to that of Franklin Del Jones, MD. Upon completion of his psychiatric specialty training at Walter Reed General Hospital in 1965, Jones was assigned as division psychiatrist with the 25th Infantry Division in Hawaii. After 5 months of familiarization time, Jones traveled with the advanced elements of the division when they deployed to Vietnam (see Chapter 3). Following his tour of duty in Southeast Asia, Jones served as the Assistant Psychiatric Consultant, Office of The Surgeon General, US Army, and 10 years later, as the Psychiatric Consultant, the senior psychiatrist in the US Army. In his field as a career military psychiatrist, Jones was as prolific as was Dr A in his area of specialization and achieved great distinction as the principle spokesperson for the heritage of military and combat psychiatry. This culminated in his becoming President, Military Section of the World Psychiatric Association and serving as senior editor and primary contributor to two landmark volumes (*War Psychiatry and Military Psychiatry: Preparing for Peace in War*) in the Army Surgeon General's series, *Textbooks of Military Medicine*. Jones retired from the US Army at the rank of Colonel in 1988 following over 26 years of active service. He was awarded the Bronze Star Medal for his service in Vietnam and the Meritorious Service Medal with Oak Leaf Cluster for his outstanding contributions to military medicine and psychiatry.

in psychiatry were not instituted until after World War II. When considering Vietnam it is more complicated. Some of the psychiatrists assigned there were trained in psychiatry in military hospitals and received some familiarization with the Army there; and some of the civilian-trained psychiatrists, although a minority, served at stateside Army posts before going to Vietnam. The latter arrangement created an optimal preparatory situation for the civilian-trained psychiatrists as they could incorporate military goals and priorities through their demonstrated utility with military populations; however, this arrangement was far more common in the

first half of the war. Overall, most of the civilian-trained psychiatrists went straight from civilian life and civilian training to service in Vietnam.

The divergence in perspective between the military-trained psychiatrists and civilian-trained psychiatrists, especially those without a predeployment military assignment—divergence that has been noted in past wars to shape clinical decision making—likely became magnified over time in Vietnam because of the growing polarization within American society regarding justification for fighting in Southeast Asia. This is illustrated in the correspondence between John

EXHIBIT 5-2. The Jones-Dr A Correspondence, continued

The following correspondence was triggered by the appearance of David Crane on the "Dick Cavett Show." At that time, Cavett had a 90-minute show on ABC that ran in the same time slot as "The Tonight Show."

DR A TO LIEUTENANT COLONEL JONES:

July 1, 1970

Dear Dr Jones:

I got so goddam mad after seeing Dave Crane [who served as division psychiatrist with the 25th ID in Vietnam] on the [Dick] Cavett show tonight that I wrote the enclosed letter to him. . . .

If you saw the show, I'd appreciate your dropping him and Dick Cavett a note. . . .

As psychiatrists and analysts, I'm sure we all have grave reservations about speaking out on public issues. But irrational rhetoric must be answered. If we, as psychiatrists who have served in Viet Nam, cannot rebut one of our own who uses national TV to preach continuation of this futile war—I think we truly deserve what we get. . . .

Yours in something constructive,

Dr A

DR A TO DR CRANE:

July 1, 1970

Dear Dave:

I [am writing] to express my disgust, anger and disappointment about the statements you made on the Cavett show tonight.

Scientific discretion, analytic neutrality, and mature skepticism—all have a place in discussing vital national issues. But Dave, if you really think there were few or minimal atrocities, if you think free fire zones are good for the country, if you think few Viet Nam returnees are exhibiting adverse opinions about the war—I think you are exhibiting the same outlandish political rhetoric that the militant revolutionaries are displaying.

If you want to join the irrational elements in American society, I suppose you have the freedom to do so—but don't lie—and don't parade yourself on National TV as a representative psychiatrist and Viet Nam veteran. Call yourself a politician, a shouter, someone who "having been there, knows the real story."

But remember, there are many psychiatrists—patriotic, not given to rhetoric and exaggeration, and trying to be truthful to ourselves, who saw and heard of atrocities, who knew and know "nationalistic" Vietnamese, and who know and treat Viet Nam returnees—who know you distort the facts.

An ego trip is quite a thing . . . but there are 17 million people who are pretty sick and tired of American ego trips— and 44,000 Americans who no longer know what that means.

Sleep well,

Dr A

EXHIBIT 5-2. The Jones-Dr A Correspondence, continued

LIEUTENANT COLONEL JONES TO DR CRANE

16 July 1970

Dear Dave:

I received an emotional and impulsive letter . . . from Dr A , seemingly urging me to castigate you for your appearance on the Dick Cavett Show. . . . I did not see the program . . . but if you expressed an unwillingness to surrender in the face of a totalitarian enemy; if you don't want another Munich; if you found, as I did, that most of the atrocities were performed by the communists; if you found that Viet Nam veterans exhibited no more adverse opinions about the war than veterans of any war express about war; and if you still hold to the conservative orientation which was present when we were in the 25th [ID] together, then I must vote "yea" on your appearance.

Sincerely,

FRANKLIN DEL JONES, LTC, MC
Asst. Chief, Psychiatry Service
[Walter Reed General Hospital]

LIEUTENANT COLONEL JONES TO DR A:

28 July 1970

Dear Dr A :

First, I took to heart your suggestion to write Dave Crane and Dick Cavett, not about what Dave said [on TV] because I missed the program, but rather my response to your letter. In general, I indicated [to them] that I would like for the U.S. to be out of Viet Nam but not by surrender. After all if the war continues, I'll likely find myself back in Viet Nam. But Dr A, don't you think our government wants this as well? If we have learned little from the lessons of World War I & II and Korea, surely one thing must be clear: weakness and conciliation to an aggressor nation is an invitation to later conflict. . . .

I admire your initiative in taking a stand on what you believe . . ., but surely you need not rely on name-calling to castigate Dave for doing the same thing. You seemed to feel that Dave was misleading people by presenting himself as a Viet Nam veteran and psychiatrist who espoused a view of the war different from your own . . . but . . . what are you doing if not the same by lending your name in endorsement of the Viet Nam Veterans Against the War . . .?

Sincerely,

FRANKLIN DEL JONES, LTC, MC
Asst. Chief, Psychiatry Service
Walter Reed General Hospital

EXHIBIT 5-2. The Jones-Dr A Correspondence, continued

LIEUTENANT COLONEL JONES TO DICK CAVETT

28 July 1970

Dear Dick:

Thank you for allowing Dr David Crane to present his view on the Viet Nam War. I was the psychiatrist who preceded Dave in the 25th Infantry Division and I got to know his views, which are in general agreement with my own. We did not see disaffection with the war different from that with any war; atrocities were mostly committed by the communists; psychiatric casualties were no different from such casualties found in any stressful environment with one exception: they tended to be fewer than in the support troops such as troops in the Continental United States. . . .

While the majority of our youth answer the call to arms at least with resignation if not enthusiasm, a pampered, vociferous few who have not known that freedom has a cost nor suffered the consequences of conciliatory policies toward aggressors would have us turn our eyes away from this unpleasantry, Viet Nam.

I want the war to end; . . . But Dick, let's end it in a way that won't lead to our return to Asia in Burma, Thailand, Indonesia or even India. Return then would find us fighting communists in those countries no doubt augmented by "volunteers" from a unified communist Viet Nam–Cambodia–Laos.

Sincerely,

FRANKLIN DEL JONES, LTC, MC
Asst Chief, Psychiatry Service
Walter Reed General Hospital
Washington, DC

A Talbott, MD, and Lieutenant Colonel Franklin Del Jones (see Exhibit 5-2, "The Jones Correspondence"). In their passionate interchange, Jones, a career military psychiatrist, argued a conser-vative, promilitary, pro-Vietnam War position, and Talbott, a drafted psychiatrist, represented the opposing perspective. Despite the charged rhetoric between Jones and Talbott, there are no certain measures of patterned clinical decision making stemming from their espoused differences in perspective about the war. Chapter 3 did suggest that Jones demonstrated a military-centered clinical conservatism regarding diagnosis, treatment, and evacuation. However, the only evidence suggesting that Talbott functioned at the other extreme came from the interview he gave upon his return from Vietnam in which he noted the rather universal opposition to the war he saw among the soldiers there and expressed his belief that although patients may have been labeled as psychiatric problems they really expressed a "widespread negative sociologic phenomenon."[20] These value

distinctions and their possible clinical effects will be explored in Chapter 11.

Professional and Military Backgrounds

Among the 85 psychiatrist participants of the WRAIR Survey, 27 (32%) received their psychiatry training in military programs, and 58 (68%) were trained in civilian programs. However, beyond this primary distinction, an additional finding pertains to the extent of formal psychiatric training. Whereas all 27 psychiatrists from military residencies had completed 3 or more years of psychiatry training, six (10%) of the 58 civilian-trained group completed only 2 years of training, and another eight (14%) completed only 1 year. The standard length of psychiatry residency training programs in both civilian and military programs was 3 years, not counting the internship year, but Army policy allowed partially trained individuals to serve in unsupervised positions of full clinical responsibility. Otherwise, the military-trained and civilian-trained

TABLE 5-1. WRAIR Survey Psychiatrist Distribution by Training and Pre-Vietnam Field Experience (N = 85)

	"EARLY" PSYCHIATRIST (40)			"LATE" PSYCHIATRIST (45)	
Military-Trained (27)	12	YES Field Experience	10	3	15
		NO Field Experience	2	12	
Civilian-Trained (58)	28	YES Field Experience	19	6	30
		NO Field Experience	9	24	

Note: "Field Experience" refers to a pre-Vietnam, post training, military assignment.

groups averaged similar amounts of elapsed time between cessation of training and assignment to Vietnam (6 and 4 months, respectively). With a few notable exceptions, on average they were assigned in Vietnam with little posttraining experience.

The data regarding practical military experience before Vietnam, apart from military residency, cut across residency type to a significant extent (Table 5-1). Twenty-five civilian-trained psychiatrists (43%) had at least 1 year of a pre-Vietnam military assignment, whereas the remaining 33 went to Vietnam as their first Army assignment. Also, 13 (48%) of the Army-trained group had a postresidency military experience before their tour in Vietnam vs 14 who did not.

Most importantly, there was a dramatic decline in preassignment military familiarity among all psychiatrists as the war lengthened. In particular, among the Army-trained psychiatrists who served in the second half of the war, there is a sharp reduction in their practical military experience base derived from a posttraining assignment compared with those who served in the first half (Figure 5-1). Furthermore, whereas psychiatrists with military residency training combined with the civilian-trained psychiatrists who had a pre-Vietnam military assignment accounted for over three-quarters (78%) of those deployed in the "early" war, they were less than half (47%) of those who served in the "late" war.

WRAIR survey data collected separately also revealed a proportional reduction in relevant background experience—though not rank—of the Vietnam theater Army Neuropsychiatry Consultants to the CG/USARV Surgeon, that is, the senior Army psychiatrist in country, in the last 3 years of the war (1970–1972) (see Chapter 4). Consistent with this finding is the following remark by Matthew D Parrish, former Chief Psychiatry and Neurology Consultant to the Army Surgeon General:

I found out that assignments of the USARV Consultants were not made on the basis of rank, and probably not on the basis of skill or of proper career development but rather on the basis of what influential psychiatrist [lobbied] to be assigned in Hawaii or to Letterman General Hospital in San Francisco, or wanted to get out of doing DA [Department of the Army] staff work. (See Parrish correspondence in Appendix 13.)

The study questionnaire did not explore psychiatrists' motives for joining the Army or serving in Vietnam. Obvious possibilities include that of volunteering versus having received an assignment to serve there. More particularly, civilian psychiatrists could have been drafted into the service or could have voluntarily entered, including under the Berry Plan (The Armed Forces Physicians' Appointment and Residency Consideration Program), which allowed draft deferment during civilian residency training. Information as to whether a psychiatrist had been a volunteer or draftee was not sought because, whether civilian-trained or military-trained, ultimately serving in Vietnam was, in most instances, the consequence of earlier and only partly related decisions. Neither accepting the Berry Plan deferment nor military residency training constituted a decision to serve in Vietnam. In fact, it was substantiated from official sources apart from the study (ie, not data from the survey) that only 22.5% of the psychiatrists who graduated from Army psychiatry training programs (Walter Reed General Hospital, Washington, DC, and Letterman Army Medical Center, San Francisco, California) during the war years were subsequently assigned there.

Combat Unit Assignment in Vietnam

Army psychiatrists serving in Vietnam can also be distinguished as to whether they were assigned to a

FIGURE 5-1. WRAIR survey psychiatrists by phase of war served (percentages of psychiatrists within the first or second half of the war), residency type, and practical military background before assignment (N = 85).

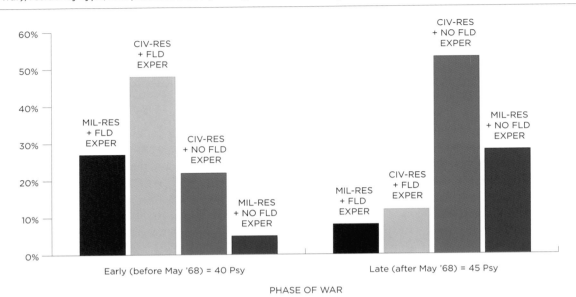

Early (before May '68) = 40 Psy

Late (after May '68) = 45 Psy

PHASE OF WAR

CIV-RES: civilian residency
FLD EXPER: military assignment before Vietnam

MIL-RES: military residency
NO FLD EXPER: no military assignment before Vietnam

combat unit vs a hospital or a psychiatric detachment; a few had nonclinical positions at some point during their tour. Psychiatric observers from previous wars have described a critical difference in clinical perspective as a consequence of this distinction,[21,22] which is similar to the distinction drawn earlier between the military-trained psychiatrist and the one who trained in a civilian setting. The psychiatrist who functions near the actual combat as a member of the combat group develops a commitment to his unit, its mission, and its welfare. He therefore more readily aligns his clinical perspective with that of force conservation than the psychiatrist who is assigned to a hospital or KO team. In this respect he is prone to see his goal as that of supporting the symptomatic soldier who has developed a "failure to adapt," that is, one who is symptomatic because his self-preservative feelings have temporarily eclipsed his commitment to the welfare of his combat unit and the achievement of its mission.[19] This is in contrast to a more civilian-based perspective, or hospital-based perspective, in which the symptomatic soldier is perceived as having an underlying psychiatric condition and who requires protection from further combat exposure.

In summarizing his experiences in World War II and Korea, Glass noted that the civilian-trained or otherwise inexperienced Army psychiatrist and the psychiatrist who has not become affiliated with the combat forces are similarly ineffective in treating the military psychiatry casualty:

Most newcomers to combat psychiatry and those psychiatrists who operate in rear areas are prone to identify with the needs and wishes of the patient. They were therefore readily made insecure when deciding that a patient was fit for return to combat duty, even though aware from a technical and intellectual standpoint that such a decision was correct. Because of anxiety from over-identification and from conscious feelings of guilt for the seeming responsibility of sending a patient to hazardous duty, the psychiatrist vacillated in his clinical judgment, thus impairing his usefulness. But as he worked in the combat zone, observed men who adjusted to battle situations, noted the usual discomforts of combat participants, and decreased his own feelings of guilt by participation, an inevitable emotional reorientation occurred, namely, [he] became identified with the welfare of the group, rather than the wishes of the individual. . . . He became convinced that it is for the best interest of the individual to rejoin his combat unit . . . to regain his confidence and mastery of the situation and prevent chronic tension and guilt. This attitude of the division psychiatrist, stemming from participation with the combat group, makes it possible for him to assume the traditional role as an exponent of reality which insists that the individual continue functioning despite anxiety rather than allowing withdrawal or a disabling neurotic compromise.[21(pp730–731)]

As a corollary, Glass also observed that until they undergo the military reorientation or indoctrination, the civilian-trained psychiatrist will also be ineffective in influencing Army commanders with psychiatric advice:

[Gradually, most civilian-trained] psychiatrists . . . became identified with the needs of the military service rather than with only the needs of the individual. In turn, line commanders came to know psychiatrists as *exponents of reality* (emphasis added) rather than as persons with impractical theories.[23(p750)]

An example of such a reorientation from Vietnam can be found in Chapter 3 in the reported experiences of Pettera, the 9th ID division psychiatrist.

Assignment Patterns in Vietnam

Over the 8 years of the war, Army personnel were individually phased in and out of Vietnam in 1-year assignments. Consequently, psychiatrists, like most other soldiers, typically joined military units that were already deployed. However, nine (11%) survey participants indicated that they had accompanied their unit into Vietnam. With the exception of one individual who stayed an additional 6 months at his own request, all the survey participants served in Vietnam no longer than 12 months. However, during the late drawdown phase of the war, a few psychiatrists, like other soldiers, received some curtailment of their tour. None of the survey participants reported serving in Vietnam for more than one tour. This is despite that fact that as the war extended, some Army personnel with specialized skills were redeployed back to Vietnam.

In terms of physical danger, by expectable combat theater standards Army psychiatrists in Vietnam functioned in a relatively safe circumstance. The sole fatality was that of Captain Peter B Livingston who died on 19 November 1968 when the helicopter in which he was a passenger crashed near Saigon as a consequence of mechanical failure.

Combat vs Hospital (Combat-Service Support) Assignments. Although it is straightforward to designate Army psychiatric positions by the previously described distinction of combat unit assignment vs hospital assignment (ie, hospital and psychiatric medical specialty detachments), the psychiatrists cannot be so easily categorized themselves. This derives from the policy of rotating psychiatrists at midtour from one to the other of these two assignment types to even the load and the hardship.[13] However, practically this was only possible for about two-thirds in any given year. For example, during the period of the greatest troop concentration (1967–1969), among the 22 Army psychiatrists assigned in Vietnam each year (excluding the position of USARV Neuropsychiatry Consultant), the seven division psychiatrist positions could only be shared by a maximum of 14 rotating psychiatrists (eg, 2 x 7); thus the remaining eight psychiatrists (one-third) would necessarily serve their year-long tour with a hospital or a psychiatric detachment.

Yet interestingly, the WRAIR data show that almost half of the survey psychiatrists served exclusively in hospital assignments (vs the predicted one-third), and only a quarter served in both types of units (vs the predicted two-thirds). There is at least a partial explanation: findings indicate that 18 (21%) psychiatrists remained in their original combat division and declined a midtour rotation to a safer, more comfortable hospital facility.[18] These individuals were almost exclusively civilian-trained and served during the first half of the war. Several volunteered that they had developed a strong allegiance to their combat units and preferred not to rotate out. This observation was confirmed by Colbach and Parrish in their review of mental health activities in Vietnam through mid-1970[18] and seems consistent with the earlier reference to psychiatrists who serve with a combat unit developing a commitment to the members of that unit and its mission. As it turned out, 38 (45%) survey participants spent at least some of their tour in Vietnam with a combat unit (Table 5-2).

TABLE 5-2. Patterns of WRAIR Study Participants' Assignments in Vietnam (N = 85)

Clinical Assignments of Army Psychiatrists	Only with a combat ("line") unit (ie, with a division or brigade)	21% (18)*
	Only with a hospital (ie, with an evacuation/field hospital or psychiatric medical specialty detachment)	49% (42)
	Alternatively with a combat unit and with a hospital	24% (20)
Nonclinical Assignments of Army Psychiatrists	Neuropsychiatry Consultant to the CG/USARV Surgeon	5% (4)
	As a medical battalion commander	1% (1)
		100%

*Three respondents served only part of their year as division psychiatrist but did not serve any time in a hospital.
CG/USARV: Commanding General, US Army Republic of Vietnam
WRAIR: Walter Reed Army Institute of Research

Otherwise, a third of psychiatrists (29) indicated that they served in more than one unit in Vietnam. Of that group, nine had a third assignment, two of whom served with yet a fourth unit.

Other Assignments of Psychiatrists. To complete the picture, 11 (13%) survey participants had assignments that deviated from the two basic psychiatric clinical roles thus described ("combat" vs "hospital"). Besides the four who served exclusively as the Neuropsychiatry Consultant to the CG/USARV Surgeon, seven psychiatrists reported serving some part of their tour in other medical or administrative assignments (eg, as a division or brigade surgeon [four], as a flight surgeon [two], or as a medical battalion commander [one]). These psychiatrists were included in the study either because they indicated that a significant portion of their tour was nonetheless spent providing clinical psychiatric services, or, as in the case of the USARV Neuropsychiatry Consultants, because they were dealing with the psychiatric problems in a secondary fashion.

Professional Activities by Type of Military Assignment

The WRAIR survey psychiatrists who had experience in a clinical assignment were asked to allocate for each of their Vietnam assignments the percentage of their professional time spent among six major activity categories. Figure 5-2 groups the means of their percentage estimates for each activity by the basic military unit type of each assignment, that is, "combat" vs "hospital."

As demonstrated in Figure 5-2, the overall trend is for survey respondents to report being most often utilized in clinical capacities, primarily those involving the provision of psychiatric care. Direct psychiatric care (patient evaluations and treatment) overshadowed indirect care (supervision of other providers and consultation with commanders), psychiatric clinical duties overshadowed general medical duties, and clinical duties overshadowed those associated with being an officer. When the psychiatrists' experiences in combat unit assignments are compared with those in hospitals or psychiatric medical detachments regarding extent of time allocated for these six basic types of duties, the following trends are also discernable:

- When psychiatrists served with combat units they reported spending somewhat more time providing *indirect care*, that is, clinical supervision and command consultation, compared to when they served with hospitals (30.4 % vs 24.2%, respectively).
- When psychiatrists served with hospitals and psychiatric specialty detachments, they reported spending somewhat more time providing *direct care*, that is, patient evaluation and treatment, compared to when they served with combat units (63.3% vs 55.2%, respectively).

Although these values are not statistically significant, as trends they are consistent with Army psychiatry's efforts to prioritize primary and secondary prevention efforts with combat troops (ie, to incorporate theories and practices of social/community psychiatry).

FIGURE 5-2. Estimates of WRAIR survey psychiatrists' percent of time devoted to professional activities by unit type, in means of percentages (N = 84 psychiatrist assignments) [modified from Camp and Carney].

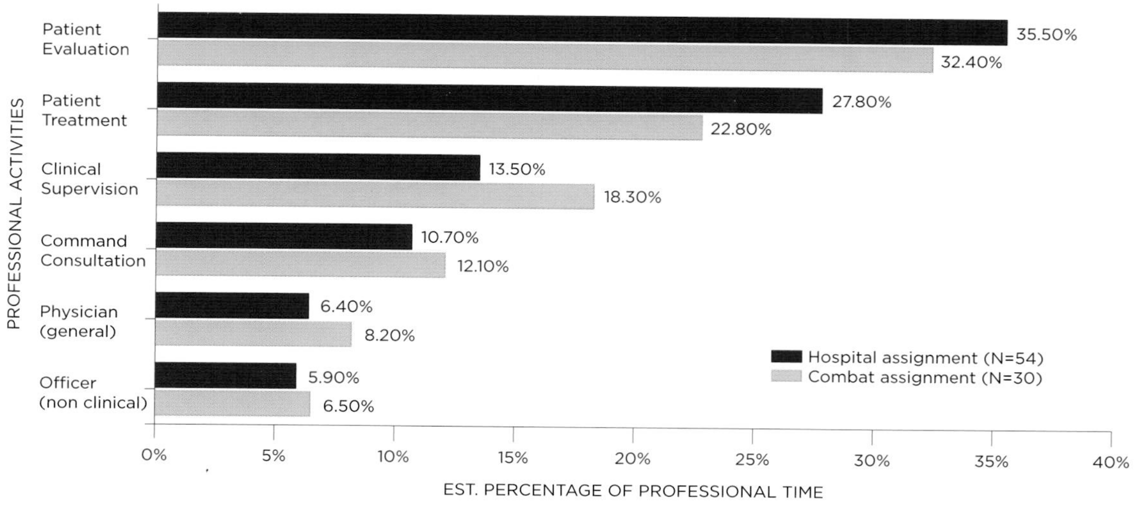

Data source: Camp NM, Carney CM. US Army psychiatry in Vietnam: preliminary findings of a survey, II. Results and discussion. *Bull Menninger Clin.* 1987;51:19–37.

WALTER REED ARMY INSTITUTE OF RESEARCH SURVEY RESULTS: CLINICAL CHALLENGES FOR ARMY PSYCHIATRISTS

This chapter begins the presentation of the WRAIR study psychiatrists' recollections of the clinical challenges they encountered in Vietnam by utilizing the more conventional diagnostic groupings. More detailed data regarding their professional involvement with combat stress reactions will follow in Chapter 6 and Chapter 7; with low morale and associated conduct and behavior problems in Chapter 8; with drug and alcohol problems in Chapter 9; and with command cadre as consultants in Chapter 10. Finally, Chapter 11 will explore operational frustrations and ethical strains associated with performing these professional duties in Vietnam.

Distribution of Clinical Conditions by Diagnosis

Survey psychiatrists were provided a list of nine psychiatric diagnostic groupings along with brief functional definitions and were asked to "estimate the percentage of the patients that you evaluated or treated during your Vietnam service that fell within

each category." Results are displayed in Table 5-3. Except for combat reaction, the groupings on the list were intended to coincide with the civilian diagnostic nomenclature that existed during the war. For simplicity purposes, the definitions for the diagnostic categories used in the survey were extracted from the *International Classification of Diseases, 9th Revision, Clinical Modification* (ICD-9-CM),[24] which was published in 1979 by the World Health Organization.

The term combat reaction was selected for use in lieu of combat exhaustion, the official military term adopted at the close of World War II and utilized throughout the Vietnam War (see Appendix IV—USARV Psychiatry and Neurology Morbidity Report—of Appendix 2: USARV Regulation 40-34). Combat exhaustion refers to a typically reversible, stress-generated psychological regression arising among combat-exposed soldiers—somewhat irrespective of predeployment psychological difficulties. In many respects it is the equivalent of civilians who are grossly affected by an extreme and emotionally traumatizing ordeal, however, there are also important distinctions, which will be discussed in Chapter 6. To avoid confusion, WRAIR survey participants were provided a spectrum of possible signs and symptoms for defining

TABLE 5-3. WRAIR Survey Psychiatrists' Estimates of Percent of Patients They Evaluated or Treated by Diagnostic Groups

Diagnostic Grouping	Mean % (N=65)	"Early" assignment mean % (N=35)	"Late" assignment mean % (N=30)	Combat assignment mean % (N=14)	Hospital assignment mean % (N=36)
Personality disorder	27.1				
Drug dependence syndrome	15.0*	8.1	19.0		
Combat reaction	12.6†			20.9	9.7
Adjustment reaction	12.1				
Schizophrenic psychosis	11.7†			4.9	13.9
Alcohol dependence syndrome	10.4				
Neurotic disorder	9.6				
Affective psychosis	7.1†			4.2	8.0
No disease found	7.0				
Organic psychotic condition	6.4				

*Statistically significant difference comparing war stage, that is, "early" and "late" refer to those served before or after mid-1968.
†Statistically significant difference comparing psychiatrist by assignment type, that is, those serving *only* with combat units vs *only* with hospitals.
Data source: Camp NM, Carney CM. US Army psychiatry in Vietnam: preliminary findings of a survey, II. Results and discussion. *Bull Menninger Clin.* 1987;51:19–37.

the combat reaction (see Table 6-1), which was drawn from a schema developed at the close of World War II.[25]

Responses of the survey participants who provided clinical care in Vietnam were compared by whether they served in the first or second half of the war in Vietnam. Also, responses of those who served *only* in combat units were compared with those who served *only* in a hospital or in psychiatric detachments. Only statistically significant subgroup findings are presented.

Predominance of Conduct and Behavior Problems Throughout the War

The findings presented in Table 5-3 appear to strongly confirm the overall impressions garnered from published theater-wide incidence measures and psychiatrists' anecdotal reports that, using the standards of World War II and Korea, Vietnam was a psychologically low (combat) intensity war. The survey respondents' mean percent of their patients seen for combat reactions was only 12.6%. In contrast, survey psychiatrists recalled that maladjustment and misconduct cases in the form of personality disorders, drug dependence syndromes, and alcohol dependence syndromes comprised over half of their diagnosable patients (52.5%). (To further verify the relatively low incidence of overt combat stress reactions, a third of the WRAIR survey psychiatrists acknowledged they had only rare exposure to combat-induced psychiatric casualties and consequently passed over the survey sections regarding combat reactions as instructed.)

Predominance of Drug Dependency During the Second Half of the War

Also quite illuminating from Table 5-3, when comparing the mean percentages of the diagnostic groups for the psychiatrists who served in the first half of the war with those who served in the second half, only drug dependence syndrome emerged as significantly more frequent in the second half. This is not surprising considering the amassed evidence, medical and otherwise, that indicates a marked upswing in the use of drugs by soldiers (especially heroin after mid-1970). What is intriguing is that it is the only diagnostic group to be elevated, considering how the sense of national purpose in Vietnam had waned and morale there plummeted. Also interesting is that alcohol dependence syndrome is relatively high throughout the war and does not correlate with the late-war demoralization and dissent.

Implementation of the Army Forward Treatment Doctrine

Subgroup analyses in Table 5-3 compared responses from 14 psychiatrists who served *only* in combat unit assignments with 36 who served *only* in hospital assignments and revealed significant differences for only three diagnostic groups:

1. Combat reactions had a higher reported caseload percentage by the "combat" psychiatrists compared with the "hospital" psychiatrists (20.9% and 9.7%, respectively).
2. Schizophrenic psychosis had a higher reported percentage by the "hospital" psychiatrists compared with the "combat" psychiatrists (13.9% and 4.9%, respectively).
3. Affective psychosis also had a higher reported percentage among the "hospital" psychiatrists compared with the "combat" psychiatrists (8.0% and 4.2%, respectively).

In themselves, these results are expectable. Even if combat reactions stayed at a low ebb over the course of the war, they should have been treated more commonly in combat units in conjunction with the military psychiatry doctrine that encouraged early diagnosis and crisis-oriented treatment of those casualties within the area of the soldier's parent unit and discouraged their evacuation out of the divisions to the hospitals. On the other hand, with respect to the two types of major psychoses, the doctrine encouraged expeditious evacuation of the more intractable cases out of the combat divisions to the more definitive treatment centers. Thus these findings are consistent with the intended clinical load differential between the combat unit (with its prioritization of primary and secondary prevention care) and the hospital (with its prioritization of tertiary prevention care). Also suggested is that they appear to validate the WRAIR study's approach to filling in the picture of Army psychiatry in Vietnam through the recollections of the participants despite their retrospective nature.

SUMMARY AND CONCLUSIONS

This chapter described the WRAIR postwar study (1982) of the Army's psychiatric activities in Vietnam using a survey of Army psychiatrists who served there. The inaccessibility of primary records tying individual soldier service records and health records from Vietnam, as well as the lack of basic epidemiological studies regarding psychiatric conditions and behavior problems in Vietnam, necessitated that WRAIR take an alternative approach to filling in significant omissions in the surviving history of Army psychiatry in the war. The survey located most of those who had been assigned in Vietnam, and it used a structured instrument to explore their: *(a)* professional training and extent of preassignment military experience; *(b)* estimates of the relative prevalence of psychiatric problems; *(c)* recollections of the psychiatric intervention efforts designed to prevent, treat, or counteract these conditions along with the degree of success obtained; and *(d)* impressions of factors perceived as pathogenic variables. The survey also inquired as to the participants' subjective reactions to their service in Vietnam and the operational doctrine of forward treatment, and it asked about ethical dilemmas inherent in the practice of military and combat psychiatry there.

Of the 115 locatable psychiatrists (of an estimated 135–140 who served), 85 (74%) responded to all or parts of the survey. Results provided some description of the psychiatrist contingent who served with the Army in Vietnam through the course of the war regarding: *(a)* phase of the war served—with assumptions as to the influence of changing military and social contexts ("early" vs "late" war); *(b)* variations in preparatory training and experience—with assumptions as to the value of military familiarity (whether through having had military psychiatry training or having a predeployment assignment after training); and *(c)* types of assignments in Vietnam ("combat" unit vs "hospital"/psychiatric detachment)—with assumptions as to the influence of combat unit affiliation and identification. The survey results also indicated patterns regarding participants' role demands and clinical challenges.

Findings from the survey presented in this chapter that were especially salient include:

- Over the course of the war, roughly 30% of the assigned Army psychiatrists had military psychiatric training and 70% had training in civilian programs; yet fewer than one in four graduates of Army psychiatry training programs during the war served a tour in Vietnam.
- In the second half of the war a much larger number of civilian-trained psychiatrists with no practical military background and a much larger number of military-trained psychiatrists with no posttraining military experience were assigned in Vietnam compared with the first half. This represents a sizeable drop in the pool of practical military expertise in the theater despite the fact that the rates of psychiatric conditions and behavior problems were climbing.

- Through the course of the war, almost half (45%) of survey respondents reported being assigned to a combat division at some time during their tour.

- Regardless of assignment type (combat unit or hospital/psychiatric specialty detachment), survey respondents reported they were most often utilized in clinical capacities, primarily those involving the provision of psychiatric care; and when they were assigned to a combat unit they more often provided indirect care (supervision of others or consultation to military leaders) than when they were assigned to a hospital/psychiatric specialty detachment.

- Frank combat reactions were reported as a more prevalent clinical challenge for the psychiatrists assigned to combat units compared to those assigned to hospitals/psychiatric specialty detachments; overall, however, combat reactions, as well as the major psychotic disorders, were distinctly overshadowed by various behavior problems (eg, personality disorders and, especially in the second half of the war, drug dependence problems). Collectively these diagnoses represented over half of psychiatric referrals.

In the chapters that follow, additional findings from the WRAIR survey will be utilized to augment data from other sources regarding the psychiatric challenge in Vietnam.

REFERENCES

1. Bey DR. *Division Psychiatry in Vietnam* (unpublished manuscript); undated.

2. Neel SH. *Medical Support of the US Army in Vietnam, 1965–1970*. Washington, DC: GPO; 1973.

3. Camp NM, Stretch RH, Marshall WC. *Stress, Strain, and Vietnam: An Annotated Bibliography of Two Decades of Psychiatric and Social Sciences Literature Reflecting the Effect of the War on the American Soldier*. Westport, Conn: Greenwood Press; 1988.

4. Personal communication, J Greenhut, Chief, Clinical History Division, Center for Military History, Washington, DC, 31 March 1983 (see Exhibit Preface 1).

5. Camp NM, Carney CM. US Army psychiatry in Vietnam: preliminary findings of a survey, I: Background and method. *Bull Menninger Clin.* 1987;51(1):6–18.

6. Camp NM, Carney CM. US Army psychiatry in Vietnam: preliminary findings of a survey, II: Results and discussion. *Bull Menninger Clin.* 1987;51(1):19–37.

7. Allerton WS. Army psychiatry in Vietnam. In: Bourne PG, ed. *The Psychology and Physiology of Stress: With Reference to Special Studies of the Viet Nam War*. New York, NY: Academic Press; 1969: 1–17.

8. Camp NM. The Vietnam War and the ethics of combat psychiatry. *Am J Psychiatry.* 1993;150(7):1000–1010.

9. Sullivan PR. Influence of personal values on psychiatric judgment: a military example. *J Nerv Ment Dis.* 1971;152(3):193–198.

10. Farrell MJ, Berlien IC. Professional personnel. In: Glass, AJ. Bernucci RJ, eds. *Neuropsychiatry in World War II. Vol 1. Zone of the Interior*. Washington, DC: Medical Department, US Army; 1966: 41–51.

11. Beaton LE, Kaufman MR. As we remember it. In: Glass AJ, ed. *Neuropsychiatry in World War II. Vol 2. Overseas Theaters*. Washington, DC: Medical Department, US Army; 1973: 739–797.

12. Glass AJ, Artiss KL, Gibbs JJ, Sweeney VC. The current status of Army psychiatry. *Am J Psychiatry.* 1961;117:673–683.

13. Baker SL Jr. Traumatic war disorders. In: Kaplan HI, Freedman AM, Sadock BJ, eds. *Comprehensive Textbook of Psychiatry.* 3rd ed. Baltimore, Md: Williams & Wilkins; 1980: 1829–1842.

14. Johnson AW Jr. Combat psychiatry, I: A historical review. *Med Bul US Army Europe.* 1969;26(10):305–308.

15. Harris FG. Some comments on the differential diagnosis and treatment of psychiatric breakdowns in Korea. *Proceedings of Course on Recent Advances in Medicine and Surgery.* Army Medical Service Graduate School. Washington, DC: Walter Reed Army Medical Center; 30 April 1954: 390–402.

16. Menninger WC. Education and training. In: Glass, AJ. Bernucci RJ, eds. *Neuropsychiatry in World War II*. Vol 1. *Zone of the Interior*. Washington, DC: Medical Department, US Army; 1966: 53–66.

17. Peterson DB. The psychiatric operation, Army Forces, Far East, 1950–1953, with statistical analysis. *Am J Psychiatry*. 1958;112(1):23–28.

18. Colbach EM, Parrish MD. Army mental health activities in Vietnam: 1965–1970. *Bull Menninger Clin*. 1970;34(6):333–342.

19. Johnson AW Jr. Combat psychiatry, II: The US Army in Vietnam. *Med Bull US Army Europe*. 1969;26(11):335–339.

20. Allerton WS, Forrest DV, Anderson JR, et al. Psychiatric casualties in Vietnam. In: Sherman LJ, Caffey EM Jr. *The Vietnam Veteran in Contemporary Society: Collected Materials Pertaining to the Young Veterans*. Washington, DC: Veterans Administration; 1972: III: 54–59.

21. Glass AJ. Psychotherapy in the combat zone. *Am J Psychiatry*. 1954;110:725–731.

22. Peterson DB, Chambers RE. Restatement of combat psychiatry. *Am J Psychiatry*. 1952;109:249–254.

23. Glass AJ. Lessons learned. In: Glass AJ, Bernucci R, eds. *Neuropsychiatry in World War II*. Vol 1. *Zone of the Interior*. Washington, DC: Medical Department, US Army; 1966: 735–759.

24. World Health Organization. *Manual of the International Statistical Classification of Diseases, Injuries and Causes of Death*. 9th ed. Volume 1, Tabular List with Inclusions [ICD-9-CM]. Geneva, Switzerland: World Health Organization. American Version: Washington, DC: National Office of Vital Statistics; 1979.

25. Bartemeier LH, Kubie LS, Menninger KA, Romano J, Whitehorn JC. Combat exhaustion. *J Nerv Ment Dis*. 1946;104:358–389.

Combat Stress and Its Effects: Combat's Bloodless Casualties

It is hard to equate our civilian experiences with fear to the combat situation. Here danger is imminent and ever present. It is a constant companion every hour of the day, every day of the week. The enormity of this fear is hard to portray and without such an experience, hard to imagine; later, dispersed with prolonged periods facing this fear, are long periods of sheer boredom and frustration—always with the knowledge that the enemy has to be faced again. Fear and its effects are cumulative . . . [t]o each experience is added another. . . . [I]f there is no chance at relief or no additional factors to sustain [the soldier], the potentiality for combat exhaustion exists. [Or alternatively] his judgment is not as good; his alertness may suffer, and his willingness to take chances may disappear. He and his men may become physical casualties long before they become psychological casualties.[1 (pp3–4)]

Lieutenant Colonel Edwin T Cooke
Psychiatrist and Faculty Member, Department of Neuropsychiatry
Medical Field Service School, Fort Sam Houston, Texas

This is a photograph of a combat fatality taken at the 15th Medical Battalion Clearing Station/1st Cavalry Division at Phouc Vinh in 1970. Although the combat intensity in Vietnam was highest during the early and middle years of the war, apprehensions about becoming a casualty remained the preeminent psychological stress factor for Army troops assigned throughout the war. Photograph courtesy of Richard D Cameron, Major General, US Army (Retired).

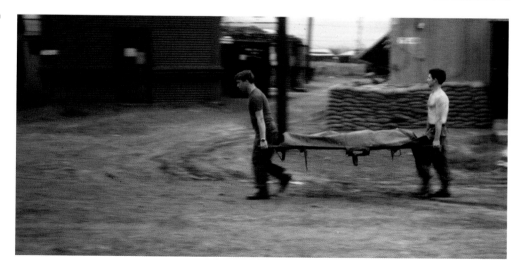

Elements of the history of Army psychiatry that addressed the importance of the prevention and timely treatment of soldiers affected by combat stress were reviewed in Chapter 2. In particular it was demonstrated that in the high intensity wars that preceded Vietnam, rates for soldier attrition and disability from the effects of combat stress could rise to levels sufficient to threaten the outcome of military engagements.

For America and its allies, the Vietnam War also started as a high-intensity, main force war. However, shortly after it began the enemy concluded that the allied forces could not be defeated in large-scale attacks, and they resorted mostly to terrorist/guerrilla tactics. What followed was a protracted, bloody, politically charged, low-intensity war that came to be bitterly opposed by the American public and the international community. In general, and especially during heightened combat activity, treatment of acute combat-generated psychiatric casualties, including what some referred to as classic combat exhaustion, was required of medical and mental health personnel at all levels of care. (In this volume, the term *combat exhaustion* is used synonymously with the terms *combat fatigue*, *combat reaction*, *combat stress reaction* [CSR], and, in some instances, *combat breakdown*.)

Compared with other psychiatric conditions, however, such combat stress reactions, at least in the forms seen in earlier wars, appeared to be well below expected levels. This does not mean that they had no clinical impact, just that their numbers did not constitute a threat to military effectiveness and success. As a result, psychiatric attention was redirected to the burgeoning behavior and disciplinary problems, especially racial tensions and incidents, challenges to military authority, drug abuse, and the number of soldiers diagnosed with character and behavior disorders (ie, personality disorders[2])—problems not limited to combat troops and thus not regarded as closely tied to participation in combat. However, these behavior problems, as well as ones that were more obviously combat-specific (ie, combat refusals and excessive combat aggression), along with psychosomatic conditions and low-grade psychiatric symptoms (anxiety, depression, and "short-timer's syndrome"), continued to arise in the theater, representing "hidden casualties"[3]—conditions that would not have been considered among the more traditional measures of the psychiatric costs of fighting in Vietnam. In fact, the greatest impact may have been among veterans. Many have argued that the proportion of Vietnam veterans with debilitating psychological and social problems greatly exceeded those from earlier American wars, but the connection between combat stress symptoms in the theater and symptoms arising after the war, including what would come to be called posttraumatic stress disorder (PTSD), has remained inconclusive.[4] (Further discussion of PTSD and the postwar adjustment of Vietnam veterans can be found later in this chapter as well as in Chapters 2, 11, and 12.)

This chapter begins with a review of the phenomenological features and etiologic assumptions associated with combat exhaustion (currently included in combat and operational stress reaction [COSR]). It also utilizes the available psychiatric literature pertaining

to the war to estimate the incidence of combat exhaustion cases in Vietnam. In addition, it explores some of the unique features of the combat ecology in Vietnam, provides case examples, and presents selected findings from the 1982 Walter Reed Army Institute of Research (WRAIR) Psychiatrists' Survey in an effort to further define the nature of combat stress there and its various symptomatic consequences.

The material presented in this chapter extends the review of the Army's forward treatment doctrine for combat stress casualties begun in Chapter 2. Management and treatment of combat reactions in Vietnam are discussed in Chapter 7. Finally, psychiatric and behavior problems in Vietnam that were not evidently associated with combat will be addressed in Chapter 8 as deployment stress reactions (currently called combat misconduct stress behavior). However, it should be noted that in many instances this distinction could be a misleading because the war was mostly a counterinsurgency/guerrilla war with no front lines and no deep, well-defended rear. Many psychiatric and behavior problems may have etiologically overlapped with overt combat reactions and belong at the other end of the spectrum of psychiatric and behavior disorders generated by the unique collection of combat-related stressors found throughout Vietnam.

BACKGROUND

The Classic Combat (Stress) Reaction: Psychosocial Regression Under Fire and the Loss of Combat Effectiveness

As indicated in Chapter 2, throughout the 20th century there was growing interest by military psychiatrists and other behavioral scientists regarding the physical and psychological limits of troops under fire and the prevention of soldier breakdown as well as its treatment.[5–19] In the wars preceding Vietnam, combat reaction symptoms were noted to be diffuse and variable and sometimes spread among soldiers by suggestion.[1] Early-stage combat reaction symptoms progressed from normal anticipatory fear and uneasiness to hyperalertness, irritability, difficulty concentrating, insomnia, somatic disturbances, and preoccupations with death and disability. Severity often increased if there was no relief or intervention, and the disorder advanced to a stage of gross disturbances in mood, thinking, and behavior[20] (Table 6-1).

TABLE 6-1. Combat Reaction Stages

	APPREHENSION "Normal Fear"	INCIPIENT Combat Reaction	PARTIAL Combat Reaction	COMPLETE Combat Reaction

Social and Behavioral	Appropriate
	Combat effective
	Close with comrades
	Shares fears with comrades
		Add: Irritability	Reclusive
			Morose
			Overdependent and
			    avoids responsibility
			Reduced initiative
			Impulsive
			Decreased interest in:
			    combat, food, letters, etc.
			Unit members alarmed
				Unstable
				Erratic
				Reckless or overcautious
				Savage irritability
				Unreasonable and defiant
				Sobbing
				Screaming
				Passive and helpless

Emotional and Cognitive	Increased vigilance
	Worries: death/mutilation
	    incapacitating fear,
	    losing caste with group
	    through fear
		Add: Startle reaction	Mild disorientation
			Reduced judgment
			Psychomotor retardation
			Affect blunting
			Depressed
			Ruminating regarding:
			    survival, combat failure,
			    excess combat aggression
				Confused
				Disorganized
				Amnestic

Somatic	Tense
	Autonomic arousal
	    (gastrointestinal disorders, etc.)
	Disturbed sleep
	    (including sleepwalking)
	Psychosomatic complaints
		Add: Major insomnia	Severe diarrhea and vomiting
			Somatic preoccupation
				Stammering and incoherent
				Tremulous and uncoordinated
				Mute and staring
				Conversation symptoms: deaf,
				    blind, paralyzed, convulsive

Drawn from observations made in the closing phases of World War II by a panel of distinguished civilian psychiatrists who visited the European theater. Data source: Bartemeier LH, Kubie LS, Menninger KA, Romano J, Whitehorn JC. Combat exhaustion. *J Nerv Ment Dis*. 1946;104:358–389.

Presenting symptoms for combat reactions were also influenced by the soldier's specific combat circumstances, that is, the "ecology" of the battlefield,[21] as well as the military's medical evacuation requirements.[7,22] They were also shaped by which symptom patterns the soldier's reference group (combat buddies) found acceptable.[23] In this regard, his condition must appear to reflect incapacitation, as opposed to unwillingness, to continue to fight so that he isn't judged to have succumbed to weakness or cowardice or to have manipulated an exit from the battlefield. Finally, obviously avoidant behaviors such as combat refusal, malingering, self-inflicted wounds, and desertion, as well as less direct ones such as alcohol and drug misuse; neglect of healthcare, weapons, or equipment; indiscipline; combat atrocities; and behaviors associated with "short-timer's syndrome" were also thought to be associated with combat stress or the threat of it.

Diagnosis of the Combat Reaction

With regard to combat reaction cases, the fully affected soldier ("Complete combat reaction" in Table 6-1) is presumed to have undergone a profound psychological regression—a mental and social decompensation—as a consequence of having had his psychological endurance, as well as his combat motivation[24,25] and adaptation, overwhelmed by the rigors, dangers, losses, or horrors of the combat situation. In other words, he has undergone psychological traumatization (for an example, see Chapter 2, Case 2-1, SP4 Delta). However, among soldiers who had little prior history of psychiatric problems or personality deficits, combat reactions have appeared to be transitory or reversible, especially when the soldier is managed with a vigorous but simple crisis-oriented regimen aimed at quickly restoring him to combat duty function—the military forward treatment

---

EXHIBIT 6-1. Phenomenological Elements in Diagnosing "Classic" Combat Reaction (Combat Exhaustion)

Five observable criteria for the diagnosis of classic combat reaction:

1. Stimulus: the affected soldier must have sustained *exceptionally stressful combat,* with the continued threat of danger as the essential element (and which is consistent with his interpretation of the threat).
2. Predisposition: distinctive by its relative absence; there is presumed *universal susceptibility* among soldiers, although individual vulnerability and coping capacities play a role in forms of presentation and severity.
3. Clinical course: there is *rapid deterioration* of the affected soldier's combat adaptation and effectiveness in the face of his personal ordeal.
4. Presentation: the affected soldier evidences symptoms of a *disabling regression* of psychological and social functions.
5. Prognosis: the affected soldier typically has a *reversible course*, especially if he gets relief from the stress or receives timely, progressive, military-centered treatment.

SOURCES:
1. US Department of Defense. *The Joint Armed Forces Nomenclature and Method of Recording Psychiatric Conditions.* Washington, DC: DoD; June 1949. Special Regulation 40-1025-2.
2. Glass AJ. Military psychiatry and changing systems of mental health care. *J Psychiat Res.* 1971;8:499–512.
3. Glass AJ. Lessons learned. In: Glass AJ, ed. *Neuropsychiatry in World War II.* Vol 2. *Overseas Theaters.* Washington, DC: Medical Department, United States Army; 1973: 989–1027.
4. Cooke ET. *Another Look at Combat Exhaustion.* Fort Sam Houston, Tex: Department of Neuropsychiatry, Medical Field Service School; distributed July 1967. Training Document GR 51-400-320, 055.

---

doctrine.[5,7,13,14] From these observations military psychiatrists have considered that the combat reaction may be a version of what is called acute stress reaction,[26] or acute stress disorder (ASD),[27,28] in civilian psychiatry.

The diagnostic criteria for the classic combat reaction are delineated in Exhibit 6-1; however, this construct may be oversimplified. For instance, with regard to stimulus and civilian patients with acute stress reactions, some psychoanalyst theorists have found it useful to distinguish between: (1) shock trauma[29] (or "catastrophic trauma"[30]) in instances of psychic disorganization and immobility following overwhelming danger, which would coincide with the classic combat reaction; (2) strain trauma[29] to allude to long-lasting stress situations causing trauma from cumulative frustration and tension; and (3) partial trauma[30] to describe a series of emotionally disturbing events, which, although failing to reach the threshold of trauma, nevertheless distort various mental functions and adaptation. Perhaps in lieu of the term classic *combat reaction*, the term *uncomplicated combat reaction* would be preferable. As will be explained, this becomes even more practical considering the history of confusion in military terminology.

Pathogenesis of the Combat Reaction

Earlier wars led military psychiatrists to believe that if the intensity of the fighting was high enough and the duration of exposure of a soldier was indeterminate, then "every man has his breaking point."[5,10,31–33] When it became evident that the average soldier's resiliency could be exceeded by combat stress, attention shifted away from the question of "who" (implying precombat susceptibility), and more toward the "when" and the "how." Earlier assumptions of faulty personality development[23] or cowardice gave way to the perspective that the combat reaction represented a normal reaction to an abnormal situation,[20] at least in its acute stage (ie, it is a matter of limits in capacity as opposed to courage). In other words, the soldier's combat motivation had been compromised by situational and environmental factors that raised his fears to intolerable levels and activated his self-preservative instincts. However, whereas this model may have broad, utilitarian applicability, it does not provide for variability at the level of the individual soldier. The following offers a more complex pathodynamic explanation.

A Bio\Psycho\Social Etiologic Model for Combat Reactions

Over the years research and systematic observation have established an extensive list of pre- and pericombat factors that strengthened the soldier's adaptation and resilience under fire and opposed the onset of combat reactions. Chief among them are indoctrination and

FIGURE 6-1. The bio\psycho\social etiological model and the combat stress reaction (CSR). The shaded figure represents an individual soldier. Vector arrows represent combat stress challenging that soldier at successive levels of mental organization.

Social Supports:
Failed social and environmental support
—immediate, for example, within the small combat group (isolated, unprotected, poorly led, estranged, depleted, etc.)
—remote, for example, that generated from home
(uncared for, blamed, etc)

Individual Psychology and Motivation:
—low commitment to mission, to comrades (socially remote)
—individual susceptibility leading to subjective distortion of the events (persecutory feelings, exaggerated fear, helplessness, rage, guilt, shame, panic, etc)

Biological Integrity:
Physical depletion (hot/cold, tired, hungry, wet, sleep deprived, over stimulated, exhausted, wounded, dehydrated) and associated organismic stress responses.

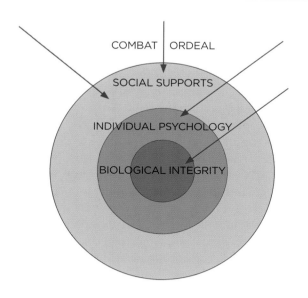

training; physical conditioning; stress inoculation[34]; efficiency of communication; quantity and quality of supplies and weapons; reiteration of the military objective; support from home; and, especially, unit morale, cohesion, and leadership.[17,20,32,35–42] (See Johnson's article, "Psychiatric Treatment in the Combat Situation," for a more complete list.[22]) With respect to social supports, according to Albert J Glass, the preeminent combat psychiatrist in the last half of the 20th century, the inadequacy of sustaining relationships within the small combat group, or their disruption during combat, was the most important factor responsible for psychiatric breakdown in World War II and Korea.[23] Elsewhere Glass wrote:

> Of special significance was the growing awareness that the stimuli of battle itself evoked a defensive process that sustained men in combat . . . the lonely, fearful battle environment forces individuals to join together for protection and emotional support . . . [W]hat began as mere instinctual huddling is crystallized into a powerful emotional bond of love and concern for comrades which deflects fear from the self and creates a compelling internal motivation for remaining with or rejoining the combat group.[43(p728)]

Further explanation for this observation came from Jon A Shaw, an Army psychiatrist and psychoanalyst. According to Shaw, the intensification of combat group cohesion/morale stems from the soldiers' need to band with, and idealize, their combat buddies, and to maintain an illusion of their unit leader's omnipotence, so as to keep out of awareness their relative helplessness in battle and primitive concerns regarding biological vulnerability.[44]

Questions regarding how much weight to give to individual predisposition have remained the more elusive variable in the combat reaction pathogenesis equation. Although it had been concluded that personality characteristics were of less importance in soldier breakdown in high-intensity combat,[45,46] they appeared to be of increasing importance in cases arising in low-intensity combat[47] as well as influence recovery[48]— observations that would have special pertinence for a counterinsurgency/guerrilla war like Vietnam.

The analysis of a specimen combat stress reaction case from World War II by Erik Erikson, the renowned psychologist and psychoanalyst, provides a useful theoretical model for intrapsychic (ie, mental or emotional) vulnerability and conflict within the affected soldier.[49] According to Erikson, apart from the traumatic potential of the combat experience itself, to fully account for the soldier's psychological and functional deterioration under fire (Erikson would refer to it as a "crisis"), one needs to assume that there have been concurrent disruptions in all three primary centers of human experience—the somatic ("bio"), the psychological ("psycho"), and the social.

Refinement of Erikson's trilateral perspective in general is provided through George Engel's bio\psycho\social model of psychiatric pathogenesis that argues for relating these levels hierarchically. According to Engel, appreciation of disturbances at the lower levels is necessary to comprehend, but not sufficient to explain, disturbances at higher levels.[50] Thus, this author [NMC] notes that in borrowing from Erikson and Engel, to fully conceptualize the pathogenesis of a case of combat stress reaction, one must not only consider the specific nature and extent of the soldier's combat ordeal (eg, its actual rigors, dangers, losses, or horrors) but also look for compounding disturbances generated from each of the levels of his mental organization, including those pertaining to his personality type and its limitations, especially his interpretation of his circumstances (ie, the personal "meaning" the events have for him alone) (see Figure 6-1).

That having been said, it should be underscored that, *in the field*, precombat susceptibility of the affected soldier can be difficult to assess because the forward treatment doctrine discourages approaches that might promote "patienthood." Based on experiences in Korea, Glass warned military psychiatrists not to focus on the soldier-patient's background features because this invites chronicity. ("Any therapy, including usual interview methods, that sought to uncover basic emotional conflicts or attempted to relate current behavior and symptoms with past personality patterns seemingly provided patients with logical reasons for their combat failure."[43(p727)])

Below is a case report from the 935th Psychiatric Detachment that illustrates features consistent with the classic, or uncomplicated, combat reaction. Relevant discussion of this and other case reports will be presented in the text.

CASE 6-1: Disorganized, Regressed, Combat Stress Reaction After Unit Was Overrun

---

Identifying information: Corporal (CPL) Foxtrot was a 21-year-old rifleman who was flown directly to the 93rd Evacuation Hospital from an area of fighting by a helicopter ambulance. No information accompanied him, he had no identifying tags on his uniform, and he was so completely covered with mud that a physical description of his features was not possible. He also was disorganized and incapable of cooperating with a formal evaluation.

History of present illness: CPL Foxtrot's symptoms developed when his platoon had been caught in an ambush and then overrun by the enemy. He was one of three who survived after being pinned down by enemy fire for 12 hours. Toward the end of that time he developed a crazed expression and had tried to run from his hiding place. He was pulled back to safety and remained there until the helicopter arrived and flew him to the hospital.

Past history: He had no history of similar symptoms or emotional disorder.

Examination: His hands had been tied behind him for the flight, and he had a wild, wide-eyed look as he cowered in a corner of the emergency room, glancing furtively to all sides, cringing and startling at the least noise. He was mute, although once he forced out a whispered "VC" ["Viet Cong"] and tried to mouth other words without success. He seemed terrified. Although people could approach him, he appeared oblivious to their presence. No manner of reassurance or direct order achieved either a verbal response or any other interaction from him. His hands were untied, after which he would hold an imaginary rifle in readiness whenever he heard a helicopter overhead or an unexpected noise.

Clinical course: The corpsmen led CPL Foxtrot to the psychiatric ward, took him to a shower, and offered him a meal; he ate very little. He began to move a little more freely but still offered no information. He was then given 100 mg. of Thorazine orally, and this dose was repeated hourly until he fell asleep. He was kept asleep in this manner for approximately 40 hours. After that he was allowed to waken, the medication was discontinued, and he was mobilized rapidly in the ward milieu. Although initially dazed and subdued, his response in the ward milieu was dramatic. This was aided by the presence of a friend from his platoon on an adjoining ward who helped by filling in parts of the story that the patient could not recall. Within 72 hours following his admission the patient was alert, oriented, responsive, and active. Although still a little tense, he was ready to return to duty.

Discharge diagnosis: Combat exhaustion, moderately severe.

Disposition: On his third hospital day he was returned to duty with his unit and never seen again at the 935th.

Source: Clinical record narrative summary. A version of the case of CPL Foxtrot was published as Bloch HS. Army clinical psychiatry in the combat zone: 1967–1968. *Am J Psychiatry*. 1969;126(3):294.

Critical Distinctions Between Combat and Civilian Stress Casualties

The US military has long operated under the assumption that the combat stress casualty must be distinguished from otherwise similar civilian and noncombat military stress cases with regard to assumptions about etiology and, by implication, treatment. Whereas the bio\psycho\social model presented above would generally apply to civilian or noncombat military situations of overwhelming stress, additional *intrapsychic* (ie, mental or emotional) dynamics are unique to the combat soldier (intrapsychic mental dynamics refers to the interaction of psychological functions in the mind, such as urges, pressure from the conscience, and the need to cooperate with the external world; intrapsychic conflict refers to clashes or tension that arise when two or more become seemingly incompatible or irreconcilable), and these may negatively influence his interpretation of the combat experience and increase his psychological vulnerability.[34,51,52] These intrapsychic dynamics include:

1. He has been *trained to kill* (the enemy, as well as accept collateral damage) and, when necessary, is expected to do this without hesitation. This is more than the fact that he was trained to use deadly force as this would also be the case for law enforcement personnel. The specific mandate under which the infantry soldier operates, that is, his duty, is "to close with and destroy or capture the enemy." This does not specify that his sole aim is to kill the enemy, but it sanctions that extreme measure as a principal tool, not one of last resort.

2. Consequent to his training to kill, he may bear substantial *moral/ethical* strain in overriding a lifetime of socialization to not be destructive, especially not to kill. (Retired Army Ranger and former professor of psychology at the US Military Academy at West Point, Dave Grossman, makes this case convincingly in his review of the extensive historical documentation substantiating the average soldier's resistance to kill. In fact, according to Grossman, the prospect that soldiers fighting in Vietnam would exhibit hesitancy in firing their weapons at the enemy was a problem the military took very seriously in conditioning troops for service in that conflict.[34]) This strain could become heightened if combat circumstances take an unfavorable turn (ie, locally, should he and his unit encounter dire combat circumstances; or more broadly, as when the moral justification for his combat participation becomes questionable secondary to public opposition to the war). According to Stewart L Baker Jr, a senior Army psychiatrist, in earlier wars the role of "guilt about killing or assailing defenseless enemy personnel, either military or civilian . . ." was found to be an important precipitating factor for some combat reaction cases. ("In such instances . . . the superimposed military code yielded to the earlier and stronger civilian prohibition against violence against others."[7(p1834)])

3. He may also become *motivationally conflicted* in instances when (1) and (2) apply or when self-preservative instincts rise to a level where they oppose his sense of his duty to perform under fire and perhaps sacrifice his life for his countrymen. While under treatment these conflicts may become elevated by the soldier's awareness that he is expected to recover and return to combat and face additional hazards.

According to Grossman, an especially pathogenic combination of factors can face a soldier and account for his becoming a combat reaction casualty (when compared to noncombatants):

Fear of death and injury is *not* (author's emphasis) the only, or even the major, cause of psychiatric casualties in combat. . . . The whole truth is much more complex and horrible. . . .

[It is man's natural] resistance to overt, aggressive confrontation, in addition to the fear of death and injury, [that] is responsible for much of the trauma and stress on the battlefield. . . .

Fear, combined with exhaustion, hate, horror, and the irreconcilable task of balancing these with the need to kill, eventually drives the soldier so deeply into a mire of guilt and horror that he [is overwhelmed].[34(p54)]

Grossman also put a high valence on a sort of combat paranoia that contributes to soldier stress. ("The soldier in combat . . . resists the powerful obligation and coercion to engage in aggressive and assertive actions on the battlefield [because] he dreads facing the irrational aggression and hostility embodied in the enemy."[34(p78)])

The following three cases from the 935th Psychiatric Detachment in Vietnam, all from the winter and spring of 1968, will serve as illustrations.

CASE 6-2: Acute Combat Stress Reaction With Fearfulness, Tremulousness, Social Withdrawal, and Aversion to More Combat

---

Identifying information: Private First Class (PFC) Golf was a 22-year-old infantryman with 5 months in Vietnam. He was brought in to the 93rd Evacuation Hospital with several casualties after a heavy firefight.

Past history: None recorded.

Examination: At the time of admission PFC Golf was described as mute, hyperalert, tremulous, and fearful. Physical exam was within normal limits.

Clinical course: He was put to sleep with Thorazine (no specifics) and mobilized the next morning. At that time he was morose, exhibited a little consciously determined posturing, and complained of stomach upset, pain, and fear of recurrence of an alleged ulcer. He talked about not wanting to fight anymore and being tired of "all the killing going on." He was alert and without evidence of psychosis. On the ward he remained quiet and somewhat seclusive. His attending psychiatrist wrote, "Although he continues to appear morose and a bit depressed, I strongly favor rapid remobilization of his functioning in an effort to prevent a more serious deterioration motivated by desire to be away from the combat situation." He was discharged back to his unit after 2 days of hospitalization.

Discharge diagnosis: Combat exhaustion, acute, moderately severe, improved. Impairment: moderate.

Disposition: Returned to full duty with a prescription for antacid medication.

Source: Discharge Summary, 935th Psychiatric Detachment/93rd Evacuation Hospital.

CASE 6-3: Acute Combat Stress Reaction With Rage After His Boat Was Ambushed

---

Identifying information: PFC Hotel was a 20-year-old married Roman Catholic infantryman with 11 months in the Army and 2 months in Vietnam. He was brought to the 93rd Evacuation Hospital from the field after the riverboat he was on was ambushed by the VC. History of present illness: During the attack an RPG [rocket-propelled grenade] round blew his buddy "to pieces," killed another, and wounded several more. PFC Hotel became angry and lost control.

Past history: None provided.

Examination: Patient was alert, tearful, and angry. He said, "We're dying for no purpose! Let me get back to my unit. I hate all VC." He was oriented and showed no signs of a thought disorder or any impairment of judgment or memory.

Clinical course: Sleep therapy for 20 hours with Thorazine. Appropriate on awakening. Able to discuss the episode. He was discharged back to his unit after an overnight stay.

Discharge diagnosis: Acute stress reaction, mild, improved. Impairment: minimal.

Disposition: Returned to duty by way of the division Mental Health Consultation Service.

Source: Discharge Summary, 935th Psychiatric Detachment/93rd Evacuation Hospital.

CASE 6-4: Acute Combat Stress Reaction With Fearfulness, Depression, Disorientation, and Mild Dissociation

Identifying information: PFC India was an 18-year-old infantryman with 8 months in the Army and 1 month in Vietnam. He was referred from the 9th Infantry Division Mental Health Consultation Service after he was evacuated by dustoff helicopter from the field.

History of present illness: When his unit came under heavy fire, he was observed to become stuporous, detached, frightened, and he removed his gear and ran around without regard for sniper fire. He kept repeating, "I didn't want to kill anyone!"

Past history: None recorded.

Examination: At the division he was reportedly disoriented. At the 935th PFC India presented as a sad, preoccupied man with shortened attention span, impaired recent memory, and depressed and diminished manifest affect. He was disoriented for time and place. There was no evidence of a thought disorder.

Clinical course: He was given an 18-hour course of sleep treatment with Thorazine and then rapidly mobilized in the therapeutic milieu. His disorientation, impoverished affect, and other manifest symptoms cleared. Though his fearfulness of returning to the field persisted, his attending psychiatrist indicated that he was ready to return to duty. He was returned to his unit after 2 days hospitalization.

Discharge diagnosis: Combat exhaustion, acute, moderately severe, improved. Impairment: mild.

Disposition: Returned to duty by way of the division Mental Health Consultation Service with the recommendation that his commander should consider whether PFC India was reliable enough for combat duty.

Source: Discharge Summary, 935th Psychiatric Detachment/93rd Evacuation Hospital.

History of the Military Classification System for Combat Stress Reactions

The military has elected to use context-specific terms to refer to the psychiatric casualties of combat while the civilian community has sought increased comprehensiveness in psychiatric diagnosis. The adoption of uniquely combat-centered terms for this new type of casualty began during World War I because the civilian diagnostic system in use was more suited to the large mental hospitals in the United States.[19] Shifts in nomenclature for combat stress casualties initially reflected revisions in assumed pathogenesis, and later, the gap between civilian-based medical priority of symptom removal versus military-based one of force conservation. The term *shell shock* was employed early in World War I because it was believed that a concussive injury to the brain was responsible. Subsequently, psychological terms like *war neurosis*, *combat neurosis*, and even *gas hysteria* were employed (the latter referred to soldiers who became incapacitated with respiratory symptoms despite there being no poison gas in the area). These labels served to characterize the affected soldier as suffering with a combat-provoked *intrapsychic* (ie, mental or emotional) conflict—an etiological proposition consistent with then popular Freudian theories.[53]

In World War II use of the terms *combat exhaustion* and *combat fatigue* represented a pragmatic decision by the military in support of force conservation. Command directives specified that such terms replace those of neurosis as the latter could encourage soldiers to imitate the bizarre symptoms of stereotypical civilian psychiatric patients in order to be exempted from further combat.[23] As Glass noted, this was a salutary shift in that "although [exhaustion was] a non-specific and non-psychological term [it] was an apt description of a temporary fluid condition resulting from physical and emotional strain of combat, regardless of manifestations or predisposition."[23(p507)] Glass also indicated that the overall manpower losses for combat stress disorders declined following this change in labeling because "psychiatric casualties became legitimized as a rational consequence of combat circumstances."[23(p506)]

At the close of World War II, *combat exhaustion* was ultimately selected as the official term for combat reactions.[54,55] The Joint Armed Forces Nomenclature (June 1949) placed "combat exhaustion" [3273] under "transient personality disorders." By definition it was intended for "previously more or less 'normal persons,'" applied to "transient," potentially reversible, reactions in which the combat soldier "may display a marked psychological disorganization akin to certain psychoses," and was "justified *only* (emphasis added) in situations in which the individual [was] exposed to severe physical demands or extreme emotional stress in combat"[55(§II[8]pp11–12)] (in other words, it satisfied all five of the observable classic combat stress reaction elements presented in Exhibit 6-1). In less clear-cut instances the nomenclature recommended "acute situational maladjustment" [3274] be utilized (also under transient personality disorders).[55(§II[8]pp11–12)] This system of categorization stood throughout the Korean War (1950–1953). In June 1963, the Armed Forces Medical Diagnosis Nomenclature and Statistical Classification (AR 40-401) became official.[56] It continued the use of "combat exhaustion" [3263] as well as "other acute situational maladjustment" [3264], and these categories carried throughout the Vietnam War (1965–1973). (Also see Exhibit 6-2, "Civilian Nosology and Combat Stress Reaction.")

However, according to Glass, as the Vietnam War lengthened, the term *classical combat fatigue*, which had originally been coined as an all-encompassing term, had ironically become a myth, despite its having been codified in official diagnostic manuals. He was concerned that it was being utilized too strictly; that is, that underlying personality defects were being dismissed as etiologically irrelevant, and the only combat casualties counted as combat fatigue cases were the "relatively few individuals who possess a theoretically healthy psychic apparatus but are temporarily overwhelmed by extraordinary circumstances of trauma and deprivation."[57(pxxv)] Finally, to complete the picture of the evolving taxonomy for combat stress reactions, it is important to acknowledge the emergence of the posttraumatic stress disorder (PTSD) diagnosis in the decade following the end of the Vietnam War. As the popularity of this new diagnosis grew among both military and civilian psychiatrists, especially those serving veterans in the Department of Veterans Affairs, many professionals, as well as lay individuals, came to assume that this diagnostic entity was synonymous with combat exhaustion; however, this was not the case[58] (see Exhibit 6-3, "The Post-Vietnam Era and Posttraumatic Stress Disorder").

VIETNAM: THE COMBAT ECOLOGY AND RELATED STRESSORS

As mentioned earlier, observation drawn from the main force wars leading up to Vietnam primarily emphasized two overlapping dimensions of modern warfare that can make it unbearably stressful and generate combat stress reactions in large numbers: (1) its intensity, that is, its lethality, which has historically been measured with the wounded-in-action (WIA) rate; and (2) how exhausting it is, that is, its strenuous and depleting nature, which has to some extent been objectively measured in terms of the duration of the soldier's exposure; but in other regards it is not measurable because it can be experienced quite subjectively (see Figure 6-1). However, Vietnam was different in many ways from the wars that preceded it, especially in becoming a counterinsurgency/guerrilla conflict; consequently, comparisons with the combat reaction model from World War II and Korea that rest on these two dimensions may be only so useful.

The Combat Intensity (Lethality) Variable in Vietnam

The designation of Vietnam as low intensity—a classification based on the low ratio of casualties to numbers of personnel deployed—appears to be somewhat misleading. Not only does the higher proportion of noncombat troops to combat troops in Vietnam alter the metric, but otherwise, as Spector, a military historian, convincingly argued using other measures, the fighting there was often as bloody as that seen in earlier wars. Combat Specimen #1: Viet Cong Ambush During the Battle of Dau Tieng (in Attachment 6-1) is excerpted from SLA Marshall's *Ambush* [59(pp138–147)] to illustrate Spector's point. (This example of the reconstruction of a small unit action by Marshall was chosen because he employed a unique method of group battle debriefing that he devised in World War II.[60(pp108–115),61(p72)])

The Combat Exhaustion Variable in Vietnam

If reduced combat intensity in Vietnam cannot account for the low incidence of classic combat reaction cases, consideration must be given to the other major variable: soldier exhaustion. To say that combat activities for the American infantry in Vietnam were not physically and psychologically arduous (and thus exhausting in the conventional sense) would also be

EXHIBIT 6-2. Civilian Nosology and Combat Stress Reaction

The civilian classification system for psychiatric disorders became increasingly complex during the second half of the 20th century and the opening years of this one. The first American Psychiatric Association *Diagnostic and Statistical Manual* (DSM-I) was published in 1952 and was based on a presumed pathogenesis for mental disturbances that emphasized intrapsychic motives and conflicts.[1] It included the entity "gross stress reaction," which more or less replicated military psychiatry's characterization of the combat (stress) reaction or CSR. This was because the establishment of the American taxonomy at that time was influenced by the many psychiatrists with military experience in World War II who had treated soldiers who developed disabling psychiatric symptoms from exposure to combat. (Later it would be the reverse, ie, that attitudes among civilian psychiatrists would come to influence the military's approach to combat stress casualties.) Gross stress reaction (54.0) was listed as a subcategory of transient situational personality disorders, as was adult situational reaction (54.1). Gross stress reaction applied to situations of reversible symptomatology occurring among otherwise normal persons who sustained "conditions of great or unusual stress." The diagnosis was considered to be preliminary and, should such cases not respond to prompt treatment, it was to be replaced with a more definitive one. Along with civilian catastrophes, DSM-I specifically included participation in combat as having the potential to produce intolerable stress. Yet it can be argued that, in lumping civilian (or noncombat military) conditions with those occurring on the battlefield, important psychodynamic assumptions regarding the pathogenesis of CSR were overlooked. Whereas gross stress reaction satisfied all five of the observable CSR criteria mentioned in Exhibit 6-1, to merge CSR with similar civilian casualties required the obviation of the unique intrapsychic features presumed to play an important role in many soldiers' breakdown (or complicate recovery), that is, *trained to kill, moral/ethical strain, and motivational conflict.*

Taxonomic matters became more confused in 1968, roughly halfway through the Vietnam War, when DSM-II as well as ICD-8 (the World Health Organization's *International Classification of Diseases, 8th Rev.*) were published following a process of synchronization. Although there had been earlier versions of the ICD, the 8th revision was the first one to include a psychiatric taxonomy to any extent.[2(p435)] No longer listed was the specific category of gross stress reaction. Consequently it must be assumed that combat reactions were to be under transient situational disturbances/adjustment reaction of adult life (307.3), described as disorders *"of any severity"* (emphasis added) in reaction to "overwhelming environmental stress" in otherwise not predisposed individuals. Regarding etiology, combat exposure is not mentioned specifically, but the DSM-II did include the following as an example of adjustment reaction of adult life: "Fear associated with military combat and manifested by trembling, running, and hiding."[3(p49)] DSM-II suggests that the treatment for these conditions lies mostly in the simple removal of the stress. By implication, combat had become lumped in with experiences in which the individual is simply the victim of an unforeseen trauma, and the proposed treatment is removal from the battlefield. Clearly by 1968, experienced military psychiatrists had faded in their influence on American psychiatry. (Also see Exhibit 6-3, "The Post-Vietnam Era and Posttraumatic Stress Disorder.")

REFERENCES
1. Mayes R, Horwitz AV. DSM-III and the revolution in the classification of mental illness. *J History Behav Sci.* 2005;41:249–267.
2. American Psychiatric Association. *Diagnostic and Statistical Manual of Mental Disorders.* 3rd ed (DSM-III-R). Washington, DC: APA; 1987.
3. American Psychiatric Association. *Diagnostic and Statistical Manual of Mental Disorders.* 2nd ed (DSM-II). Washington, DC: APA; 1968.

misleading. Combat Specimen #2: Patrolling the Rong Sat Zone, also provided by Marshall in *Ambush* [59(pp187–192)] (in Attachment 6-2), describes conditions faced by Army troops operating in lowlands of the Mekong River delta in Vietnam. Clearly by that example, the task of eliminating the Viet Cong threat in the Mekong River delta was outrageously physically demanding, and thus psychologically challenging. However, it is noteworthy that, compared to their enemy counterparts, at least the American soldiers were regularly rotated out

of those conditions in order to recover body and spirit. And that is to the point: on the whole, soldiers fighting in Vietnam were less frequently exposed to *sustained* fighting than was typical in previous wars (Figure 6-2).

American technological superiority and the enemy's inability to deliver precision-guided indirect fire as with artillery and combat aircraft dramatically reduced the dimension of fatigue for committed troops as they were less likely to get pinned down for prolonged periods (with the special exception in early 1968 of the 76-day siege

EXHIBIT 6-3. The Post-Vietnam Era and Posttraumatic Stress Disorder

As noted in Chapter 2, combat stress reaction (CSR) is often confused with posttraumatic stress disorder (PTSD).[1] In the decade following the end of the Vietnam War, the *Diagnostic and Statistical Manual of the Mental Disorders*, 3rd edition (DSM-III)[2] (1980) and the *International Classification of Disease*, 9th edition, Clinical Modification (ICD-9-CM)[3] (1979) were published and included the new category "Posttraumatic Stress Disorder" (PTSD), which was initially referred to as "post-Vietnam syndrome."[4]

According to DSM-III, PTSD (309.81) referred to "symptoms *following* (emphasis added) a psychologically traumatic event."[2(p236)] It applied to individuals who had experienced an event outside the range of usual human experience, which was accompanied by intense fear, terror, and/or helplessness, and which would be markedly distressing to almost anyone; and it included adverse combat events as having this potential. By these criteria alone, the new PTSD resembled the gross stress reaction of DSM-I. PTSD symptoms included variations of: (*a*) reexperiencing the traumatic event; (*b*) avoiding stimuli associated with the trauma or experiencing a numbing of general responsiveness; and (*c*) symptoms of increased arousal (eg, sleep difficulties, irritability, hypervigilance, exaggerated startle response, or increased physiological arousal upon exposure to events that symbolize or resemble an aspect of the traumatic event).

Notably, the revised version of DSM-III clarified that the PTSD diagnosis was not intended for individuals whose symptoms remitted within 1 month after the event.[5(p435)] Thus, as defined by DSM-III, PTSD satisfied two of the aforementioned CSR diagnostic criteria: (1) exposure to *exceptionally stressful* (combat) *events*, and (2) *universal susceptibility*. However, the diagnosis of PTSD did not explicitly include *rapid deterioration* and *disabling regression* as associated phenomena. Furthermore, by excluding individuals whose symptoms lasted less than 1 month it explicitly did not satisfy the *reversible course* criteria for CSR. In other words, by these terms alone it was evident that PTSD was distinct from CSR.

Further distinguishing PTSD from CSR, DSM-III referred to delayed and chronic PTSD. Delayed PTSD was to be used when symptoms emerged after 6 months following the traumatic event; and chronic PTSD applied if the symptoms persisted 6 months beyond it. The first of these stipulations would negate the *rapid deterioration* criteria for CSR, and the second one would negate the *reversible course* criteria (presuming the individual had timely treatment in the field without effect). DSM-III was also confusing in that it assigned PTSD the number 309.8, which placed it in the category of adjustment disorders (which would satisfy the *universal susceptibility* condition for CSR); however, in the arrangement of psychiatric conditions in the schema, PTSD was placed among the "anxiety disorders" (or anxiety and phobic neuroses), which would suggest the opposite, that is, psychological predisposition.

of 5,500 defenders of the Marine base at Khe Sanh[62]). Combat engagements with the enemy were more often intermittent, relatively brief (lasting minutes to hours; rarely days), and staged from well-defended enclaves that were easily resupplied by helicopter. Troops were also well supported through the tactical use of heliborne maneuver and artillery/air support.

On the other hand, the new heliborne capability of rapid, vertical assaults may have added a new means of exhaustion as it allowed troops to become engaged in more frequent contacts with the enemy over time compared to the soldiers from earlier wars who would get to the fight over the ground. It also meant that units could be sustained in place during intense, prolonged combat, which resulted in elevated combat stress levels. Air-mobile insertions in Vietnam were also very dangerous. The troops typically had to deploy from a hovering aircraft and make an exposed assault across an open clearing large enough for several helicopters.[63] (See Chapter 1 for an overview of the shifting stress-generating and stress-mitigating factors that comprised the physical, social, and psychological combat "ecology" affecting ground forces in Vietnam.)

Additional Features Comprising the Combat Ecologies in Vietnam

As mentioned in Chapter 1, the United States and its allies faced a two-fold enemy in South Vietnam, each of whom employed different tactics and weapons: (1) the indigenous Viet Cong guerrilla forces employed harassment, terrorism, ambush, and psychological warfare (see Exhibit 1-1, "The Viet Cong Strategy of Terror"), and (2) the regular units of the North Vietnam Army (NVA) staged more conventional attacks from behind the safety of the 17th parallel/demilitarized zone (DMZ). Combat Specimen #1 may serve as an example of the former, but the variations in the sub-(combat) ecologies in South Vietnam should also be considered as each brought unique challenges for US forces. Colonel Matthew D Parrish, the third Neuropsychiatry

EXHIBIT 6-3. The Post-Vietnam Era and Posttraumatic Stress Disorder, continued

Peculiarly, DSM-III did not initially include the alternative to PTSD—acute stress reaction—that was listed in ICD-9-CM. However, DSM-III did include brief reactive psychosis, with combat listed as an etiologic event. This omission was rectified in the later iterations when DSM-IV[6] (1994) and DSM-IV-TR[7] (2000) added acute stress disorder or ASD (308.3) for symptoms in conjunction with intense fear, helplessness, or horror, that arise *"while experiencing or* after experiencing the distressing event" (emphasis added). Although the military nosology has conceptually embraced the acute stress disorder diagnosis, the doctrine for combat deployed troops has continued to utilize the term *combat stress* (currently *combat and operational stress reaction* [COSR][8]).

REFERENCES
1. Kentsmith DK. Principles of battlefield psychiatry. *Mil Med.* 1986;151:89–96.
2. American Psychiatric Association. *Diagnostic and Statistical Manual of Mental Disorders.* 3rd ed (DSM-III). Washington, DC: APA; 1980.
3. Centers for Disease Control. *International Classification of Disease-9th ed-Clinical Modification.* Available at: http://www.cdc.gov/nchs/icd/icd9.htm. Accessed 11 August 2011.
4. Shatan CF. The grief of soldiers: Vietnam combat veterans' self-help movement. *Am J Orthopsych.* 1973;43:640–653.
5. American Psychiatric Association. *Diagnostic and Statistical Manual of Mental Disorders.* 3rd ed (DSM-III-R). Washington, DC: APA; 1987.
6. American Psychiatric Association. *Diagnostic and Statistical Manual of Mental Disorders.* 4th ed (DSM-IV). Washington, DC: APA; 1994.
7. American Psychiatric Association. *Diagnostic and Statistical Manual of Mental Disorders.* 4th ed, text rev. (DSM-IV-TR). Washington, DC: APA; 2000.
8. Brusher EA. Combat and Operational Stress Control. In Ritchie EC, ed. *Combat and Operational Behavioral Health.* In: Lenhart MK, *The Textbooks of Military Medicine.* Washington, DC: Department of the Army, Office of The Surgeon General, Borden Institute; 2011: 59–71.

Consultant to the Commanding General, US Army Republic of Vietnam (CG/USARV) Surgeon (senior Army psychiatrist in South Vietnam), summarized some of the fundamental adaptational requirements:

[Under optimal circumstances] the infantry unit welds itself into a cohesive and effective team [while training for deployment in the United States]. These men maneuver and practice together until they are familiar, trusting, and nicely coordinated with each other. They study and do exercises needed for Viet Nam, [for example], in tunnel warfare, night infiltration, special fire discipline. They learn all about mines, punji sticks, booby traps, ambushes and enemy ruses. Only upon deployment in Vietnam and infused into its own target area, does the infantry team reach final maturity. Once there it seeks to become symbiotic with the jungle. Its individual soldiers coordinate quickly with each other in their response to communication with natives, to a change of jungle and village smells and sounds, or to the reactions of their dog and his handler. The jungle becomes an extension of the men's, of the team's, organs of sense and locomotion, and the team becomes an extension of the jungle.

The brigade deploys now in forested plains north of Saigon. There one of the soldiers, who knows all about booby traps, finds a cigarette lighter, and it blows his hand off. His buddies, also trained in such matters, rush to his aid and a Claymore mine booby trap kills five of them. A soldier jumps across a ditch and onto a set of punji sticks under the leaves. A little girl walks in among the Americans in their camp. She is carrying a satchel charge. A company completely surrounds a village and fights its way in, but it finds only women and children. The Viet Cong [VC] has escaped by a tunnel or a little string of underbrush. Farmers, seemingly on freedom's side by day, are VC by night. All of this the brigade already learned in the [United States], but they learn much of it again the hard way.

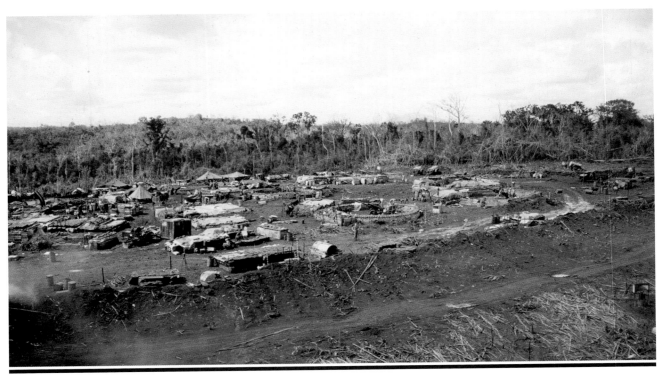

FIGURE 6-2A. Close aerial view of a fire support base of the 1st Cavalry Division, 1970. Such forward bases as this provided artillery support for combat operations and served as staging areas for ground maneuver elements that were typically moved around the battlefield by helicopter. Photograph courtesy of Richard D Cameron, Major General, US Army (Retired).

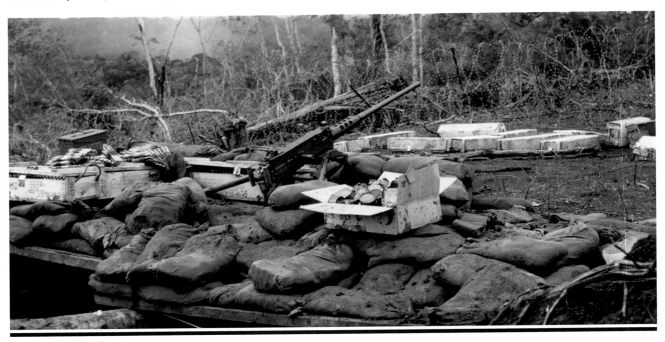

FIGURE 6-2B. Perimeter defenses of a 1st Cavalry Division fire support base. This photograph illustrates both passive (concertina wire and cleared vegetation) and active (.50 caliber machine gun emplacement) components in the perimeter defense of a firebase in 1970. Although the machine gun appears to be unmanned, undoubtedly the crew was close by. This reflects the Viet Cong practice of using the cover of darkness to initiate mortar and rocket attacks and attempts at infiltration using sappers (stealth commandos). Photograph courtesy of Richard D Cameron, Major General, US Army (Retired).

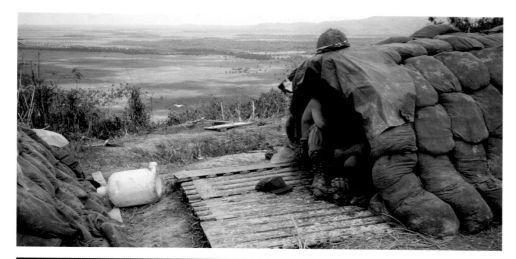

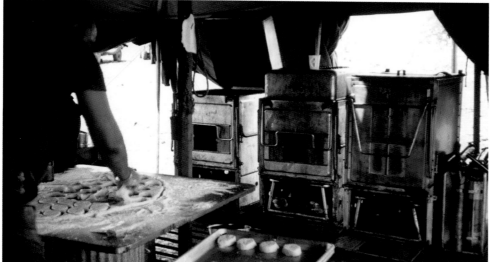

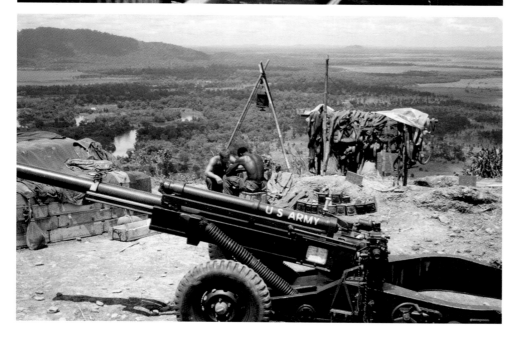

[Top] FIGURE 6-2C. Primitive living conditions on a 1st Cavalry Division forward fire support base, 1970. The high heat and humidity, persistent threat of enemy attack, confined living quarters and limited personal amenities, and episodes of continuous operations combined to create high stress for those assigned to such isolated outposts. Photograph courtesy of Richard D Cameron, Major General, US Army (Retired).

[Middle] FIGURE 6-2D. Mess tent on a 1st Cavalry Division fire support base, 1970. The Army made every effort to make life on these remote outposts as tolerable for troops as possible. As food is always a critical morale-bolstering element, this especially included the provision of hot meals whenever possible. Photograph courtesy of Richard D Cameron, Major General, US Army (Retired).

[Bottom] FIGURE 6-2E. Soldiers playing chess during a lull in activities on a 1st Cavalry Division fire support base, 1970. This photograph illustrates how the dangers and sparse living conditions found on these isolated forward bases meant that troops had limited means to ward off long stretches of boredom and loneliness. Perhaps also insinuated by the picture is that the racial tensions of the era were less problematic in the field, where the shared goal of fighting a common enemy promoted cooperation and tolerance. Photograph courtesy of Richard D Cameron, Major General, US Army (Retired).

Having cleaned up the plains, it moves confidently to the central highlands. There the weather is colder, wetter; the malaria is of a far more deadly type. The natives are mostly Montagnard, with ways of living and thinking completely different from the majority of Vietnamese. The enemy is not the VC but mostly the North Vietnamese regular army. There are few booby traps or tunnels. Many of the things the brigade is alert to no longer apply. One day an American company is following down a steep mountain trail. The platoons are fairly well spread out in a manner okay for the southern plains. Suddenly, in the thick woods, a North Vietnamese force fires into them. The Americans can't concentrate their platoons. The second company is too far back to move up through the mountainous forest. Air support is called in but the individual Americans have insufficient markers to show their position in this terrain. They're pinned down by their own air fire. Reinforcements come, but this enemy does not evaporate as the VC would. The Americans simply aren't with it yet in the central mountains. A few weeks later we find these same Americans traveling in different formation, alert to different clues, carrying more ammunition and more air signals. The NVA [North Vietnam Army] is getting hard to find. The brigade has begun to take over this terrain. They've become a part of it. If the brigade is now moved to the Delta they begin a new system, a fourth system. They must forge themselves into yet a different weapon.[64(pp6–7)]

The Strain on Troops Fighting an Irregular War in Vietnam

Although Parrish portrayed a range of challenges facing combat troops under differing conditions, the psychological strain on conventional ground troops associated with fighting a mostly irregular type of warfare was never systematically addressed in Vietnam (Figure 6-3), at least not by military psychiatry. Such considerations would include the overall feature of serving in a combat zone in which there were no front lines, no deep rear area, and no location that was completely safe. It especially would include the challenge of chasing elusive insurgents, often repeatedly over the same ground, who nonetheless killed and wounded US troops using mines, booby traps, ambushes, sappers (infiltrating commandos), rocket and mortar attacks, or "the little girl with the satchel charge"—a strategy

specifically designed to demoralize combatants and noncombatants. Recall from Chapter 1 that fewer than 1% of US patrols conducted in 1967 and 1968 resulted in contact with the enemy—while the US casualty count steadily mounted.

Psychiatric observers underscored the fact that troops in Vietnam were not pinned down for long periods by artillery or automatic weapons fire, and that this spared them the depletion of soldier morale seen in earlier wars; however, it could be argued that a more subtle debilitation came from the steady attrition of troops from a mostly invisible and unpredictable enemy. Quoting Navy Lieutenant Stephen Howard, a Marine battalion surgeon, "Where [is there frank acknowledgement] of the blood, the death and pain, the fear in men tracking other men through an unknown jungle, and the stark terror of walking into an ambush or some other fierce danger?"[51(p124)]

Doyle, Weiss, et al described the morally corrosive stressors affecting US combat troops in the theater as follows:

> The strategy of terror employed by the Communists raised the level of savagery with which the war was fought and made the population of rural South Vietnam that much more negligible in the eyes of many who had come from so far away to protect them. Young and inexperienced, without adequate leadership, American fighting men encountered . . . an alien culture, a ruthless opponent, and a frequently indifferent, if not hostile, population. Instead of grateful civilians happy to be liberated, soldiers met sullen, suspicious people who regarded them as intruders and often seemed to conspire in their destruction. . . . For many men the source of terror became not simply the VC (Viet Cong) or NVA (North Vietnam Army), but "Nam" itself.[65(pp155,157)]

As a corollary, the challenge for US troops to contain the urge to retaliate under these circumstances could be enormous. "For some men the pressure to act could become so unbearable that eventually any Vietnamese they encountered would serve as a necessary target."[65(p155)] According to Balkind, a military historian, fighting an unconventional/counterinsurgency/guerrilla war naturally breeds a "habit" of undisciplined violence. Specific examples in Vietnam may be found in the periodic "mad minutes" (indiscriminate firing of weapons from the perimeter), reports of soldiers "zippoing" villages (soldiers commonly carried Zippo cigarette lighters to the field), some soldiers decorating their uniforms with body parts of dead enemy as trophies, and instances of brutality toward civilians who were suspected of harboring the enemy or being their informants.[66(p235)] More broadly, according to Spector, the casual abuse of designated "free-fire zones," the high frequency of "unobserved" artillery and air support missions (areas where no specific target had been identified), and a general tendency for military overreaction all contributed to unacceptable and potentially counterproductive levels of collateral damage in Vietnam.[67(p202)]

Individual Expressions of Excessive Combat Aggression in Vietnam

Excessive combat aggression refers to acts of violence that violate the principles of military necessity, discrimination, proportionality, and humanity, which are the basis of the law of war. In a survey conducted in 1989, 12% of Vietnam veterans reported they witnessed or participated in excessive combat aggression.[67(p202)] In contrast, over the entire span of the war, there were only 242 US Army personnel formally accused of war crimes, with only 32 convictions. Additionally, 201 soldiers were convicted of serious crimes against Vietnamese civilians, including murder, rape, assault, mutilation of a corpse, and kidnapping.

These incidents were more common in the later years of the war, but otherwise, only about a quarter occurred during combat operations.[65] However, there is evidence to suggest that the problem was substantially underreported.[65,67(p202),68–71] In their especially balanced historical review Doyle, Weiss, et al provided extensive corroboration ("atrocities did take place . . . from the casual to the deliberate, from horsing around to mass murder"[65(p150)]). They also catalogued a broad collection of circumstances and stressors that promoted callousness among US combat troops. These can be roughly divided as to whether they were: (*a*) elements of the combat ecology in Vietnam; (*b*) structurally induced elements from outside the theater, which in turn influenced the combat ecology in Vietnam; or (*c*) a mixture of both:

(a) *Elements of the combat ecology in Vietnam*
- Encountering evidence of the systematic brutalization of Vietnamese civilians and officials by Viet Cong guerrillas

- Regular loss of combat buddies by mines, booby traps, snipers, sappers, rocket attacks, and ambushes
- The difficulty in distinguishing combatants from civilians
- Vast cultural differences between US troops and the rural population, which led to mutual mistrust and hostility
- Deteriorating morale as the war prolonged and resultant confusion among soldiers regarding what they were fighting for
- A "mere gook rule" in the field, that is, a belief shared by many that the deaths of Vietnamese did not matter, which helped justify a "shoot first and ask questions later" attitude
- A deficient reporting system for war crimes and a tendency to overlook them in the field

(b) *Structurally induced elements from outside the theater*
- Fielding mostly conscripted and very youthful troops ("Vietnam was a dangerous place to be struggling with issues of manhood and identity. Late adolescence is typified by recklessness, instability, and sexual uncertainty . . . and the war provided all too many opportunities for violent self-assertion."[65(p153)])
- Chronic personnel shortages
- The gradual lowering of the physical and intellectual induction standards consequent to retaining peacetime draft deferments (until 1970) and the military serving as "the employer of last resort"
- Abbreviated training cycles
- Boot camp indoctrination that encouraged racial hatred of Asians (referred to as "gooks," "slants," and "dinks")

(c) *Mixed external and internal influences*
- Employing a strategy of enemy attrition versus one that pursued territorial control and pacification (through the first half of the war, combat success was measured in body counts and kill ratios, and many commanders employed both positive and negative incentives to increase their tally)
- Excessive turnover of experienced leadership personnel in the field, especially officers
- A cursory training in the Geneva Convention and casual enforcement of the theater Rules of Engagement

Nonetheless, Doyle, Weiss, et al did not conclude that US forces engaged in widespread brutality toward the Vietnamese nationals. ("For every instance of illegality and cruelty there were thousands more of courage and compassion. Heinous conduct was the exception, not the rule, taking place most often in poorly led units and in direct violation of existing policy."[65(p150)]) They suggested that the worst offenders brought to the situation limitations in their intellect and personality or found themselves in unusual combat unit circumstances. (It should be further recognized that at least half of the items in their list of morale-depleting influences applied to all US troops serving in Vietnam, not just combat troops.)

THE PSYCHIATRIC LITERATURE FROM VIETNAM: OBSERVATION AND INTERPRETATION

The Apparent Low Incidence Level for Combat Stress Reaction Cases in Vietnam

The incidence rate for frank combat reaction cases appears to have remained low for the Army throughout the war. The first psychiatrist to indicate this trend was John A Bowman, who served early in the buildup phase (1966) as the first commander of the 935th Psychiatric Detachment. Although he reported that his KO team treated an array of anxiety-based symptoms, including conversion ("hysterical") symptoms, combat exhaustion was rarely seen (less than 2% of referrals). He attributed this to the fact that morale was high, combat was usually short-lived as the enemy typically did not choose to "stand and fight," adequate food and rest were usually available for the troops, and most cases were uncomplicated and effectively treated at the battalion aid stations.[72] He also credited the fact that the troops (then) were "primarily Regular Army professional soldiers who were well-motivated and skillfully led."[73(p59)] Bowman had little to say about the nature of the combat stress apart from the expectable fears of death or disfigurement. Soon, psychiatrists assigned to the Army combat divisions indicated that they also were seeing a low incidence for combat reaction, at least for classic combat exhaustion. They reported a range from seeing none[74] to treating only four to 12 per month,[75] with the higher numbers arising in 1967 and 1968.

Proposed explanations for the apparent low combat reaction incidence rate in Vietnam observed during the first half of the war ranged across a list of stress-reducing preventive and operational features that were credited with making combat operations in Vietnam more psychologically tolerable despite the remote and challenging tropical setting and the enemy's terrorist/guerrilla tactics and tenacity [7,62,76–81]:

- the relative low intensity of the fighting, including its intermittent nature;
- the practice of staging combat activities from fixed, relatively secure and easily resupplied bases;
- the abundance of supplies, equipment, and support, including medical and psychiatric support;
- the relative low proportion of soldiers in Vietnam actually engaged in combat;
- American technological superiority, especially heliborne mobility;
- the professionalism of the troops;
- high-quality leadership; and
- fixed, 1-year assignments in the theater.

Problems in Documenting the Impact of Combat Stress in Vietnam

However, in reality the psychiatrists serving in the field were in a poor position to measure overall incidence rates for combat reaction because of the varying troop movements and evacuation procedures and the likelihood that many cases were effectively treated at the unit level or at the battalion aid stations and never seen by them.[72,82–84] Harold SR Byrdy (1st Cavalry Division [Airmobile], 1965–1966) was the only division psychiatrist to report a combat reaction incidence rate for his division (1.6/1,000 troops/year). He commented:

> Some cases of combat exhaustion were taken directly to the clearing hospital or to an evac hospital. For the less seriously disturbed, referrals often came when the units were recouping in the base camp. Referrals directly from the field were often for anxiety while from the base camp they mostly were characterological, as you'd expect. My point is, what gets referred [to the division psychiatrist] depends on the tactical situation of the unit involved, [consequently], one is hard-pressed to know what a real incidence is.[85(p50)]

In the spring of 1967, Arnold W Johnson Jr, the second Psychiatry Consultant to CG/USARV, announced that combat fatigue cases had remained infrequent for the initial 2 years of the war, with most being handled by the corpsmen and the battalion surgeons.[86] Parrish, his successor, concurred. He noted the attrition by combat-generated casualties in the theater was light, and that the combat stress symptoms seen were not the acute, disabling conditions seen in earlier wars but were more often milder, that is, tremulousness, insomnia, nightmares, severe somatic complaints, and startle reactions (between the normal combat reaction and the incipient/mild combat exhaustion in Table 6-1).[87]

In fact, numbers for Army combat exhaustion cases were never systematically collected and analyzed, or at least the figures were not released, despite the fact that the deployed psychiatrists and the medical treatment facilities were explicitly required to forward monthly counts for inpatients with a combat exhaustion diagnosis to USARV HQ [See Appendix IV: USARV Psychiatry and Neurology Morbidity Report, in Appendix 2, "USARV Regulation 40-34"]. Regarding outpatients, William S Allerton, Chief, Psychiatry and Neurology Consultant Branch, Office of The Surgeon General (at the Pentagon), indicated that records of psychiatric outpatient contacts, irrespective of diagnosis, were not being collected in Vietnam,[6] but this appears disputable based on a later psychiatric overview from the war.[76] More specific to combat exhaustion cases, following the war Stewart Baker indicated that, "There are no epidemiological projections for the number of [combat stress reaction (CSR)] cases not reaching [3rd echelon treatment facilities in Vietnam] or that have remained untreated [following the war]."[7(p1837)] What seems evident in retrospect is that, at a central level, the Army Medical Department lost interest in the prevention, diagnosis, treatment, or management of combat reaction casualties in Vietnam, evidently because of their low numbers.

The only published summary of the US Army medical experience in Vietnam, which was limited to the first two-thirds of the war, did not include rates for combat exhaustion cases; in fact, it did not explicitly mention combat-generated psychopathology in any form or context.[88] The semiofficial overview of Army psychiatric experience in Vietnam, which was published after the war by Jones and Johnson, stated that the combat fatigue incidence rate throughout the war was "extremely low"; however, the authors provided no supporting data. Besides the fact that combat exhaustion incidence numbers were low, they acknowledged that

disagreements regarding diagnostic criteria impeded the collection and comparison of combat exhaustion statistics. (As an aside, Franklin Del Jones and Arnold W Johnson added some ambiguity by referring to *all* hospitalized psychiatric patients in Vietnam as "combat psychiatric casualties."[76]) This is consistent with William Hausman and David McK Rioch, both senior Army psychiatrists, who noted that during the Korean War, the term *combat exhaustion* was intentionally used to designate all combat-generated psychiatric casualties in order to minimize the damage to evacuees who might read their diagnoses.[89])

An alternative approach to measuring the impact of combat stress in Vietnam has been through noting the proportion of combat stress casualties found within total psychiatric diagnoses. The preliminary, semiofficial overview of Army mental health activities in Vietnam by Edward M Colbach and Matthew D Parrish, which also was limited to the first two-thirds of the war, reported that only 7% of all psychiatric admissions had been diagnosed as combat reaction. Unfortunately their report did not include data sources either.[87] This figure was very near to that of field research psychiatrist Peter G Bourne, who compared US Army psychiatric hospitalization rates in Vietnam with those of the Army of the Republic of Vietnam during the first year of the war and found 6% of psychiatric admissions to the Army hospitals in Vietnam (3rd echelon treatment facilities) were diagnosed as combat exhaustion.[90] (And Bourne bolstered his findings with a comment that "comparing the diagnostic compilation among the different Army facilities did not produce any marked inconsistency in diagnostic criteria."[91])

This figure for combat reaction, that is, 6% to 7% of all hospital psychiatric diagnoses, was reassuringly low; however, the metric could be misleading because it compared combat exhaustion casualties with other psychiatric disorders—conditions whose incidence could be based on different pathogenic variables (for example, the upsurge in use of illegal drugs in the second half of the war did not correlate with the overall decline in combat activity). It also understated the combat reaction attrition rate by only including cases hospitalized at 3rd echelon facilities in Vietnam (Army-level hospitals). Because, by definition, combat exhaustion is typically a reversible, stress-generated psychological regression that, when treated early and effectively, typically remits within a couple of days, many cases would be treated early and at lower echelons of medical care by primary care physicians (general medical officers [GMO]) and thus not be included in psychiatric statistics.[6,82,92]

The exceedingly low number of soldiers who warranted out-of-country medical evacuation for combat exhaustion was also a form of measurement of the low medical impact on the force for combat stress casualties. Among Army soldiers evacuated through Travis Air Force Base, California, between January 1967 and June 1967, 6.7% had psychiatric transfer diagnoses, but only one case of combat exhaustion was reported.[93] Similarly, Rorschach testing was administered to 1,500 soldiers with psychiatric diagnoses who were evacuated from Vietnam to the US Air Force Hospital, Clark Air Force Base, Republic of the Philippines, over a 2-year period early in the war. Only two of these cases produced results unambiguously consistent with a diagnosis of traumatic neurosis (defined by the author as a syndrome originating in an adequately functioning person and contracted acutely while the soldier was engaged in combat and in realistic danger of losing his life).[94]

Estimating the Army Combat Reaction Incidence Rate in Vietnam for 1967

One approach for estimating the incidence rate for combat stress reaction (CSR) cases for the Army in Vietnam, at least for 1967, is through utilizing the only two reports that include theater-wide data regarding CSR cases (Table 6-2):

1. The 1967 incidence rates for CSR cases treated at 1st and 2nd medical echelon levels can be roughly estimated using William E Datel and Arnold W Johnson Jr's survey of outpatient psychotropic drug prescription patterns in Vietnam[95] (3.8 and 1.3 CSR cases /1,000 troops/year, respectively). (A description and summary of the Datel and Johnson study is in Chapter 7.)
2. The CSR incidence rate for cases treated at 3rd echelon medical treatment facilities (Army-level hospitals) in Vietnam in 1966 can be reasonably calculated using the aforementioned Bourne study.[90,91] The resultant rate of 0.66 CSR cases per 1,000 troops per year for 1966 provides a basis for a rough estimation of the CSR incidence rate for 3rd echelon medical treatment facilities for 1967 by comparing the combat intensity in 1966 against that for 1967 (as measured by the wounded-in-

action rate—the traditional measure of combat intensity). The result is an estimated rate for 3rd echelon hospitals for 1967 of 0.89 CSR cases per 1,000 troops per year.
3. Summing the two CSR rate figures from (1), that is, 1st echelon care as 3.8 and 2nd echelon care as 1.3, and the 3rd echelon CSR rate figure from (2), that is, 0.89, provides a reasonable estimate of the incidence rate for CSR cases among Army troops in Vietnam in 1967: 6 CSR cases per 1,000 troops per year.

Thus, by these estimates, for every case of combat stress reaction in 1967 there were 17.5 soldiers wounded in action (ie, the wounded-in-action rate of 105.1/1,000 troops/year divided by the estimated CSR incidence rate of 6 CSR cases/1,000/year). It can be further noted that this ratio, 1 CSR:17.5 WIA, is far lower than the predicted rate of 1:4, which was based on pre-Vietnam combat experience.[1]

Estimating the Overall Army Combat Reaction Incidence Rate in Vietnam

Although it requires successive approximations, the 1967 theater ratio of 1 CSR per 17.5 WIA can be used to approximate the Army CSR incidence rates in Vietnam for each year of the war. Table 6-3 presents the Army WIA rates for each year of the war and applies the ratio of 1 CSR per 17.5 WIA to calculate the corresponding annual CSR rate estimates. The mean for these eight yearly CSR incidence rates is 5.4 cases per 1,000 troops per year.

Despite the paucity of actual CSR incidence data, ambiguities as to how combat exhaustion was defined by Army physicians in Vietnam (most of whom were not trained in psychiatry), and shortcomings in the data used in these calculations, 5 to 6 CSR cases per 1,000 troops per year for the war represents a crude but reasonable estimate of the overall CSR incidence rate for the Army in Vietnam. Still, if the ratio of 1 CSR per 17.5 WIA approximates the reality in Vietnam, and if, in fact, Army Medical Department planners applied the 1 CSR:4 WIA rule of thumb from the pre-Vietnam high-intensity wars, they would have overestimated the actual CSR incidence rate for Vietnam by a multiple of 4 to 4.5 (17.5 divided 4). As a corollary, by these estimates, the risk to any one soldier of developing CSR in Vietnam was 22% to 25% of that found in the high-intensity wars preceding Vietnam.

TABLE 6-2. Estimated and Predicted Combat Stress Reaction Rates in Vietnam, 1966 and 1967

ESTIMATED CSR RATES IN VIETNAM	1966	1967
1st Echelon Care Settings: Treatment by nonspecialized battalion surgeons and medics (at Battalion Aid Station, Dispensaries)	[No data]	Derived from Datel and Johnson[1]: Cases treated in June = 44 "Soldiers-at-risk" = 138,900* Estimated 1st echelon CSR rate = 3.8 (44/138.9 X 12 months)
2nd Echelon Care Settings: Specialized treatment by division psychiatrists and allied psychiatric personnel at the division clearing company	[No data]	Derived from Datel and Johnson[1]: Cases treated in June = 9† "Soldiers-at-risk" = 85,700* Estimated 2nd echelon CSR rate = 1.3 (9/85.7 X 12 months)
3rd Echelon Care Settings: Specialized treatment at evacuation or field hospitals and psychiatric specialty detachments (KO teams)	Data derived from Bourne[2]: CSR cases hosp in 1st 6 mo. = 46 Mean Army strength in 1st 6 mo. = 138,900[3] Estimated 3rd echelon CSR rate = 0.66 (46/138.9K X 2)	[No data] Extrapolated from 1966 Bourne data[2]: 1966 hospital level CSR rate = 0.66 Estimated 3rd echelon CSR rate = 0.89 (0.66 X 1.35‡)
PREDICTED CSR RATE FOR VIETNAM	1966	1967
WWII/Korea Rule of thumb: "1 CSR to 4 WIA"[4]	US Army in Vietnam = 239,000[5] Army WIA = 18,568[6] WIA rate (ie, combat intensity) = 77.7	US Army in Vietnam = 319,500[5] Army WIA = 33,572[6] WIA rate (ie, combat intensity) = 105.1 Predicted CSR rate = 26.3 (.25 X WIA rate)

Note: US Army combat stress reaction incidence rate in Vietnam as estimated for 1967 and compared with a predicted rate derived from World War II and Korea. All rates are per 1,000 troops per year.

*"Soldiers-at-risk" refers to investigators' estimates of the population of soldiers cared for by the Army 1st echelon primary care physician study participants; and by the Army psychiatrist study participants who provided 2nd echelon, that is, outpatient, care.

†Nine represents three-fourths of the 12 CSR cases treated. Of the eight psychiatrist respondents, six were Army psychiatrists (thus deleted were the three cases estimated to have been treated by the two Navy psychiatrists assigned to the Marines in Vietnam).

‡1.35 is the 1967 WIA rate (105.1) divided by that for 1966 (77.7)

Data sources: (1) Datel WE, Johnson AW Jr. *Psychotropic Prescription Medication in Vietnam.* Alexandria, Va: Defense Technical Information Center; 1981. Document No. AD A097610; (2) Bourne PG, Nguyen DS. A comparative study of neuropsychiatric casualties in the United States Army and the Army of the Republic of Vietnam. *Mil Med.* 1967;132(11):904–909.; (3) US Department of Defense. *Number of Casualties Incurred by US Military Personnel in Connection With the Conflict in Vietnam as the Result of Actions by Hostile Forces (January 1, 1961—December 31, 1973).* Washington, DC: OASD (Comptroller), Directorate for Information Operations; 15 March 1974; (4) Cooke ET. *Another Look at Combat Exhaustion.* Fort Sam Houston, Tex: Department of Neuropsychiatry, Medical Field Service School; distributed July 1967. Training Document GR 51-400-320, 055; (5) US Department of Defense. US Military Personnel in South Vietnam 1960–1972. Washington, DC: OASD (Comptroller), Directorate for Information Operations; 15 March 1974; (6) US Department of the Army. *Active Duty Army Personnel Battle Casualties and Non-Battle Deaths Vietnam, 1961–1979.* Washington, DC: Office of The Adjutant General Counts, US Army Adjutant General, Casualty Services Division (DAAG-PEC). 3 February 1981.

CSR: combat stress reaction
WIA: wounded in action
WWII: World War II

TABLE 6-3. Estimated Annual Combat Stress Reaction Incidence Rates Utilizing US Army Vietnam Wounded-in-Action Incidence Rates and the Estimated Rate for 1967 (Table 6-2)

	1965	1966	1967	1968	1969	1970	1971	1972
US Army WIA rates (ie, combat intensity)*	30.1	77.7	105.1	166.3	152.9	100.7	65.0	52.6
Estimated CSR rates (WIA rate/17.5)	1.7	4.4	6.0	9.5	8.7	5.8	3.7	3.0

Data sources: (1) US Department of the Army. *Active Duty Army Personnel Battle Casualties and Non-Battle Deaths Vietnam, 1961–1979.* Washington, DC: Office of The Adjutant General Counts, US Army Adjutant General, Casualty Services Division (DAAG-PEC); 3 February 1981; (2) US Department of Defense. *US Military Personnel in South Vietnam 1960–1972.* Washington, DC: OASD (Comptroller), Directorate for Information Operations; 15 March 1974.

CSR: combat stress reaction
WIA: wounded in action
*Calculated from: Total WIA numbers[1] divided by annual Army troop strength in Vietnam.[2] All rates are per 1,000 troops/year.

Although these calculations are based on the best available data, they could be misleading for the following four reasons:

1. There may have been some overestimation of the CSR incidence rate in Vietnam because of the possibility of case duplication, that is, during the month time frame for the Datel and Johnson study, some cases seen in lower echelons may have been passed up the evacuation chain and counted again. At the level of primary echelon care (versus secondary echelon care), this error seems minor as the Datel and Johnson study reported that 97% of combat exhaustion cases treated by primary care physicians responded satisfactorily to treatment. With regard to secondary echelon care (vs tertiary echelon care, ie, hospitals), this error may have been larger because, although the survey was limited to outpatients, Datel and Johnson indicate that they were not certain the six Army psychiatrists in the survey always limited their responses to experiences with outpatients.

2. Alternatively, some underestimation of the CSR incidence rate may have occurred because, whereas in past wars casualty rates (whether physical or psychiatric) have been calculated using overall Army troop strength in the theater, in Vietnam combat support and service-support troops outnumbered combat arms troops by perhaps as much as 3 to 4:1.

3. There may have also been some underestimation of the CSR incidence rate because these calculations only pertain to soldiers who were seen by Army physicians, including psychiatrists. There were undoubtedly many soldiers with degrees of combat reaction who were effectively treated by buddies, unit cadre (including chaplains or enlisted corpsmen), or who simply withstood their symptoms, pressed on, and were never counted.

4. The fact that the psychiatrists and other Army physicians deployed in Vietnam were not provided operational guidelines for making the diagnosis could also contribute to a measurement error. The USARV regulation governing the provision of mental health care in Vietnam did indicate that combat exhaustion was a stress reaction, but it referred ambiguously to civilian texts for specific diagnostic criteria (see Appendix IV—USARV Psychiatry and Neurology Morbidity Report, in Appendix 2, "USARV Regulation 40-34"). This omission is similar to the vagueness in a handout distributed to newly inducted physicians on combat exhaustion during their 5-week training at the Army's Medical Field Service School (MFSS). The MFSS faculty defined combat exhaustion as "an acute situational reaction from the stress of battle that renders the soldier ineffective," and they alluded to the "wide range and intensity of symptoms" seen in combat exhaustion—based primarily on etiologic assumptions of "fear and exhaustion" and driven by the natural tendency for soldiers to manifest symptoms as a "passport" to the rear—but the training participants were

EXHIBIT 6-4. Progressive Stages of Combat Exhaustion

1. *Normal combat reaction:* applied to soldiers who could tolerate stress reaction symptoms. Danger signs indicating a soldier was reaching his tolerance limit were lack of appetite, inability to sleep, increasing irritability, and a decrease in judgment capability.

2. *Mild combat exhaustion:* applied when he could no longer function as an adequate combat soldier (predicted to be 80% of combat exhaustion cases referred to the battalion aid stations).

3. *Moderate combat exhaustion:* applied when he could no longer assume the responsibilities of a soldier in any capacity, much less in combat (predicted to be 15% of combat exhaustion cases referred to the battalion aid stations).

4. *Severe combat exhaustion:* applied when he could no longer function as a person, much less as a soldier (predicted to be 5% of combat exhaustion cases referred to the battalion aid stations).

Adapted from: Cooke ET. *Another Look at Combat Exhaustion.* Fort Sam Houston, Tex: Medical Field Service School, Department of Neuropsychiatry; 1967: 156. Training document GR 51-400-320, 055.

evidently expected to seek out diagnostic criteria on their own. ("The . . . symptoms noted in soldiers with combat exhaustion would fill many additional pages. Any standard reference will give a multitude of examples. The delineation of specific patterns will not receive further attention."[1(p9)]) However, MFSS did include a simplified, albeit very general, set of operational criteria regarding combat reaction stages (Exhibit 6-4)[1]—a taxonomy that coincided with the combat reaction symptom spectrum from World War II presented in Table 6-1.

The fact that these potential errors appear to be offsetting may help to reinforce this belated approach to the measurement of the clinical impact of combat stress for the Army troops fighting in Vietnam.

Challenges in Making the Diagnosis of Combat Reaction in Vietnam

As noted, complicating the measure of the incidence rates in Vietnam for combat reaction were apparent variations in diagnostic criteria used by the Army psychiatrists in the field (Table 6-4). In fact, to diagnose combat exhaustion in Vietnam the psychiatrists and primary care physicians would have had to draw upon their pre-Vietnam experiences with acute stress reactions or extrapolate from the civilian taxonomy represented in the American Psychiatric Association's *Diagnostic and Statistical Manual* (DSM-I, succeeded by DSM-II in 1968—see Exhibit 6-2, "Civilian Nosology and Combat Stress Reaction").

There is one exception regarding the dearth of military-centered combat reaction diagnostic guidelines in the theater: in early 1967, Johnson published a timely article in the *US Army Vietnam Medical Bulletin* ("Psychiatric Treatment in the Combat Situation"[22]) that reviewed the combat reaction diagnostic criteria and the Army's forward treatment doctrine. This may have been disseminated in Vietnam in 1967 when it was published; however, it was not systematically distributed to those who were subsequently assigned over the next 5 years.

Observations Regarding Combat Reaction Presentations and Pathogenesis in Vietnam

The following review of the reported experiences of the Army psychiatrists deployed in Vietnam is extracted from the material presented in Chapter 3 and Chapter 4.

Division ("Combat") Psychiatrists

Table 6-4 presents a summary of the various diagnostic taxonomies for combat reaction that were pragmatically devised by the division psychiatrists who provided 1st and 2nd echelon specialized care in Vietnam (ie, those who saw such cases and who provided a record). In addition it includes their impressions regarding pathogenic influences.

It is evident that the division psychiatrists had diverse experiences and that they were drawn to highlight differing diagnostic features among psychiatrically affected combat troops. It is also apparent they were not generally able to distinguish between the

TABLE 6-4. Summary Of Division Psychiatrists' Combat (Stress) Reaction Diagnostic Groupings, Criteria, and Impressions Regarding Pathogenic Factors

Psychiatrist Unit and Year	Combat Stress Reaction (CSR): Categories and Criteria	Pathogenic Factors
Byrdy 1st Cavalry Division 1965–1966	Combat exhaustion: Disorganizing anxiety in reaction to combat situation (not in anticipation of combat). Symptoms must remit under the CSR treatment doctrine in order to retain diagnosis	Cumulative combat stress over time Comorbid psychiatric conditions Breakdown in combat group integrity Green sergeants leading seasoned troops "Short-timer's"
Bostrom 1st Cavalry Division 1967–1968	1. Normal combat syndrome—included "realistic anxiety" with increased physiological arousal but without degraded effectiveness 2. Precombat syndrome—included greater anxiety, sleep problems, psychosomatic complaints (nausea, tension headache, exaggerated musculoskeletal symptoms, reduced combat effectiveness) 3. Combat exhaustion—included psychosis or near psychosis, with gross loss of combat effectiveness	No specifics
WL Baker 9th Infantry Division 1967	1. Transient (combat) anxiety reaction—with hyperventilation and functional GI symptoms; in early months; in light combat 2. Classic combat fatigue—increased anxiety, regression (some with brief psychosis), and some degraded effectiveness 3. Modified combat stress reaction—disabling anxiety, GI disturbances (anorexia, nausea, "dry heaves"), hypervigilance, insomnia, combat trauma dreams, "short-timer's" syndrome (feels impending doom, "outlived the odds")	Increased combat activity/intensity, cumulative over time Traumatizing turning point (buddy lost; wounded) Breakdown in combat group integrity (from heavy combat losses; command transferred soldiers to other units to spread DEROS dates ["infusion"]) "Short-timer's" and 10 mo. veteran
Pettera 9th Infantry Division 1967–1968	1. Transient (combat) anxiety reaction—"nebulous, ill-defined"; recovered with supportive therapy 2. Combat fatigue—acute, severely incapacitating psychological reaction: anxiety, uncontrollable crying, hyperventilation, "clutching and freezing" 3. Vietnam combat reaction/"combat neurosis"—severely incapacitating psychophysiologic reaction: anxiety, tremulousness, GI disturbances (anorexia, nausea, vomiting, diarrhea), insomnia, combat trauma dreams, survivor guilt or shame for loss of control	1. "Little or no specific etiology" 2. Consequent to emotional and especially, physical fatigue from sustained combat exposure 3. Always developed from: repeated, severe combat trauma; a serious wound; or unit overrun. Only seasoned combat soldiers approaching DEROS were affected.
Motis 4th Infantry Division 1967–1968	Acute combat reaction—Types: Dazed, disoriented, exhausted, unresponsive, flat affect, hypokinetic ("I can't take it any more.") Hysterical, panicky, as if reliving a traumatic experience Anxious secondary to near-miss	Sustained, fierce fighting Extreme physical fatigue Surviving a near-miss
Bey 1st Infantry Division 1969–1970	1. Situational (combat) reaction—treatable at battalion aid station 2. Combat exhaustion—combat trauma dreams, anorexia, problems with concentration 3. Conversion/dissociation reaction	Individual: Posttraumatic reaction; Frightful reaction to first firefight Group: Unit rejects new member
Alessi 23rd Infantry Division 1970–1971	Nonpsychiatric emotional problem—"normal anxiety": headaches, abdominal cramps, sleep disturbance, poor appetite, fear of the field, combat refusal Psychophysiologic reaction—panicky, hyperventilation, syncope, vomiting, incontinence, headaches, freezing up, sleepwalking, "nerves," conversion pains	No specifics

GI: gastrointestinal
DEROS: date expected return from overseas

pathogenic variables outlined in Figure 6-1. Moreover, the available record suggested that so-called classic or uncomplicated combat exhaustion cases were overshadowed by those that were pathogenically more involved. Although the reporting psychiatrists did not provide full case examples, the following case material was provided by Specialist 6th Class Dennis L Menard, an enlisted social work/psychology specialist, who served with the 1st Infantry Division (1967) and treated the patient in collaboration with the battalion surgeon.[96(pp51–52)]

CASE 6-5: Tanker With Anxious Incoherence (Acute Stress Reaction) After His Tank Was Hit by an RPG

Identifying information: PFC Juliet is a 21-year-old, single enlistee who was dusted off via a medical evacuation helicopter from a forward area after a rocket-propelled grenade hit his tank. Upon arrival at the clearing station he was somewhat incoherent and hyperventilating and repeating, "I'll be all right." At first it was thought that he had physical injuries, but upon examination it was concluded that he was in an anxiety state. He was treated with an injection of 50 mg of Thorazine, IM. In the morning he was sent to the MHCS [mental health consultation services] in full uniform.

History of present illness: The patient vaguely recalled yesterday's incident. He remembered seeing a flash, hearing shrapnel fly by his head, and seeing his tank commander attempt to pull him out of the crippled vehicle. This patient has been on line for approximately 7 months as a tank crewman and driver and has functioned well thus far. However, over the past months he has been under considerable strain as his unit has been having enemy contact daily. As a result of the physical hardships of constant moves, lack of sleep, and hard work, the entire troop was keyed up and was "nothing but a bundle of nerves." Regarding yesterday's action, the patient indicated he had been through "much worse." For example, he has run over a few mines, has been sniped at frequently, and was in a 7-hour battle once in which his tank was immobilized on a hillside slope. After expending all the tank's ammunition, the patient and his crew fought off the hostile force with .45 caliber pistols until help finally arrived.

Past history: PFC Juliet was born and raised in the upper Midwest as the oldest of five children. The domestic environment was described as stormy and chaotic. His mother, a cancer victim, and his father, a diabetic, fought constantly. At age 16, while attending the 11th grade, he left home and began a life of crime. Ultimately he was apprehended and offered the choice of joining the Army or going to jail. His troubled past notwithstanding, he adjusted well to Army life and completed both BCT [basic combat training] and AIT [advanced individual training] satisfactorily. He was assigned to Fort Benning as a weapons instructor where he stayed for 9 months before coming to Vietnam. He adjusted well in Vietnam and did his job with no qualms. After the above-mentioned firefight he was demoted because he failed to unload his pistol upon returning to base camp. Otherwise he has gotten along well with his crew, subordinates, and superiors.

Examination: At the mental health consultation service he presented as alert, attentive, coherent, and oriented with no signs of suicidal ideation, depression, hallucinations, or a thought disorder. He was mildly anxious and apprehensive. Insight and judgment appeared adequate.

Clinical course: The patient was reassured that he had sustained a normal reaction to having been in prolonged combat, and that it would be temporary with no lasting effects.

Discharge diagnosis: Combat exhaustion syndrome, moderate, manifested by an acute anxiety attack. Taken in consideration is his sustained combat performance and the fact that his unit has been under prolonged hostile harassment resulting in everyone sustaining physical and mental exhaustion.

Disposition: He was returned to full duty following his interview. [Addendum: Because of his injuries he was awarded the Purple Heart. It was reported that in the 4 months until his DEROS (date expected return overseas) he continued to function well.]

Source: Adapted from Menard DL. The social work specialist in a combat division. *US Army Vietnam Med Bull.* 1968;March/April:51–52.

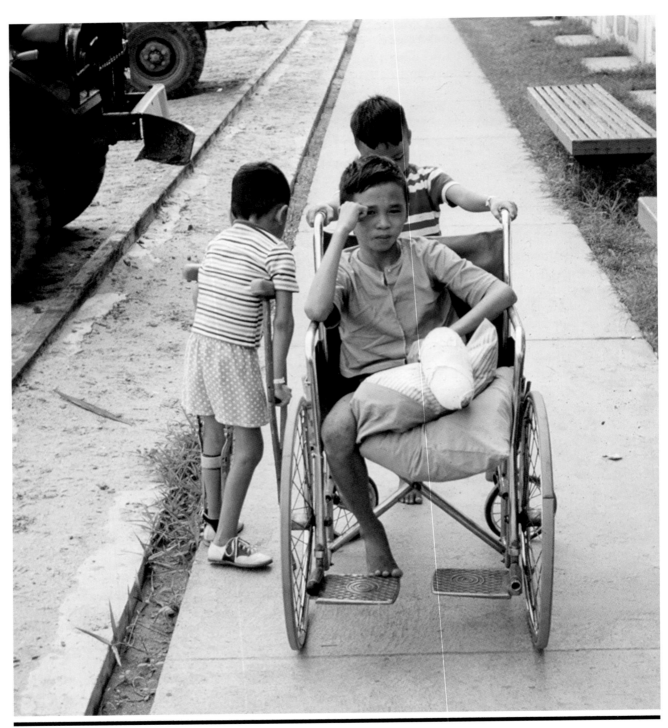

FIGURE 6-3. Wounded Vietnamese children at a US Army hospital in Vietnam, 1970. These children, who are undergoing treatment for war wounds, are a reminder of how the Viet Cong utilized a strategy of terror that included systematic, deliberate attacks on South Vietnam civilians resulting in the death or injury of tens of thousands of noncombatants. From the standpoint of the war's psychological impact on the conventional US troops who fought there, the strain of engaging in irregular psychological warfare against determined guerrillas who employed such tactics apparently included a high potential for demoralization and associated psychiatric and behavioral problems (and in some instances, provoking retaliation and atrocities). Photograph courtesy of Norman M Camp, Colonel, US Army (Retired).

[Author: In retrospect it seems evident that a possible contributing etiologic factor would be that of a traumatic brain injury.]

Hospital and KO Team ("Hospital") Psychiatrists

Evacuation and Field Hospitals Without a Psychiatric Detachment. Overall, the available reports from psychiatrists assigned to the field and evacuation hospitals without psychiatric specialty detachments suggest they treated relatively few fresh combat reactions. They also offered little about diagnostic criteria or contributory stresses. This is not surprising because these facilities were not organized to serve as the definitive treatment settings for soldiers in the combat units. Robert E Huffman (8th and 3rd Field Hospitals, 1965–1966) noted that 8% of his patients had combat stress as an etiologic factor; however, his greater numbers most likely stemmed from the fact that he was assigned in Vietnam before the psychiatric specialty detachments arrived to serve as 3rd echelon treatment facilities. John A Talbott (3rd Field Hospital, 1968) was equally anomalous. He reported seeing six combat reactions among 100 consecutive referrals, but these were primarily service-support troops reacting to fighting in and around Saigon during the Tet offensives. Neither Huffman nor Talbott commented on diagnostic criteria or contributory stresses. William F Kenny (17th Field Hospital, 1966) and Arthur S Blank Jr (3rd Field Hospital, 1966), both of whom were located in Saigon, said that they saw almost none. Gary L Tischler (67th Evacuation Hospital, 1966–1967) indicated that he saw some soldiers affected by combat stress, short-timer's syndrome, and combat aversion, but his catchment area (Qui Nhon) was mostly composed of noncombat units too, and his report primarily centered on general patterns of stress and adaptation. The one case vignette of a combat soldier provided by Tischler does not include the element of exhaustion. Although he was an airborne soldier who had seen heavy enemy action over his 7 months in Vietnam, his disabling anxiety and paranoid symptoms arose on his return from R & R (rest and recuperation) and centered on his apprehension about resuming his combat role ("killing and being killed"), guilt from having survived several of his buddies, and feeling estranged from his unit's new commanding officer (CO) and recent replacements (ie, as "the only old timer").[47]

Psychiatric Specialty Detachments/KO Teams. The Army's two specialized psychiatric detachments were intended to serve the combat units (along with noncombat units); however, they were not organized to treat large numbers of direct admissions from the field because they were primarily expected to provide secondary and tertiary echelon care. CSR cases should have been treated first at 1st and 2nd treatment echelons within the divisions (battalion aid stations and brigade clearing companies), with the specialized psychiatric detachments serving as backup for soldiers who failed to recover. Bowman, the first commander of the 935th KO team (Long Binh post near Saigon), reported that fewer than 2% of their referrals in 1966 received a diagnosis of combat exhaustion (as mentioned earlier). His staff used two criteria for making the diagnosis: (1) actual exposure to combat, that is, under hostile fire, and (2) the presence of fatigue, whether produced by physical causes such as exertion, heat, dehydration, diarrhea, and loss of sleep, or by psychological causes such as anxiety and insomnia. Louis R Conte, the first commander of the 98th KO team (Nha Trang, 1966–1967) around the same time indicated that they saw even fewer.

Two years after Bowman and Conte, combat intensity in Vietnam rose sharply and, as H Spencer Bloch reported, 5.7% of the caseload of the 935th KO team was diagnosed with combat exhaustion. Bloch defined combat exhaustion as a syndrome that represented a stress-induced psychotic reaction with both external precipitating factors (including sleep deprivation, traumatic events, and possibly poor nutrition) and internal predisposing factors (including the inability to tolerate hostile feelings, anxiety associated with increased responsibility, or a strict conscience). In other words, he advocated the bio\psycho\social etiologic model alluded to earlier. However, because he and his team were working in a 3rd echelon treatment facility, they were often treating the more intractable cases, which would include soldiers with a greater degree of contributory personality susceptibility. The following case exemplifies a relatively uncomplicated combat exhaustion case that was a direct admission from the field to an evacuation hospital/KO team:

CASE 6-6: Acute Combat Stress Reaction With Psychomotor Retardation, Fearfulness, and Traumatic Dreams

---

Identifying information: PFC Kilo was a 20-year-old rifleman with 9 months in the Army and 3 months in Vietnam. He volunteered to serve in Vietnam.

History of present illness: On the day of his admission, two friends were killed. Also, he was to get on a dustoff flight but didn't, and the helicopter crashed. He has since become fearful of returning to the field. He was referred to the 935th Psychiatric Detachment/93rd Evacuation Hospital.

Past history: He reported having had prescient dreams of the deaths of an uncle and some friends in the past.

Examination: PFC Kilo presented as stunned and fearful. He had marked psychomotor retardation and fearfulness. In a monotonous voice he repeated, "Charlie killed my buddies," and cried and moaned without tears. He was fully oriented and acknowledged being more frightened than angry or sad. He told of having dreams of his own death and that of others, although he denied being superstitious. Physical exam was unremarkable.

Clinical course: The patient was encouraged to ventilate and then put to sleep with Thorazine for 18 hours, after which he was mobilized in the therapeutic milieu. He socialized well in the ward activities. He was held another day and began to express the desire to rejoin his unit, although he remained apprehensive about his dreams.

Discharge diagnosis: Combat exhaustion, acute, moderately severe. Stress: loss of buddies in combat. Predisposition: mild. Condition at discharge: recovered.

Disposition: Returned to full duty after 2 days of hospitalization; to be followed by the division psychiatrist.

Source: Narrative Summary, 935th Psychiatric Detachment/93rd Evacuation Hospital.

The next case is etiologically more complicated and the length of the hospitalization is greater. The therapeutic milieu is the primary treatment modality, along with time. Although the discharge diagnosis was that of a neurotic dissociative reaction, contemporary thinking would wish to rule out a traumatic brain injury as well despite the negative neurological evaluation.

CASE 6-7: Dissociative/Factitious Disorder Following a Friendly Fire Near Miss

Identifying information: Sergeant (SGT) Lima was a 21-year-old with 3 years service in the Army and 24 months in Vietnam who was hospitalized at the 935th Psychiatric Detachment/93rd Evacuation Hospital.

History of present illness: The patient was initially kept overnight at his brigade clearing company after he developed a stunned, mute state in conjunction with a friendly fire incident in which an American bomb landed close to his position. A neurological exam was within normal limits. The following day he appeared coherent but indicated a retrograde amnesia, including for the events of the previous day.

Past history: The record only indicates that he had similar episodes previously (no details).

Examination: SGT Lima complained of a mild, frontal headache, spoke slowly, and generally stared straight ahead. He was cooperative and complained of being frightened because of his inability to recover his memory. He claimed that he did not know his full name, where he was, nor the time or year. He demonstrated some right-left confusion, inability to name common objects, didn't know what a book was (Question: "What is meant by 'You can't tell a book by its cover?'") or what a president is. Short-term and recent memory tested as adequate. Social judgment through hypothetical questioning was poor.

Clinical course: The patient was hospitalized for 7 days, treated with milieu therapy and group therapy, and progressively regained his memory. He received no psychoactive medications. He was seen and cleared for duty by the neurologist.

Discharge diagnosis: Psychoneurotic dissociative reaction, acute, severe. Predisposition: moderate, hysterical personality features.

Disposition: Returned to duty.

Source: Narrative Summary, 935th Psychiatric Detachment/93rd Evacuation Hospital.

The following case is even more complex regarding pathogenesis, diagnosis, and treatment.

CASE 6-8: Treatment-Unresponsive Rifleman With Headache and Auditory Hallucinations

---

Identifying information: PFC Mike was a 20-year-old rifleman with 14 months service in the Army and 9 months in Vietnam who was hospitalized at the 935th Psychiatric Detachment/93rd Evacuation Hospital.

History of present illness: He was admitted to the brigade clearing station for what was eventually labeled combat exhaustion [the record did not include circumstantial substantiation]. His complaints at that time were of hearing "screeching, shrieking noises" as well as hallucinated voices warning him that people around him were his enemies. He also reported "shooting headaches" and a sleep disturbance. He was held at the clearing station for 2 weeks and treated with Thorazine but without significant improvement. He was then transferred to the 935th KO unit.

Past history: His record only noted that "auditory phenomena have been present for at least 3 years and antedated his induction into the Army."

Examination: When seen he complained bitterly about his auditory symptoms and expressed intense anger that no one had found the cause and treated it. Besides noting that he was anxious and intense, his mental status examination did not reveal a disorder of his thinking or mood. Psychological testing revealed extensive conflict about aggressive impulses.

Clinical course: The examining psychiatrist wrote, "he is clinically non-psychotic, and I suspect his symptoms are primarily hysterical . . . I can't be sure that he doesn't have an underlying thought disorder." He was prescribed a "diagnostic-therapeutic trial of Stelazine" and returned to his combat unit. Five days later he was again referred to the 935th for persistence of his auditory hallucinations and inability to sleep. When examined, he was calmer, but otherwise he appeared as before. He was again hospitalized and received more Stelazine and analgesics. He participated passively in ward work, recreational, and group therapy programs. His auditory complaints disappeared by the second day, but the complaints about headaches persisted. On his eighth hospital day he was told that his headaches would have to be "lived with" and that he would be returning to duty. Soon thereafter he began to complain of his original set of symptoms. Nonetheless he was returned to his unit.

Discharge diagnosis: Psychoneurotic reaction, moderate impairment.

Disposition: Return to duty; continue Stelazine and Valium, along with analgesics for headaches. His unit was told that he was fully responsible for his behavior. It was also recommended that he be reassigned to a noncombat unit. He was given an appointment at the 935th KO Detachment in 3 weeks.

Source: Narrative Summary, 935th Psychiatric Detachment/93rd Evacuation Hospital.

See also Bloch's case #4 in Appendix 12, "Some Interesting Reaction Types Encountered in a War Zone."

US Marine Corps/Navy Experience in Vietnam

Robert E Strange, a Navy psychiatrist, provided etiologic information regarding combat stress reaction cases evacuated off the coast to the USS *Repose* between mid-February and December 1966. Fifteen percent of psychiatric admissions (raw numbers were not provided by the authors), representing both Navy and Marine personnel, were designated as "classic" combat fatigue (ie, "situational reaction to combat"). These were individuals who had typically been in Vietnam for 6 or more months, sustained "lengthy and harrowing" combat experiences, and, although being junior noncommissioned officers, had shouldered considerable responsibility, such as that of squad leader or corpsman. Their military records were excellent, and they showed healthy pre-Vietnam social histories. Of these cases, following physiological restoration, limited psychopharmacological support, and "supportive-directive" psychotherapy, 78% were returned to duty function, usually with less than 2 weeks of treatment.

In contrast, approximately a quarter of psychiatric evacuations to the ship were also admitted following combat exposure and exhibited similar symptoms of anxiety or depression with psychophysiological manifestations. However, these individuals were ultimately loosely referred to as "pseudocombat fatigue" because they primarily had personality disorders (or in some instances, psychoneurotic disorders). They were more likely to have background characteristics of impulsivity, poor stress tolerance, tenuous emotional control, and histories of previous psychiatric contacts and poor adjustment. According to Strange, they showed inadequate motivation and poor identification with their military group. Whereas they initially responded to the same treatment as the combat fatigue cases, their symptoms recurred when they were confronted with the prospect of returning to duty in the combat environment ("the crucial test"). Although 50% of the pseudocombat fatigue cases were nonetheless returned to duty, some required rehospitalization and evacuation out of the theater. Several cases of "combat neurosis" were also described. These presented similarly to the "classic" combat fatigue and the pseudocombat fatigue cases. They were otherwise competent individuals who had chronic premorbid but subclinical neurotic symptoms, such as patterns of compulsivity, and whose symptoms were exacerbated by combat.[48,97]

Special Problems Among Combat-Exposed Troops in Vietnam

Negative Effects From the 1-Year, Individual, Troop Replacement System

As previously noted, maintenance of unit cohesion has been found to be a critical variable in protecting soldiers against combat-generated psychiatric disabilities because of the vitally interdependent relationships required in a successful combat unit. Nevertheless military planners implemented a random, individualized, troop replacement system throughout the war, perhaps assuming that staggering replacements would be less disruptive to mission accomplishment than unit replacements.[64] They also limited tours of duty in Vietnam to 12 months (US Marine Corps was 13 months), and most soldiers served only one tour. Although the 1-year tour was initially felt to contribute to stress-mitigation, over time it resulted in excessive personnel turbulence and appeared to critically interfere with combat unit morale.[87] Furthermore, as discussed in Chapter 2, as the war dragged on the Army of necessity had to increasingly rely on relatively inexperienced officers and noncommissioned officers, young draftees, and volunteers.[98] The impact of this system on the performance and mental health of the troops in Vietnam

was never systematically studied by the Army, but its more general negative effects on individual soldiers was often noted by mental health personnel (see Appendix 8, Byrdy's account as division psychiatrist during the first year of the war with the 1st Cavalry Division).

Douglas R Bey, the 1st ID division psychiatrist (1969–1970), explored the question of impaired group bonding when individual soldiers, especially soldiers new to Vietnam, joined already functioning combat units. Bey described how the unit's members ritualistically hazed the initiate while encouraging him to diminish his ties to home, embrace the group, and, especially, to adopt the group's psychological defenses of denial and counterphobic bravado. He indicated that this was a precarious process, and, for some, obstacles such as a new member's social, cultural or language handicap threatened the group's homeostasis and provoked their harsh and even violent reactions toward him, which in turn resulted in higher psychiatric referrals. Bey and his team developed a program in which they sought to help unit commanders reduce the stress and foster the unit's integrity and continued effectiveness through empathy for the initiate, admission of more than one replacement at a time, improved orientation, and assigning him a sponsor.[99] However, in general no measures of the effects of this program were available.

Short-Timer's Syndrome

The so-called short-timer's syndrome—a low-grade form of emotional and behavior disability exhibited by combat soldiers as they approached the date they were to rotate back to the United States (date expected return overseas or DEROS)—was regularly observed by commanders and treated at all medical care levels. Symptoms especially included reduced combat efficiency; preoccupation with fears about being killed; sullen, irritable, or withdrawn behavior; and opposition to further combat participation. It was also common for noncombat troops to experience a version of this upon nearing their DEROS,[47] evidently because of absence of clearly defined rear areas and a lack of sense of safety. One must remember that for the combat soldier who was getting "short," the individual rotation policy guaranteed that his inevitable anxiety about leaving Vietnam alive and in one piece would be greatly fueled by his awareness that, simply based on longevity, he was literally the last man. He had witnessed the gradual disappearance of the cohort of soldiers he joined when he arrived by their having become casualties, through sickness, or as a consequence of their DEROS. The reality that many members of his unit left unscathed may not have modulated his tendency to envision that when his turn arose, it might come in the more adverse form (ie, killed or wounded).

The emergence of this type of psychological disability was also consistent with professional observations regarding the psychological defenses employed by combat troops to keep their fears and anxieties under control. Because, as observed in Bourne's studies of combat stress,[90] soldiers commonly used the mental defense of denial in order to tolerate the high risks of combat, the individual soldier's belief from early in his tour that his odds were favored because of the spread of risk over time and among the combat group would gradually erode because of the steadily diminishing time and numbers. Short-timer's symptoms were only so preventable—recall from Chapter 3 that Jones (25th Infantry Division) observed that commanders who established a policy of exempting soldiers from combat exposure within a month of their DEROS found these symptoms arose even sooner among the other troops. Similarly, Byrdy (1st Cavalry Division) reported that such a policy resulted in so much bitterness within the unit that the concession had to be rescinded. (Short-timer's syndrome will be explored in general in Chapter 8.)

Evidently, low-grade short-timer's pathology was so common in the combat units and relatively manageable that most of the deployed psychiatrists felt it unnecessary to publish case examples. However, for some individuals approaching their DEROS could awaken more serious psychosocial conflicts pertaining both to Vietnam and to what was waiting in the United States. The following case record from the 93rd Evacuation Hospital/935th KO Detachment serves as illustration:

CASE 6-9: Acute Stress Reaction in an Infantryman Within 2 Weeks of Going Home

---

Identifying information: Specialist 4th Class (SP4) November is a 20-year-old, single, white infantryman with over 2 years in the Army and 11 1/2 months in Vietnam (ie, within 2 weeks of DEROS).

History of present illness: He was taken to his battalion aid station at 2000 hours after he jumped off his track and ran into the jungle muttering something about getting "Charlie" (Viet Cong) because Charlie had killed several of his buddies. His unit was setting up a night perimeter at the time. He had had 5 or 6 beers before the episode. Upon being seen at the clearing station, a diagnosis of combat fatigue was made, and he was given Thorazine and restrained. The next day he was transferred to the 93rd Evacuation Hospital.

Examination: Upon arrival at the 935th he was noted to be somewhat withdrawn, staring at the ceiling, and answering questions tersely and in a monotone. After being admitted to the ward, he slept through the night. The morning after admission he was alert, oriented, and without complaint. He was described as a sober, somber, somewhat sad-faced young man with a reticent, though cooperative, manner. He denied a history of psychotic symptoms or those of severe neurosis or suicidal or homicidal intent. He had good immediate and past memory, general fund of information, social judgment; proverbs were interpreted concretely. He acknowledged unresolved feelings about his dead buddies and was hesitant to discuss these, but he noted that it would take time for these feelings to become settled. There was no evidence of severe depression. He reported an earlier episode of "blacking out" subsequent to drinking alcohol several months earlier. He denied past or recent use of drugs, including marijuana. His physical exam was within normal limits.

Past history: SP4 November was one of eight children. His father was permanently hospitalized following an injury when SP4 November was 1 year of age. Shortly thereafter his parents divorced. Following his mother's remarriage, he was raised by a stepfather toward whom he had mixed feelings. His mother died when he was 16, and an older brother committed suicide last year. He denied neurotic symptoms in childhood, though he always had a penchant for solitary activity. He quit school at 16 and joined the Army.

Clinical course: Unremarkable. The clinical record does not indicate that additional medications were prescribed. He was discharged after day 2.

Discharge diagnosis: Adult situational reaction—acute, moderately severe; manifested by dissociative-type symptoms. Stress: alcohol; unresolved feelings about lost buddies; preparation to leave the war zone. Predisposition: moderate. Condition at discharge: recovered.

Disposition: Return to duty. Recommendation: Consider keeping him in company area until DEROS.

Source: Narrative Summary, 935th Psychiatric Detachment/93rd Evacuation Hospital.

Chronic Combat Stress Reaction

Overlapping symptomatically with short-timer's syndrome were some soldiers who had previously withstood extensive combat but who became severely disabled in the last couple of months of their tour, apparently consequent to cumulative stress. William L Baker, the division psychiatrist for the 9th Infantry Division, referred to them as the "ten month veteran (syndrome)," and his successor, Robert L Pettera, referred to them as the "Vietnam combat reaction" (he also referred to them as "combat neurosis"). Early in the war Strange and Ransom J Arthur, also a Navy psychiatrist, similarly noted a second incidence peak for combat stress casualties treated aboard the USS *Repose*, a Navy hospital ship. According to them, some Marines who were highly conscientious, if somewhat anxious and "neurotic," developed incapacitating symptoms after approximately 10 to 11 months of combat duty in Vietnam.[100(p285)]

The following is Baker's description of the "ten month veteran" (syndrome):

Its symptoms are so nearly uniform from one man to another, and different from the classic combat fatigue syndrome, that I feel it is a syndrome produced by the [unique] stress encountered here. The typical case is an infantryman who had been with the division since training in the [United States] and in Vietnam for ten months. His past history indicates good-to-superior duty performance and social adjustment. He had a normal degree of fear and anxiety during most of that time [in Vietnam]. Recently there has been a considerable increase in anxiety, to a degree markedly impairing his ability to function, often in spite of continued motivation. Referral notes from battalion surgeons often indicated that the man repeatedly went in the field

and was non-effective and had to be evacuated because of symptoms. He complains of all the usual "short timer" feelings, in other words, a sense of impending doom. He fears he will "get someone killed" by making a mistake, sleeps poorly, has recurrent bad dreams in which he sees again some specific horror. He has functional anorexia, nausea, and often "dry heaves" or cramps. Some have been evacuated with a diagnosis of appendicitis. Often there is a fear of artillery noise, even outgoing, which seems to be more of a conditioned response than rational fear. The patient is often more distressed by his recurrent dreams than by fear of returning to combat. He says he will return to combat willingly if only he could sleep without "those dreams." Usually the dreams are not a fantasy of what may happen, but are "re-runs" of something that did happen (ie, being splashed with a friend's brains, etc).[75(p6)]

These cases combined elements of the "old sergeant syndrome" of World War II (described in Chapter 3) and the short-timer's syndrome. Affected individuals seemed to especially illustrate what Richard Rahe later came to describe as a chronic combat reaction. This refers to a state of psychophysiological hypoarousal with attendant psychological depression and withdrawal secondary to continuous exposure to high stress demands. In contrast, the temporarily disabling acute combat reaction would apply to soldiers experiencing an abruptly arising physiological hyperarousal, that is, panic reaction (so-called battle shock[101]).[102] The following case example is illustrative of the chronic combat stress reaction:

CASE 6-10: Chronic Combat Stress Reaction in a Battle-Hardened Track Commander

Identifying information: SP4 Oscar is a 21-year-old, single, white infantryman with 2 years in the service and 11 months in Vietnam. He was transferred to the 935th Psychiatric Detachment on 1 June after a 3-day stay at his brigade medical clearing station for "combat fatigue," which did not clear with rest and sedation.

History of present illness: Patient has performed well throughout his tour, but over the past 2 months became increasingly preoccupied with and upset by the gore, wounding, and chaos. He has been having nightmares, became emotionally labile, and expressed that he has "had it!" He noted that he had become socially withdrawn in an effort to avoid hearing about killing. He expressed guilt about surviving while many buddies had died. Two weeks prior he was taken off the line and given a job at the base camp.

Examination: SP4 Oscar presented as "tearful, earnest, disheartened, disconsolate, though not despondent young man." His mood was depressed and his affect was labile. He spoke vehemently, though without pressured speech; his associations were relevant; he was not homicidal or suicidal; there was no evidence of psychosis or intellectual impairment. In addition, his attending psychiatrist included the following observation, apparently suggesting the patient was in a psychologically regressed state, "[He] presents himself as a bit helpless, which I suspect is not typical for him.")

Past history: The clinical record contained no details regarding his past history. He denied use of drugs or alcohol.

Clinical course: According to the record, "The patient's reconstitution had begun before he arrived at the 935th." Once he was at the 935th, he was put to sleep with Thorazine for 20 hours. Subsequently he reported feeling better and wished to return to duty. He was discharged on the second day of hospitalization.

Discharge diagnosis: Adult situational reaction, acute, moderately severe; Stress: chronic battle exposure; severe; Predisposition: none; Impairment: none; his emotional lability, fatigue, and guilty ruminations were in remission.

Disposition: Returned to duty (noncombat).

Source: Narrative Summary, 935th Psychiatric Detachment/93rd Evacuation Hospital.

Behavioral and Psychosomatic Symptoms Among Combat Troops

The psychiatric literature from Vietnam was mostly silent on soldiers exhibiting specific maladaptive behaviors associated with combat risk and exposure, that is, malingering, desertion, absent without leave (AWOL) in the field to avoid combat duty, combat refusal, and neglect of healthcare, weapons, or equipment. Jones,[103] who served very early, and Bey, who served midwar,[104] both commented that few self-inflicted wound cases were seen. However, according to Raymond M Scurfield, an Army social work officer, Blank (1966–1967) had told him about a soldier who shot himself in the chest with his rifle to manipulate a transfer from Vietnam. Also, Scurfield reported that when he was assigned to the 98th KO Detachment (1968–1969) they saw several self-inflicted wound cases.[105] Larry E Alessi, who served with the 23rd ID during the drawdown phase, mentioned that combat refusal had become a problem (Appendix 9), and Harry C Holloway, a research psychiatrist, reported that early in the war, units with poor morale were lax in malaria discipline, with some soldiers indicating that they purposefully exposed themselves to mosquito bites in an attempt to get relief from the field.[106] Soldiers with less conspicuous behavioral expressions of resistance to combat exposure (in the language from earlier wars, the "goldbricks" and "stragglers,"[7] and in Vietnam, "shammers"), as well as those with factitious medical/psychiatric disorders or exaggerated psychosomatic problems who hoped for exemption from combat, that is, for "secondary gain," also got little explicit acknowledgment by the reporting Army psychiatrists. Undoubtedly such behaviors were widespread, and if such soldiers received psychiatric attention they were most likely labeled as either a character and behavior disorder or an adjustment disorder. More likely is that they were treated symptomatically by the primary care physicians or other medical specialties and not referred.

Regarding exaggerating physical symptoms to avoid duty, especially combat duty, Allerton, who did not serve in Vietnam, provided the following statement in his 1969 overview, "[Because] there is no area within the country that is without danger . . . there is little merit in developing secondary gain type symptoms which might consciously or unconsciously be utilized to extricate oneself from a dangerous situation."[6(p16)] However, this may have been a naïve assumption. SP5 Paul A Bender, an enlisted social work/psychology technician, indicated that "iatrogenically aggravated," functional psychosomatic symptoms were among the most intractable cases seen in the 11th Infantry Brigade in early 1968,[107] and Carden and Schramel, US Air Force psychiatrists stationed at Clark Air Force Base in the Philippines who treated soldiers evacuated from Vietnam, felt that even during the first year of the war, the war's unpopularity contributed substantially to secondary gain as motivator for certain types of psychiatric disability in Vietnam.[108] (See Chapter 8 for more on the findings of Carden and Schramel.)

As for soldiers presenting with psychophysiological symptoms and conditions, it seems likely that large numbers of unrecognized combat stress cases were represented in this population. In general, the psychiatrists who produced reports from Vietnam said little about this group. One exception is Blank (3rd Field Hospital), who reported early in the war that 20% of his inpatients were "psychosomatic" cases, and that he suspected there were many additional cases being treated by other physicians. However, he did not explicitly tie these cases to combat stress. Also early, Byrdy (1st Cavalry Division) reported that 4.8% of his referrals received as their primary diagnosis that of "psychophysiological reaction," but he did not link their symptoms to combat stress either. Late in the war, Alessi (23rd Infantry Division) was very explicit that psychophysiologic symptoms had become the most common combat-generated psychiatric reaction, and he advocated that the battalion surgeons prescribe the neuroleptic tranquilizer Mellaril for these soldiers. Intriguingly, in the follow up to his study of outpatient psychotropic drug prescription patterns in Vietnam (with Datel),[95] Johnson reported that Compazine, also a phenothiazine neuroleptic, which was mostly prescribed for gastrointestinal irritability, accounted for 45% of all psychotropic prescriptions written by the primary care physicians in Vietnam. Furthermore, it was his assumption that most of these cases were generated by combat and related stress.[81]

The subject of alcohol and drug use by combat troops will be addressed in Chapter 9. Overall, there are ample data to indicate that use, abuse, and dependency were widespread problems with respect to alcohol throughout the war, marijuana beginning early in the war, and for heroin from mid-1970 until combat troops were withdrawn in 1972. However, in general there are not sufficient data available to indicate greater use of drugs or alcohol among combat troops or that the use of these substances was an additional risk factor in the pathogenesis of combat-related conditions. On the other hand, a number of commentators posited that both marijuana and later heroin were commonly used in the field by troops to calm down after combat engagements.

Otherwise, there were undoubtedly many psychiatrically disabled soldiers with complex etiologies that included at least the prospect of combat risks or a history of combat exposure but without evidence of acute combat stress, or certainly not combat exhaustion, per se. As such they defied neat categorization of combat versus noncombat stress. Probably it should be suspected that any significant psychiatric symptom or problematic behavior in the theater might be etiologically linked to combat stress or an experience of combat traumatization (as suggested by Bruce Boman, an Australian psychiatrist[8]). The following case example, extracted from a report from the 1st Infantry Division Mental Health Consultation Service (April 1969–April 1970), involved a corpsman who was facing charges for combat refusal. It demonstrates how SP5 Walter E Smith, an enlisted social work/psychology technician, provided effective therapeutic counseling to the patient for his underlying traumatic experiences and effective consultation to his unit cadre and battalion surgeon.[109(p365)]

CASE 6-11: Field Medic Accused of Combat Refusal

Identifying information: SP4 Papa is a 19-year-old Puerto Rican combat medic who was seen by the psychiatric technician after referral from his battalion surgeon in anticipation of his being court-martialed for combat refusal.

History of present illness: The patient had been experiencing increasing internal and external stress from combat exposure for some time. Two months prior to referral he had been wounded during an ambush in which his company commander and several friends were wounded or killed. During the confusion following a retreat, several wounded men were apparently left in the field. The patient had returned under fire to aid them but was unable to save the life of a friend. After being seriously wounded, he attempted to carry the company commander (whom he later said he respected and admired "like a father") to safety, but he was unable because of his own small stature and his wound. When ordered to the rear, he became hysterical and was "dusted off" (evacuated by helicopter) prior to men whom he considered to be more severely wounded. In the clearing station the patient became depressed and self-critical. When he was returned to his unit several weeks later, he refused to go to the field because he felt he had proven he was a failure as a medic and did not want to cause further harm to his platoon because of his inadequacy. The platoon was later ambushed and, because of his refusal to participate, the patient further blamed himself for their casualties. All this was compounded because the patient's immediate superior was an "old Army" Mexican American NCO [noncommissioned officer] who reacted to the patient's depression and combat refusal by insisting that he "be a man" or else be punished for cowardice.

Past history: None provided.

Examination: During the initial interview and in consultations with his superiors and peers, it became apparent that SP4 Papa had an excellent record after 7 months in the field and was admired by his company for his capabilities and dedication as a combat medic. The referring battalion surgeon noted that the patient appeared to be under stress, but he failed to fully appreciate the extent of the problem due to a breakdown in communication with him.

Clinical course: The social work/psychology technician allowed the patient to talk about his situation and his feelings, and a trusting relationship was developed. Counseling was directed toward helping him to be less critical of himself in order to rebuild his self-esteem and confidence, while permitting him to mourn the loss of his friends. In addition, the technician met with the patient's NCOIC [noncommissioned officer in charge] and the battalion surgeon to facilitate their understanding of his dynamics, especially the "homeostatic necessity" [Author: meaning it served to preserve self-esteem rather than represented an adaptive failure] for his seemingly "cowardly" behavior.

Discharge diagnosis: None provided.

Disposition: As a result of these interventions, the patient regained his previous level of functioning and completed his tour of duty in the field.

Source: Adapted with permission from Bey DR, Smith WE. Mental health technicians in Vietnam. *Bull Menninger Clin*. 1970;34(6):365–366.

The next case example demonstrates the prophylactic recommendation of noncombat assignment for a combat soldier with demonstrably low intelligence and education.

CASE 6-12: Depressed Machine Gunner With Low Self-Confidence

Identifying information: PFC Quebec is a 19-year-old, white machine gunner with 1 year in the Army and 3 months in Vietnam. He was referred to the 935th Psychiatric Detachment for evaluation and treatment for anxiety and depression.

History of present illness: He reports he always "messes up" and is fearful that he would mess up in his machine gunner job if the column were to be attacked. He intimated to a friend that he might commit suicide as a solution (allegedly the friend removed the firing pin from his weapon after he tried to shoot himself). The division psychiatrist feels he is fit for duty, but the commanding officer and the battalion surgeon feel he is not.

Past history: PFC Quebec is the fourth of five children. He left school after the 4th grade and worked as a cow-puncher. He later got a 6th grade equivalency education. He was denied entry into the Army on three previous tries. He completed truck-driving training as well as became an expert machine gunner.

Examination: His IQ [intelligence quotient] measured at 86. He is not psychotic but does present with low self-esteem secondary to low education and intelligence.

Clinical course: Unremarkable over a 2-day hospital stay.

Diagnosis: Chronic, mild depression.

Disposition: Returned to duty; recommended transfer to a combat support unit.

Source: Narrative Summary, the 935th Psychiatric Detachment/93rd Evacuation Hospital.

US Army Combat Stress Research in Vietnam

The historical debate between external stress versus individual predisposition as the best explanation for combat breakdown took a turn toward the latter as a consequence of a pair of studies conducted in Vietnam in early 1966 by the Neuropsychiatry Division of WRAIR, which were directed by Rioch and conducted in the field by Bourne and his associates. Over a 3-week period the investigators measured physiological stress levels and emotional states in members of an elite combat unit (Special Forces "A" team) under threat of attack. They repeated this approach with members of a noncombat unit (helicopter ambulance medics) who were intermittently subjected to great combat risks. The research protocol involved collecting 24-hour urines to measure steroid excretion levels (urinary 17-hydroxycorticosteroid [17-OHCS]) and analysis of self-reports of emotional states (using the daily form of the Multiple Affect Adjective Check-List [D-MAACL]).[110]

The Special Forces team (N = 11) was camped in the central highlands in territory controlled by the Viet Cong during a phase when an enemy attack was predicted. Over the course of the study the authors found no significant daily increases in steroid excretion levels except for the two officers. However, on the day of the anticipated attack, the commanding officer and the radio operator showed significant elevations. These results suggested that stress levels increased for those who were more knowledgeable of the real risks or were among those in positions of greater responsibility.[111] Administrations of the D-MAACL were obtained during the same time frame and were compared for anxiety, depression, and hostility levels. Scores and participant observations corroborated that hostility was the dominant affect expressed.[112]

Regarding the helicopter ambulance medics (N = 6), steroid excretion levels showed little variation from the overall mean and did not correlate to objective measurement of danger. In fact, on the basis of weight alone, the chronic mean level for each subject was lower than predicted.[113] However, anxiety scale scores from the D-MAACL (high, middle, and low) were significantly correlated with type of daily activity (combat mission, work, or day off). Interviews revealed that subjects used an extensive range of psychological defenses to perceive risk situations as less dangerous, thus enhancing feelings of omnipotence and invulnerability and allowing a high level of adaptability to the unit mission.[114]

Bourne interpreted the overall results as:

Among psychological defenses utilized by fighting men are religious faith, a statistical conclusion that the chances of being killed or injured on any one day are small, inordinate faith in one's own ability to stay alive, and a restructuring of reality to avoid facing the danger. In the process of ignoring danger . . . there can be a generalized suppression of affective arousal as reflected by normal, or even below normal, urinary 17-OHCS levels.[115(p10)]

Glass added that these results validate clinical impressions that "an event is only stressful for the individual when he perceives it as such,"[57(pxxviii)] and that the individual's characteristic defenses serve to mitigate the stress (ie, his individual psychological style, especially denial, suppression, reliance on others, religious faith, and compulsive activities).[57]

However, it is uncertain how much to generalize to the average soldier from studies of combat adaptation among members of elite units. For example, in their study of Special Forces veterans of Vietnam (over 10 years after service in Vietnam), Neller et al found them to be somewhat immunized from combat stress, at least while in the theater. This was presumed to be the product of their being volunteers and several years older than the average soldier, their repeated pledges of mutual support, and the extensive specialized training they received, especially in the use of guerrilla warfare tactics, which afforded them a resistance to the tactics guerrilla forces use to try to psychologically separate troops from their base of support.[63,116]

The Role of Demoralization and Psychological Conflict in Combat Reactions: Postwar Considerations

Disabling Psychiatric Conditions as a Function of Demoralization

In the aftermath of the Vietnam War, references to combat-risk avoidance as a primary motivation for combat reactions still appeared in the military psychiatry literature, even if not implying the moral judgments from earlier times. Harry R Kormos, a Navy psychiatrist, provided a thorough review of combat-related psychiatric casualties in American wars from World War I through Vietnam, which ranged from psychotic disorganization to drug abuse and assassination of superiors, and posited that "refusal to fight" was a central dynamic in these conditions.[16(p11)] Scientific support for this model from the Vietnam theater came from Bourne, who summarized his own findings and those of others: "A slowly shifting emphasis, culminating in the Vietnam experience, has led to a conceptualization of the psychiatric casualty as an adaptive failure of a basically temporary nature rather than a disease entity."[9(p229)] Furthermore, according to Bourne, although the majority of hospitalized soldier-patients in Vietnam were categorized as character and behavior disorders, the actual presenting symptoms, which in earlier wars could have taken the form of a hysterical paralysis or a self-inflicted wound, have been socially or culturally shaped and mask the critical issue—that the soldier has ceased to cope and function in the combat environment, with their "manipulative" goals being to pursue a socially permissible means for opting out of combat risk. He concluded that healthy men only succumb to combat stress under exceptional circumstances, and that psychiatric attrition is mostly limited to those with predeployment, including subclinical, personality susceptibility, that is, deficits[9] (see next section).

Corroboration also came from Noy, who drew upon later Israeli military experience. He noted the correlation between combat intensity and all forms of "exits" from the battlefield, that is, not only combat reactions and other psychiatric conditions, but also disciplinary exits and medical exits for disease and nonbattle injury. According to Noy,

> Combat reaction [is] one of a family of stress syndromes with various expressions, including psychiatric, medical and disciplinary . . . [which] can be understood in terms of a clinical entity, a social entity, and a communication of "I can't take it any more."[117(p84)]

Jones basically agreed but argued for combat avoidance as a secondary motivation. Still, he reiterated the traditional view of military psychiatrists that, when a soldier becomes a combat reaction type of casualty and is not managed with the forward treatment doctrine, there is a significant risk that his condition will become intractable because it affords him an honorable means

for escaping additional combat risk while salvaging his self-esteem and warding off guilt.[5] However, there were no studies conducted during the war to confirm this assumption.

Regrettably, also not measured in Vietnam was the effect of sagging overall morale in the theater over time and consequent impairment of combat effectiveness and psychological resilience and durability of combat-exposed troops. As senior Army social psychologist FJ Manning compellingly argued: whereas in earlier wars "commitment and cohesion" within the small combat unit were found to be crucial in mitigating individual combat stress (a finding that linked with the historic observation that "ideology [only] serves to get soldiers into battle"[40(p7)]), there is ample evidence to indicate that this was contradicted in Vietnam where the lack of widespread agreement on the necessity for, and the value of, the war effort in America severely undermined the morale and *esprit de corps* of US forces.[40]

Disabling Psychiatric Conditions From Psychological Disturbances Within the Individual Soldier

Despite advances in the psychoanalytic structural model and other, more general, enhancements in so-called ego psychology, the literature from the Vietnam War era contained little to further the understanding of the contributions of *intrapsychic*, or mental/emotional, conflicts in the pathogenesis of combat stress disorders among individual soldiers (a model advocated by Bloch with the 935th Psychiatric Detachment). However, findings of three psychoanalysts (mental health professionals with additional extensive training in psychological infrastructure) who treated veterans from Vietnam permit, by extrapolation, development of a model of pathogenesis for some combat reactions that arose there. Generalizability of their findings and conclusions to soldiers affected in the theater is, of course, limited because the subjects were veterans and because they were patients. There were no nonsymptomatic controls, and undoubtedly patient presentations were affected by the passage of time and by shifts in their status (active service to civilian) and context (Vietnam to stateside).

Effects of the Interaction of Predisposing Psychological Disturbance and Combat Events

Army psychiatrists PM Balson and CR Dempster described results from their evaluation of 15 combat veterans using hypnosis. They interpreted their findings as arguing for a psychodynamic etiology of "combat neurosis," representing the conjunction of a "chance traumatic reality stress" with an "internal affectual experience." For the soldier-patient, the symptom selection may serve to symbolically express his "disordered self-perception." In other words, the authors believed they verified a theory of internal conflict and "compromise formation" (as advocated by Erikson), at least among some casualties, in which a combat trauma causes a strong regressive response that is qualitatively specific for that soldier.[118]

Combat-Associated Guilt as a Principle Source of Psychologically Disturbance

Corroborating and extending their conclusions were the observations of Harvey J Schwartz. Schwartz reported on his experience conducting analytic psychotherapy with Vietnam veterans—an approach that permitted a deeper appreciation of the "personal meaning" of the veteran's combat experience. In particular Schwartz studied his patients' verbal associations, dreams, and transference reactions to him (as subjectively derived distortions), with a primary focus on the role of unconscious guilt (a chief element in intrapsychic conflict) in the pathogenesis of their combat-centered adjustment difficulties. His rich, nuanced description of his therapeutic process with Patient B serves as a model of care that took into account his unconscious motives and defenses, effectively restoring a psychologically wounded soldier-veteran. ("The patient served in Vietnam in continuous combat for 10 months. He was the point man for his unit which brought him into intimate contact with the most violent and dangerous aspects of guerrilla warfare. Death and mutilation were an everyday encounter, and most of his friends were either maimed or killed."[119(p61)]) Notably, there is no reference to the patient developing symptoms in the theater, and his symptoms as a veteran proved primarily to be grounded in his pre-Vietnam personality organization and in his reported excessive combat aggression in the field (he killed a defenseless civilian).

With regard to the effects of predisposition, Schwartz argued for a common sense, "bifocal" approach for understanding posttraumatic psychological disturbances and disability:

> Regression, the inevitable response to massive stress, can, in and of itself, lead to altered [mental] functioning. To claim that all regression derives from [predeployment] predisposition is . . . to misunderstand the organism as a physiological entity whose primary motive is survival. On the other hand, to state that [soldiers'] emotional conflicts begin only at the moment of trauma and that they bring none of their past distortions to that event is . . . to be naïve about psychological functioning. Stressful events can only be perceived through the veil of [ones past].[120(ppxvi)]

The Potential for Widespread Guilt Among Troops Fighting in Vietnam

Nadelson, a psychiatrist who spent much of his professional career evaluating and treating veterans at the Boston DVA Hospital, ultimately synthesized his impressions in his book, *Trained to Kill: Soldiers at War*[121] (elaborated with verbatim interviews with Vietnam veterans in a companion publication, *Attachment to Killing*[122]). In contrast to the hypnotherapeutic methodology of Balson and Dempster,[118] or Schwartz's utilization of psychoanalytic theory in the treatment of individual cases,[119] Nadelson's approach[121,122] centered on interpreting vignettes from veterans of World War II, Korea, and especially Vietnam, through the various lenses of the history of war, philosophy, social anthropology, ethology, neurobiology, social psychology (both macro and micro), and biopsychodynamic developmental theory.

According to Nadelson, a fundamental precombat susceptibility to psychological disorder in troops arises from the innate characteristics and anxieties within all young males. The effect is that to a certain degree they welcome participation in the lethal, winner-take-all experience of war as the quick and sure path to establish a confident masculinity ("The myth of maleness . . . "[121(p3)]). Not only does combat permit the expression of such masculine traits as daring, impetuousness, and male-bonding, but since sanctioned killing in the service of the nation's protection is honorable (and "a male duty"[121(p42)]), the young soldier may be forced, as well as permitted, by the immediacy of combat to fully exercise the primal male drive to possess and dominate (with killing as its highest form), while at the same time "rejecting all that is civilian and soft."[121(p24)] However, it is unmistakably a harsh test. ("Men's self-esteem has been strongly shaped by evolutionary and cultural pressures toward use of counterforce rather than surrender. . . . Failing to do so, even if the possibility of successful response to overwhelming force to save oneself or a comrade is slim or nonexistent, is psychologically devastating, and the memory is haunting."[121(p88)]) At stake is the misery of being a failed male. ("You're pussy."[121(p24)])

However, this can be a slippery slope: killing can become addictive. According to Nadelson, "Killing the man who would kill you while escaping injury is electrifying ("a hyperaroused, excited emotional state"[121(p79)]). Soldiers in contact with the enemy become enthralled. They risk death focusing only on destroying the enemy. The reflex to defend against mortal harm results in lust and freedom—no thought, only action."[121(p6)] He also, like other psychiatric observers in Vietnam, commented on the potential for the sexualization of killing. ("Men at war experience intense excitement—orgasm pushed up a notch, an automatic weapon on 'rock and roll.' In its momentum toward absolute force, war can engage some of its participants in savage amusement—which defines the perverse. . . ."[121(p70)])

Given these features, it is not a stretch to appreciate how the combat-required killing can spiral into unconstrained use of force and atrocity (with societally unsanctioned killing referred to as "murder"). According to Nadelson, "[With respect to Vietnam] the danger of being overrun—the enforced passivity before engagement—agitates men beyond comparison and demands assertion of mastery. Such feelings, especially if leadership is poor or weak, can move the susceptible to atrocity. Once the killing started [in Vietnam], soldiers could not break cohesion with friends—they killed together. Love . . . can also pull soldiers into evil."[122(p60)]

As discussed in Chapters 1 and 2, the Vietnam War brought with it several novel features that appear to have greatly magnified the potential for these types of conflicts within the soldier: (1) the great expansion in firepower under the control of the individual soldier compared to his earlier counterparts; (2) the enemy's terrorist/guerrilla tactics encouraged equivalent, more brutal responses from US troops; (3) the failed US strategy of enemy attrition employed there ("The Vietnam War stretched the envelope of 'just' rules designed to control the actions of soldiers. . . . The war's incoherence affected the men on the ground, lessened the claim of rules and standards, and, in that, further demeaned them. Killing—the body counts—became command's purpose because they had no other, and for many ordinary soldiers, killing became their purpose,

too."[121(p59)]); and (4) effects from the reversal of the American public's approval for the war. According to Nadelson, "[T]he soldier's real work is killing. The soldier's [societally granted] privilege to kill is unlike anything most other individuals have ever experienced, and the soldier who kills is permanently changed, fixed to the death he has made."[121(p38)] When the "privilege" was revoked by a disheartened America ("There were none of those customary and necessary 'expiatory rituals' . . . "[121(p52)]), combat troops were left holding the (moral) bag.

As for the clinical effects of this rich combination of psychologically disturbing factors, it appears that it is Nadelson's legacy to serve as an eloquent witness to what all this did to the more susceptible troops in Vietnam (and it would seem to be naïve to assume that this only pertained to veterans no longer in the theater, see Case 6-1, PFC Foxtrot; Case 6-2, PFC Golf; and Case 6-3, PFC Hotel.). The following are selected examples from Nadelson:

- For many of the boys who fought in Vietnam, combat lifted a corner of the expected universe. They experienced a world in war moved only by uncompromising necessities, where life and death were regulated by immediacy (or accident), stripped of the rules and conventions. Some boys achieved a precocious manhood, conferred on them by the intensity of the experience, the power of their brotherhood and weapons. Many felt strong, exultant, and empowered after survival in Vietnam in the fellowship of their comrades.[121(p21)]
- When the brain reward systems are firing, everything feels right, and there is no need for an external moral sanction; the good feeling speaks only of the rightness of the moment. With your brain buzzed, the feeling of flow, of one's control and certainty amid the unpredictable, sometimes carries a person with it [to excess]. . . . [121(p115)]
- Combat veterans said of themselves that in Vietnam as adolescents they were "lords of death," "kings," "gods."[121(p59)]
- For many, a constant dark shadow of guilt about the satisfaction of and charge in killing in successful counterforce lingers.[121(p92)]
- For some soldiers, the nature of the war in Vietnam and, they fear, their own nature, carried them beyond defined civilized limits, and they cannot find those limits within themselves again.[121(p48)]

- Some still are deeply troubled by the thought that [perceived excess aggression] rose out of a profound defect in their own character. Many register deepest sadness about what they became . . . and also speak with great clarity about what the availability of force did to them.[121(p59)]

In conclusion, although Nadelson's review and analysis is rich and liberally illustrated with clinical vignettes, unfortunately he did not provide detail regarding his methodology or data. Nonetheless, it is a compelling essay by a distinguished psychiatrist and psychoanalyst on the wrenching effects of war based on his innumerable clinical encounters with combat veteran-patients spanning two decades. In particular his findings also appear to coincide with some of the clinical examples and other professional observation from the Vietnam theater. If not serving hypothesis testing, certainly his observations and conclusions regarding a generally taboo subject, the sometimes damaging (to self or others) pleasure soldiers often derive from participation in combat, deserves more attention.

USMC/Navy Studies of Combat Stress Treatment and Combat Effectiveness

USMC/Navy Experience at Khe Sanh

As has been previously noted, this work does not attempt a full review of the psychiatric experience of the Marines and Navy personnel deployed in Vietnam. However, a unique opportunity for the study of combat stress in Vietnam among ground troops pinned down by enemy fire arose during the 76-day siege of the 5,500 Marines and Naval personnel located on the Marine base at Khe Sanh in early 1968. Lieutenant Commander Stephen W Edmendson, a Navy psychiatrist, and Lieutenant (Junior Grade) Donald J Platner, a Navy psychologist (both of whom were attached to the 3rd Marine Division), reported that the percent of personnel who received psychiatric evacuation to either the 3rd Medical Battalion at Phu Bai or to the hospital ship, USS *Repose,* during the two-and-a-half month siege (1.3% [67 cases]) did not represent an increase over the percent who received psychiatric evacuation during the relatively quiet month before it began (26 cases). They credited high morale and confidence among the Khe Sanh defenders and the excellent field treatment provided by battalion surgeons and corpsmen ("sedation and tranquilization in a relatively safe place"). However,

they also acknowledged the hazards associated with air transport off of the base, suggesting that this may have discouraged evacuations and distorted the metric. Perhaps more important, "situational reactions," mostly of the anxious type, that is, combat stress reactions, went from 4% of evacuees (one case) before the siege to 34% (23 cases) during the siege. Also, as a sidebar, because of special stresses, Navy corpsmen were overrepresented in the psychiatric evacuees during the siege (10 cases). (Strange also found corpsmen overrepresented in Marine combat fatigue cases earlier in the war.[97]) Finally, 60% of all evacuated psychiatric cases from the base (40) were ultimately returned to duty in the theater.[62]

Correlation Between Background Features and Combat Performance

On the side of prevention, background qualities contributing to enhanced combat effectiveness (and which presumably serve to buffer against combat breakdown) were studied among Marines by Jack L Mahan and George A Clum. They examined the records of 831 first-enlistment Marines who served in Vietnam early in the war (1964–1965) and sought to correlate their field supervisor's rating of their combat performance in Vietnam (a single rating on a 7-point scale) with pre-Vietnam predictor variables. Overall the group achieved a mean rating of 4.99. One-third had ratings of either 6 or 7, and only 3% had ratings of 1 or 2. Of the predictor variables, 40 (of 70) were significantly correlated with combat effectiveness. These described the effective combat Marine as older, better educated, and white, with more siblings and fewer arrests. In the recruit processing, he had measurably higher intelligence and aptitude, especially in the areas of general information, mechanical aptitude, and arithmetic reasoning. In recruit training, he showed good drill instructor ratings. Higher second year ratings for performance, personal relations, and overall adjustment were also predictive of later combat effectiveness.[123] Although these findings make intuitive sense, it is regrettable that they were only collected very early in the war. It can be assumed that the number of Marines who brought these qualities into the theater would have decreased as the war prolonged because of the 13-month tour limits and the rapid turnover of personnel (see section on excessive combat aggression).

Additional observations regarding Marines and combat stress-related psychiatric conditions are found in the summaries of the report by Ted D Kilpatrick, who was assigned to the 3rd Marine Division in 1967 (Chapter 3), and the reports by Strange and Arthur, who served aboard the hospital ship USS *Repose* off the coast of Vietnam in 1966 (Chapter 4). Summaries of reports by Howard, Herman P Langner, and John A Renner Jr regarding excessive combat aggression follow. Perhaps of special note, Howard W Fisher, the division psychiatrist with the 1st Marine Division (March 1970–February 1971), made no specific mention of combat stress in his account of the avalanche of personality disorder referrals he saw later in the war (Chapter 2).[124]

Excessive Combat Aggression and Atrocities

Reports Regarding Army Troops in Vietnam

This subject has been left for last because of its only tangential connection to military psychiatry (compared to military authority). In fact, although the war saw increasing concerns in the United States about excessive combat aggression in Vietnam, including atrocities (Figure 6-5), the psychiatric literature from the Army psychiatrists in the theater did not address this behavior. For example, midway through the war, 1st Infantry Division psychiatrist Bey (July–December, 1969) conducted a study of 43 soldiers referred because of violent behavior, but in none of the incidents studied were Vietnamese the targets.[125] One exception came from Jones (25th Infantry Division), who served in the first year of the war. He described a junior officer who was distraught because he had witnessed soldiers desecrating the body of an elderly Vietnamese civilian who was apparently killed when it was assumed that he was a Viet Cong sympathizer (the body was repeatedly dragged behind a jeep through the village) and felt powerless to intercede because he wasn't confident that his superiors would agree that this was wrong.[21] The apparent absence of psychiatric attention to the subject could be accounted for by the paucity of publications by the psychiatrists assigned in Vietnam after 1968 to 1969 when, as suggested earlier, these incidents may have been more common. It is even more likely that such behaviors were not being brought to the attention of the deployed psychiatrists, at least as clinical matters, because command did not see them as pertaining to mental health. (In the WRAIR survey data, psychiatrist respondents estimated their involvement with excessive combat aggression as infrequent, and there was no significant difference in comparing respondents by

phase of the war in which they served [see Chapter 8, Table 8-4].)

Below are summaries of two hospital case records from the 935th Psychiatric Detachment that include such possible war crimes:

CASE 6-13: Psychomotor Regression Following Combat Losses and Responsibility for a Civilian Casualty

---

Identifying information: PFC Romeo was a 24-year-old, Mexican-born rifleman with 6 months in the Army and 2 1/2 months in Vietnam.

History of present illness: The patient was sent directly from the field to the 93rd Evacuation Hospital for "possible appendicitis and choking."

Examination: Upon his arrival at the hospital, his abdominal complaints had abated, and he was observed to be lying in a fetal position, distracted, and repeatedly rhyming, "La-la-la."

Past history: None recorded.

Clinical course: PFC Romeo was given an opportunity to get cleaned up, to ventilate, and then was put to sleep with Thorazine. In the morning he mobilized easily and was symptomatically much improved. He described several recent incidents in which platoon members had been killed, and he expressed anger that the ineptitude of his platoon leader was largely responsible. He also described an episode the previous evening in which he (and his platoon sergeant) went after a buddy who was wounded, heard something moving in the bushes, and shot into the bushes, only to find that he had killed a Vietnamese child who had previously befriended members of his platoon. He felt anguish about this. There was no evidence of psychosis.

Discharge diagnosis: Combat exhaustion, acute, moderately severe, manifested by somatic symptoms and regressive behavior. Stress: death of friends, anger at platoon leader. Predisposition: mild.

Disposition: Returned to duty following his overnight stay. He was referred to his division psychiatrist.

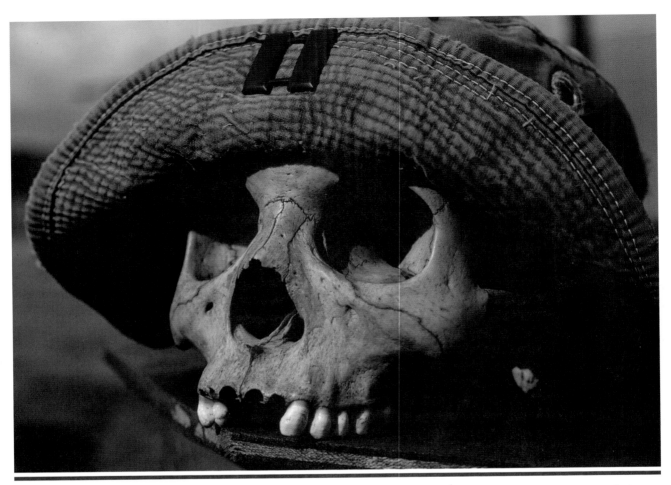

FIGURE 6-5. Human skull wearing a US Army captain's hat. This photograph was taken somewhere in Vietnam in 1970, during the drawdown phase, and serves as a reminder of the sometimes thin line between combat-appropriate aggression and excessive combat aggression. Whereas it was evidently someone's attempt at ghoulish humor, it suggests the creator's, and perhaps his reference group's, deeper feelings of moral tension regarding participation in America's (by then) discredited war. By placing an American hat on what is most likely an enemy skull, he has obliterated the distinction between the soldier and his dead enemy. This could express feelings of victory (and even revenge), or it could represent an effort at atonement, or both. Regardless, it would have been against military regulations and the law of war. Photograph courtesy of Richard D Cameron, Major General, US Army (Retired).

Source: Narrative Summary, 935th Psychiatric Detachment/93rd Evacuation Hospital.

___

CASE 6-14: Sergeant With Preexisting Emotional Instability

Identifying information: SGT Sierra is a 22-year-old white soldier with 5 years of Army service and 4 months service in Vietnam. He was assigned to the 11th Armored Cavalry Regiment.

History of present illness: He was admitted to the 93rd Evacuation Hospital following an incident in which he threatened the driver of his track with his weapon and fired it in the air. Over the previous 2 months the patient was repeatedly abusive and angry, physically attacking others in his unit. In addition, he increased his alcohol intake. In a recent incident he became intoxicated and waded out into an unsafe river, requiring rescue by nearby ARVN rangers. He also bragged that he had a "fascination with pain," which, on one occasion, prompted him to grab strands of barbed wire to prove he was unfazed. On another occasion he decapitated two enemy corpses and threatened to hang their skulls in the track in order to repulse members of his crew. The patient also complained of increasingly severe headaches that would produce double vision and blackout spells.

Past history: SGT Sierra was the sixth of seven children. Early development was reported as unremarkable, but his family members were adamant segregationists. He joined the Army following high school. He was arrested three times for drinking and disorderly conduct. Although distinguishing himself in his Army training (an honor graduate at NCO school and performing well in Drill Sergeant school), he also received four Articles 15 and was court-martialed for drinking, speeding, and destroying government property. He has had a stormy marriage with his wife of 2 years. She is German with an African American stepfather, and they have had numerous arguments over racial issues. He reported that his family treats him as the "black sheep" and rejects his wife because of her background.

Examination: The patient was noted to be anxious and smoking heavily. He had pressured and rambling speech, but he demonstrated relevant and coherent thinking. He acknowledged numerous obsessional rituals (counting), but these were not evident in the exam. There was no evidence of hallucinations or delusions. He repeatedly spoke of his fear that he had ruined his life, and that he was "going down hill." He also expressed intense, prejudicial feelings about African Americans, which bordered on the bizarre.

Clinical course: He participated in group therapy, work therapy, and recreational therapy, as well as individual therapy. He was not a management problem although he tended to stay to himself and often complained of headaches. He was treated with a tapered regimen of Mellaril (begun at 200 mg/day) until the 6th day of his 7-day hospitalization.

Discharge diagnosis: Emotional instability. Stress: mild, exposure to normal military and combat conditions. Predisposition: severe; long history of immature behavior, inability to handle racial attitudes. Impairment: marked. Condition on discharge: unchanged; his condition existed prior to service.

Disposition: Returned to duty.

Source: Narrative Summary, 935th Psychiatric Detachment/93rd Evacuation Hospital.

The first case insinuates that it was accidental. The second suggests that a major contributor was the patient's personality disorder. In neither case does the record indicate that there was command interest regarding excessive combat aggression. This does not mean there was none. It is puzzling that the list of precipitating stressors listed in the first case did not include the reported murder of the Vietnamese child, and that both clinical records seem to overlook questions regarding war crimes.

The following is a record of a forensic evaluation of a soldier referred to the 935th Psychiatric Detachment by his commanding officer in conjunction with several counts of assault on US personnel with a deadly weapon. (The requirements for conducting forensic psychiatric evaluations are in Appendix III—Format for Psychiatric Report of Sanity in Appendix 2, "USARV Regulation 40-34.") It is likely that the Army's psychiatrists in Vietnam were periodically required to provide forensic evaluations for a wide variety of misconduct, including violent behaviors and threats. In this case it is interesting that there was apparently no prosecutorial attention devoted to the alleged murder of the Vietnamese child.

CASE 6-15: Helicopter Door Gunner Facing Charges for Threatening Behavior While Drunk

Identifying information: E-4 Tango underwent a pretrial psychiatric evaluation conducted at the 935th Psychiatric Detachment. E-4 Tango is a 20-year-old E-4 with 28 months of active duty service and 19 months in Vietnam.

History pertaining to the charges: EM's [enlisted man's] service record, including in Vietnam, had been favorable, and he was allowed to extend in Vietnam in order to become a helicopter door gunner. Leading up to the events in question was: (1) the death of a friend and fellow door gunner, a loss for which the EM felt responsible because he had not flown on that mission (because of a recent hand injury resulting from fighting while drunk); (2) [a] few weeks later EM allegedly shot an infant out of its mother's arms. [Author: whereas the report included no additional information regarding this incident, it suggested that it was assumed the child's death was accepted as collateral damage associated with combat activity.] As a consequence he felt intense guilt and was no longer willing to fire his weapon. ([T]he examining psychiatrist speculated that this incident coincided with displaced hostile feelings he had for the infant of another Vietnamese woman whom he believed he had impregnated); (3) [h]e was removed from flying and given a noncombat assignment; he was urged to curtail his drinking; and he was told he was being reassigned. The charges facing the EM arose after he got drunk, went to the flight line, and apparently threatened several individuals with a weapon, events for which the EM claimed compete amnesia [results of the criminal investigation were not available for this review].

Past history: EM had been "a rather headstrong boy who was somewhat spoiled" before the birth of his siblings. He reported that in his early development he demonstrated difficulty tolerating frustration and controlling hostile, sadistic impulses. Ultimately he managed to cope by rigidly controlling himself and becoming a loner.

Examination: Aside from presenting as somber, anxious, agitated, and tense, the mental status findings were unremarkable. Intelligence, social judgment, and conceptual ability were deemed within normal limits. Psychological testing was negative for psychosis.

Clinical course: Not applicable.

Final diagnosis: No psychiatric disease.

Disposition: EM was psychiatrically cleared for administrative or judicial proceedings. At the time of the examination he met Army retention standards and was deemed mentally responsible. Regarding the incidents in question, the evaluating psychiatrist indicated that the EM was "probably drunk," and that, although he had an earlier amnestic incident when he assaulted a friend while drunk, he was not subject to such episodes when sober. He concluded that the EM had been having increasing difficulty managing hostile, violent impulses, as well as guilt and remorse, regarding his actions as a door gunner; and that alcohol served to [disinhibit him].

Source: Report of Psychiatric Evaluation, 935th Psychiatric Detachment/93rd Evacuation Hospital.

Reports From the US Marine Corps/Navy

Several of the Navy physicians who provided care for Marines in the theater published material bearing on the subject of excessive combat aggression in Vietnam. Howard served as a Marine battalion surgeon in 1968 and pursued psychiatric training shortly after returning to the United States. The combination of his close proximity to the troops and the fighting (he reported getting wounded) and his subsequent specialization training allowed him to have a unique vantage point for observation and interpretation regarding the connection between the challenges in adapting to combat stress at that time in Vietnam and the development of excessive combat aggression. According to Howard, the Marines of 1968 had to contend with fear and terror regarding the combat mixed with intense feelings of isolation from home and the familiar (causing feelings of "unreality," "adrift"); alienation from their surroundings (provoking "contempt toward Vietnam and its people"); and despair and hopelessness regarding the mission (stemming from their feeling the war was "futile and senseless"); and a "glaring absence of good leadership."

Furthermore, the real and frequent danger they faced not only fueled their combat motivation, but it also provoked their most primitive urges. ("Under the overwhelming threat of annihilation, our priorities regress to the survival state; all higher priorities, all ethical and moral considerations lose relevance, and only the survival of the individual and the immediate group retain significance."[51(p133)]) Embedded in his reference to moral considerations Howard includes: (a) their anger at being sent far from home and isolated from "something real and human"—especially warm and desirable women (thus they reverted to the local prostitutes); and (b) that they relished the opportunity to satisfy a wish to kill (according to Howard, an almost universal desire but one that is generally repressed). Serving as a remedy, combat activity permitted them to "prove themselves," especially to their comrades, through the crudest myth of masculinity, "fighting and f--king," ("[thus] blurring the distinction between gun and phallus, to the extent that orgasmic release is sometimes experienced in the very act of committing violence"[51(p128)]). Howard also described some of the psychological and social defenses utilized by the Marines as they struggled to maintain their personal equilibrium: heavy reliance on slang and empty euphemisms to refer to the enemy and emotionally charged subjects (ie, kill, danger, fear, death); counterphobic, almost psychotic, denial of danger and a quasidelusional belief in one's invulnerability; and intense ("pseudointimate") love for one's comrades. (These observations and reconstructions pertaining to troops in the field appear to validate the aforementioned impressions by Schwartz and by Nadelson derived from DAV veteran patients.)

Finally, Howard recommended some temperance of judgment of Marines regarding accusations of excessive combat aggression in Vietnam. "It is important not to distinguish too strongly between 'normal' combat killing on the one hand, and murder and atrocity on the other."[51(p133)] He also suggested that understanding these psychosocial dynamics can help to explain readjustment symptoms in some returnees whose suspension of civilian morals in Vietnam collapsed into guilt upon return to stateside life (the "real world") and facing society's repudiation of the troops who served there.[51]

Langner, a Navy psychiatrist who served aboard the hospital ship USS *Sanctuary* (1967–1968) at about the same time as Howard, published a report ("The Making of a Murderer"[126]) that provided some corroboration of Howard's observations. In Langner's opinion, the My Lai massacre by Army troops was not unique because the problem of poorly controlled aggression, even toward fellow Marines, was endemic in Vietnam while he was there. According to Langner:

[M]any other such brutalities were reported to me by different individuals . . .

 . . . Often a young man came in or was sent to me with the fear or threat of killing one of his superiors who he felt had harassed him or treated him unfairly. Others were sent to me after shooting holes through their "hootches" or throwing grenades around. On occasion such cases turned into incidents involving the indiscriminate killing of comrades. Fighting and "accidental" shootings among the men were frequent; they represented another way of discharging aggressions that were reaching unmanageable proportions. It should also be noted that many [of these] problems were dealt with through disciplinary rather than psychiatric channels and therefore did not come to the psychiatrist's attention.[126(p951)]

Langner used a specimen case of a young Navy corpsman, "Bob," to explore the concatenation of circumstance and personality that led Bob to murder a defenseless farmer, in front of an officer. Bob originally came to psychiatric attention after he apparently tried to take his own life in a morphine overdose. This was ostensibly brought about from survivor guilt following the death of a fellow corpsman in a firefight. However, when Langner conducted an amobarbital interview to facilitate Bob's cathartic relief of what was assumed to be unrealistic guilt, Langner was surprised at the outpouring of guilt and sorrow associated with Bob's participation in an earlier military action ("a bloody military operation . . . during which his unit had swept through a village, killing all living things, including men, women, children, and livestock. [Bob] described setting fields of rice ablaze 'with my Zippo lighter' and watched peasants shot down as they ran from their burning homes."[126(p950)]) Langner referred to these incident as "mayhem" and "a massacre." He also noted that in the course of the narcosynthesis, Bob exhibited "fascination and pleasure."[126(p951)] These events preceded the death of the corpsman friend by several weeks and included the incident of his killing the farmer.

With respect to pre-Vietnam susceptibility, Bob, himself a son of a farmer, had always been mild-mannered and nonaggressive and wanted to become a corpsman to help others. However, according to Langner, Bob's violent behavior flowed from repressed rebellious and destructive urges toward his passive but demanding father and his domineering mother, which led to lingering doubts about his masculinity and late-adolescent instability and instinctual recklessness (perhaps it was implied that Bob had used a reaction-formation defense against these urges in choosing to be a noncombatant corpsman). Once in Vietnam the breakthrough of these urges (ie, a "regression") arose when Bob became increasingly insecure, frightened, frustrated, and angry as a consequence of the aggregate stressful circumstances he faced:

- enduring the hardships and misery associated with serving in an inhospitable and distant land;
- participating in an unpopular war;
- fighting against an elusive enemy that took its toll gradually and indirectly, thereby avoiding open

combat that would have allowed US troops to vent their anger and frustration;

- sacrificing for an indigenous people who were unwelcoming, ungrateful, suspicious, and often cooperated with the enemy;
- operating in a war-torn culture where death was common and the value of life had been cheapened;
- influenced by a group-sanctioned, killing mind-set that "swept away" the moral restraints of civilized society;
- enabled by a military authority that relinquished its traditional duty as "in loco parentis"; and
- encountering a specific releasing situation during which a mob mentality prevailed.

Similar to Howard's theory, Langner surmised that Bob's barbaric conduct gratified primitive destructive urges as well as sexual ones. (According to Grossman, a professor of military psychology, this is an underlying temptation within every soldier.[34]) In the final analysis, however, Langner concluded that "Bob was in many ways an American Everyman." By that he meant that, in explaining Bob's brutality his preservice risk factors were far overshadowed by the "pathological circumstances" in Vietnam at that time. There is nothing in his report to indicate whether Langner notified military authorities about Bob's confession or whether Bob was formally accused of war crimes.[126]

Also from the vantage point of providing 3rd echelon care, Renner, also a Navy psychiatrist, offered his impressions regarding the epidemiology of psychiatric and related difficulties in Vietnam from his contact with over 1,200 Marine and Navy referrals. He served aboard the hospital ship USS *Repose* (1969) roughly a year after Howard and Langner and at the beginning of the American drawdown. Renner cataloged the numerous circumstantial features affecting the combat troops (then) that served to seriously erode social (military) structures, psychological defenses, mission identity, and associated military comportment, what he referred to as "hidden casualties" (drug abuse, disciplinary problems, and the numbers diagnosed as character and behavior disorder). These included the moral and ethical ambiguity consequent to the political upheaval in America; hostility toward the apparently ungrateful South Vietnamese; the individual rotation system, which accentuated preoccupation with each individual's welfare and reduced ties to unit members to "superficial" ones based on "sharing a primitive

struggle for survival"; and the enemy's "unacceptable" and "deliberate" terrorism, which ostensibly justified revenge, dehumanization of the enemy, and primitive aggression. According to Renner:

> For the majority of soldiers these drives are not dominant, and the men are not personally aggressive. However, some men derive a vicarious and sometimes unconscious pleasure out of their involvement in the impersonal killing of war. . . . It reduces existence to its vital essentials, life or death. One can escape the boring details of civilized life and act out childhood fantasies of valor, power, and indestructibility. These fantasies are necessary to keep soldiers functioning under the terrible real dangers of combat.[3(p174)]

In these remarks, Renner appears divided. Initially he was clear that these attitudes and behaviors were pathological, but then he reverted to arguing that they were necessary for adaptation. He also noted that for some, psychological conflicts arose when they sensed (in the theater or afterward) that their drives for survival, revenge, and aggression conflicted with their moral standards; and they became plagued with guilt for having participated in the violence (a "degrading and amoral struggle").[3] (Renner's observations and reconstructions also appear to validate the aforementioned impressions of Schwartz and Nadelson.)

To conclude this section, from a historical standpoint it is fortunate to have available for study the reports by Howard, Langner, and Renner. Their clinical perspectives and impressions of the stressors affecting their patients and fellow Marines should not be dismissed because they are frankly disturbing, they seem too impressionistic, or they may be limited because of the prevailing medical, particularly the military medical and psychiatric, mind set and methodologies of the 1960s and early 1970s. In fact, they offer uniquely valuable insights because they were from a set of professionally trained observers of human nature who were actually working in the theater. Whereas their conclusions are sometimes ambivalent, they are mostly consistent with each other and give eyewitness testimony as to the deleterious effects of a mounting collection of bio\psycho\social-environmental stressors on combat-committed troops in Vietnam; the degrading effect the stressors had on overall military morale, order, and discipline; and the corrosive effects they had on

FIGURE 6-4. WRAIR survey psychiatrists' recollections of prevalence of specific symptoms or syndromes among combat-exposed troops above "uncommon"

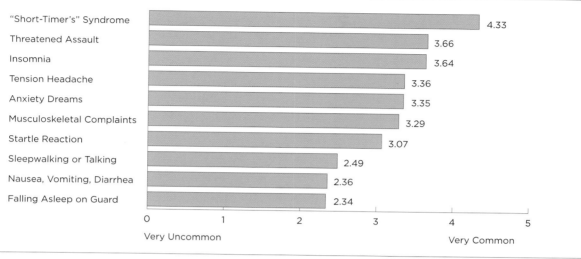

Means of recollections of the prevalence of specific symptoms or syndromes among combat-exposed troops (presumes absence of a primary physical cause) along a 1–5 point scale with 1 = very uncommon to 5 = very common (N = 45). Values falling in the "uncommon" range are not included. They are hysterical amnesia (1.93), hysterical deafness and/or aphonia (1.78), narcolepsy (1.68), hysterical seizures (1.64), nocturnal enuresis (1.64), hysterical stuttering (1.61), and hysterical blurred vision (1.53).

the measured application of military aggression in the field, that is, within the constraints of the official rules of engagement—observations that were not limited to psychiatrically impaired individuals.

Reports of Veterans Regarding Excessive Combat Aggression

As the war lengthened, some corroboration of these observations came from psychiatrists and other mental health professionals who wrote about veterans they had evaluated, treated, or encountered who admitted responsibility for excessive combat aggression or acknowledged they witnessed it by others.[68,127–132] Summarized below are the more data-centered reports that offer some illumination on the prevalence and causes of excessive combat aggression in Vietnam.

Joel Yager, an Army psychiatrist, reported on clinical evaluations of a subset of 31 Vietnam combat veterans who had a history of at least one self-confirmed kill in Vietnam (their service in Vietnam was 1966–1971 [most in 1968–1969], and they were evaluated 2 to 18 months after their return). These soldiers were still on active duty and were referred because of either symptoms or conduct problems. Participants were questioned about acts of violence against persons at

close range that were unnecessary from a military point of view, and almost half (14) reported they had engaged in such "personal violence." Another nine (30%) reported witnessing such behavior. All the personal violence participants had volunteered to go to Vietnam, and significantly more personal violence participants reported killing four or more persons in Vietnam than did nonparticipants. They also more frequently had a history of arrest prior to military service and could be distinguished from nonparticipants by the average number of items acknowledged in each of several groupings of negative pre-Vietnam variables.[68]

Based on his clinical contacts with Vietnam returnees, William B Gault, an Army psychiatrist, seemed to corroborate the earlier observations in the field by Howard and Langner regarding the Marines and the intersection of the prevailing military culture with specific individual, circumstantial, and mechanical features to produce excessive violence against civilians. Gault specifically found the following factors as contributing to excessive violence in Vietnam: (*a*) adaptational paranoia ("The weary [soldier] realistically perceives threat from every quarter . . . he feels that the country itself may murder him at any moment"[131(p451)]); (*b*) dehumanization of the Vietnamese ("the image of

TABLE 6-5. WRAIR survey psychiatrists' recollections of professional involvement with specific behavior problems among combat troops

Behavior problem	Overall mean	Combat (only) assignment mean	Hospital (only) assignment mean
Individual combat avoidance (malingering, self-inflicted wound, etc.)	2.83*	3.36	2.49
Excessive combat aggression (to civilians, prisoners, souvenirs of the dead)	1.76		
Group combat refusal	1.28		

Means of recollections along a 1-to-5 point scale with 1 = "very uncommon" to 5 = "very common" (N = 60–65).
*Statistically significant difference comparing 14 "combat" (only) psychiatrists with 36 "hospital" (only) psychiatrists (p < .05).
Modified from Camp NM, Carney CM. US Army psychiatry in Vietnam: Preliminary findings of a survey: II. Results and discussion. *Bull Menninger Clin.* 1987;51:19–37.

a degraded enemy is essential to the psychology of any robustly homicidal combat team"[131(p451)]); (c) blurred responsibility ("the individual infantryman often has the sense that responsibility for the specific slaughter of a specific victim is not precisely his but that it is shared [both with higher ups and with combat buddies]"[131(p452)]); (d) the need for action ("repudiation of passivity and the desire for vengeance"[131(p452)]); (e) the situational preeminence of those with psychopathic tendencies; and (f) the ready availability of firepower ("Terrified and furious teenagers by the tens of thousands have only to twitch their index fingers, and what was a quiet village is suddenly a slaughterhouse"[131(p453)]).

Similarly from the Marine Corps, Richard P Fox, a Navy psychiatrist, reported on a cross-sectional study of 106 Vietnam returnee clinical referrals (service in Vietnam was 1967–1969, and they were seen weeks to months after their return) that had severe reentry psychiatric symptoms and behavioral problems. Two-thirds showed evidence of difficulties handling their hostile and aggressive feelings in Vietnam; 16% reported continuing violent behavior in the United States; and 52% acknowledged being fearful of destructive outbursts. By their own account, while in Vietnam these Marines had exhibited a psychological deviation from the group-controlled and group-sanctioned "adaptive aggression," which is the norm for a member of a functioning combat team. They had regressed to a state of "hostile aggressiveness," a vengefulness that was motivated by a narcissistic rage. Fox posited that

the intense buddy relationships that typically develop between combat soldiers involves a range of narcissistic "mirror transferences" that, to varying degrees, leave each individual vulnerable to this regressive process should his "other self" be killed. Furthermore, in seeking to avenge this loss, he becomes devoid of concern for the victim and thus capable of atrocity. Most importantly, that act does not provide relief but instead leads to new anxieties related to fear of retaliation. According to Fox, although this has undoubtedly been a common battlefield process in past wars, the troops in Vietnam were more narcissistically vulnerable because of the political storm surrounding the war and the withdrawal of the public support for those sent to fight.[132]

Obviously the reports by Yager, Fox, and Gault cannot be generalized to conduct in the theater because they are drawn from clinical populations who had returned to the United States. Late in the war, Bourne sought to explain the reported rise in combat atrocities by American soldiers in Vietnam through drawing on his multifaceted field research early in the war and his 1965 study of adolescent identity transformation occurring in Army basic training. He posited that excessive combat aggression represented the soldier's abandonment of his preservice values and beliefs as a result of the combination of: (a) the "militarization process" resulting from basic training—a training designed to force the new soldier to reject his civilian identity—an identity that had emphasized personal initiative—to be replaced with the obedient institutional identity of the military

TABLE 6-6. WRAIR survey psychiatrists' perceptions as to the etiological relevance of major risk factors in the pathogenesis of combat breakdown cases in Vietnam

Combat Environment Dimension	Mean N = 45	No. of Subjects Who Chose Item as Leading Factor (N = 43)
Noxious combat events specific to soldier: buddy killed, unit overrun, guilt about combat aggression or inactivity, helplessness under fire, new to combat	4.53	9
Combat magnitude: intensity, combined with duration, of individual's combat ordeal (general)	4.38	12
Combat intensity: the life-threatening circumstances faced by the individual (general)	4.02	2
total =		23
Personal Dimension		
Precombat personality traits: psychological susceptibility contributing to the soldier's adaptive failure or incapacitation under fire	3.94	12
Life circumstances: anxieties apart from combat events including regarding home, new baby, etc.	3.26	1
total =		13
Unit/Social Dimension		
Limited bonding: low acceptance by combat unit members due to limited intellect or social skills, atypical background, or newness to the unit	3.67	7
total =		7

Psychiatrists were queried on a 1-to-5 point scale with 1 = "not very relevant" to 5 = "very relevant" (N = 45).

organization; and (*b*) the brutalizing socialization to the war, especially the killing, which only occurred once he was in the theater.[133] (Several other Vietnam-era authors also complained about the dehumanization of American troops stemming from basic combat training, but they indicated they were voicing objections of the antiwar activists.[134-136] However, later the same points were made articulately and dispassionately by Grossman.[34])

Notably, none of these physician/psychiatrists addressed the prospect that, overall, many American troops had developed a "habit of undisciplined violence"[66] that is seen among troops fighting an unconventional war against a guerrilla force that utilizes psychological warfare and the tactics of terrorism and violence against noncombatants (mentioned earlier); but perhaps it was implied. In a parallel fashion, it should be recalled that, as the war progressed there were increasing incidents of soldiers and Marines assassinating their military leaders, although such violence was apparently equally or more common in noncombat units.

Only Gary K Neller, an Army psychiatrist, and his colleagues addressed the insidiously corrosive psychological effects this type of warfare had on American combat troops. Their conclusions stemmed from their 1983 study of Special Forces veterans as well as from Neller's experiences as a Special Forces medic in Vietnam (1967). According to these authors: "Guerrilla warfare is essentially a political war, and its area of operation always exceeds the territorial limits of conventional warfare."[63(p13)] Because of the guerrilla's smaller numbers and inferior equipment, it is self-defeating for him to hold territory. Thus the minds of individuals (in the case of Vietnam, the Vietnamese civilians and the allied troops) become the target, and psychological warfare is the means (ie, a series of actions—political, military, economic, and ideological— whose goal is to defeat the enemy by influencing their attitudes, opinions, emotions, or behavior). In general, there are four distinct phases seen among victims of guerrilla/terrorist violence: (1) initial denial, shock, and disbelief; (2) which becomes overwhelmed by reality—

producing frozen fright, clinging, and compulsive talking [sic]; (3) followed by depression and self-recrimination; (4) which in turn stirs attempts to prevent further victimization—the victim divests himself of his property and such sentiments such as feeling, caring, loving, and intimacy.

Neller et al posited that many of the soldiers and Marines serving in Vietnam were affected by a version of this process: "It is easy for the [soldier] to feel that his people at home, and his government, are indifferent to his fate. He embraces his feelings of rage and injustice; he then seeks reparation and revenge for his victimization to such an extreme that, often, he becomes psychologically disabled."[63(p28)] More specific to patients seen by military psychiatrists, the authors held that the guerrilla/terrorist warfare in Vietnam contributed to the initiation of combat stress symptoms, and for many, they became severe enough to become lifelong patterns.[63]

WALTER REED ARMY INSTITUTE OF RESEARCH PSYCHIATRIST SURVEY FINDINGS: CHARACTERIZATION OF COMBAT STRESS REACTION CASUALTIES IN VIETNAM

The following is a summary of selective findings from the Walter Reed Army Institute of Research postwar survey (1982) of Army psychiatrists who served in Vietnam that bear on questions surrounding combat stress-generated psychiatric and related symptoms. In Chapter 5 it was reported that almost one-third (24) of the psychiatrist participants in the survey indicated that they saw combat reaction cases very infrequently in Vietnam. However, when the overall group of respondents (excluding the four USARV Psychiatric Consultants) were asked to apportion their clinical activities—treating cases or supervising their treatment by others—combat reaction cases accounted for 12.6% of their cases among the 10 diagnostic groupings, which ranked as the third most common group requiring clinical attention. Furthermore, the 14 psychiatrists who served *only* with combat units reported significantly higher estimates (21%) than the 36 who served *only* with hospitals/psychiatric specialty detachments (9.7%) [see Chapter 5, Table 5-3]. These data suggest that management of combat stress symptoms constituted more of a psychiatric challenge than previously recognized.

Prevalence of Specific Symptoms Associated With Combat Stress

Apart from formal diagnostic groupings, overall clinical challenges for the mental health professionals and paraprofessionals in Vietnam included a wide variety of psychological and physical symptoms or problematic behaviors. Regarding these, the 50 WRAIR survey participants who reported they saw combat reaction cases more often than very infrequently were asked to estimate the prevalence for 17 specific symptoms or syndromes among combat-exposed troops and to identify the medications they found useful in their treatment. Figure 6-4 presented means for the prevalence estimates for 10 items that exceeded "uncommon," that is, a mean score above 2. The full set of responses is presented in Chapter 7, Table 7-6.

The 10 most common symptoms seen by the survey participants are consistent with the psychiatric literature from Vietnam and appear to corroborate the observation of Parrish, who indicated that the combat stress symptoms being seen in Vietnam in 1967–1968 were often milder than the more acute, disabling conditions seen in earlier wars. This suggests there was a substantial prevalence for psychological and psychophysiological disturbances that represented an insidious, low-grade, but only partially disabling stress on combat troops. Also noteworthy is the especially high prevalence of the short-timer's syndrome, which, as discussed, evidently became more common in Vietnam as a consequence of the staggered, 1-year, individual troop replacement system.

Prevalence of Specific Behavior Problems Associated With Combat Stress

Survey participants were also asked to indicate the extent to which they became professionally involved in the evaluation and diagnosis of soldiers manifesting problematic behaviors in 17 categories. The full set of these responses will be presented in Chapter 8, Table 8-4; however, Table 6-5 presents the results for the three items that were specific for combat-exposed troops. Overall the means did not exceed the intermediate level (ie, above 3), and there were no statistically significant differences when comparing "early" war (30) and "late" war (35) survey participants for these items. The only mean that exceeded 3 was for individual combat avoidance, and that was a modest increase among the subset of 14 survey psychiatrists who only served with combat units. Evidently, these behavior problems were not

TABLE 6-7. WRAIR survey psychiatrists' perception of etiological relevance of group factors in the pathogenesis of combat breakdown cases in Vietnam

Circumstances Degrading Combat Group Morale, Bonding, and Commitment			
Counterinsurgency/guerrilla warfare*	3.84	Combat was brief, intermittent, intense, and fluid	2.96
Fragmentation of the unit by competing subgroups (re: race, drugs, or status)	3.42	Racial tensions and conflicts	2.93
Tactical errors by unit leaders led to loss of confidence	3.41	Soldiers generally antagonistic regarding combat objectives and risks	2.88
Retaking the same combat objectives perceived as "meaningless" missions	3.39	Minor unit losses cause exaggerated perception of impaired unit capability	2.81
Physically depleting combat: prolonged exposure to arduous field/combat conditions	3.39	Combat operations were in rugged, hot, tropical environment	2.79
Excessive rotation of officers (between field and staff after 6 months)	3.36	The unprecedented proportion of teenage soldiers	2.78
Combat leader perceived as incompetent or uncaring about welfare of his troops	3.30	Soldier alienation to the military and its values	2.78
Soldiers pessimistic about chances of strategic success (war's outcome)	3.26	Some soldiers disavowed national pride, felt United States was hopelessly divided	2.66
Individual rotation schedules in/out of Vietnam reduced unit bonding	3.23	US combat strategy of enemy attrition (body count vs territorial control)	2.63
Excessive combat losses to unit	3.21	1-year tours impaired soldier commitment to combat and unit objectives	2.54
Combat loss of a soldier-leader	3.08	Some soldiers disapprove of excessive aggression by unit members	2.26
Soldiers were pessimistic about chances of tactical success (local)	3.08	Concerns that weapons, equipment, and tactics were not suitable for Vietnam	2.20
Drug or alcohol use (general): unit health degraded by regular or excessive use	3.00	Some adopted a passive personal credo congruent with some civilian peers	2.00
Drug or alcohol use before or during combat by some soldiers	2.98	Doubt regarding medical care available under combat circumstances	1.49

Note: Means of perceptions concerning the etiological relevance of group factors in the pathogenesis of combat breakdown cases in Vietnam (N = 45). Survey psychiatrists were asked extent of relevance on a 5-point scale with 1 = "not very relevant" to 5 = "very relevant."
*Counterinsurgency/guerilla warfare was defined in the survey questionnaire as, "Combat was rarely conducted in conventional set piece battles with clearly delineated lines of engagement in which allied forces fought with an identifiable enemy; but instead it consisted of fragmented combat with an enemy who blended in with civilians and took its toll with surprise attacks by his initiative with unconventional weapons and tactics."

pressing clinical challenges for the deployed psychiatrists. However, there is little reason to presume that the values in Table 6-5 necessarily reflected the real prevalence for these behavior problems. Command's involvement of psychiatrists would have been a predictably less common disposition compared to administrative or judicial ones.

Pathogenesis of Combat Breakdown in Vietnam

The 50 WRAIR survey psychiatrist participants who reported they saw combat reaction cases more often than very infrequently were further queried as to the etiologic factors they perceived as contributing (ie, "relevant") in the development of combat reaction symptoms. For this purpose they were asked to indicate the extent of their agreement with a series of forced-choice questions divided into: (1) six *individual* stress factors that may have undermined the psychological resiliency of an individual soldier and (2) 28 *group* stress factors that may have degraded the morale and commitment of small combat units and consequently

explored in Chapter 7, but it can be considered that, whereas these medications may have effectively reduced stress levels in combat troops, or served to suppress symptoms and therefore limited combat stress-related psychiatric disability, there were no systematic outcome studies conducted that would reveal whether the medication in question would have enhanced or degraded combat performance or led to adverse long-term effects.

- **Additional data suggest higher soldier dysfunction secondary to cumulative combat stress.** Other evidence suggests that combat-related circumstances in the theater were more broadly pathogenic than has been assumed, that is, that soldiers faced a more insidiously cumulative set of stressors, and that a wider spectrum of combat-centered psychiatric and behavior disorders resulted. Documentation includes not only that pertaining to the increased drug use among combat troops as the war progressed, which paralleled that for noncombat troops, but also anecdotal reports, data from the WRAIR survey of Army veteran psychiatrists, the Datel and Johnson drug prescription study, and the findings by US Navy physicians regarding excessive combat aggression among Marines. In other words, evidently far more combat troops in Vietnam suffered with low-grade psychiatric, behavioral, and psychosomatic symptoms (partial trauma and strain trauma) in Vietnam compared to the relative few who became overwhelmed with combat exhaustion as in earlier wars. The higher prevalence of these more diffuse conditions and behaviors may have also corresponded with the war's depletion of soldier morale and fitness over its course.

- **Combat troops fighting in Vietnam sustained a unique collection of stressors.** Apart from the expectable challenges and privations associated with combat operations a long way from home and in a very foreign and unforgiving environment, it can be theorized that additional, overlapping stress-inducing features applied to combat troops in Vietnam that went mostly unrecognized by military leaders and the mental health personnel at the time:

  - **The requirement that conventional troops fight a counterinsurgency/guerrilla war.** The impact on conventional troops engaged in "psychological warfare" against determined counterinsurgent guerrillas apparently included a high potential for demoralization and associated psychiatric and behavioral disorders (in some instances resulting in excess combat aggression). Although the data presented from the WRAIR survey of veteran Army psychiatrists did not clearly isolate specific etiologic factors operating at the level of the group, it is noteworthy that the leading one was that of counterinsurgency warfare.

  - **Effects of the new, widespread use of the helicopter.** Although not applicable to all combat engagements, the frequency and dangers associated with heliborne assaults apparently greatly increased the stress levels for airmobile troops. Helicopter mobility also meant that units could be sustained in place during intense, prolonged combat with concomitant rise in stress levels.

  - **Compromised combat unit cohesion from the policy of individualized troop rotations, which was further aggravated by the USARV practice of rotating commanders out of the field after 6 months.** Soldier commitment (to military structure, leaders, and mission) and cohesion (within small units) have been found to be critical for mitigation of combat stress. These processes became greatly impaired in Vietnam by the personnel churning resulting from these two policies.

  - **Overall depletion of combat leaders and skills secondary to the 1-year tour limitations.** In planning for Vietnam, it was anticipated that the combat there would be less stress-inducing if combat tours were limited to 1 year. Because the war became protracted, the pool of experienced and professional soldiers, officers, and NCOs was gradually depleted; induction and promotion standards were relaxed; and replacements were less skilled, less confident, and less effectively led.

  - **Withdrawal of national approval for the war.** The repudiation of those sent to fight in Vietnam by those at home also severely demoralized service personnel, especially the ones doing the killing and bearing the greatest burdens. From a different vantage point, it was also especially challenging for citizen soldiers fighting in Vietnam—the growing and ultimately preponderant numbers of drafted and draft-motivated volunteers whose growing resistance to serving in the theater was unprecedented. As a consequence, it can be reasonably speculated that, for many soldiers who served there, their moral tension was evidently raised to unbearable limits, with a consequent weakening of soldier confidence and combat effectiveness.

From this list of stress-inducing features it can be said that, whereas the overall combat ecology may have been less "exhausting" than earlier conflicts because of reduced demands for continuous combat operations, American ground troops fighting in Vietnam were nonetheless exposed to a more diffuse collection of stressors—variables not represented in the classic combat exhaustion model. It is especially notable that only the first two items on the list pertain to combat conditions in Vietnam: fighting a counterinsurgency/guerrilla war, and the effect of the new heliborne maneuver capability; the others are stressors generated in the United States: political and military decisions regarding force selection/deployment, how the armed forces pursued their objectives in Southeast Asia, and the nation turning on its troops.

Finally, the data collected in this chapter do appear to verify the earlier impression that the incidence levels for the more extensive forms of combat stress-generated disability were much lower than were produced in the wars that preceded Vietnam. However, they suggest that, when all forms of combat stress-generated psychosocial disorders are considered, covert and overt, the psychological cost of fielding the Army in Vietnam was much greater than has been previously recognized. In other words, although combat exposure is often traumatic (ie, psychologically daunting, even overwhelming at the time), psychiatry's experience in Vietnam, particularly with regard to cumulative stress, indicates that the profession is still shy of understanding the full set of variables that predict disability, whether in the theater or as a veteran. The data also suggest that the etiologic model of combat stress and disability must be broadened, to include extracombat variables (such as those pertaining to personnel selection and mobilization), and deepened, to recognize that there are certain limits as to how low the nation's approval for the war can dip before fighting it becomes markedly more difficult from the standpoint of lowered morale, psychological

repercussions among combat troops, and consequent impediments to accomplishing military objectives.

REFERENCES

1. Cooke ET. *Another Look at Combat Exhaustion.* Fort Sam Houston, Tex: Department of Neuropsychiatry, Medical Field Service School; distributed July 1967. Training Document GR 51-400-320, 055.

2. American Psychiatric Association. *Diagnostic and Statistical Manual of Mental Disorders.* 2nd ed (DSM-II). Washington, DC: APA; 1968.

3. Renner JA Jr. The changing patterns of psychiatric problems in Vietnam. *Compr Psychiatry.* 1973;14(2):169–181.

4. Bryant RA, Creamer M, O'Donnell ML, Silove D, McFarlane AC. A multisite study of the capacity of acute stress disorder diagnosis to predict posttraumatic stress disorder. *J Clin Psychiatry.* 2008;69(6):923–929.

5. Jones FD. Psychiatric lessons of war. In: Jones FD, Sparacino LR, Wilcox VL, Rothberg JM, Stokes JW, eds. *War Psychiatry.* In: Zajtchuk R, Bellamy RF, eds. *Textbooks of Military Medicine.* Washington, DC: Department of the Army, Office of The Surgeon General, Borden Institute; 1995: 1–33.

6. Allerton WS. Army psychiatry in Vietnam. In: Bourne PG, ed. *The Psychology and Physiology of Stress: With Reference to Special Studies of the Viet Nam War.* New York, NY: Academic Press; 1969: 1–17.

7. Baker SL Jr. Traumatic war disorders. In: Kaplan HI, Freedman AM, Sadock BJ, eds. *Comprehensive Textbook of Psychiatry.* 3rd ed. Baltimore, Md: Williams & Wilkins; 1980: 1829–1842.

8. Boman B. The Vietnam veteran ten years on. *Aust N Z J Psychiatry.* 1982;16(3):107–127.

9. Bourne PG. Military psychiatry and the Vietnam war in perspective. In: Bourne PG, ed. *The Psychology and Physiology of Stress: With Reference to Special Studies of the Viet Nam War.* New York, NY: Academic Press; 1969: 219–236.

10. Dean ET Jr. *Shook Over Hell: Post-Traumatic Stress, Vietnam, and the Civil War*. Cambridge, Mass: Harvard University Press; 1997.

11. Gabriel RA. *No More Heroes: Madness & Psychiatry in War*. NY: Hill and Wang; 1987.

12. Ingraham L, Manning F. American military psychiatry. In: Gabriel RA, ed. *Military Psychiatry: A Comparative Perspective*. Westport, Conn: Greenwood Press; 1986: 25–65.

13. Johnson AW Jr. Combat psychiatry, I: A historical review. *Med Bull US Army Europe*. 1969;26(10):305–308.

14. Jones FD, Hales RE. Military combat psychiatry: a historical review. *Psych Annals*. 1987;17:525–527.

15. Keegan J. *The Face of Battle: A Study of Agincourt, Waterloo and the Somme*. New York, NY: Penguin Books; 1978.

16. Kormos HR. The nature of combat stress. In: Figley CR, ed. *Stress Disorders Among Vietnam Veterans: Theory, Research and Treatment*. New York, NY: Bruner/Mazel; 1978: 3–22.

17. Marlowe DH. The human dimension of battle and combat breakdown. In: Gabriel RA, ed. *Military Psychiatry: A Comparative Perspective*. Westport, Conn: Greenwood Press; 1986: 7–24.

18. Marlowe DH. *Psychological and Psychosocial Consequences of Combat and Deployment, With Special Emphasis on the Gulf War*. Santa Monica, Calif: National Defense Research Institute/RAND; 2001.

19. Shephard B. *A War of Nerves*. Cambridge, Mass: Harvard University Press; 2000.

20. Bartemeier LH, Kubie LS, Menninger KA, Romano J, Whitehorn JC. Combat exhaustion. *J Nerv Ment Dis*. 1946;104:358–389.

21. Jones FD. Traditional warfare combat stress casualties. In: Jones FD, Sparacino LR, Wilcox VL, Rothberg JM, Stokes JW, eds. *War Psychiatry*. In: Zajtchuk R, Bellamy RF, eds. *Textbooks of Military Medicine*. Washington, DC: Department of the Army, Office of The Surgeon General, Borden Institute; 1995: 37–61.

22. Johnson AW Jr. Psychiatric treatment in the combat situation. *US Army Vietnam Med Bull*. 1967;January/February:38–45.

23. Glass AJ. Military psychiatry and changing systems of mental health care. *J Psychiat Res*. 1971;8(3):499–512.

24. Peterson DB, Chambers RE. Restatement of combat psychiatry. *Am J Psychiatry*. 1952;109:249–254.

25. Bey DR, Chapman RE. Psychiatry—the right way, the wrong way, and the military way. *Bull Menninger Clin*. 1974;38:343–354.

26. World Health Organization. *International Classification of Diseases-10*. 2007 rev. Available online at: http://apps.who.int/classifications/apps/icd/icd10online2007/. Accessed 8 July 2013.

27. American Psychiatric Association. *Diagnostic and Statistical Manual of Mental Disorders*. 4th ed (DSM-IV). Washington, DC: APA; 1994.

28. American Psychiatric Association. *Diagnostic and Statistical Manual of Mental Disorders*. 4th ed, text rev. (DSM-IV-TR). Washington, DC: APA; 2000.

29. Kris E. The recovery of childhood memories in psychoanalysis. *Psychoanalytic Study of the Child*. Vol 11. New York, NY: International Universities Press; 1956: 54–88.

30. Krystal H. Trauma and affects. *Psychoanalytic Study of the Child*. Vol 33. New York, NY: International Universities Press; 1978; 81–116.

31. Swank RL, Marchand WE. Combat neuroses: development of combat exhaustion. *Arch Neurol Psychiatry*. 1946;55:236–247.

32. Grinker RP, Spiegel JP. *Men Under Stress*. New York, NY: McGraw-Hill; 1963.

33. Shaw JA. Unmasking the illusion of safety. Psychic trauma in war. *Bull Menninger Clin*. 1987;51(1):49–63.

34. Grossman DA. *On Killing: The Psychological Cost of Learning to Kill in War and Society*. New York, NY: Little, Brown; 1995.

35. Glass AJ. Lessons learned. In: Mullens WS, Glass AJ, eds, *Neuropsychiatry in World War II*. Vol 2. *Overseas Theaters*. Washington, DC: Medical Department, United States Army; 1973: 989–1027.

36. Stouffer SA, DeVinney LC, Star SA, Williams RM. *The American Soldier*. Vol 2. Princeton, NJ: Princeton University Press; 1949.

37. Belenky GL. Varieties of reaction and adaption to combat experience. *Bull Menninger Clin.* 1987;51(1):64–79.

38. Glass AJ, Artiss KL, Gibbs JJ, Sweeney VC. The current status of Army psychiatry. *Am J Psychiatry.* 1961;117:673–683.

39. Stouffer SA. *Studies in Social Psychology in World War II: The American Soldier.* Vol 2. *Combat and Its Aftermath.* Princeton, NJ: Princeton University Press; 1949.

40. Manning FJ. Morale and cohesion in military psychiatry. In: Jones FD, Sparacino LR, Wilcox VL, Rothberg JM, eds. *Military Psychiatry: Preparing in Peace for War.* In: Zajtchuk R, Bellamy RF, eds. *Textbooks of Military Medicine.* Washington, DC: Department of the Army, Office of The Surgeon General, Borden Institute; 1994: 1–18.

41. Marshall SLA. *Men Against Fire.* New York, NY: William Morrow; 1950: 54–58.

42. Rioch DMcK. Problems of preventive psychiatry in war. In: Hoch PH, Zubin J, eds. *Proceedings of the Annual Meeting of the American Psychopathological Association, Vol. 1954.* Orlando, Fla: Grune and Stratton; 1955: 146–165.

43. Glass AJ. Psychotherapy in the combat zone. *Am J Psychiatry.* 1954;110:725–731.

44. Shaw JA. Comments on the individual psychology of combat exhaustion. *Mil Med.* 1983;148(3):223–225, 229–231.

45. Glass AJ. Observations upon the epidemiology of mental illness in troops during warfare. In: *Symposium on Preventive and Social Psychiatry.* Washington, DC: Walter Reed Army Institute of Research; 15–17 April 1958: 185–198.

46. Noy S. Stress and personality as factors in the causation and prognosis of combat reaction. In: Belenky G, ed. *Contemporary Studies in Combat Psychiatry.* Westport, Conn: Greenwood Press; 1987: 22–29.

47. Tischler GL. Patterns of psychiatric attrition and of behavior in a combat zone. In: Bourne PG, ed. *The Psychology and Physiology of Stress: With Reference to Special Studies of the Viet Nam War.* New York, NY: Academic Press; 1969: 19–44.

48. Strange RE. Combat fatigue versus pseudo-combat fatigue in Vietnam. *Mil Med.* 1968;133(10):823–826.

49. Erikson E. *Childhood and Society.* New York, NY: WW Norton; 1950: 23–47.

50. Engel GL. The clinical application of the biopsychosocial model. *Am J Psychiatry.* 1980;137(5):535–544.

51. Howard S. The Vietnam warrior: his experience, and implications for psychotherapy. *Am J Psychother.* 1976;30(1):121–135.

52. Goderez BI. The survivor syndrome. Massive psychic trauma and posttraumatic stress disorder. *Bull Menninger Clin.* 1987;51(1):96–113.

53. Freud S. Psychoanalysis and the war neurosis (introduction). In: Strachey J, ed. *The Standard Edition of the Complete Psychological Works of Sigmund Freud (1919).* London: Hogarth Press; 1955; Volume 17: 205–215.

54. War Department. *Nomenclature and Method of Recording Diagnoses.* Washington, DC: War Department; October 1945. Technical Bulletin Med 203.

55. US Department of Defense. *The Joint Armed Forces Nomenclature and Method of Recording Psychiatric Conditions.* Washington, DC: DoD; June 1949. SR 40-1025-2.

56. US Department of the Army. *Armed Forces Medical Diagnosis Nomenclature and Statistical Classification.* Washington, DC: DA; June 1963. Army Regulation 40-401.

57. Glass AJ. Introduction. In: Bourne PG, ed. *The Psychology and Physiology of Stress: With Reference to Special Studies of the Viet Nam War.* New York, NY: Academic Press; 1969: xiii–xxx.

58. Brusher EA. Combat and operational stress control. In: Ritchie EC, ed. *Combat and Operational Behavioral Health.* In: Lenhart MK, ed. *The Textbooks of Military Medicine.* Washington, DC: Department of the Army, Office of The Surgeon General, Borden Institute; 2011: 59–74.

59. Marshall SLA. *Ambush.* New York, NY: Cowles Book Company; 1969: 187–192.

60. Marshall SLA. Conducting the interview after combat. In: *Island Victory: The Battle of*

Kwajalein Atoll. Lincoln, Neb: University of Nebraska Press; 2001: Appendix.

61. Marshall SLA. *Bringing Up the Rear: A Memoir.* San Rafael, Calif: Presidio Press; 1979.

62. Edmendson SW, Platner DJ. Psychiatric referrals from Khe Sanh during siege. *US Army Vietnam Med Bull.* 1968;July/August:25–30.

63. Neller G, Stevens V, Chung R, Devaris D. Psychological Warfare and Its Effects on Mental Health: Lessons Learned From Vietnam (unpublished); 1985.

64. Parrish MD. Man-team-environment systems in Vietnam. In: Jones FD, ed. *MD Parrish: Collected Works 1955–1970.* Alexandria, Va: Defense Technical Information Center; 1981. Document No. AD A108069.

65. Doyle E, Weiss S, and the editors of Boston Publishing Co. *The Vietnam Experience: A Collision of Cultures.* Boston, Mass: Boston Publishing Co; 1984.

66. Balkind JJ. *Morale Deterioration in the United States Military During the Vietnam Period* [dissertation]. Ann Arbor, Mich: University Microfilms International; 1978. [Available at: *Dissertations Abstracts International,* 39 (1-A), 438. Order No. 78-11, 333.]

67. Spector RH. *After Tet: The Bloodiest Year in Vietnam.* New York, NY: The Free Press; 1993.

68. Yager J. Personal violence in infantry combat. *Arch Gen Psychiatry.* 1975;32(2):257–261.

69. Schell J. *The Military Half: An Account of Destruction in Quang Ngai and Quang Tin.* New York, NY: Alfred A. Knopf; 1968.

70. Norden E. American atrocities in Vietnam. In: Falk RA, Kolko G, Lifton RJ, eds. *Crimes of War.* New York, NY: Random House; 1971: 265–284.

71. Vietnam Veterans Against the War. *The Winter Soldier Investigation: An Inquiry Into American War Crimes.* Boston, Mass: Beacon Press; 1972.

72. Bowman JA. Recent experiences in combat psychiatry in Viet Nam (unpublished); 1967. [Full text available as Appendix 11 to this volume.]

73. Bowman JA. In: Johnson AW Jr, Bowman JA, Byrdy HS, Blank AS Jr. Panel discussion: Army psychiatry in Vietnam. In: Jones FD, ed.

Proceedings: Social and Preventive Psychiatry Course, 1967. Washington, DC: GPO; 1968: 41–76. [Available at: Alexandria, Va: Defense Technical Information Center; 1980. Document No. ADA 950058.]

74. Jones FD. Experiences of a division psychiatrist in Vietnam. *Mil Med.* 1967:132(12):1003–1008.

75. Baker WL. Division psychiatry in the 9th Infantry Division. *US Army Vietnam Med Bull.* 1967;November/December:5–9.

76. Jones FD, Johnson AW Jr. Medical and psychiatric treatment policy and practice in Vietnam. *J Soc Issues.* 1975;31(4):49–65.

77. Tiffany WJ Jr, Allerton WS. Army psychiatry in the mid-'60s. *Am J Psychiatry.* 1967;123(7):810–821.

78. Bourne PG. Military psychiatry and the Viet Nam experience. *Am J Psychiatry.* 1970;127(4):481–488.

79. Hays FW. Psychiatric aeromedical evacuation patients during the Tet and Tet II offensives, 1968. *Am J Psychiatry.* 1970;127(4):503–508.

80. Westmoreland WC. Mental health—an aspect of command. *Mil Med.* 1963;128(3)209–214.

81. Johnson AW Jr. Combat psychiatry, II: The US Army in Vietnam. *Med Bull US Army Europe.* 1969;26(11):335–339.

82. Bloch HS. Army clinical psychiatry in the combat zone: 1967–1968. *Am J Psychiatry.* 1969;126(3):289–298.

83. Johnson AW Jr, Bowman JA, Byrdy HS, Blank AS Jr. Panel discussion: Army psychiatry in Vietnam. In: Jones FD, ed. *Proceedings: Social and Preventive Psychiatry Course, 1967.* Washington, DC: GPO; 1968: 41–76. [Available at: Alexandria, Va: Defense Technical Information Center; 1980. Document No. AD A950058.]

84. Bostrom JA. Management of combat reactions. *US Army Vietnam Med Bull.* 1967;July/August:6–8.

85. Byrdy HSR. In: Johnson AW Jr, Bowman JA, Byrdy HSR, Blank AS Jr. Panel discussion: Army psychiatry in Vietnam. In: Jones FD, ed. *Proceedings: Social and Preventive Psychiatry Course, 1967.* Washington, DC: GPO; 1968: 41–76. [Available at: Alexandria, Va: Defense Technical Information Center. Document No. AD A950058.]

86. Johnson AW Jr. In: Johnson AW Jr, Bowman JA, Byrdy HS, Blank AS Jr. Panel discussion: Army psychiatry in Vietnam. In: Jones FD, ed. *Proceedings: Social and Preventive Psychiatry Course, 1967*. Washington, DC: GPO; 1968: 41–76. [Available at: Alexandria, Va: Defense Technical Information Center. Document No. AD A950058.] [Full text of Johnson's remarks available as Appendix 7 to this volume.]

87. Colbach EM, Parrish MD. Army mental health activities in Vietnam: 1965–1970. *Bull Menninger Clin*. 1970;34(6):333–342.

88. Neel SH. *Medical Support of the US Army in Vietnam, 1965–1970*. Washington, DC: GPO; 1973.

89. Hausman W, Rioch DMcK. Military psychiatry. A prototype of social and preventive psychiatry in the United States. *Arch Gen Psych*. 1967;16(6):727–739.

90. Bourne PG. *Men, Stress, and Vietnam*. Boston, Mass: Little, Brown; 1970.

91. Bourne PG, Nguyen DS. A comparative study of neuropsychiatric casualties in the United States Army and the Army of the Republic of Vietnam. *Mil Med*. 1967;132(11):904–909.

92. Allerton WS, Forrest DV, Anderson JR, et al. Psychiatric casualties in Vietnam. In: Sherman LJ, Caffey EM Jr. *The Vietnam Veteran in Contemporary Society: Collected Materials Pertaining to the Young Veterans*. Washington, DC: Veterans Administration; 1972: III: 54–59.

93. Hays FW. Military aeromedical evacuation and psychiatric patients during the Viet Nam War. *Am J Psychiatry*. 1969;126(5):658–666.

94. Bersoff DN. Rorschach correlates of traumatic neurosis of war. *J Proj Tech Pers Assess*. 1970;34(3):194–200.

95. Datel WE, Johnson AW Jr. *Psychotropic Prescription Medication in Vietnam*. Alexandria, Va: Defense Technical Information Center; 1981. Document No. AD A097610.

96. Menard DL. The social work specialist in a combat division. *US Army Vietnam Med Bull*. 1968;March/April:48–57.

97. Strange RE. Effects of combat stress on hospital ship psychiatric evacuees. In: Bourne PG, ed. *The Psychology and Physiology of Stress: With Reference to Special Studies of the Viet Nam War*. New York, NY: Academic Press; 1969: 75–93.

98. Crowe RR, Colbach EM. A psychiatric experience with Project 100,000. *Mil Med*. 1971;136:271–273.

99. Bey DR. Group dynamics and the 'F.N.G.' in Vietnam: a potential focus of stress. *Int J Group Psychother*. 1972;22(1):22–30.

100. Strange RE, Arthur RJ. Hospital ship psychiatry in a war zone. *Am J Psychiatry*. 1967;124(3):281–286.

101. Belenky GL, Noy S, Solomon Z. Battle stress: the Israeli experience. *Mil Rev*. 1985:29–37.

102. Rahe RH. Acute versus chronic psychological reactions to combat. *Mil Med*. 1988;153(7):365–372.

103. Jones FD. Psychological adjustments to Vietnam. Presentation to the Medical Education for National Defense Symposium; 18 October 1967; Walter Reed General Hospital, Washington, DC.

104. Bey DR. *Division Psychiatry in Vietnam* (unpublished); no date.

105. Scurfield RM. *A Vietnam Trilogy: Veterans and Post Traumatic Stress: 1968, 1989, 2000*. New York, NY: Algora Publishing; 2004.

106. Holloway HC. Vietnam psychiatry revisited. Presented at the American Psychiatric Association Annual Meeting; 19 May 1982; Toronto, Ontario, Canada.

107. Bender PA. Social work specialists at the line battalion. *US Army Vietnam Med Bull*. 1968;May/June:60–69.

108. Carden NL, Schamel DJ. Observations of conversion reactions in troops involved in the Viet Nam conflict. *Am J Psychiatry*. 1966;123(1):21–31.

109. Bey DR, Smith WE. Mental health technicians in Vietnam. *Bull Menninger Clin*. 1970;34(6):363–371.

110. Bourne PG. Urinary 17-OHCS levels in two combat situations. In: Bourne PG, ed. *The Psychology and Physiology of Stress: With Reference to Special Studies of the Viet Nam War*. New York, NY: Academic Press; 1969:95–116.

111. Bourne PG, Rose RM, Mason JW. 17-OHCS levels in combat. Special Forces "A" team under threat of attack. *Arch Gen Psychiatry*. 1968;19(2):135–140.

112. Bourne PG, Coli WM, Datel WE. Affect levels of ten Special Forces soldiers under threat of attack. *Psychol Rep.* 1968;22(2):363–366.

113. Bourne PG, Rose RM, Mason JW. Urinary 17-OHCS levels. Data on seven helicopter ambulance medics in combat. *Arch Gen Psychiatry.* 1967;17(1):104–110.

114. Bourne PG, Coli WM, Datel WE. Anxiety levels of six helicopter ambulance medics in a combat zone. *Psychol Rep.* 1966;19(3):821–822.

115. Bourne PG. Psychiatric casualties in Vietnam, lowest ever for combat zone troops (interview). *US Med.* 15 May 1969:10–11.

116. Chemtob CM, Bauer GB, Neller G, Hamada R, Glisson C, Stevens V. Post-traumatic stress disorder among Special Forces Vietnam veterans. *Mil Med.* 1990;155(1):16–20.

117. Noy S. Combat psychiatry: the American and Israeli experience. In: Belenky G, ed. *Contemporary Studies in Combat Psychiatry.* Westport, Conn: Greenwood Press; 1987: 70–86.

118. Balson PM, Dempster CR. Treatment of war neuroses from Vietnam. *Compr Psychiatry.* 1980;21(2):167–175.

119. Schwartz HJ. Unconscious guilt: its origin, manifestations, and treatment in the combat veteran. In: Schwartz HJ, ed. *Psychotherapy of the Combat Veteran.* New York, NY: Spectrum Publications Medical & Scientific Books; 1984: 47–84.

120. Schwartz HJ. Introduction: an overview of the psychoanalytic approach to the war neuroses. In: Schwartz HJ, ed. *Psychotherapy of the Combat Veteran.* New York, NY: Spectrum Publications Medical & Scientific Books; 1984: xi–xxviii.

121. Nadelson T. *Trained to Kill: Soldiers at War.* Baltimore, Md: Johns Hopkins University Press; 2005.

122. Nadelson T. Attachment to killing. *J Am Acad Psychoanal.* 1992;20:130–141.

123. Mahan JL, Clum GA. Longitudinal prediction of Marine combat effectiveness. *J Soc Psychol.* 1971;83:45–54.

124. Fisher HW. Vietnam psychiatry. Portrait of anarchy. *Minn Med.* 1972;55(12):1165–1167.

125. Bey DR, Zecchinelli VA. GI's against themselves. Factors resulting in explosive violence in Vietnam. *Psychiatry.* 1974;37(3):221–228.

126. Langner HP. The making of a murderer. *Am J Psychiatry.* 1971;127(7):950–953.

127. Haley SA. When the patient reports atrocities. Specific treatment considerations of the Vietnam veteran. *Arch Gen Psychiatry.* 1974;30(2):191–196.

128. Borus JF. Reentry, I: Adjustment issues facing the Vietnam returnee. *Arch Gen Psychiatry.* 1973;28(4):501–506.

129. Lifton RJ. *Home From the War: Vietnam Veterans: Neither Victims Nor Executioners.* New York, NY: Simon & Schuster Inc; 1973.

130. Shatan CF. The grief of soldiers: Vietnam combat veterans' self-help movement. *Am J Orthopsych.* 1973;43(4):640–653.

131. Gault WB. Some remarks on slaughter. *Am J Psychiatry.* 1971;128(4):450–454.

132. Fox RP. Narcissistic rage and the problem of combat aggression. *Arch Gen Psychiatry.* 1974;31(6):807–811.

133. Bourne PG. From boot camp to My Lai. In: Falk RA, Kolko G, Lifton RJ, eds. *Crimes of War: A Legal, Political-Documentary, and Psychological Inquiry Into the Responsibility of Leaders, Citizens, and Soldiers for Criminal Acts in Wars.* New York, NY: Random House; 1971: 462–468.

134. Eisenhart RW. You can't hack it little girl: a discussion of the covert psychological agenda of modern combat training. *J Soc Issues.* 1975;31(4):13–24.

135. Shatan CF. Bogus manhood, bogus honor: surrender and transfiguration in the United States Marine Corps. *Psychoanal Rev.* 1977;64(4):585–610.

136. Regan DJ. *Mourning Glory: The Making of a Marine.* Old Greenwich, Conn: Devin-Adair; 1981.

ATTACHMENT 6-1. COMBAT SPECIMEN #1: Viet Cong Ambush During the Battle of Dau Tieng

SLA Marshall, the noted combat historian, reconstructed the following combat action from Vietnam.

By the time Starr and Carter emerged into the open, the lead files in the column were two-thirds of the way across and stepping out briskly. That they had moved far better than they had scanned became apparent that instant.

In the lead was Pfc. Hawatha Hardison, a burly twenty-year-old Negro from Winston-Salem. He stopped dead in his tracks and stared, not believing what he saw.

Standing 10 feet away, directly in front of him, and unseen until that moment, were three uniformed figures, stock still and with their backs turned. They were togged in green pants and brown shirts, wore camouflaged pith helmets, and carried rifles at shoulder. So dressed, they had blended into the background.

Getting that sweet picture in one flash, Hardison's mind had room for one thought only: "We sneaked up on them and we've got them." In the nature of things, that would have been impossible. Yet Hardison and his mates had never heard that the Vietcong put out human lures, wittingly risking their lives to suck innocents into an ambush. It is a concept in any case too diabolical for ready acceptance by Western minds.

Before Hardison could manually react, the three figures darted away rightward toward the tree line at the rounded end of the clearing. It was a hot sprint. Still, Sgt. Ray Dickerson had time to shoulder his M-79 and fire three rounds while they were in sight. The explosions came just as they hit the trees and Dickerson thought he saw two of them stagger and fall. Maybe. Inevitably, the front half of the column, giving chase, became spread out broadside to the dense forest growth on the far side of the clearing, the precise effect for which the three stooges had risked their lives. The name of the game was Follow Me. Hardison had his own technical term for this random and spontaneous deployment: "We went at once into an overmatched formation."

Starr and Carter were six paces into the clearing when Dickerson fired. Neither said a word to the other. Busy with his own thoughts, Carter was not at once jolted into action by the M-79 rounds and later could not remember that he had heard them. Starr left him instantly and ran forward about 30 meters. Before he could flop down, automatic fire broke out from the far tree line directly against the platoon front. The hidden positions could not have been more than 20 to 25 meters from the uneven line of skirmishers. By now Carter was on radio to Bravo Battery: "We're in it, so stand by." The question was where to fire.

Where he lay, Hardison was being buzzed by bullets from his front, and he thought, from his left. It wasn't healthy. He decided to swing as far over as possible to the right, toward the point where the three VC had hit the tree line. He squirmed on his belly in that direction; and six or seven other riflemen followed him. It seemed, at first, like a fair hunch. Although that corner was not exactly quiet, to Hardison's anxious ear it sounded as if the bullet fire "was more thinned out there."

Private First Class Eugene Hicks, a twenty-year-old Negro from Forrest City, Arkansas, had been bringing along the M-60 machine gun in the second half of the column. A good soldier, on the quiet side, Hicks rushed the gun forward into the clearing on hearing the firing. It wasn't given to him to stay long, which was his good luck.

Sergeant Dickerson saw him and yelled, "Take that gun and get back to the trail opening! We're drawing fire from the rear."

Hicks might have let that go, but here came a reenforcing [*sic*] yell from Starr: "Get on the rear with that machine gun!" Hicks started to move. However, Dickerson, reacting compulsively to Starr's order, ran over and grabbed the M-60 from Hicks, then legged it for the trail mouth, with Hicks following along.

Dickerson flopped down as he came to the tree line and opened fire down trail. There were only 20 bullets in the M-60 (of which fact Dickerson was unaware) and within seconds the gun sputtered out. The sergeant wasn't given time to determine what had happened; a bullet hit him and he slumped over.

Hicks' ammo bearer had dropped his load 15 meters back along the trail. Being there on the spot, before Hicks could stop him, he picked up the gun and carried it back to the ammunition deposit. Hicks simply followed along. No one was present to give him orders, and besides, he was not the assertive type. Dickerson crawled along after them just to be near someone. No one was offering first aid and he wasn't asking for it.

The other machine gun was somewhere forward. Hicks didn't know just where; in his less than one-half minute on the open fire field he'd had little chance to see anything. What his ears told him was that the forward gun wasn't firing. He took that as a bad sign. Muffled by the forest, as if far off, he heard cries of "Medic, medic."

Seldom has a soldier had reason to feel lonelier than Hicks at this time. He did not know the platoon. He had joined it 30 days before. On his first morning, he had been hard wounded while on patrol. There followed 29 days in hospital. He had returned the prior evening, a stranger, and a stranger he stayed. It shouldn't happen to a dog.

ATTACHMENT 6-1. COMBAT SPECIMEN #1: Viet Cong Ambush During the Battle of Dau Tieng, continued

They now were drawing continuous fire from all around the clearing, in heavy volume and without a single break. Except for that growing rattle, the silence of surprise still hung heavily over the place. All the riflemen had gone flat, and for these minutes only, the depth of the elephant grass gave them a little hold on life. The enemy, too, showed signs of being plagued by nerves; most of the bullet fire was going high.

Hugging his radio in the center of the clearing, Carter heard Starr sing out above the rising whine of the metal, "Where's the goddamn artillery?"

"On the way, sir!" Carter yelled back.

And it was truly on the way; he had just called for it and had less than 30 seconds to wait for the first round. Starr was on the PRC-25 (lightweight infantry field radio) again. This time he was begging higher command for mortar fire. Carter could hear him yelling, "You got to give me the 81s right now!"

But he was wasting time and breath. Back came the answer, "We can't help you. You're out of range."

Seconds later, he was pleading for gunships (rocket-armed helicopters). The anguish in his voice startled Carter. A minute before, artilleryman Carter had supposed that the infantry platoon would be getting the upper hand in short order. Now he sensed that the situation was becoming fully desperate, or at least he knew Starr thought so.

Starr was putting it over the radio to his company commander, Captain Crain:

"We must have help. There's more than a company against us. We're already hurting and we can't withdraw."

But Starr's estimate was pure guess, reckoned from the sound and fury of the enemy fire. So far, he personally had seen not one VC. Nor had Carter. It does not necessarily follow that there was no visible enemy movement. The grass still stood high and their heads were low; they had to be.

Carter asked himself, "What does it mean?" Continuous VC fire at almost measurable intervals would blaze higher from quadrant to quadrant, as if there were suddenly five or six automatic weapons working where one had been before. The movement was clockwise. Every half-minute or so the fusillade would swing to a different quarter. Carter thought he had it figured out: There must be fixed positions all around the clearing. The VC were clustering their weapons and swinging their killer groups from one fire bunker to another. Now if he could catch them during movement in the open—.

Carter had already made two adjustments. The first shells had landed far off. Now he had them coming where he felt they might check the rotary movement of the VC firers, provided he could lay the rounds on thick.

This was his message to the guns: "Give us continuous fire, not just a shell now and then."

A more pitiful request in the circumstances is beyond imagination. The 105-mm. battery had only three tubes firing in support. There was never any chance that artillery used in such weak numbers could influence the outcome, irrespective of how accurately the fire was adjusted.

And the last chance for adjustment died with Carter's words. In that split second, as the FO [forward observer] quit speaking, a bullet shot his radio's cord away. An earlier bullet had already shattered the microphone and Carter had put on a spare; at the same time another enemy slug snubbed the PRC-25 aerial one foot above his head. With that, Carter was dead as a communicator and could only witness the results. The friendly shells kept falling along the flanks of the clearing; there was no change in the volume of the enemy fire except that it steadily built upward. In these moments Carter lost his belief in the magic of artillery.

In these moments also Hardison was lying near one other member of the platoon whom he did not know. Between them was an ant hill about three feet high and looking as if it were made of concrete loosely poured into a weathered conical form. Both riflemen, firing, were using the base of the ant hill for protection, nothing in sight looking better.

There was an explosion, and quite suddenly, the ant hill was gone. Hardison was blown into a spin, and coming to rest, bruised but otherwise unhurt, said, "It looks like Charlie is using mortars, or was it a grenade?"

No answer was returned. His unknown friend, his body badly battered, was dead.

Hicks, low man on the totem pole, at the tail end of the formation, and well out of the fuss and fury, or so he thought, was under fire from both sides. Bullets were kicking up the dirt and clipping the leaves from the vines on his left and right. He guessed that there were two or three VC both ways from him, not more than 15 to 20 meters off, and he decided that their shooting was much too personal. Not wishing to make an issue of it, he got as close as possible to earth and said a few prayers.

Prayers were not for Hardison, he not being the praying type. He noticed that no yelling was rising from the American side, except for the cry, "Medic! Medic!" which rose close at hand, but he could hear it only faintly, almost as an echo at greater distance. His rifle jammed. Beating the M-16 on the ground, Hardison yelled, "Goddamn that weapon!" The impact, rather than the profanity, partly broke the block, but the rifle would no longer fire full automatic.

Another bullet smashed through the center of Carter's radio, and metal fragments from the instrument slashed him

ATTACHMENT 6-1. COMBAT SPECIMEN #1: Viet Cong Ambush During the Battle of Dau Tieng, continued

through the shoulder and left arm. Still, he felt no pain, and although he bled profusely, for the moment he did not notice it. He was too busy harkening to the voice of Starr and trying to catch a glimpse of him.

The infantry platoon leader was not more than 10 meters from Carter and directly to his left. He was scrabbling around in the buffalo grass, feeling for M-79 rounds, and finding a few of them. One of the thump gunners had died next to him from a bullet through the heart, and Starr had picked up the launcher. At top voice, he was calling out, "Squad leaders and machine gunners, hear me! Keep firing! But wait till you see targets. I'll tell you when to move."

It was a gallant effort and no less futile. The fight was then about 10 minutes along. Already the small plot where Starr and Carter were sprawled had been bracketed by mortar rounds. Carter reflected idly that there were no targets to be seen, and he wondered dully if anyone save himself was listening to Starr.

Then he heard Starr shout, "Bring the artillery closer!" Carter thought to himself, "Dear God, if I only could," and sensibly held back from singing out to Starr that he no longer had any control over the guns. "It's better that he not know," he thought to himself.

It was forbearance wasted. As he glanced toward the direction of the voice, he saw Starr rise to his knees with just the top of his head showing. In that split second, a bullet swarm hit him in the face and Carter knew from the motion as the body was lifted and thrown back that Starr was dead.

The artillery was not slowing down the VC attack one bit. The few who ultimately survived could all feel it was so. At his roost where the platoon had entered the clearing, Hicks could hear many enemy voices. But it was not the usual taunting chatter and laughter. It was steady and rhythmic: They were chanting directions to one another as they moved from bunker to bunker within the tree line. Hardison followed the beat, also. The VC were deploying more people around the clearing and the fire intensified in an ever-widening circle.

The ammo bearer, Private First Class Flagg, later killed, lay motionless within arm's length of Hicks. He became hysterical, and repeated over and over, "I know the sound. It's Chinese assault weapons." The litany jangled Hicks' nerves till, sickening of it, he snapped, "You shut your big mouth. Who doesn't know the sound?" The man quieted for only a few seconds.

Starr's RTO, Specialist 4 White, was already dead from a bullet burst. The forward machine-gun crew had been given no chance to open fire; as they went into position behind a fallen tree, about one rod ahead of Starr, that spot was fairly swarming with bullets.

One of the rifleman scouts, Private First Class Welch, tried to warn them. Having flattened, Welch rose on his haunches and yelled, "Get away from that spot. They're coming over. They're all around us!"

It was too late for them and for Welch. He was cut down by bullets before he could flatten and the same enemy machine gun, traversing, scythed the crew and wrecked the M-60.

Of that, very early in the game, had come the elimination of the platoon aid [sic] man, Specialist 4 Harrison. Cries arose from the forward ground, "Medic, medic! Doc, come help us!" There was never a more willing aide man and it was given to Hardison to see him die. Harrison rose from the grass a few feet from Hardison and started running toward the log, made not more than a few strides, and pitched over, dead from a bullet burst.

Carter's RTO, Private First Class Strong, was also down, although not yet unconscious. There were multiple wounds in his head, both shoulders, back, and both arms, some caused by bullets and others from the propelled fragments of the PRC-25. He lay there, eyes open but not speaking, and Carter also maintained silence.

From forward in the clearing, an unidentified rifleman came running toward Strong and Carter. His right sleeve streamed blood. "We're all that's left," he shouted. "Everybody's dead." Then he flopped down between the two of them. Neither said a word. They made no protest that the fight was still going; possibly they could not think on it. The unknown picked up the M-16 that Carter had dropped, relieved Strong of his Colt .45, and started firing them alternately. He did not bother to aim. Blood pulsing from his head, Strong turned slowly to stare at the newcomer as if not understanding. He was still saying nothing. This bizarre scene endured not more than two minutes. The stranger suddenly slumped over and died; his was not quite the last fire from the American side.

Carter, gradually dulling to all sensation from pain and loss of blood as his wounds took over, looked that way to see why the firing had stopped and noted for the first time, without shock or any reaction, that another wounded American was stretched out just beyond the diehard rifleman.

Flagg, the ammo bearer next to Hicks, had ceased muttering about Chinese assault weapons. A bullet had drilled him through the head. The fire seemed to slow a little. Hicks looked about for the first time. Two other U.S. dead lay face down within less than a body length to his left. He had no idea how and when they had been killed, nor could he sense how the fight was going in the clearing.

ATTACHMENT 6-1. COMBAT SPECIMEN #1: Viet Cong Ambush During the Battle of Dau Tieng, continued

Hardison, from his position in the center of the bulge at the extreme right of the clearing, knew more about that. He had wormed his way to another ant hill and intended to use it as a buffer till the finish, if given a chance. Five other rifleman still lived on that far flank, although none was firing. Hardison reckoned this was all that was left of the platoon. But he had no desire to go to them; he preferred the ant hill.

One of them, Private First Class Haskell, in his last moment of panic, arose shouting, "They're coming on!" and started on a dead run for the mouth of the trail. As he dashed past Hardison, he reached down, grabbed his M-16, and sped on. He almost made it to Hicks before he was cut down by a machine-gun burst.

It "scared the hell" out of Hardison, not so much the snatching for this last weapon as the wild expression on Haskell's face when he passed. One of the rifleman Haskell had quitted rose halfway as if to follow him. Before he could straighten, a bullet swarm hit him around the head and shoulders and toppled him. Hardison crawled over belly down, grabbed his rifle, an M-16, and wiggled back to the ant hill.

Snuggled behind it, Hardison checked the magazine. There were 10 bullets. Somehow he had lost his own extra magazines as the fight opened. Still seeing no human targets, he took deliberate aim, firing nine rounds toward the ground level of the tree line on the far side of the clearing.

Then he held his fire. Almost instantly, the clearing was silent, or at least free of lethal noises. Hardison heard men moaning and a few feeble cries of "Medic, medic." There was no one to respond; not one American on the field had been given first aid.

The loud silence did not exactly awe Hardison; a phlegmatic Negro, surly by nature, uncommunicative except with himself, he knew what it meant, and continued to hug ground. There no longer remained one American armed and in condition to fight.

He grunted, then checked to make sure that the last bullet was still there. It was. He had his moment of bitter satisfaction that he had hoarded it.

Hicks heard the roar and rattle cease in these same moments and wondered what was happening. Not more than 45 meters from Hardison, he was still unaware that the platoon had died, never really having been in the fight. Even a little distance may make a vast difference.

Carter knew that something had changed. The noise was gone. Physically, mentally, he was too weak to interpret what it meant. He was not resigned to death. He was not even thinking about it. To think at all had become an intolerable strain. He lay motionless.

During these minutes, General Rogers and his party in the Huey had at last made their fix. They were bucketing back and forth above the clearing and viewing it as if from an upper-gallery seat. Of the enemy, they saw nothing. They saw the forms of the Americans, sprawled in the grass, motionless, apparently lifeless. The Huey orbited over the curved end of the clearing, flying just above the trees. Rogers tried to count bodies. The Huey lifted again. Then Rogers could see "a few of the kids down below beckoning to me with their arms."

Over the radio, he heard the battalion commander (who was also somewhere aloft) say, "I've got Charley Company on the road in APCs coming fast to relieve the platoon." It stunned Rogers. Relieve the platoon? It was already too late. Via the road? Rogers knew that the bridge was out a mile or so short of the forest. He had seen it while circling. Someone had blundered.

Moments later, Hardison regretted that he hadn't kept all 10 bullets. Five enemy soldiers, uniformed in khaki and conical hats, entered upon the clearing at his end; the central figure was carrying a machine gun. It was Hardison's first sight of any enemy figure or weapon. As the five men advanced, the VC gunner dusted the foreground with his weapon, blasting in short bursts. They walked straight toward Hardison, on the way spraying bullets into the three riflemen who still lived, as well as the dead men.

Hardison kept wiggling around the ant hill, hoping (not praying) that by some fluke he would stay out of sight.

Fate was on his side, intervening in the strangest possible way. Suddenly, there was a smell of chemical in the air. Hardison got it faintly, and his eyes smarted. A slight wind carried it in Carter's direction, and he coughed heavily; it came to him that the enemy must be gassing the area to finish the fight, and that was still his impression days later. But Hardison had seen the thing happen. One of the dead riflemen near him had been carrying a gas grenade hitched to his belt. In blasting him, the gunner had put a hole through the container. The VC party turned and headed back toward the tree line to escape the drifting gas. Hardison lived on. All other Americans in the semicircular end of the clearing were now dead.

Reproduced with permission from Marshall SLA. *Ambush*. New York, NY: Cowles Book Company; 1969: 138–149.

ATTACHMENT 6-2. COMBAT SPECIMEN #2: Patrolling the Rong Sat Zone

The following description is provided by SLA Marshall, the noted military historian.

There was a common saying among the swamp rats who paddled and patrolled through the Rong Sat Zone night and day that anything seen moving there except the tide was bound to be Vietcong [VC] and a man had better shoot first and question later. . . .

All Americans who went into the Rong Sat [the great tidal bog south of Saigon] agreed that it was the worst possible place to fight a war, more fearsome than the jungle, gloomier than the rubber plantations, and made the Delta seem like a picnic ground by comparison. To patrol in the Rong Sat, soldiers either plodded through calf-deep slime, waded through the tide, or swam. There was no solid earth anywhere. The tree cover was mainly mangrove, with an occasional outcropping of banyan. The rare vegetated and green hummocks high enough to form an island at high water were dressed in grasses that cut the flesh. In a warfare conspicuous for its lack of uncomplicated terrain, operations in the Rong Sat Zone were bizarre beyond all other military experience.

. . . For man or beast, there is no relief from living strain in the Rong Sat. Eighty percent of its land mass is under water at high tide. The VC, who out of misfortune are detailed there . . . [endure] a debilitating, enervating existence beset by fever, fatigue, and fear.

Then why not leave them there alone to stew in their own juice? The explanation is elementary. Through the Rong Sat Zone twists and turns the main commercial channel of the Saigon River. Should that channel become blocked through enemy action, or should the shipping suffer constant harassment and heavy loss, the damage to Saigon and to the war effort could be enormous. Any such threat has to be parried methodically, however great the difficulty.

Operations by the [American] invaders have two familiar forms: the ambushing of sampans, usually by night, and prowling the swamp in search of enemy base camps, usually by day. Only by carrying out these movements regularly can the Vietcong be kept off balance and fighting defensively.

The Americans who go on patrol there do not stay longer than 72 hours. Such a stretch is enough to wear them down. Should they risk a longer tour in the swamp, the medical people figure, losses from jungle rot, foot infection, carelessness, fear, and drowning might become excessive. . . . After their 72-hour stint, the swamp rats are normally whisked to a nearby high-and-dry peninsula for a brief R & R. When deemed ready, they then go at it again.

Patrols in the Rong Sat go as light as possible. Each man perforce carries a poncho and a nylon hammock. The unit takes along a one hundred-foot nylon rope for stream crossings. Three air mattresses go with each squad. They are used to float nonswimmers across the deep-water passages; on an average, about one-third of the men in any American patrol are in that category. Four canteens of water are carried by each soldier; the only fresh water to be found in the Rong Sat are the stores in the VC base camps, brought in by sampan. . . .

When night coincides with high water, the game is that one squad or so of the patrol goes on ambush next to the deepest slough. Any VC base camp area is preferred for bivouac. The men not on ambush try to set their hammocks high enough to ride dry above the surging water. But [sometimes]...sleepers [are]warned only when their bottoms [are] wetted.

Although they [Charley Company, First Battalion, 18th Infantry, 1st Infantry Division] were a weapons platoon, they could not carry their mortars into the swamp. The weight was too much. So they had gone armed as a rifle unit. There was trouble enough with the M-16's and the ammo. Salt from the seawater built up around the metal and the rifle malfunctioned unless they were careful to keep rubbing the piece with vaseline. The ammo had to be lugged along in boxes or it would also corrode speedily. Such claymore mines as they toted were cased in waterproof bags.

To get across the mud flats at low tide, they would cut mats of foliage with their machetes, palm fronds being especially useful. Where the front runners stumbled through the ooze during the cutting, the last man in the column stayed dry-footed, walking along on a carpet. In this way, hacking as they went, they could move about three hundred meters in an hour. Three thousand meters of distance were rated as a long day's march.

Helicopters could not be used for resupply; there was not enough dry, flat ground anywhere to serve as a pad. So what they required for maintenance during the three days, they carried along.

Reproduced with permission from Marshall SLA. *Ambush*. New York, NY: Cowles Book Company; 1969: 187–192.

CHAPTER 7

Treatment of Combat Reaction Casualties: Providing Humanitarian Care While "Protecting Peace in Southeast Asia"

Looking at the matter from a military point of view alone, one might ask whether it is not desirable to send home all "shell-shock" cases—in whom so much effort results in so few recoveries. Such a decision would be as unfortunate from a military as from a humanitarian standpoint. Its immediate effect would be to increase enormously the prevalence of the war neuroses. In the unending conflict between duty, honor, and discipline, on the one hand, and homesickness, horror, and the urgings of self-preservation on the other, the neurosis—as a way out—is already accessible enough in most men without calling attention to it and enhancing its value by the adoption of such an administrative policy.[1(pp526–527)]

Dr Thomas W Salmon
Director of the Psychiatric Program
American Expeditionary Force, World War I

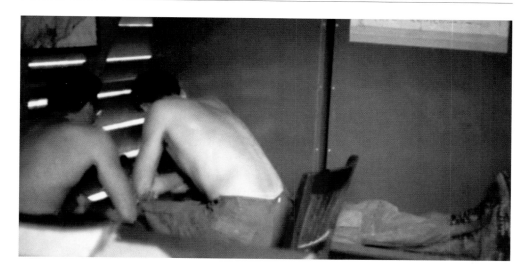

"Psych techs" interviewing a mock combat exhaustion casualty. In this photograph enlisted social work/psychology technicians simulated a sodium amytal interview of a peer portraying a combat exhaustion casualty, all under the supervision by the division psychiatrist. This was a training exercise conducted sometime between April 1969 and April 1970 at the 1st Infantry Division mental hygiene clinic. Photograph courtesy of Douglas R Bey.

The US Army went to war in Vietnam for the purpose of "supporting freedom and protecting peace in Southeast Asia."[2(p3)] And the Army went with a battle-tested set of principles for the management and treatment of combat stress-generated symptoms and conditions—the forward treatment doctrine.[3] In general this doctrine advocated that Army psychiatrists lead deployed medical personnel in providing field treatments that would quickly restore soldiers disabled by combat stress (ie, rest, replenish, reassure, and return affected soldiers to their units to resume their duty function[4]). It also meant that they should advise commanders regarding the preservation of the psychological fitness of their troops. Whereas this approach was principally designed to support the accomplishment of the military mission, it had long been noted that alternative treatments, specifically the rapid evacuation of psychiatric casualties from the field, or even the provision of more elaborate and prolonged treatments there, were counterproductive in that they both eliminated capable soldiers from the fighting force and led to higher disability rates. Thus the doctrine was not only in the service of the collective (ie, for military success and the survival of the nation), but it was also intended to serve humanitarian values (ie, treatment for the sake of the individual's welfare).

Chapter 6 presented data suggesting that the incidence of acute combat exhaustion cases in Vietnam was roughly 25% of that seen in the preceding wars, and that the soldiers who required treatment often had less severe symptoms. However, it still appears that the treatment challenges for these conditions were substantial in many circumstances. Yet documentation of the use and effectiveness of the doctrine in Vietnam remains incomplete because the record is mostly anecdotal. This is regrettable because the fighting there evolved into irregular/counterinsurgency warfare—a new circumstance for US forces that, to some degree, foreshadowed similar conflicts to come. Compounding this omission, the Vietnam War provided military medicine with its first set of physicians—especially psychiatrists—routinely trained in the use of neuroleptic (antipsychotic), anxiolytic (antianxiety), and tricyclic (antidepressant) psychotropic medications. These drugs had revolutionized psychiatric care in general and were reported to be widely used in Vietnam for the treatment of combat exhaustion and other combat reaction symptoms; however, there was no systematic study of their use and impact over the course of the war, nor was a protocol established incorporating them in the forward treatment doctrine. Also unaddressed was the impact on the deployed mental health professionals of the mounting ethical objections to the forward treatment doctrine that were based on concerns that it sacrificed humanitarian values for the sake of military and political expediency.[5]

This chapter summarizes the salient features of the combat psychiatry doctrine as it was brought to Vietnam for the prevention, treatment, and management of these conditions. It also reviews the relevant professional literature from the war, selected clinical case examples, and the findings from the Walter Reed Army Institute of Research (WRAIR) survey of Vietnam veteran Army psychiatrists, to fill in the blanks regarding efforts to adapt it to the novel features encountered there, including the availability of the new psychiatric medications. The material presented in this chapter extends the review of the various clinical presentations and evident pathogenic influences for combat stress reactions in Vietnam provided in Chapter 6. Later, Chapter 9 will review the various efforts by Army psychiatrists to respond to the rapidly developing drug abuse problem later in the war—a problem that was not unique to combat-exposed troops but which apparently did jeopardize the maintenance of combat strength and effectiveness. The subject of command consultation, which could prove invaluable in prevention of these as well as other types of psychiatric casualties in the combat zone, will be explored in Chapter 10.

BACKGROUND

From the outset, Army medical and psychiatric leaders in Vietnam had confidence in the utilization of the historically validated doctrine for the care of soldiers with combat stress symptoms. This section will extend the presentation of the doctrine's rationale, which was begun in Chapters 2 through 4, and summarize its management and treatment principles as they were represented in the post-Korean War professional literature and specific Army training documents and technical manuals.

The Pre-Vietnam Rationale for the Traditional Combat Psychiatry Forward Treatment Doctrine

Over the course of the wars leading up to Vietnam, combat psychiatrists empirically established a set of treatment and management principles designed to quickly identify and restore large numbers of psychiatrically disabled combat soldiers, so-called secondary and tertiary prevention, thereby salvaging a vital source of military manpower. Three cardinal publications by senior Army psychiatrists—Glass,[6] Artiss,[7] and Hausman and Rioch[8]—plus Army Technical Manual (TM) 8-244, *Military Psychiatry*,[3] served to distill the observations and assumptions that established the doctrine's rationale and treatment/management elements. These can be condensed as follows (with some elaboration).

The Doctrine as Serving the Military Mission Through Force Conservation

- The soldier who becomes incapacitated by combat has undergone a transient psychological regression—a failure of adaptation—that is otherwise similar to the (now) civilian acute stress disorder.

- This follows the depletion of his personal resources resulting in lowered self-confidence as a soldier and rising doubt that his combat group can prevail in combat (and thereby guarantee his protection). More specifically he has undergone:

  - *disruption of his physical and psychological defenses*—his dysfunction represents the final common pathway produced by the stress of his ordeal in interaction with his physical and personal limitations; and
  - *breakdown of his morale*—his dysfunction correspondingly represents a failure in social support (ie, the soldier sustains a loss in his sense of bonding with his unit and its mission, *esprit de corps*, or belief in the war's rationale[9]).

- The net effect is that "fear for the self" comes to dominate his mental functioning. In essence, he becomes convinced that he has reached his limits ("loss of the will to fight"[10]).
- This in turn activates an overriding motivation to psychologically withdraw from battle and welcome any exit from the battlefield (psychiatric, medical, or disciplinary[11]).
- This condition can usually be reversed if he is provided physical and psychosocial support and given an opportunity to recover in a situation of relative safety—but as near as possible to his unit and accompanied by sustained encouragement to quickly resume his military duties.

The Doctrine as Serving Humanitarian Treatment

The earlier combat psychiatrists also observed that, seemingly paradoxically, the extent of disability (among recoverable soldiers) could be dramatically reduced through restricting the scope of the treatments to physical and psychological replenishment and limiting the length of reprieve from combat to a few days. Most of those who are returned to duty under this regimen—often despite their initial protests—do not apparently incur a performance decrement nor require further psychiatric treatment. Alternatively, among those who are ultimately evacuated out of the area of the fighting, few are recovered for further military service, least of all combat duty, and many of those remain disabled.[12,13]

The Traditional Combat Psychiatry Forward Treatment Doctrine

Chapter 6 reviewed the array of commonly presenting symptoms seen among acute combat reaction casualties (a psychiatric casualty is defined by the Army as a soldier missing 24 hours or more of duty for psychiatric reasons[14]). The traditional combat psychiatry doctrine for the care of these soldier-patients can be summarized using two dimensions:

1. *Management of casualties.* This refers to the application of four principles to structure the treatment to both coincide with military requirements and bolster the soldier's recovery of duty function: proximity, immediacy, expectancy, and simplicity (PIES). These will be explained more fully below. The salutary effects associated with these management principles especially rely on the soldier's bond with the members of his unit and its leaders and his commitment to their welfare.

2. *Treatment of casualties.* This refers to the timely provision of elementary, mostly recuperative, measures for affected soldiers such as safety; rest, physical restoration, and wound care; peer support; and psychologically supportive assistance, including in recounting their disturbing combat experiences. It may also necessitate the judicious use of psychotropic medications. The beneficial effects of these treatment elements especially rely on the resiliency of soldiers and their natural ability to recover mind and spirit, as well as their military motivation, if provided a timeout from the battle and recuperative assistance.

Principles in the Management of Acute Combat Reaction Casualties

Although the PIES management principles are interwoven with the treatment principles and are overlapping and mutually reinforcing, the following provides some elaboration of each from the pre-Vietnam viewpoint (presented in their logical order as opposed to the acronym sequence).

Immediacy. As already noted, acute combat reaction cases tend to be florid, amorphous, fluid, and potentially reversible psychiatric states stemming from the soldier's having been psychologically overwhelmed or worn down by his combat experiences. Especially prominent among the symptoms are vague anxiety, personality disruption, and, important for treatment purposes, marked suggestibility. The latter is believed to be the consequence of the soldier's still ongoing internal struggle between his emotional investment in his primary combat group and his heightened self-protective impulses. Consequently, the rapid provision of military-oriented, crisis intervention measures increases the likelihood of his having a favorable outcome, primarily through resuming his duty functioning.[6]

Proximity. Affected soldiers are also more likely to recover when they are treated as if they have developed a common, temporary reaction to combat stress and thus as near their units as is practical ("forward treatment"). The latter encourages the maintenance of ties with unit comrades, which in turn bolsters unit identity and the urge to rejoin them and contribute to the accomplishment of the unit's mission. As Glass noted from World War II and Korea, absent or disturbed relationships with combat unit members is the primary factor responsible for the development of the combat reaction.[15] Immediacy and proximity are best accomplished by the unit's field medics and the medical personnel operating at the 1st echelon of care, the battalion aid station.

Simplicity. Optimally, the soldier's recovery follows a brief period of rest and recuperation and, with the psychiatric team's assistance, ventilation of his psychologically disturbing combat experience. However, according to Glass, one-on-one therapy, in fact even interview methods that seek to uncover basic emotional conflicts or attempt to relate combat stress symptoms with past personality patterns, can be counterproductive. The results of such explorations suggest logical explanations for the soldiers' combat exhaustion and tend to convince them, as well as their therapists, that they have reached the limits of their combat endurance as a consequence of psychological susceptibility. This is especially true regarding the application of specialized methods, including barbiturate interviews and hypnosis, to encourage catharsis and abreaction of traumatic, and in some instances repressed, battle events. While these approaches may help relieve anxiety, soldiers treated through these means are rarely recovered for combat duty. They commonly plead or insist they should not be sent back, and therapists, who have become impressed by all the stories of trauma they have heard, identify with their distress and promise exemption from future combat exposure. According to Glass, a simplified "repressive or suppressive" therapy is preferable, whereas uncovering

depth techniques and other abreaction methods should be reserved for "severe or resistant cases where the therapeutic goal was either recovery for non-combat status, or the relief of regressive or other grossly incapacitating symptoms."[6(p727)]

Similarly, the doctrine advises that specialized psychiatric treatment in 2nd and 3rd echelon treatment settings (division clearing stations and hospitals in the theater) should mostly come from the clinical milieu there, that is, the prorecovery culture of the psychiatric unit, especially that fostered by the enlisted social work/psychology techs. Moreover, the psychiatrists should have a less conspicuous presence. According to Hausman and Rioch:

> Personal attention from the psychiatrist, except on a clearly routine basis, may well imply special attention and, consequently, more serious illness. Thus, it may impede recovery. . . . Consequently, the enlisted specialists may take a *routine* [authors' emphasis] social history, but the physician only deals with the precipitating events and the current responses.[8(p733)]

In addition, discrepant messages should be avoided, such as telling a man he has no illness and then prescribing medication, or treating a man for exhaustion but inquiring as to his childhood experiences as though his present response was due to some long-standing "weakness."[8] (This admonition had considerable implication regarding the ubiquitous use of psychotropic medications in Vietnam.)

Expectancy. This refers to an overarching clinical attitude that has long been recognized to be essential in restoring combat soldiers and returning them to duty. The treatment team's collective attitude of expectancy shapes the various physical, psychological, and environmental interventions to reinforce the patient's self-confidence as a soldier, discourage self-protective feelings, and reduce the secondary gain wish for medical exemption from further combat. Overall, the soldier is managed more as a soldier and less as a patient. Despite being under medical care, the quasimilitary treatment environment encourages him to believe his condition is a natural reaction to stress and fatigue, and that he can and will recover quickly, rejoin his comrades, resume his military job, and regain his self-respect—even if his job is dangerous or he still has some of the symptoms that brought him to medical attention.

Shaw described the requisite exhortative approach:

Reinforcement is given to the soldier's softly heard voice of conscience, which urges him to stay with his buddies, not to be a coward, and to fulfill his soldierly duty. Encouragement is given to patriotic motivation, pride in the self and the unit, and to all aspects of one's determination to go through with one's commitment.[16(p131)]

In summary, the traditional forward treatment doctrine for combat reactions advocates a push/pull approach. The "push" is from the medical/psychiatric personnel who offer temporary safety, compassion, and restoration, but who are simultaneously unwavering in urging the soldier to return to his unit and his duties as soon as possible. (This is consistent with the indoctrination provided new Army physicians at the Medical Field Service School [MFSS] at Fort Sam Houston, Texas, during the Vietnam War in which they were advised to adopt the clinical attitude of "studied indifference," as opposed to "aggressive concern."[17]) The "pull" is from the soldier's comrades who are nearby and expect him to relinquish his patient status and rejoin them in their brotherhood and achievement of the mission (ie, by promoting what has historically been referred to as "concurrence" [of the group] and "commitment" [to its task][8]). According to Glass, this approach, along with physiological restoration, serves best to reactivate the soldier's previous defenses and return him to his premorbid state; it allows him to "regain confidence and mastery of the situation and prevents chronic tension and guilt."[6(p730)]

Ethical Strain Sometimes Associated With the Doctrine and "Expectancy"

In some instances combat psychiatrists (as well as allied medical and mental health personnel) can be subjected to exquisite moral and ethical strain in the course of implementing the Army forward treatment doctrine, especially the principle of expectancy.[5] The subject of ethical conflicts and the psychiatric treatment provided in Vietnam will be more fully explored in Chapter 11.

Army Technical Manual 8-244: Pre-Vietnam Guidelines for Management and Treatment of Combat Reaction Cases

A functional blueprint for the adaptation of the psychiatric forward treatment doctrine to the three-echelon system of combat medical care implemented in Vietnam was contained in Army Training Manual (TM) 8-244, *Military Psychiatry*.[3] It was published in 1957 and served as a practical distillation of the military psychiatry experience obtained during the Korean War. This section will summarize the more salient features of the manual and provide some elaboration.

Psychiatric Care and the Three Echelons of Army Medical Care System

According to TM 8-244, primary psychiatric care is to be provided at the battalion aid station level, specialized psychiatric care at the brigade/division clearing station level, and more extensive, specialized psychiatric care in the hospitals with psychiatric specialty detachments. However, early care of combat stress-generated problems should come through psychological "first aid" by members of the soldier's platoon or company. An especially good example of such care can be found in an article written for *Army Digest* in 1968 by William O Woolridge,[18] Sergeant Major of the Army (Exhibit 7-1). In his article, "So You're Headed for Combat: How to Get Ready and What to Expect," Woolridge provides the soldier-reader with education, reassurance, exhortation, justification for the Army's engagement in combat, and encouragement to bond with fellow soldiers as a crucial countermeasure against the loss of morale and self-confidence.

In addition to help by combat buddies, officers and noncommissioned officers (NCOs) should provide reassurance and counseling, firm discipline, modified job assignments in suitable cases, and "expect the best from their men." The Medical Field Service School recommended REV: rest (only a few hours); exhortation (reinforcing the necessity of the soldier's resumption of duty); and ventilation (of his recent combat ordeal or anticipatory fears).[19] The overall objective is to mitigate the soldier's stress as well as preclude his becoming a psychiatric casualty, that is, requiring formal medical attention at the battalion aid station. According to TM 8-244:

As combat approaches, palpitation, nausea, tremulousness, and other somatic manifestations of the usual fear reactions appear. [In the absence of support and reassurance] the soldier becomes alarmed and, interpreting these symptoms as those of heart disease, gastrointestinal disease, or some other physical disorder, he reports to his medical

EXHIBIT 7-1. Soldier-to-Soldier Counseling for the Normal Combat Reaction

These comments by Sergeant Major of the Army William O Woolridge are excerpted from an article published in 1968 in Army Digest *for soldiers bound for Vietnam.*

We have an Army for one reason—to fight. And we fight only to preserve the things we American people believe in. That's why all your training is aimed at making you ready to fight. Training is tough because combat is tougher. You must be physically tough, mentally alert, and skilled in the care and use of your weapons. These plus your eagerness to use them for the good of the team add up to what we call military discipline.

How do the conditions—confusion, noise, waiting, and weather—affect the individual [anticipating combat]? You'll be afraid. The most outstanding reaction is FEAR. Don't ever let anyone kid you about this. Every normal man has a fear of battle. There are few, if any, men who really relish combat. But in your first fire fight, you are likely to have mixed feelings. In a way, you'd just as soon avoid the whole business. On the other hand, you want to mix it up a bit and find out how good you are. You wonder how you'll stack up with the other men in your unit. Will you do the right thing? Will you have the courage to carry through with the job? Nearly every man who ever went into combat pondered these questions. Chances are your reaction to battle will be the same as theirs. You're going to be scared—and you're going to have lots of company.

What are the signs of fear? You may experience all or any one of these, or some we won't mention. Your throat and chest feel tight. Your mouth is dry. You try to swallow but you don't succeed very well. Your hands shake and perhaps your palms are sweaty. You repeat some meaningless act such as checking the time or patting the rounds in your magazine pouch. Veteran soldiers also experience these reactions caused by fear. The difference is that veterans have learned to control their fears better than green troops. Fear is not altogether undesirable. It is nature's way of preparing your body for battle. As a consequence, the body automatically undergoes certain changes. You may temporarily lose a sense of fatigue, no matter how tired you are. Your heart pumps faster and sends more blood to your arms, legs, and brain. Your blood pressure goes up. You breathe faster. Your adrenal glands are stimulated and their strength-giving secretion is poured into your blood stream. More sugar, which is fuel for your body, is released into the blood. If you're wounded, your blood clots more easily to stop the bleeding. Surprisingly enough, action or "doing something" will also help you overcome the initial paralyzing effect of fear in combat. This is especially true when you're waiting for battle and the suspense is bothering you. Put your fears aside by doing something—even if you have to make work for yourself. The man who controls his fear and goes about his business despite it is a courageous man. There's no limit to what courage can accomplish on the battlefield. A worthy goal is to become a responsible, dependable soldier who doesn't let his fear stop him from doing his job.

One of the easiest things to do is talk to someone. Talk is a convenient way to relieve your tension—and it also helps the men you are talking to. Talk helps before, during, and after the battle. It has been said that the battlefield is the most lonesome place men share together. Talking with your buddies helps overcome this lonesomeness. It's a reminder that the rest of the team is with you. Your confidence goes up and your fear goes down when you think of the coming fight as a team job.

[Once the fighting begins, remember,] you're not in battle to pass a requirement. You're in battle to kill the enemy and the way you do that is to shoot your weapon. Even if you don't actually see him, and most of the time you won't, fire where you think he is. Another thing which helps you to overcome fear in combat is to fire your weapon with the rest of the team. It also helps defeat the enemy. This sounds like obvious advice. You'd be surprised how many men disregard it.

We could talk for days about what combat is like, but one thing is evident. . . . SURVIVAL IN COMBAT IS NOT SOLELY A MATTER OF LUCK. Doing things the right way is more important than luck in coming through a battle alive.

Source: Woolridge WO. So you're headed for combat: how to get ready and what to expect. *Army Digest.* 1968;23(1):6–11.

officer . . . [because this is] a culturally acceptable manner of . . . communication.[3(p71)]

1st Echelon Psychiatric Care: Nonspecialized Management and Treatment at the Battalion Aid Stations

Recommendations for Care. First echelon care encompasses basic medical and psychological treatment provided by nonspecialized medical personnel assigned

to the battalion aid station, that is, field medics and the battalion surgeon, who functions as a general medical officer. According to TM 8-244, treatment for combat stress-generated symptoms at this level would begin with a proper evaluation, especially regarding physical complaints. It may also include pharmacologically assisted sleep/rest (using sodium amytal, 0.4–0.6 grams, or the equivalent in other barbiturates). The supportive psychotherapy provided requires that the therapist be calm, confident, understanding yet firm, and expect early resumption of duty function. TM 8-244 furthermore specified that:

1. For normal fear syndromes (ie, manifested by palpitation, nausea, tremulousness, and other somatic manifestations of the usual fear reaction, along with somatization and preoccupation with organic symptoms), the soldier should be provided explanation and reassurance that physical manifestations of fear are normal.

2. For mild/moderate anxiety syndromes (ie, manifested by anxiety associated with varying degrees of exposure and exhaustion), he should be treated with sedation and measures designed to counteract physical depletion as well as provide reassurance, explanation "of the realities involved," and support.

3. For severe neurotic syndromes/psychotic syndromes (ie, manifested by severe agitation and tension, acute panic reactions, marked hysterical symptoms, or acute psychotic reactions), sedate and evacuate him to 2nd echelon care facility.

4. For behavior and attitudinal problems (the unwilling, inadequate, malingerer, symptom exaggerator, or straggler), treat him with uncompromising firmness, including references to administrative and judicial consequences, or refer him to his commanding officer.

Unresponsive Cases. In general, if the soldier's psychiatric symptoms extend beyond roughly 24 to 48 hours, he should be transferred further from the area of the fighting to the clearing station, which is located at the division or brigade base (2nd echelon treatment facility), for specialized psychiatric treatment.[3] According to the Korean War experience, roughly 20%[20] to 40%[3] of combat-affected soldiers did not respond to 1st echelon care interventions. Some demonstrated persisting tension and feelings of helplessness, severe ego constriction and depression, noise sensitivity (especially in reacting to ordinary stimuli as if they were battle stimuli), explosive outbursts of rage, and battle nightmares. Jones indicated that these resemble civilian traumatic neuroses and represent the combination of the battle trauma with predisposing personality vulnerability. However, clouding this picture is the general observation that, in the theater of combat operations, "gain in illness" may contribute to the

"fixation" of combat stress symptoms among soldiers; thus, for any particular soldier, it is difficult to distinguish between circumstantially determined symptoms and irreducible limitations in his personality. In other words, under sufficiently adverse field circumstances, predisposition may be just one of a host of variables contributing to the reluctance of soldiers to "give up their symptoms" because they permit an honorable medical exemption from further combat risk.[21]

2nd Echelon Psychiatric Care: Specialized Management and Treatment at the Division Clearing Company

Recommendations for Care. According to TM 8-244, soldiers requiring care at this level should be those in categories (2) and (3) above. Treatment would be provided by the division psychiatrist and his staff, that is, the division social work officer and the enlisted social work/psychology technicians. They were expected to maintain a small treatment facility at the brigade or division's base camp in conjunction with the clearing company. Although hospital-like, it was not technically a hospital, but it offered a broader range of support and treatment than what was available in the field. According to TM 8-244, "Every possible step is taken to foster the patient's expectation of return to full duty after a brief rest."[3(Chap6,§4,No97,p75)] This included operating in a tent and the administration of care by enlisted specialists in regular uniform. It also meant that soldier-patients would sleep on folding cots with neither mattress nor sheets, remain ambulatory and wear their regular uniform, serve themselves meals and go to the latrine unassisted, and perform work details when asked. Otherwise, the psychiatrist "avoids suggestion of organic or psychiatric illness. He maintains an attitude of firm kindness, and avoids display of oversympathy and concern."[3(Chap6,§4,No97,p75)] However, for soldiers still affected by fatigue and exposure, TM 8-244 included the provision of "rest under sedation" and the "alleviation of deprivations" (both physical and psychological).

TM 8-244 also called for individual therapy of combat reaction casualties at this echelon, both psychologic and pharmacologic. These are spelled out in Exhibit 7-2. In the division clearing stations (and even more so in the 3rd echelon psychiatric treatment facilities), an additional treatment focus becomes helping soldiers manage the guilt they experience as a result of feeling they let their combat buddies down. Still,

EXHIBIT 7-2. Korean War Era Treatment for Soldiers With Combat Reaction

The following list of psychotherapeutic and pharmacologic techniques for the specialized field treatment of soldier-patients with combat reactions is excerpted from the post-Korean War (1957) Army Technical Manual, Military Psychiatry [TM 8-244].

1. The patient–physician relationship: This combines an attitude of respect and sympathy for the patient and "qualities of firmness, decisiveness, and realism." History taking can be a therapeutic intervention when "the examiner hears the patient out, and the patient feels he has received an adequate hearing." Also, the psychiatrist should not ask leading questions. These soldiers are "extremely responsive to suggestion, whether for illness or health. . . . Every effort should be made not to lose a potential therapeutic factor within the resources of the soldier himself."

2. Ventilation: Alludes to allowing them to express their fears, hopes, and resentments. "While it is being produced, the psychiatrist strives to remain interested and attentive, utilizing only the amount of verbal or nonverbal activity necessary to maintain this type of communication."

3. Support for the superego: This entails the strengthening of the soldier's "loyalties to his buddies . . . and pointing out to him the implications of his duty to support and defend his family."

4. Suggestion: In general, this refers to a positive suggestion that is "implanted in the mind of the patient—that he is not seriously ill, that his symptomatology will be markedly alleviated, and that he will return to full combat duty." It may also be used specifically to eliminate specific hysterical symptomatology (eg, a tic, blindness, or paraplegia).

5. Sedation: Patients who have been on the battlefield within a few hours of admission often require initial sedation (usually oral sodium amytal, 0.4–0.6 grams or its equivalent in Nembutal). Overall, its purpose is to facilitate one night's sleep. Continuous heavy sedation is contraindicated. Sedation with barbiturates is also contraindicated for patients who are confused and disoriented. Also, "the more experienced the psychiatrist, the less he relies on sedation."

6. Uncovering therapy: This is primarily directed at recovering repressed traumatic battlefield experiences. It is usually accomplished with a firm suggestion and often brings about the release of strong emotion, ie, abreaction. Uncovering therapy using intravenous barbiturates (pentothal or amytal), that is, narcosynthesis, may be utilized in extreme cases. Hypnosis may serve as an alternate approach. Whereas these may be useful in relieving symptoms, they are rarely effective in returning individuals to combat duty.

7. Explanation: Soldier-patients commonly derive great benefit from learning about the causation of their symptoms, especially regarding the "normal battle reaction," that is, the predictable psychologic and somatic symptoms accompanying battle fear.

8. Reassurance: Soldier-patients also greatly benefit from being assured that, after a proper physical examination, they have no serious illness, their condition will be short-lived, and it is not the consequence of "insanity."

9. Manipulation of secondary gain: "Symptoms will often be markedly ameliorated following a firm disposition decision to return the soldier back to duty."

10. Manipulation of the environment: This includes suggestions made to the soldier's commander as to temporary alterations in his work assignment or regarding the attitudes of others toward the soldier.

11. Utilization: This refers to an array of means that can be employed to maintain the soldier's identification with, and proximity to, his primary combat group.

expectancy of return to duty—perhaps to a noncombat unit in the division, or at least in the theater—should be the overriding attitude of the treatment team. This outcome permits the soldier some recovery of his self-esteem through functioning in a military role.

Unresponsive Cases. If, following this treatment, the soldier failed to recover his functioning within roughly 3 to 5 days from the onset of symptoms, he should be evacuated out of the operational area of the division to one of the Army-level hospitals in the theater, that is, a 3rd echelon treatment facility/neuropsychiatric

detachment. By one report summarizing the Korean War experience, roughly 25% of combat-affected soldiers referred to the division psychiatric facility will not respond to the treatment provided there.[22]

3rd Echelon Psychiatric Care: Extended Management and Treatment at the Psychiatric Specialty Detachments

Recommendations for Care. The same treatment elements that were applied at the division clearing stations would be expanded for soldier-patients who were hospitalized in the specialized psychiatric treatment facilities. The obvious beneficial difference is that these units provided a greater level of protection by being more remote from the fighting, an increased length of time for treatment, and the utilization of an augmented staff with specialized training. However, according to the forward management principles in the doctrine, these same features also mitigate against the soldier recovering his premorbid military functioning. In this regard, TM 8-244 specifically advocated that soldier-patients in these treatment facilities remain in regular uniform, participate in rigorous combat training, and not be allowed "to hibernate." The staff should maintain the "proper therapeutic atmosphere," avoid the suggestion of serious psychiatric illness, and emphasize early return to duty. ("When they learn that they are expected, as normal individuals, to perform either routine combat or noncombat duties, the vast majority improve rapidly."[3(Chap6,§4,No98,p88)])

Unresponsive Cases. It was assumed that most soldier-patients at this level could still be treated and returned either to full duty or to noncombat duty within their division. However, if they continued to manifest disabling symptoms after 30 or more days of treatment and rehabilitation, they were to be either evacuated out of the combat theater to an Army general hospital in the communications zone (out of the combat theater but still in the rear part of theater of operations, which contained communications, supply and evacuation networks, and means for supporting the field forces) or to one in the United States. It was furthermore assumed that those requiring evacuation out of the combat theater would mostly be individuals with persistent psychotic conditions, and they could be evacuated sooner than 30 days if the clinical staff concluded that they were not likely to recover within that time span or if they were unlikely to be returned to duty within the combat zone.[23]

Use of Psychotropic Medications for Combat Reaction Symptoms

Through the ages the extreme physical and emotional demands of combat naturally led warring states to experiment with various psychoactive substances to limit excitement and fear and reduce exhaustion and dysfunction among their warriors.[24] In the American wars leading up to Vietnam, the use of medications in the treatment of combat-generated psychiatric casualties was generally limited to sedatives,

especially chloral hydrate and bromides in World War I and barbiturates in World War II.[25] American psychiatrists in World War II commonly used sodium amobarbital and pentobarbital for nighttime sedation in the treatment of acute combat stress cases, and British psychiatrists advocated continuous narcosis for 4 to 10 days utilizing both insulin and barbiturates. Sodium amobarbital was also thought to be useful in facilitating the abreaction (emotional release) of repressed traumatic combat experiences—the "Amytal" (amobarbital) interview.[26] However, as already noted, there could be a problem with functional impairment associated with use of sedating drugs; also, their use could contribute to soldiers' believing that they had a combat-exempting psychiatric condition.[25] Finally, and apparently quite important, TM 8-244 indicated that, "the more experienced the psychiatrist . . . , the less he relies on sedation."[3(Chap6,§4,No97,p78)] This suggests the experienced combat psychiatrist would be more conservative in prescribing medication and thus reduce the risk of problematic side effects because he had confidence in the other treatment elements, the soldier's capacity for recovery without medication, and the necessity of his resuming full military function.

Challenges in Measuring Management/ Treatment Outcomes for Combat Reactions

From the standpoint of the military mission, the inherent metric that serves to validate these principles for the management and treatment of combat reaction cases is the percent of psychiatrically disabled soldiers who can be restored and returned to duty, especially combat duty. Of course this objective includes the proviso that, upon release from medical control, they perform their duties capably. Thus military medical and psychiatric leaders have historically placed a premium on limiting the time that soldiers are excused from duty because of combat stress-generated symptoms, and they have monitored the proportion of admitted soldiers who are returned to duty status. In fact, the overall goal with respect to all forms of psychiatric attrition—measured in evacuation rate from the theater—has been to approximate the apparent irreducible minimum, one to two per 1,000 deployed troops, which equals the Army's worldwide rate for psychosis through periods of war and peace.[3,27]

However, comparisons between Vietnam and the earlier wars have been difficult because of ambiguities in diagnostic criteria. For example, Hausman and Rioch claimed that Army psychiatrists were successful in the Korean War because the lessons drawn from World War I and World War II were utilized to the fullest by division psychiatrists and allied mental health personnel: 65% to 75% of soldiers diagnosed as combat exhaustion at the division level or forward were returned to duty, and 70% of referrals to 3rd echelon care hospitals were returned to duty, although typically to noncombat units; however, the authors hasten to add that the term *combat exhaustion* was used to designate *all* (emphasis added) psychiatric casualties. Still, of those returned to duty status in the divisions, only 10% required additional psychiatric attention. And of the soldiers evacuated beyond the division, 70% were successful at duty in noncombat assignments.[8] Also, as reported by Johnson, Rioch (with Harris) queried the superiors of men returned to duty in Korea following psychiatric hospitalization and found that 80% to 90% of them were functioning satisfactorily. Regarding long-term negative effects, Rioch indicated that the patients treated utilizing these principles in World War II and in Korea were not overrepresented in clinical populations in the Veterans Administration related to their combat stress and treatment.[27]

VIETNAM: OBSERVATION AND INTERPRETATION

Inconsistencies in Disseminating the Combat Psychiatry Treatment Doctrine in Vietnam

As noted, during the planning for the war in Vietnam, Army medical and psychiatric leaders assumed that the combat troops fighting there would face stressors similar to those found in earlier wars, and they advocated the replication of the structure for the prevention and treatment of psychiatric casualties that had previously proven so effective. However, similar to the absence of uniformly disseminated diagnostic criteria for combat reactions in Vietnam, there was also unevenness regarding the dissemination of a treatment protocol there. For example, whereas the Army regulation governing the provision of psychiatric care at the time, Army Regulation (AR) 40-216, *Medical Service: Neuropsychiatry*,[28] provided some guidance as to the traditional management principles for combat reactions, it did not specifically address treatment:

In combat, treatment will be instituted early, as near the front as practicable, and in a military rather than a hospital atmosphere. Less severe cases should be treated at the Battalion Aid Station level whenever the tactical situation permits. Early return to duty is the desired objective and intrinsically therapeutic for the majority. This can be accomplished only if the medical officer accepts his full responsibility to make this often difficult decision objectively and without temporization. Psychiatric patients other than those treated at the aid station will be channeled to the division psychiatrist or when appropriate to the neuropsychiatric treatment facility in direct support of the combat unit to avoid loss of men to the rear.[28(§1,¶4b,p3)]

Newly inducted Army physicians assigned directly to Vietnam did receive some pre-Vietnam didactic familiarization with the Army's stress and fatigue model of combat breakdown ("[t]he two most important ingredients that make up the source of combat exhaustion are fear and physical exhaustion"[22]). In conjunction, they were instructed to manage combat breakdown cases early, conservatively, and with restraint with regard to prolongation of care or evacuation. However, as the following from Training Document GR 51-400-960—"Organization of Psychiatric Services at Division Level"[20]—indicates, the recommendations they received for treatment were brief, and the only reference to psychopharmacology was that of "mild sedation."

The initial detection of the Combat Reaction casualty is usually by the unit leader. In many situations the company aid man can be expected to assist in both detection and treatment. As a result of early detection, simple measures within the unit may be sufficient to return the soldier to duty. If the illness becomes more severe, the soldier is seen in the battalion aid station [1st echelon care]. . . . At this level, the soldier is held as a patient not more than 24 hours [depending] on patient load and tactical situation. Treatment measures are simple and usually easily applied. Such things as reassurance, ventilation, relief from physical discomfort; when necessary, mild sedation, a good night's sleep, a hot meal, and understanding, and firm handling are all most soldiers need. . . . Some soldiers require a temporary change in assignment, but most are able to return to duty. Keeping them with their unit if at all possible is the most beneficial action medical personnel can take.[20(pp4–5)]

Most puzzling, TM 8-244, *Military Psychiatry,*[3] which was reviewed in the previous section, was not systematically distributed to the Army medical officers who deployed to Vietnam, including psychiatrists. (This omission was confirmed by data gathered from the veteran Army psychiatrists in the WRAIR survey.) As mentioned in Chapter 6, this lack of available information might have been somewhat rectified in 1967, 2 years into the war, when Arnold W Johnson Jr, the second US Army Republic of Vietnam (USARV) Neuropsychiatry Consultant in Vietnam, published "Psychiatric Treatment in the Combat Situation" in the *US Army Vietnam Medical Bulletin.* In this excellent review, Johnson spelled out the diagnostic criteria for the combat reaction and elucidated the Army's field principles for its prevention and treatment. He also included an account of the doctrine's evolution from earlier wars and the pragmatic observations that validated its effectiveness, both in the acute battlefield situation and in reducing morbidity.[27] It is uncertain if Johnson's synopsis was disseminated in the theater in 1967, but it is even more doubtful regarding the five annual cohorts of replacement physicians, including psychiatrists, who would follow (1968–1972). Still, overall, the published record of the psychiatric care provided for combat reaction cases by Army psychiatrists and their mental health colleagues does suggest that at least knowledge of the doctrine's management principles was widespread in Vietnam, even if they were not uniformly applied.

Missing, however, is evidence that efforts were made at a central level in Vietnam to incorporate the new generation of psychotropic drugs in the doctrine as the war progressed. For example, Johnson's other-wise thorough 1967 review recommended "mild sedation" for soldiers with combat reaction, whereas, evidently even in the first years of the war, some division psychiatrists, such as Byrdy and Bostrom, had been confidently prescribing anxiolytic or neuroleptic tranquilizers.

Documentation of the Care of Combat Stress Reaction Cases in Vietnam

The following summarizes the available professional literature regarding the care provided for troops in Vietnam who had combat-induced psychiatric conditions and symptoms, including combat stress reaction (CSR).

Mental Health First Aid

There is no available information in the professional literature that would serve to document the psychological first aid that may have been provided within the small combat units serving in Vietnam, but it was likely ubiquitous. After the war, Stewart L Baker Jr, a senior Army psychiatrist, reported that Vietnam was unique among American conflicts in that unit commanders had been trained to use common sense to "size up" soldiers with psychiatric complaints; appreciate the value in psychiatric first aid supplied by members of their own combat unit, especially the medics; and not evacuate soldiers with relatively minor problems. He also maintained that the division psychiatrists in Vietnam routinely indoctrinated newly assigned line officers in the principles of forward area psychiatric treatment.[26]

Battalion Aid Station/1st Echelon Care of Combat Stress Reaction Cases in Vietnam: Treatment by Battalion Surgeons and Field Medics

Army psychiatric leaders expressed satisfaction in the 1st echelon psychiatric care directed by the battalion surgeons (Figure 7-1). For example, William S Allerton, Assistant Chief, Psychiatry and Neurology Consultant to the Army Surgeon General, summarized the Army psychiatry experience through the first half of the war and indicated that primary care physicians had managed the lion's share of the combat reaction cases. He credited their having been indoctrinated in military psychiatry at the MFSS, Fort Sam Houston, Texas, and that they had more exposure to psychiatry in their medical training compared to the physicians who served in earlier wars. However, he remained vague regarding specifics as to their use of psychopharmacology. He only acknowledged "occasional sedation and sometimes tranquilization"—less than what would be prescribed for a comparable population in the United States.[23]

Anecdotal reports from psychiatrists who served in Vietnam also suggested that the treatment provided at the 1st echelon care level was effective in reducing soldier attrition from combat stress. During the first year of the war, John A Bowman, with the 935th Psychiatric Detachment, observed that uncomplicated combat exhaustion cases not only had a low incidence, but most were effectively treated by field medics and battalion aid station personnel within the combat divisions.[29] The following year, Bostrom, division psychiatrist with the 1st Cavalry Division, reported that over a 3-month

FIGURE 7-1. Battalion aid station, 1st Cavalry Division, 1970. A medical treatment facility such as this one would typically be located forward of the division base camp in the battalion's area of operations. Its staff would consist of a battalion surgeon, who is a primary care physician, and medical corpsmen. They would provide 1st echelon medical care for the battalion's sick and wounded soldiers. Combat stress casualties would also receive their initial care here, which would coincide with the combat psychiatry management and treatment doctrine (proximity, immediacy, expectancy, simplicity). Photograph courtesy of Richard D Cameron, Major General, US Army (Retired).

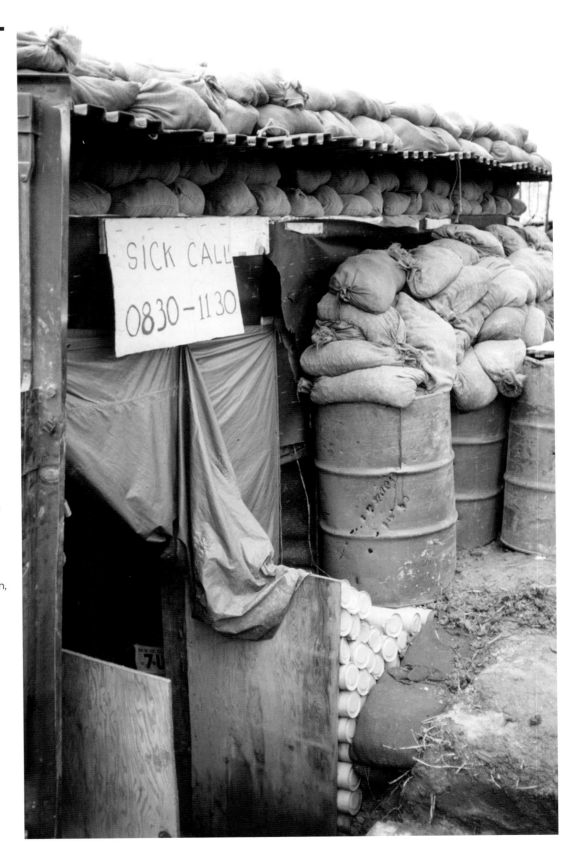

span, only 11 precombat syndrome cases and four combat exhaustion cases were referred to him from the battalion surgeons.[30] The same year, William L Baker, division psychiatrist with the 9th Infantry Division (ID), indicated that most combat fatigue cases in the 9th ID were managed by the battalion surgeons using rest and sedation "as they had been taught at Ft. [Fort] Sam [Houston] and by my instruction."[31(p5)] Robert L Pettera, who followed Baker at the 9th ID, confirmed his observation. "A great number of these soldiers are treated at the battalion aid station now, and are not seen in mental hygiene unless the doctor is not satisfied that his patient is responding."[32(p674)]

Further illustration from the field came from the USARV Psychiatry Consultant, Johnson, who offered the following:

> I've talked with [battalion surgeons] who understand this process very well and need little help from psychiatrists or social workers. The 1st Infantry Division at Di An is perhaps the division that has seen more combat fatigue than any other. They've had some lengthy operations in which the fellows stayed out in the jungle for long periods of time, and right along they've had maybe up to 6 or 8 combat fatigue cases a month—not a large number, but a steady trickle—which have gotten back to the [division] psychiatrist. However, there have been many more that have been taken care of in the medical companies, sometimes by the social work technicians in conjunction with the [battalion surgeons].[33]

Forward Treatment of Combat Stress Reactions by Enlisted Social Work/Psychology Technicians

However, Johnson's statement also illustrates the difficulty in distinguishing between 1st echelon, nonspecialized mental health care, and care provided there by personnel with specialized training. This is because, as noted in Chapter 3, division psychiatrists commonly attached one or two of their enlisted psychiatric technicians to the forward clearing stations and medical companies of the brigades in support of the battalion surgeons and the other forward-operating medical personnel (Figure 7-2); however, organizationally these enlisted specialists belonged to the division medical battalion and functioned under the technical supervision of the division psychiatrist (2nd echelon care). For example, Gerald Motis, who

saw numerous combat stress casualties as the division psychiatrist with the 4th ID in 1967–1968, indicated that his forward-deployed enlisted social work/ psychology technicians were crucial in reducing the attrition of these soldiers. He described how these psych techs applied "time-honored" treatment techniques, that is, support in abreaction, encouragement, and exhortation, and, as a consequence, the majority of soldier-patients were eager to rejoin their units within 24 hours. He also noted that the use of intramuscular Thorazine by the battalion surgeons served as a valuable adjunct in aiding rest and restraint. Two years after Motis was in Vietnam, Douglas R Bey, a division psychiatrist, similarly indicated that most combat stress-generated casualties arising in the 1st ID were "treated by their unit corpsman, the battalion surgeons, or our nearest social work/psychology technician"[34(ChapIX,p2)]; however, by that time in the war there were apparently fewer cases requiring treatment.

Johnson provided this commendable example of the work of one of the semiautonomous social work/ psychology technicians:

> Operation Attleboro was one of the big operations last fall [1966] . . . there were two companies of the 25th Division up in that area who got hit rather hard. They worked hard during that period but they sustained a lot of casualties and a lot of people's buddies got killed. At the medical clearing company of the 196th Brigade at Tay Ninh there's a social work specialist by the name of Mann, the only mental hygiene-kind of personnel [there]. He has operated in such a manner that the medical people have gained great confidence in his ability to screen and work with psychiatric patients. Specialist Mann submits monthly reports to me on the patients he sees . . . , and I talked with him about what happened during Operation Attleboro. Inside of a couple of days or so, Mann processed about 12 or 14 soldiers from these two companies who were essentially a form of combat fatigue or combat exhaustion. The way Mann described it, these were rather typically "shook up" and anxious, frightened and exhausted kids. He treated them in conjunction with the doctors there in the classical textbook fashion for combat exhaustion with a little rest, a little ventilation, a little reassurance, a little food, and sleep overnight. After 24 hours they all went back to duty and, as far as he could tell, they all

TABLE 7-1. A Summary of Division Psychiatrists' Management and Treatment for Combat Reactions in Vietnam

Psychiatrist Unit and Year	Treatment Provided for Combat Reaction Cases	Medications Utilized
Byrdy 1st Cavalry Division 1965–1966	"Hospitalized" two-thirds of referrals; treated the remainder as outpatients who were on light duty Provided brief, simple treatments Adhered to principles of "immediacy, proximity, expectancy" Pharmacotherapy Evacuated unresponsive patients out of division after 3 days	Inpatients: Librium and Thorazine Outpatients: Librium
Bostrom 1st Cavalry Division 1967–1968	Encouraged decentralized, forward treatment Provided simple treatment, that is, "limited indulgence" (rest, empathy, food) Emphasized expectancy of return to combat duty	For combat exhaustion: Thorazine, also *dauerschlaf**
WL Baker 9th Infantry Division 1967	Most were housed at base camp, rested, and treated as outpatients over 2–3 days Provided counseling ("ventilation" and supportive psychotherapy), recreation, and pharmacotherapy, especially for disturbed sleep and trauma dreams Recommended noncombat duty for those with persisting symptoms	For anxiety: Seconal as sedation For sleep: Hypnotics (ie, Seconal 100 mg–200 mg) For GI upset: Combid spansules (Prochlorperazine 10 mg and isopropamide 5 mg), Compazine, Pro-Banthine, or Donnatal
Pettera 9th Infantry Division 1967–1968	For *combat exhaustion*: provided sleep-inducing medication (no specifics) For *Vietnam Combat Reaction*: provided 3 days of "R & R" at base camp plus ventilation, reassurance, pharmacotherapy, and exhortation of return to combat	*Vietnam Combat Reaction:* For anxiety: Librium (20 mg qid) For GI upset: Combid spansules, 1–2 b/ meals For sleep: Seconal (200 mg) or Doriden (500–1000 mg)
Motis 4th Infantry Division 1967–1968	Provided initial forward treatment at brigade clearing stations "Hospitalized" unresponsive cases with other casualties for 2–3 days Provided rest, pharmacotherapy, hot meals, and "a few luxuries" Counseling included "invitation to ventilate" their combat ordeal, exhortation, and encouragement	For rest and, for some, restraint: IM Thorazine For selected cases of conversion hysteria: sodium amytal interview
Bey 1st Infantry Division 1969–1970	24-hour "hospitalization" Provided supportive psychotherapy and pharmacotherapy, including for disturbed sleep and trauma dreams	For combat exhaustion: Thorazine (100 mg qid), also *dauerschlaf** For selected conversion cases (rare): sodium amytal interviews

Data extracted from psychiatrists' reports reviewed in Chapter 3 of this volume.

*Dauerschlaf is a treatment protocol involving the administration of sufficient Thorazine to induce arousable sleep for about 24 hours. This treatment approach was also used by Navy psychiatrists treating Marines with combat exhaustion.[1]

Reference: Strange RE. Combat fatigue versus pseudo-combat fatigue in Vietnam. *Mil Med*. 1968;133(10):823–826.

did fine. So it isn't that these cases don't happen; it's that to some extent they are being handled perhaps better than they have at times in the past. This is a credit to the other physicians in the area, too, that they understand this process and are able to cooperate with it.[33]

Matthew D Parrish, who succeeded Johnson as USARV Psychiatry Consultant and who later (with Edward M Colbach) published a review of the Army psychiatry experience in Vietnam through 1970, described the collaboration that would optimally take place between the medical personnel assigned to the battalion aid stations, the enlisted social work/psychology technicians borrowed from the division, and the soldier's unit-based medical personnel and leaders:

> The general medical officer, who works in the field at the battalion or dispensary level, has proven to be quite sophisticated in mental health principles. He has often been the first real line of defense against psychiatric casualties.
>
> . . . [M]ost patients have been seen first by the enlisted [social work/psychology] technicians, right where the problem has arisen, and medication given, if needed, by the unit general medical officer. Often others in the patient's unit have been called upon to help in getting him back to good functioning. This may take the form of the technician having a private conference with the sergeant, or of an impromptu group meeting with the patient and some of his buddies.[14(pp334–335)]

The exceptionally capable service provided by forward-functioning enlisted social work/psychology technicians in Vietnam was represented by Specialist 5th Class Paul A Bender in an article written for the *US Army Vietnam Medical Bulletin*. Bender was attached to a battalion aid station with the 23rd ID (American), 11th Light Infantry Brigade, in 1968, and he offered his perspective on the challenges he faced in treating soldiers for combat stress-generated symptoms (Exhibit 7-3). In particular, Bender suggested opposing the combat soldier-patient's regressive, "egoistic" leanings by using: empathy; reassurance (of normalcy and that the soldier will eventually overcome his symptoms and return to duty); explanation (of mental mechanisms); reflection (on how the soldier may be contributing to his own problems by defensive maneuvers such as isolation from

peers); and support for his adaptive behaviors (as in encouraging his return to his unit and peer group—the classic combat psychiatric principle of expectancy).[35]

The Division Psychiatrist and the 2nd Echelon Care of Combat Stress Reaction in Vietnam: Treatment by Specialized Clearing Company Personnel

Table 7-1 summarizes the treatment elements that could be extracted from the published reports by the six division psychiatrists who specifically described their care of combat stress casualties in Vietnam. Although quite variable, collectively they suggest that the treatments more or less conformed to the doctrine, that is, all treatment elements centered on promoting the soldier's rapid recovery of previous function and reintegration into fighting units. It should be underscored that most of the actual psychiatric treatment within the combat divisions was provided by the enlisted psychiatric/social work technicians (an estimated, 75%[36]–90%[37] of the direct care of referred soldier/patients). In Chapter 6, Case 6-5, PCF Juliet served as an example of the straightforward treatment of a combat reaction case, and Case 6-11, SP4 Papa illustrated the treatment of a more complicated case of chronic combat stress; both were by enlisted social work/psychology technicians.

The few published reports by individual psychiatrists that provided follow-up data on combat stress casualties returned to duty following treatment suggest that the treatments provided by the division mental health personnel were generally effective in minimizing soldier attrition. For example, Motis noted that 18 of 23 soldiers (78%) treated for combat stress-related difficulties at the 4th ID forward clearing station were returned to duty within 1 to 3 days; and of the remaining five who were sent to the base camp for additional treatment by him and his staff, two returned to the field, while the other three were given profiles (a medically determined duty restriction) to limit their duties to the rear area of the division. Also, Pettera reported that, while combat exhaustion was rare in the 9th ID, most of the cases they treated referred to as "Vietnam combat reaction" (a "psychophysiological disturbance") were successfully returned to combat duty from the battalion aid stations. Among those who were not and who were referred to him, 85% returned to combat duty and the remainder served in noncombat positions within the division. As an interesting side note with respect to Pettera, in some instances when

EXHIBIT 7-3. Counseling the Soldier With Combat Stress Symptoms in Vietnam

The US Army in Vietnam relied heavily on decentralized mental healthcare provided by specialized enlisted corpsmen—social work/psychology technicians who had received additional behavioral science training from the Army (so-called psych techs). In the combat units, they typically operated out of a mental hygiene clinic at the clearing company medical facility (clearing station), which was located with the division's medical battalion at a brigade, or the division's, base camp. However, it was also common for enlisted social work/psychology technicians to be attached to medical units closer to the fighting to provide timely, specialized support of the battalion surgeons and other 1st echelon medical personnel. The following, excerpted from Specialist 5th Class (SP5) Paul A Bender's article, "Social Work Specialists at the Line Battalion," illustrates the perspective of the forward-functioning enlisted neuropsychiatric technician working with soldiers with combat stress reactions. SP5 Bender was deployed with the 11th Light Infantry Brigade to South Vietnam in early 1968 and assigned to its base camp at Duc Pho on the northern coast where he functioned under the technical supervision of the American Division psychiatrist who was based elsewhere with the division's other two brigades and divisional support units. (See also Exhibit 3-2, in Chapter 3, "Problems Associated With One-Session Counseling," derived from the same article.)

THE ANXIOUS COMBAT SOLDIER WITH SOMATIC SYMPTOMS

The usual treatment is to provide insight into the cause of the physical symptoms and to deemphasize their seriousness. An explanation [is offered as to] just how this seeming physical illness (e.g., general weakness, headache, lack of appetite, vomiting, and constant nervousness) may result from the body's attempt to mobilize for action. This provides both reassurance and insight to the patient as to how his physiology affects his capabilities in certain positive ways instead of merely the negative way he had surmised.[1(p64)]

COMBAT EXHAUSTION

[These were] our most acute cases. This type of case enlightened me as to the actual will of the soldier to surmount his difficulties. In such a breakdown the patient is overcome by the continuous strain and tension under which he has been functioning for a period of time. The symptoms usually include irritability, hypersensitivity, insomnia, anxiety, and over-reactivity. A treatment program provides sedatives, food, psychological ventilation, and therapy. The therapy consists of reassurance, understanding and explanation—all underlined by the pervasive aim of returning the patient to duty. In more serious cases, patients may be suffering from [psychological] shock, disorientation, fear, and recurring nightmares. At first, I doubted that such a condition could be reversed in a short period. . . . An exemplary case changed my thinking and gave me a more optimistic outlook on the power of the individual to overcome his difficulties:

The patient was a medical aid man suffering from an acute battle fatigue syndrome as a result of the shock he experienced at seeing four traumatic amputations on his first patrol. Despite rest and medication, the patient remained quite fearful of returning to the field and also suffered from recurring nightmares of the initial shock. However, within three days he recovered a genuine desire to return to duty. Because he was convinced that it was the only way to rid himself of these nightmares, and also to prove to himself that he would be able to function effectively in the field, he became motivated to place himself in the same situation which caused his breakdown. He then had a genuine desire to return to duty. He was hospitalized only three days.[1(p64)]

he sought to have soldiers that he felt were no longer capable of performing under fire assigned to noncombat duty, he was overridden by command; ultimately he concluded that he had inadvertently prolonged these soldiers' disability by being protective.

. . . [W]e found that many cases [for whom we recommended noncombat duty] were actually quite effective in combat upon their return . . . , and that the battalion surgeon and unit commanders were in a much better position to make an objective judgment. . . . As our experience grew, we began

to find that our direct intercessions only served to crystallize the neurotic symptoms in these soldiers [such that] they continued to remain relatively ineffective.[32(p675)]

Otherwise it was difficult to confirm the treatment outcomes of other division psychiatrists for combat stress casualties because their reports of generally high return to duty rates and low evacuation rates included other types of psychiatric disorders.

The impression of generally successful treatment of combat reaction casualties by the 2nd echelon/division

EXHIBIT 7-3. Counseling the Soldier With Combat Stress Symptoms in Vietnam, continued

CASES WITH FUNCTIONAL SOMATIC SYMPTOMS

A big obstacle in handling psychosomatic cases in Vietnam is the patient's tendency to prolong his symptoms, consciously or unconsciously, since these symptoms are keeping him in a relatively safe area. This is not to downgrade the individual since it is entirely natural behavior to want to preserve one's security. The patient's ambivalent feelings about any alleviation of symptoms impairs his motivation toward recovery. Motivation must be maximized to effect recovery of psychological symptoms.[1(p66)]

[These were] undoubtedly the most perplexing cases. They are referred from the various hospitals and clinics who have ruled out an organic etiology and indicated a functional basis. Two poignant problems are encountered in these cases.

1. [T]he soldier has been out of combat for an extended period in order to take all the necessary examinations and has now lost his commitment to his field unit. He resists return to duty.
2. Even more of an obstacle to therapy is his impression that his somatic complaints are the result of his nervous condition and therefore that he has a medical malfunction. He confidently assumes that the mental hygiene specialist will recognize this and will provide a solution or 'magic cure' for his complaint. Therapy would be greatly facilitated by the patient's prior realization that mental hygiene can ferret out the causes only through his cooperation and desire to get well. I think the medical doctor referring him should present the patient with a basic understanding of his problem and not extend to him just another source to which he can be referred.[1(p65)]

COUNSELING THE FIELD SOLDIER

How do you prepare a soldier to return to the field? This can be a very difficult session. The pervading atmosphere of such a session should be constantly aimed in one direction: The patient is to return to duty. He must realize this will be his ultimate destination and although much resistance is met the technician should not permit the discussion to become argumentative. He must continue to delve into the patient's feelings until the patient himself has ventilated all his superficial emotions and begins to realize and plan his return to his unit. At this point the technician has certain elements he may stress to reassure the patient. By pointing out that he has functioned previously in a combat unit, the technician can make him aware that he is capable of functioning again. The man himself will tend to underrate his own abilities and his inner and acquired capabilities. The technician must also impress upon him that the situation will not be as traumatic as [he] is imagining it to be since in most cases the human organism will adapt to the environment it finds itself in. Probably the most vital commitment played upon is the individual's peer group. When the patient begins to concentrate on thinking [about his buddies], he coordinates and cooperates with combat and turns away from his own egoistic strivings; he will create a feeling of security and confidence within himself which is really an outgrowth of the past emotional ties established within his unit.[1(p65)]

PREPARING THE UNIT FOR A SOLDIER'S RETURN

The technician should follow-up each patient restored to duty by a visit to his unit. At this time the technician must explain to the patient's superiors why he developed combat exhaustion, that he is now fit for duty, and impress upon them that this man is best used in the capacity in which he had functioned previously and in the same peer group if it was a favorable one. The preemptory impression to be left with his unit is that this man's condition was not too different from a combat wound in that he has been treated and is now ready for duty.[1(p65)]

SOLDIERS UNSUITABLE FOR COMBAT DUTY

In some combat exhaustion cases the individual personality involved may not be [suited] for field duty. In this instance it is not just a non-battle casualty precipitated by long fatigue or one traumatic event but it is the result of a basic character disorder in the patient. In such cases the technician must candidly inform the unit of the man's capabilities and potentialities for further duty in a most candid appraisal so that the unit may exercise appropriate administration and leadership.[1(p66)]

Reference: (1) Bender PA. Social work specialists at the line battalion. *USARV Med Bull.* 1968;May/June:60–69.

mental health personnel was verified by Johnson, who noted the high rates of return to combat duty and low rates of evacuation by the division psychiatrists in Vietnam through the first couple of years of the war:

When they have reached the division [psychiatrist], he takes care of them for 2 to 5 days in the medical battalion back at his headquarters, and then he returns them to duty. Very rarely are they evacuated as far back as the [neuropsychiatric KO team] at Long Binh, although there have been a few.[33]

Likewise, according to Allerton, Johnson's successor, Parrish, indicated that between mid-1967 and mid-1968, each division had only evacuated an average of four patients per month to the KO teams[38]—a rate that was reassuringly low.

Regarding treatment of the individual soldier at the 2nd echelon of care (the division psychiatric service), Bey provided a vignette demonstrating effective counseling of a combat stress casualty by one of his social work/psychology technicians.[39(p229)]

CASE 7-1: Infantryman With Combat Exhaustion, Anorexia, and Combat Aversion

---

Identifying Information: Corporal (CPL) Uniform, an infantryman, was evacuated from the field by helicopter to a division clearing station with symptoms of combat exhaustion. At the time his symptoms included anorexia, difficulty concentrating, strong aversion to returning to the field, and especially combat nightmares that resembled his earlier experience of being wounded.

History of present illness: Leading up to his evacuation from the field, he had been recovering from having been wounded while on ambush patrol.

Past history: None provided.

Examination: None provided.

Clinical course: CPL Uniform was "hospitalized" for 24 hours and treated with Thorazine (100 mg QID). In addition he also received counseling by the social work/psychology technician who presented him with the observation that, as his wound had healed, his

psychological problems seemed to have increased. He pointed out to CPL Uniform that the dreams were probably his way of gradually working out anxieties about his stressful experience—anxieties that would have immobilized him had he experienced them at the time he was wounded. The psych tech also commented that, just as the infantryman had done the right thing during the crisis and at the end of the dream, he could be assured that he would do the right thing in future times of stress.

Discharge diagnosis: Combat exhaustion.

Disposition: "The soldier went back to the field, and subsequent follow-up from his unit indicates he has been on patrol and is functioning effectively."

Source: Adapted with permission from Bey DR. Division psychiatry in Viet Nam. *Am J Psychiatry*. 1970;127(2):229.

Bostrom, a division psychiatrist, offered an intriguing model for counseling the soldier with combat stress symptoms. He recommended a careful blending of two, seemingly opposing, approaches: (1) the "maternal" one ("be careful—don't take chances—you are more important than anything else in the world") and (2) the "paternal" one ("the battle must be won at any cost—so fight furiously—even into death"). According to Bostrom, the paternal side must always dominate, while the maternal can be included but only at a "nonregressive level." ("We will give you food, drink, and sleep—so that you can keep fighting. . . . I know how you feel, it's a tough war. . . . It takes real men to put up with all this."[30(p6)]) With respect to psychosomatic complaints, he recommended the battalion surgeon see his role as helping soldiers have an easier time "out there fighting," not primarily one of eliminating symptoms (ie, "make the mother work with the father, instead of against him"[30(p7)]).

The following account by Specialist 6th Class (SP6) Dennis L Menard, a social work/psychology technician in the 1st ID (1967–1968), illustrated how environmental manipulation would have been the treatment of choice for some soldiers. The case example suggested that the management of this anxious, "trigger happy" squad leader did not center on a formal psychiatric diagnosis, and that no additional treatment was provided. Timely advice to command encouraging them to reassign the soldier to a noncombat position apparently served as the primary therapeutic element. However, it must be acknowledged that such a remedy would have to be weighed against the countervailing pressure to maintain combat unit strength.

CASE 7-2: Sergeant With Paranoid Anxiety

Identifying Information: Staff Sergeant (SSGT) Victor is 28 years old, married, and has 11 years of active service and 2 months in Vietnam. He is assigned as an infantry squad leader and was referred by his command for evaluation of his fitness for line duty.

History of present illness: The patient was referred following a series of difficulties. In one incident he fired M-16 rounds at a fellow soldier who had allegedly tried to get a beer out of the patient's refrigerator and threatened him when he objected (for which the patient received Article 15 punishment and was demoted). Also, while on night patrol he became fearful and tried to fire at his own men because he believed they were VC [Viet Cong]. He also attempted to throw a grenade at a fellow soldier who was urinating to the rear of his position. One night at base camp he imagined his bunkmate was a VC and tried to strangle him.

Past history: SSGT Victor was born in the Midwest. He was the youngest of three siblings. When he was 15 his mother died of cancer and his father was robbed and beaten to death, both on the same day. Although his earlier years were described positively, he acknowledged that his father was a heavy drinker who would abuse his mother. He made average grades in school. Following graduation, he enlisted. He served tours in CONUS [continental United States], Germany, and Korea, and his service record was mixed. Over his 11 years in the Army, he received various punishments for minor infractions. In one instance, he received a Summary Court Martial for fighting in the NCO club.

Examination: He presented as alert, attentive, and oriented, but mildly anxious. He also appeared mildly depressed. There was no evidence of a thought

disorder, but he did reveal some paranoid ideation. Insight and judgment appeared lacking. The patient explained the incidents for which he was referred as stemming from his extreme fearfulness. He acknowledged that while in the jungle on [patrol], he would become extremely tense and apprehensive, feel "paranoid," and have illusions of VC, and fear his imminent death. As a result he would become unable to function and worried he might accidently harm someone.

Clinical course: Contact was made with his unit cadre and fellow squad members. They acknowledged they were afraid of the patient ("trigger happy") and would avoid going on patrol with him. They observed him to be highly tense and preoccupied with fearful thoughts, believing all movements were hostile.

Final diagnosis: No official diagnosis was provided. The impression included, "Due to the stress of the combat situation, (the patient) is apparently exhibiting many paranoid tendencies that are increasingly causing him to become ineffective as a combat soldier."

Disposition: Upon the advice of the psych tech, command elected to have the patient reassigned to a rear area pending further evaluation by the division psychiatrist who ultimately concurred with this disposition. The patient completed his tour in Vietnam in a noncombat assignment without further incident.

Source: Adapted from Menard DL. The social work specialist in a combat division. *US Army Vietnam Med Bull*. 1968;March/April:49–51.

Finally, although Colbach and Parrish reported that sodium amytal had not been used in Vietnam, Bey and Motis, both division psychiatrists, acknowledged its occasional use for amytal interviews (Figure 7-2). Motis (with West), who served with the 4th ID, described the effective use of a well-trained, well-supervised, social work/psychology technician as a primary therapist in the field treatment of a soldier who had developed combat stress-related conversion symptomatology. The interaction of the soldier's susceptible personality and his combat risks produced a hysterical mutism, and the

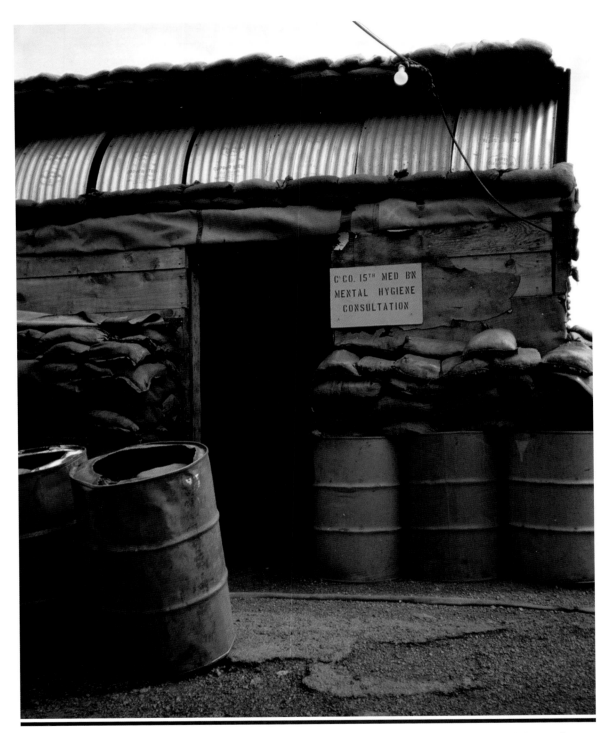

FIGURE 7-2. Brigade-level mental health treatment facility, 1st Cavalry Division, 1970. In Vietnam the US Army advocated a doctrine of psychiatric care for acute casualties among combat troops that included the provision of safety, replenishment, support in assimilating their combat ordeal, and encouragement to soon resume their military function—in some instances utilizing psychotropic medication. This was applied as rapidly as possible and as close to their unit and the fighting as feasible. Enlisted social work/psychology technicians staffed forward mental health treatment facilities such as this one and operated with the support of the battalion surgeons (primary care physicians). Indirect supervision came from the division psychiatrist or social work officer who typically worked out of the division's base camp. Photograph courtesy of Richard D Cameron, Major General, US Army (Retired).

treatment centered on the use of an amytal interview to bypass his symptom. Although the soldier-patient recovered the use of his voice, the account made evident that this was only accomplished because he was allowed a noncombat duty assignment within the division.[36] In fact, Bey indicated that in the 1st ID they were unable to return most of the soldiers to combat duty who had been treated with amytal interviews, even though they gave up the hysterical symptoms with suggestion[40] "The sodium [amobarbital] interviews we did were, for the most part, quite dramatic in terms of the outpouring of emotion by the patients and quick recoveries. However, most cases of conversion reactions in the 1st [ID] were cured by medics and battalion surgeons without any specialized techniques."[40(p189)]

Some mention should also be made of the psychiatrists who served in solo, hospital-based positions, that is, in the field and evacuation hospitals without attached specialized psychiatric units. As described in Chapter 4, these facilities were established to provide inpatient, primarily 2nd echelon medical care, and their catchment population mostly consisted of noncombat support and service-support troops; however, at times these facilities did care for combat troops. As it turned out, among the five Army psychiatrists who provided a record of their experiences with these facilities, only two, Gary L Tischler with the 67th Evacuation Hospital and John A Talbott with the 3rd Field Hospital, mentioned combat stress casualties per se; and neither was specific about treatments provided or outcome.

Psychiatric Specialty Detachment/3rd Echelon Care of Combat Stress Reaction Cases

Chapter 4 presented the structure and staffing of the two neuropsychiatric specialty detachments ("KO teams") deployed in Vietnam as well as summaries of the overviews provided by three psychiatrists who served in these detachments. Only two of them, Bowman ((December 1965–October 1966) and H Spencer Bloch (August 1967–August 1968), referred specifically to the treatment of combat reactions; but even their reports did not distinguish clearly between treatments provided for combat troops as opposed to noncombat troops.

Bowman and the 935th Psychiatric Detachment.

According to Bowman, after the 935th had deployed to Vietnam there were relatively few classic, uncomplicated, combat exhaustion cases requiring treatment. The low combat exhaustion referral rate at the 935th Psychiatric Detachment could be partly explained by the fact that it was early in the buildup phase of the war. It also could be because effective treatment was provided at lower echelons of care as previously indicated. Even though Bowman provided an extensive list of seriously disabling symptoms seen among combat-exposed troops at the 935th, these represented fewer than 2% of their referrals. The majority of combat troops were referred for either behavioral disturbances or functional somatic complaints. Bowman made the following observations with regard to the latter:

> The somatic complaints were usually such that they temporarily removed the soldier from the stresses he was experiencing in an honorable way, [in that he avoided receiving] an Article [15] or court-martial. Stress symptoms such as headaches, sleep-walking, dizziness, nausea were frequently presented. Occasionally a soldier was given tranquilizers to help bind his anxiety so that he could return to his previous satisfactory level of performance and functioning.[41(p2)]

Bowman implied that many of the soldiers they treated for combat stress-generated conditions at the 935th Psychiatric Detachment were brought directly in from the field after having bypassed the division clearing stations and the psychiatric personnel there. This was likely because the Army medical and psychiatric care system was still in flux and especially because of the expanding role for heliborne transport. A general description of Bowman's specialized inpatient treatment environment at the 935th Psychiatric Detachment was provided in Chapter 4.

Bowman did not provide clinical examples of their treatment of combat stress reaction cases; however, he included the following general comments pertaining to the specific challenges they faced in treating these casualties:

> The [combat] soldier was allowed to ventilate feelings, especially fear of death or fear of derangement [sic] of his body image. . . . The KO Team personnel would work to the best of their abilities to help the soldier with his problem, but the presenting symptom was rarely considered sufficient reason to evacuate [him] from Viet Nam

unless, of course, the soldier proved to be frankly psychotic. . . . Occasionally mild sedatives were used, but tranquilizers were seldom prescribed. It was the staff's feeling that tranquilizers would tend to reinforce the soldier's concept of being ill.

. . . After a period of grief, catharsis, or rest we found many of the soldiers ready for duty. In spite of mild to moderate anxiety, the soldiers for the most part did function effectively when returned.[29(pp4–5)]

Still, even at this early point in the war, evidence of the ethical strain associated with the Army treatment doctrine can be seen in Bowman's account.

Occasionally a soldier asked forthrightly to be relieved from combat because he was 'too nervous.' Some were vehement and demanding, some tearful, some agitated, and some emotionally labile. Too, some pleaded to be given a non-combatant assignment. . . . Indeed it was difficult to return to duty a soldier who had seen considerable combat, or had been wounded, or a soldier who had seen his best friend killed. . . . Frequently the members of the KO Team turned to each other for support when we returned a soldier to duty who may have narrowly escaped death or injury and was now reluctant to go back to combat. Without our own intra-group support a firm policy on evacuation could not have existed.[29(pp4–5)]

Bloch and the 935th Psychiatric Detachment. By the time Bloch (August 1967–July 1968) was assigned to the 935th Psychiatric Detachment, combat intensity in Vietnam had tripled over that of the first year; but as he reported, relatively few patients with combat exhaustion were hospitalized there—a phenomenon he, like Bowman, also attributed to the effective treatment they received at the 1st and 2nd medical care echelons within the divisions. The 935th Psychiatric Detachment did treat the more complicated cases of combat fatigue that were transferred from the division psychiatrists. They also treated fresh casualties flown in directly from the battlefield. Overall, their treatment regimen incorporated the principles of the Army forward treatment doctrine.[42] According to Bloch, the average stay for combat exhaustion cases was 3 days, and 100% of the 34 hospitalized cases over the course of a year

were returned to duty (Bloch does not indicate if these soldiers returned to combat duty per se).

However, in contrast to Bowman's conservative philosophy regarding the use of tranquilizing medications, Bloch and his colleagues regularly employed both major and minor tranquilizers for a broad range of psychiatric conditions.[43] In particular, they utilized a protocol of Thorazine-induced narcosis (24–48 hours of sleep treatment—*dauerschlaf*—a term of German derivation that roughly translates into long-lasting sleep but which has been adopted over the years for "sleep therapy") for severely disorganized and uncontrollable patients (114 over a year), not just those with combat exhaustion.[43] (As noted in Chapters 3 and 4, this treatment approach was also used by both division psychiatrists and hospital psychiatrists.) Bloch described the 935th Psychiatric Detachment's *dauerschlaf* protocol as follows:

The patient was told he would be given medicine which would enable him to sleep for a day or even a little longer after which his condition would be much improved. He was then administered oral or intramuscular doses of Chlorpromazine [Thorazine] every hour until a sound narcosis was achieved and thereafter as necessary when he awoke to maintain sleep. Treatment was initiated and maintained with oral doses of 100–400 mg. or IM doses of 50–100 mg. and occasionally 200 mg. when oral medication was refused. Physical restraints were sometimes used if necessary until sleep was achieved. [Medically monitored] Chlorpromazine narcosis was maintained for 24–48 hours and never longer than 72 hours.[43(p348)]

Bloch took pains to justify their approach as other than just "snowing" objectionable patients or subduing those perceived as dangerous. "[It] capitalizes on the as yet poorly understood psychologically restitutive powers of sleep or [Thorazine]-induced sleep. . . ."[43(p351)] In his experience, this treatment proved to be especially efficient and effective for a cross-section of severely disordered soldiers who, by necessity, had to be hospitalized in an open, crisis-oriented, milieu ward. With regard to acute and transient psychotic stress states, it also seemed to serve diagnostic ends by helping to differentiate (and treat) such conditions in contrast to the less responsive schizophrenias.[43] Case 2-1, SP4 Delta in Chapter 2;

Case 6-1, CPL Foxtrot; Case 6-6, PFC Kilo; Case 6-10, SP4 Oscar; and Case 6-13, PFC Romeo, all in Chapter 6, serve as illustrations. They are suggestive of 2nd echelon care, that is, that that would ordinarily be provided by the division psychiatrists, and all had a rapid, and apparently full, recovery of duty functioning. (Bey and Bostrom, both division psychiatrists, also reported utilizing the *dauerschlaf* method.)

More central to the mission of the 935th Psychiatric Detachment was the provision of more extensive, 3rd echelon, psychiatric care. Bloch indicated that treatments for combat troops in their inpatient unit varied widely, depending on the pathodynamics of each case. However, befitting the highly charged psychosocial context of a military organization involved in combat operations a long way from home, Bloch and his staff favored an interpersonal treatment orientation, that is, toward interventions in the social and military dimensions of the patient's problems (versus one representing an intrapsychic or internalized emotional conflict). The following case is illustrative of a more involved treatment approach at a 3rd echelon care facility.

CASE 7-3: Withdrawn, Noncommunicative Soldier Following the Death of His Platoon Leader and Radio Operator

Identifying information: Private First Class (PFC) Whiskey is a 20-year-old, married infantryman who was evacuated to the 93rd Evacuation Hospital/935th Psychiatric Detachment following 4 days of psychiatric treatment in his division clearing station.

History of present illness: EM [enlisted man] was initially dusted off [transported by helicopter] to the division clearing station after developing bizarre behavior (crying, incoherent, and biting his fingers) immediately following a mine explosion that resulted in the death of his platoon leader and radio operator. It is unclear if he was medicated in the field, but when seen by the division psychiatrist he was mute and stuperous. While at the 25th ID, Thorazine (100 mg. QID) was administered, and, although he "maintained contact with the environment," he remained uncommunicative with some psychomotor retardation. Two Methadrine interviews (intravenous administration of an amphetamine derivative to promote alertness and activity) followed by an Amytal-Methadrine interview (sodium amytal was added for disinhibition) brought forth "considerable abreaction" ("[h]e began to cry and shout out about the deadly mine explosion"), and he spoke of his guilt in not preventing the deaths. He also talked about his wife and the death of their child 6 months previously. However, following the interviews, he again regressed and required transfer to the 935th Psychiatric Detachment.

Past history: None provided.

Examination: Upon arrival at the 935th Psychiatric Detachment, PFC Whiskey was noted to be appropriate and cooperative, but when asked questions, he contorted his face and remained mute. His affect was depressed and anxious.

Clinical course: On the ward he was treated with Thorazine (50 mg TID) and group therapy. Gradually he became more comfortable speaking to individuals, but he remained anxious when expected to speak to the group. Ultimately this abated, and he was able to confide in the group about his traumatic combat experiences. After 3 weeks of hospital care, he was considered fit to return to duty.

Discharge diagnosis: Acute situational maladjustment, severe, improved. Stress: moderate, sight of buddies injured and dying. Predisposition: unknown. Impairment, none.

Disposition: Returned to unit with 10-day supply of Thorazine (50 mg TID).

Source: Narrative Summary, 935th Psychiatric Detachment/93rd Evacuation Hospital.

Still, some combat reaction cases warranted an emphasis on intrapsychic mental dynamics. For example, Bloch presented a case of a young combat soldier with disabling anxiety and suicidal ideation who was not only treated with milieu therapy and nighttime sedation, but he also was given individual, crisis-oriented, supportive/interpretive psychotherapy.[42(pp295–296)]

CASE 7-4: Newly Arrived Soldier With Neurotic
Anxiety and Suicidality

Identifying Information: Private (PVT) X-ray was a
20-year-old artillery observer, who had 6 months
of Army service but only 1 week in Vietnam. He was
transferred to the 93rd Evacuation Hospital/935th
Psychiatric Detachment after spending a night at the
division clearing station for anxiety reaction.

History of present illness: He indicated that he had
always been anxious, but this had become worse
after he joined the Army and received his assignment
to Vietnam. He additionally complained of recently
developing phobic symptoms along with obsessional
thoughts and nightmares in which his mother, his
fiancé, and his brother died violently. These worries
made his separation from them seem unbearable and
led him to suicidal thinking.

Past history: PVT X-ray was the middle child raised
by a nervous and histrionic mother and a much-
loved stepfather. At age 13 his stepfather suffered an
accidental death, followed by his mother slashing her
wrists. These events resulted in the patient harboring
strong feelings of guilt and led him to become "a
model, compliant lad" who could never experience
anger, only "nervousness." The patient also reported
that, as he prepared for his assignment in Vietnam, his
mother began to behave in a fashion similar to when
she went "out of her mind" following the death of his
stepfather.

Examination: He initially presented at the 93rd
Evacuation Hospital as tremulous, hyperventilating,
rocking, tearful, and uncommunicative. However,
in response to "a firm approach," the patient
soon calmed and became cooperative with the
hospitalization and treatment.

Clinical course: The patient was "worked with
intensively in the ward milieu" and given occasional
sleeping medication. He was also provided individual
psychotherapy that centered on a supportive
interpretation of his pre-Vietnam psychic conflicts
(". . . that his concerns were like those of the phobic
patient with separation anxiety who could not let
persons toward whom he felt much unconscious rage

out of his sight for fear that they would die because
of his own hostile impulses"), which had become
heightened by anxieties associated with being new
to combat. After a couple of days of this combined
treatment approach, his social isolation began to
abate, he became responsive to the milieu, and he
reported that his anxiety had modulated and his
sleeping had improved. He returned to duty on day 4.

Discharge Diagnosis: Anxiety reaction.

Disposition: Returned to duty with follow-up
reevaluation arranged with the division psychiatrist.

Source: Adapted with permission from Bloch HS.
Army clinical psychiatry in the combat zone: 1967–
1968. *Am J Psychiatry*. 1969;126(3):295–296.

Finally, Bloch noted that some combat reaction
cases were especially difficult in that they presented
with extremely protean clinical findings, which required
active collaboration between the psychiatrists operating
in the field and those in the specialty unit. Not only
might a patient's symptoms worsen when he was
closer to combat risks, but also, as has been discussed,
important differences in psychiatrist values and priorities
may derive from these differing professional contexts.
By way of illustration, see Case #4 in Bloch's paper[44(p8)]
(provided in Appendix 12, "Some Interesting Reaction
Types Encountered in a War Zone").

Preventive Psychiatry and Combat Stress

All clinical activities of Army psychiatrists have
been conceptualized as falling into three functional levels
of prevention: "primary prevention" (ie, minimization
of psychiatric conditions through advice to military
leaders regarding morale and stress reduction—true
prevention); "secondary prevention" (ie, early detection
and intervention to minimize symptoms for individual
soldiers); and "tertiary prevention" (ie, the treatment
of affected soldiers who require removal from duty
status, as in hospitalized). With regard to primary
prevention, except for Bey with the 1st ID (April 1969–
April 1970),[45] there is little published evidence that
Army psychiatrists in Vietnam were able to influence
commanders regarding stress-inducing factors affecting
combat units. On the other hand, there also is no
evidence that the commanders were accessible for

TABLE 7-2. Estimated Percent of Combat Stress Reaction (CSR) Cases Treated Among the Three Army Medical Care Echelons in Vietnam in 1967 Compared With the Korean War

Army Medical Care Echelons	Reported Treatment Provided in Korea*	Estimated Treatment Provided in Vietnam (1967)†
1st echelon care of CSR cases: Treatment provided by nonspecialized battalion surgeons and medics (at battalion aid stations, dispensaries)	80%	63%[1]
2nd echelon care of CSR cases: Treatment provided by division psychiatrists and allied psychiatric personnel (at division clearing companies)	15%	22%[2]
3rd echelon care of CSR cases: Treatment provided at evacuation or field hospitals and psychiatric specialty detachments ("KO" teams)	5%	15%[3]

Data source:

*Cooke ET. *Another Look at Combat Exhaustion*. Fort Sam Houston, Tex: Department of Neuropsychiatry, Medical Field Service School; distributed July 1967. Training Document GR 51-400-320, 055.

†Percentages in this column are derived from the estimated combat stress reaction (CSR) incidence rates for 1967 presented in Table 6-2 in this volume (all rates are /1,000 troops/year).

    1. CSR incidence rate for this echelon [3.8] divided by the total CSR incidence rate for all echelons [6].
    2. CSR incidence rate for this echelon [1.3] divided by the total CSR incidence rate for all echelons [6].
    3. CSR incidence rate for this echelon [0.89] divided by the total CSR incidence rate for all echelons [6].

primary prevention interventions, or that the assigned psychiatrists believed they possessed the requisite expertise. There is, however, ample documentation of secondary and tertiary prevention activities on the part of the division psychiatrists and their staffs, as in establishing a liaison between the symptomatic soldier and his unit cadre to minimize disability, or in the treatment of disabled soldiers. Chapter 10 provides a broader review of command consultation in Vietnam.

Estimating Treatment Outcomes for Combat Stress Cases in Vietnam

In their medical officer's basic training newly commissioned Army physicians bound for Vietnam were taught that, based on experiences in Korea, primary care physicians could expect to effectively treat four combat stress reaction cases for every one that required referral on to the division psychiatrist; and for every three cases effectively treated by the division psychiatrist and his staff and returned to duty, one would require evacuation out of the division and on to a neuropsychiatry specialty center in Vietnam.[20] Unfortunately the Army's failure to define and track combat stress reaction cases in Vietnam made it impossible to realistically compare the Vietnam experience with that in Korea.

However, CSR treatment outcomes in Vietnam can be surmised from the estimate of the combat stress reaction (CSR) incidence, at least for 1967, presented in Table 6-2, which drew from findings from the Datel and Johnson survey of outpatient psychotropic drug prescription patterns in 1967 in Vietnam[46] and Bourne's 1966 study of US Army psychiatric hospitalization rates in the theater.[47] Table 7-2 presents the proportions of CSR cases treated at the three medical echelons in Vietnam compared to Korea. As the second column indicates, by these measures it can be roughly estimated that primary care physicians and other nonspecialized personnel in Vietnam effectively treated only two combat reaction cases for every one referred on to the division psychiatrists. In turn, division psychiatrists effectively treated only three cases for every two referred on to the psychiatric specialty centers (KO teams) in Vietnam. These figures suggest that the care provided within the combat divisions in Vietnam (ie, 1st echelon treatment success by nonspecialists and 2nd echelon treatment success by division psychiatrists) effectively treated only 85% of combat exhaustion cases, versus 95% for Korea. In other words, the treatment success rate for combat stress reaction cases within the combat divisions in Vietnam (at least for 1967), that is, cases not requiring evacuation to the two KO teams for more extensive, 3rd echelon, specialized treatment, appears to be lower, or at least the evacuation rate was higher, than was the case in Korea. However, apart from the extremes to which the data have been stretched, a conclusion of lower treatment effectiveness in Vietnam is arguable if one takes into account that TM 8-244, *Military Psychiatry,* suggested that only 60% of combat reaction cases in Korea were successfully treated by 1st echelon, nonspecialized personnel[3] (vs Cooke's 80% in the first column in Table 7-2). Furthermore, the Datel and Johnson survey found that primary care physicians reported treating four combat fatigue cases for every one treated by psychiatrists.

Also, regarding 3rd echelon care, the 3 times higher figure for Vietnam over Korea noted in Table 7-2 (ie, 15% vs 5%) could be misleading because the source of the estimate for Vietnam, that is, Bourne's study, was conducted during the first year of the war—early in the development of the Army's medical care delivery system. However, if, in fact, a greater proportion of combat reaction cases was treated by the KO teams in Vietnam compared to Korea, this could be explained simply by the ubiquity of helicopter medical transport. In Vietnam, evacuation and field hospitals commonly received direct admissions of casualties from the battlefield, including psychiatric casualties.[48] It also may represent the fact that the KO teams were often required to provide 2nd echelon care for the four independent combat brigades fighting in Vietnam that had no assigned psychiatrists.

As for measures of success for combat reaction treatment at the psychiatric specialty detachments (KO) in Vietnam, the data are scant. In his summation of the first half of the war, Allerton indicated that the two KO teams had contributed to the "lowest [out of the combat zone] evacuation rate for psychiatric reasons in the history of the Army Medical Service."[23(p7)] To this end he partly credited their role as evacuation choke points in that they held the final authority for psychiatric patients exiting Vietnam.[23] However, Allerton was referring to all psychiatric conditions, not just combat stress reactions. Also, recall from Chapter 6 that numbers of combat stress cases evacuated to Travis Air Force Base in California during the first half of 1967 were negligible, and there were very small numbers of cases with a diagnosis of traumatic neurosis evacuated through Clark Air Force Base in the Philippines early in the war.

Finally, in March 1969, almost 2 years after Johnson collected his survey data, BH Balser, a civilian psychiatrist who was a consultant to the US Army, visited all echelons of Army psychiatric care in Vietnam, beginning with the 1st echelon medical care of four combat divisions. There he noted how the basic cathartic care of the "emotionally disturbed and upset soldier" was provided primarily by trained mental health technicians under supervision of the battalion's physician, who, at times, prescribed augmenting neuroleptic or anxiolytic tranquilizer medications. He described this care as extremely effective, returning 80% of affected soldiers back to their units and to combat duty. According to Balser, intractable cases passed through increasingly sophisticated treatment areas so that those who required evacuation to Japan were, with few exceptions, seriously ill.[49]

In conclusion, using the best information available it appears that effective treatments, as well as conservative evacuation policies, were implemented in Vietnam. Among various implications, these data especially appear to generally validate the combat psychiatry doctrine as serving force maintenance under the conditions found there. They also underscore the value of familiarizing the primary care physicians in the doctrine's principles. On the other hand, the data do not necessarily make the case for broader or more effective use of the newer psychiatric medications, even if anecdotal reports suggest that it was so.

Mixed Reviews on the Use of Psychoactive Medications for Combat Reaction Cases in Vietnam

The availability of recently discovered neuroleptics, anxiolytics, and tricyclics in the Vietnam theater represented powerful new tools in the armamentarium of combat psychiatrists. From material already presented it is evident that the new tranquilizers were commonly prescribed by psychiatrists and primary care physicians and had displaced the sedatives from the Korean War era in the treatment of a wide variety of conditions, including those affecting combat-exposed troops. Yet officially, at least early in the war, the role of pharmacotherapy was debatable. Allerton summarized the Army's Vietnam experience through mid-1968 as:

[Although] phenothiazines have often been used where barbiturates previously might have been [in World War II and Korea], it has been observed that fewer drugs of any type are being used by psychiatrists in their combat psychiatric experiences in Vietnam. . . . Evidence tends to show that the temporary removal from [combat exposure] coupled with the fostering of an expectation of early return to duty is a much more meaningful part of the therapeutic regime than any of the drugs (barbiturate or tranquilizers) that have been or are being used.[23(pp13–14)]

Unfortunately, Allerton supplied no data to support this conclusion. However, it did coincide with the impression held by Peter G Bourne, an Army research psychiatrist, who reported from the field from the first year of the war that these medications had a "relatively slight impact" in prevention and treatment of psychiatric conditions.[50] However, this was contradicted by Johnson who was the USARV Psychiatry Consultant in the second year of the war and the principal investigator in the Datel and Johnson survey.[46] "It may very well be that the use of tranquilizing medications is one of the most important factors in keeping the psychiatric rates in Vietnam at a low level."[51(p339)]

More specific to the combat soldier, in their summary of the first 4 years of Army medical experience in Vietnam, Colbach, who had served as an Army hospital psychiatrist there (November 1968–November 1969), and Parrish, who had been the USARV Psychiatry Consultant during the third year of the war, commented that

[t]his is the first war in which the new phenothiazines have been available, and they have been widely used in all kinds of conditions. They have been safely used to control excessive anxieties in combat infantrymen without any apparent interference in duty performance.[14(p340)]

Navy physicians similarly advocated prescribing major tranquilizers for Marine combat stress casualties.[52,53] For example, Strange and Arthur reported broad use of Thorazine ("very heavy doses"), along with nighttime sodium amobarbital, for acute combat syndromes.[54]

But the possible dangers in prescribing psychotropics for combat troops in Vietnam were not entirely overlooked. In a pained postscript after the war, Colbach offered a more confused perspective on the use of these medications in Vietnam:

. . . [In Vietnam] we did not like to use the minor tranquilizers and barbiturates and related

compounds because of their abuse potential. We rarely used anti-depressant medication. Our main psychotropic weapons were the major tranquilizers, primarily the phenothiazines. We used these not only for the psychoses but for all kinds of anxiety and psychosomatic states. Many soldiers went into the field with Thorazine or Mellaril in their pockets. Among ourselves we debated whether this was really a good idea. Obviously the medication made people less alert. At the same time, though, excessive anxiety could be very harmful to functioning also. Again it was a balancing act, trying to weigh the benefits of medication against its drawbacks. In civilian life there are all kinds of cautions about what a person on psychotropic medication can and cannot do. . . . Yet in Vietnam risks of the sort were regularly taken. Our job was to keep the Army functioning.[55(p261)]

Also, regarding potential adverse long-term consequences, Holloway conjectured that for some veterans, taking psychotropic medications in Vietnam might have contributed to postwar adjustment problems if the drug disrupted critical cognitive functions to the effect that they "could not achieve an integration of their overseas and combat experience."[56] In fact, concerns for both short- and long-term effects from the use of these medications were consistent with a larger set of ethical questions regarding the military psychiatry treatment doctrine in Vietnam that were raised as the war progressed and after its conclusion.[5]

Many years after the war, as if to quell contentions that psychotropics were injudiciously prescribed in Vietnam, Franklin Del Jones, former division psychiatrist there and distinguished historian of military psychiatry, offered the following regarding the use of such medications for combat troops (but without referring to Vietnam per se or his experience serving there):

. . . All drugs are potentially double-edged swords. All will have side effects and overdose effects. Some may produce additional effects upon withdrawal or elimination of the drug. Some interact dangerously with environmental factors, diet, other drugs, or specific diseases. All drugs may have idiosyncratic effects on some individuals. It is unwise to dispense any drug lightly, without first evaluating the recipients and briefing them (and their support group) on what to expect and what to be alert for. It is then wise and ethical to follow them up periodically. For these reasons, any use of pharmacologic agents should be kept under appropriate medical supervision if not necessarily medical control.

. . . After analysis of the risks, some drugs may be judged safe enough for "over the counter," self-administered use. Other drugs may be judged safe for routine prescription use with periodic followup. Other drugs still may be so risky that they should be prescribed only in urgent, carefully defined situations.[25(pp124–125)]

. . . [Finally,] the neuromuscular, autonomic nervous system, and cognitive impairments produced by [Thorazine] make it a particularly questionable choice on the battlefield.[25(p126)]

Missing Information Regarding Combat Stress Treatment in Vietnam

The foregoing observations regarding the management and treatment of combat stress-related conditions in Vietnam essentially came from the first half of the war. The only documentation of the character of combat reactions in the theater during the second half came from Larry E Alessi's communiqué to the battalion surgeons of the 23rd Infantry Division (American) (see Appendix 9, "Principles of Military Combat Psychiatry"). As Alessi indicated, burgeoning psychophysiologic reactions and "non-psychiatric emotional problems," including anxiety, fear of the field, and refusal to go to the field, were the dominant patterns seen among the division's combat troops in the fall of 1970 despite the dropping combat intensity. Evidently combat stress was still a factor for some. He advised battalion surgeons to regard them as having natural aversion to combat risks and to manage greater numbers at the battalion aid stations though the use of reassurance, peer support, and firm opposition to claims of psychiatric impairment—along with judicious use of Mellaril. If nothing else, it is startling that Alessi found it necessary to reiterate the need for battalion surgeons to oppose default by combat soldiers and that he recommended the neuroleptic Mellaril for this purpose. (For use with outpatients, Mellaril was apparently preferred because it was less sedating compared to Thorazine, the other widely available neuroleptic.)

Also, the material in this section on psychiatric treatments for combat-exposed troops in Vietnam has been rather exclusively centered on symptomatic

disorders. There were many other soldiers in Vietnam who exhibited behavior and discipline problems, including drug and alcohol abuse, in response to excessive combat stress—problems that were not generally considered to be exclusively medical/psychiatric ones but instead expressive of low morale or faulty attitudes. As such, these soldiers would have primarily been the responsibility of their military leaders, who may have resorted to various judicial and nonjudicial punishments or recommended that they be administratively discharged from the Army. The psychiatric literature from Vietnam did not systematically address any treatments for these problems. It did, however, indicate that large numbers of such soldiers were referred for a psychiatric evaluation, many of whom received a diagnosis of character and behavior disorder (ie, personality disorder[57]). This may have constituted a remedy, if not a treatment per se, in permitting them to receive an expeditious separation from the Army through a less punitive type of discharge. According to John A Renner Jr, the Navy psychiatrist who treated Marines there in 1969, these were the "hidden casualties" of Vietnam.[58]

Byrdy, with the 1st Cav, offered this observation from the first year of the war that alluded to the awkward line between behavior and discipline problems and evident psychiatric disorders:

By and large, COs [commanding officers] and XOs [executive officers] were very glad and relieved to discuss patients. . . . They saw the psychiatrist as functioning in a capacity mostly to rid them of problems at hand in a manner, I'm sure, no different from any other operating division. These problems usually involved someone who was disturbed or someone against whom it was hoped that a characterological case could be built because administrative grounds for action were lacking. In a combat situation one certainly becomes sympathetic with their wishes to be relieved of troublesome personnel. However, there were many cases in which they wanted the psychiatrist to be simply the "hatchet man."[59(p50)]

Byrdy also noted that:

Familiarization with the situation in the field brings the realization that the kinds of referrals depend on the tactical situation. [For example,] homosexuals and discipline problems are rarely referred in from units which are under engagement.[60(p4)]

Distinctions between diagnosable psychiatric conditions and misconduct/behavior/discipline problems in general will be explored in Chapter 8.

RESEARCH AND ANALYSIS

Although there was very little systematic research into the patterns of care and outcomes for combat stress conditions in Vietnam, two studies warrant special attention: (1) the 1967 survey of psychoactive medication prescriptions for soldiers (outpatients) by Datel and Johnson, and (2) the postwar epidemiologic review of the Marine casualty data by Palinkas and Coben.

The Datel and Johnson Survey of Patterns of Outpatient Psychotropic Pharmacotherapy for US Army Troops in Vietnam

The survey of psychotropic drug-prescribing patterns of Army physicians in Vietnam, including psychiatrists, which was mentioned in Chapter 6, was not limited to combat-exposed troops; nevertheless, it serves as the sole source for epidemiologic data regarding the psychiatric disability secondary to "combat fatigue" in the theater. It also provides the only data regarding the dominant patterns of pharmacologic treatment of combat fatigue, at least among outpatients.[46]

Description of the Study

In July 1967, as combat intensity in Vietnam was nearing its peak, Johnson, senior Army psychiatrist in Vietnam (the USARV Psychiatry Consultant), surveyed Army primary care physicians and psychiatrists in Vietnam regarding the psychotropic drugs they had prescribed for outpatients during the previous month. The primary care physician target group (233) consisted of all Army physicians in Vietnam who were serving in 1st echelon medical roles, for example, as battalion surgeons in combat units, or in dispensaries providing care for support and service-support troops. These physicians had undergone a range of general and specialized medical training before assignment in Vietnam. The psychiatrist target group consisted of all Army psychiatrists assigned in Vietnam (21).

It also included two Navy psychiatrists who were providing specialized care for Marine combat divisions because their role was analogous to the Army division psychiatrists. One-hundred and ten (47%) primary care physicians and eight (35%) psychiatrists participated in the study.

Selected Study Findings

There were many important findings from this survey that pertained generally to treatment of stress in the Vietnam combat zone in mid-1967. For instance, the overall outpatient psychotropic drug prescription rate for Army troops treated by the two respondent groups was 126 per 1,000 troops year (ie, one of every eight soldiers assigned in Vietnam). However, when the prescriptions written for Compazine (for "gastroenteritis") and Serpasil (for hypertension) are removed from the analysis—medications not utilized primarily as psychotropic agents—the psychotropic prescription rate drops to 86.4 per 1,000 troops per year (ie, one of every 11.5 soldiers assigned in Vietnam). The most frequently treated psychiatric condition was anxiety, which was mostly treated with minor tranquilizers (ie, anxiolytic medications: Equanil/Miltown, Librium, Valium, Vistaril, and Atarax). Insomnia was next in frequency, treated with sedatives/hypnotics. At the other extreme, depression was surprisingly low in frequency. (Selected survey findings not exclusively pertaining to combat fatigue will be presented in more detail in Chapter 8.)

Combat fatigue, which was not defined in the study, was regarded as a subgroup of the anxiety category and accounted for 56 (12%) of the 464 cases of anxiety treated between the two groups of respondents during the month of the study. Notably, primary care physicians treated 44 (79%) of them. The pharmacologic agents preferred by both psychiatrists and primary care physicians for treatment of this condition were the major tranquilizers, primarily Thorazine (Mellaril and Stelazine were also available); 64% of combat fatigue cases were treated with this family of medications. The daily dosages of Thorazine ranged from 20 mg to 300 mg—usually limited to a 3-day period, but six cases were treated on a "take as needed" basis. Minor tranquilizers were next in preference for combat fatigue, but no information was provided on the percent of combat fatigue cases receiving these medications. The most commonly prescribed was Librium, with the daily dose ranging from 30 mg to 40 mg. The typical

EXHIBIT 7-4. Use of Pharmaceuticals to Bolster Combat Performance

During the Vietnam War, the growing popularity of the new tranquilizing drugs for the reduction of combat stress symptoms ultimately provoked interest in the prophylactic use of those and other psychoactive compounds under combat circumstances—the so-called brave pill. But should the pharmacologic reduction of hyperarousal in anticipation of enemy contact, or even in response to it, be regarded as a compromise of medical ethics? For the military physician in the field, the boundary between prescribing a drug for clinical purposes versus for the enhancement of soldier performance in battle is not easily determined. Franklin Del Jones, a senior Army psychiatrist, provided the following commentary regarding these challenges in his 1995 chapter, "Psychiatric Principles of Future Warfare," in *War Psychiatry*.

If a drug can help [soldiers] sustain unit cohesion, good training, and good sense in the face of otherwise over-whelming fatigue or arousal, with an acceptable risk of other harmful effects, is it ethical to withhold it? Undoubtedly alcohol was the first drug [in modern times] to be utilized for such purposes. When Holland became a major source of gin, the widespread use of this alcoholic beverage by soldiers led to the expression "Dutch courage" to express the desired effect. [However] the ancient Assyrians, Egyptians, and Greeks reportedly utilized opiates before and during battles to sustain or enhance bravery and courage.[1]

Edmund G Howe and Jones, in their 1994 chapter, "Ethical Issues in Combat Psychiatry," in *Military Psychiatry: Preparing in Peace for War*, also noted that

. . . Vikings of the first millennium often fought after being intoxicated on mead (beer made from honey), and during the middle ages, armies often went into battle intoxicated. As late as World War II, Japanese troops sometimes prepared themselves for final, desperate banzai charges with saki. A medieval Moslem sect gave the word "assassin" to the English language because of its members' use of hashish (they were called "hashishim") before they were sent to kill their leader's critics. Like alcohol, cannabis can seriously impair combat performance, and it is unclear whether the hashishim were still "stoned" as they committed the assassinations or just convinced that they had experienced, briefly, the paradise that was to be their eternal reward.[2]

prescription length for Librium for combat fatigue was 2 or 3 days, and it was not prescribed on a "take as needed" basis. Primary care physicians were generally more satisfied regarding treatment outcome; they rated the result on 75% of their combat fatigue treatments as excellent/good, 22% as fair/satisfactory, and only 3% as no improvement. In contrast, the psychiatrists rated treatment outcome only 25% as excellent/good and 75% as fair/satisfactory. Some of this difference would be expected because the psychiatric specialists should be treating the more difficult cases.

Study Conclusions

Among its many findings, the study indicated that primary care physicians served a major role in the first line of defense against psychological breakdown of combat troops (they reported treating four combat fatigue cases for every one treated by psychiatrists, which mirrored the Korean War estimate in Table 7-2), and that pharmacotherapy was perceived as very effective (97% received at least satisfactory

improvement designation). More generally, neuroleptic and anxiolytic medications, which were prescribed by both groups, appeared to be instrumental in soldier recovery and return-to-duty function.

However, some survey results led Datel and Johnson to a peculiar conclusion: whereas they reported that "across condition and across drug, the prescribing physicians were of the opinion that psychotropic drug treatment was by and large quite influential in reducing the problems,"[46(p10)] in a separate publication Johnson acknowledged that the study demonstrated that much of the prescribing of psychoactive drugs was unwitting as these medications were frequently prescribed "for apparently emotional conditions even when this was not immediately obvious to the patient *or the physician* [emphasis added]."[51(p339)] He was especially referring to the finding that Compazine, a phenothiazine neuroleptic that accounted for 45% of all psychotropic prescriptions written by the primary care physicians, was for reported gastrointestinal irritability, which Johnson assumed was generated in large part by combat and deployment

EXHIBIT 7-4. Use of Pharmaceuticals to Bolster Combat Performance, continued

Jones discussed this further, noting that:

... Other drugs studied or used to enhance combat performance include ergot alkaloids, cannabis, amphetamine and other stimulants; Dramamine and other antihistamines; benzodiazepines; and L-tryptophan. It is the author's contention that the most extensive modern use of performance enhancing drugs occurred among Soviet personnel during World War II shortly after amphetamine was synthesized. Amphetamine was useful not only to stave off fatigue and drowsiness but also to improve memory and concentration, particularly among Soviet pilots.

During the Vietnam conflict, methylphenidate (Ritalin) and sometimes dextroamphetamine (Dexedrine) were standard issue drugs carried by long-range reconnaissance patrol (LRRP) soldiers. The LRRPs found the most efficacious use to be upon completion of a mission when fatigue had developed and rapid return to the base camp was desirable. Other than mild rebound depression and fatigue after the drug was discontinued, no adverse effects were reported. Other investigators studying the drug abuse problem later in the Vietnam conflict reported problems with abuse of these stimulants. Although there was no documented abuse of the morphine syrettes, commanders suggested such abuse might be occurring, causing them to be withdrawn from the soldiers.

Sedatives have also been studied as a method to improve performance in anxiety-producing situations such as paratroopers making low-altitude jumps or for reducing the emotional tension of young soldiers during the firing of guns. Reports of improved target accuracy through use of the ß adrenergic blocker, propranolol, and the anxiolytic, diazepam (Valium), have resulted in a US Army ban on use of these drugs by soldiers engaged in marksmanship competition because they would confer an unfair advantage.

[On the side of psychopharmacology for therapeutic use] the most consistent symptom of combat stress, whether occurring early in exposure to combat or after cumulative exposure, is anxiety. Such anxiety may be manifested by [excessive] fear, hysterical conversion or dissociation, tremors, and similar symptoms. In the past, these conditions have been treated with sedatives ranging from chloral hydrate and bromides in World War I to barbiturates in World War II and even self-prescribed alcohol, cannabis, and heroin in Vietnam. These drugs often not only produced unwanted sedation but also decreased the probability of return to combat due to the fixation of a sickness role suggested by taking medication. In the Vietnam conflict, neuroleptics (antipsychotic or major tranquilizer drugs) were widely utilized for psychotropic effects, but benzodiazepines were also used. But are such drugs safe, especially in the highly unpredictable and unstable physical, logistical, and emotional context of combat?[1]

REFERENCES
1. Jones FD. Psychiatric principles of future warfare. In: Jones FD, Sparacino LR, Wilcox VL, Rothberg JM, Stokes JW, eds. *War Psychiatry.* In: Zajtchuk R, Bellamy RF, eds. *Textbooks of Military Medicine.* Washington, DC: Department of the Army, Office of The Surgeon General, Borden Institute; 1995: 125–126.
2. Howe EG, Jones FD. Ethical issues in combat psychiatry. In: Jones FD, Sparacino LR, Wilcox VL, Rothberg JM, eds. *Military Psychiatry: Preparing in Peace for War.* In: Zajtchuk R, Bellamy RF, eds. *Textbooks of Military Medicine.* Washington, DC: Department of the Army, Office of The Surgeon General, Borden Institute; 1994: 121.

stress.[51] In other words, by these measures many soldiers were affected by combat stress- and combat theater-generated psychophysiologic disorders, but the specific nature of their difficulties remained obscure to the clinicians. Although the investigators failed to distinguish between combat and noncombat troops (this obviously was not a problem in the analysis of the data regarding combat exhaustion), their findings appear to bolster the speculation that there may have been large numbers of combat-exposed troops in Vietnam who sustained unrecognized, low-grade, psychiatric and psychosomatic symptoms (ie, suggesting partial trauma or strain trauma).

Study Limitations

Although Datel and Johnson acknowledged that their study had many shortcomings, their findings are the best data available in confirming the overall popularity of the new psychotropic medications for the outpatient treatment of various psychiatric and related conditions in the Vietnam theater, including combat-generated ones. In addition to its failure to include an operational definition of combat fatigue, the study's other limitations included that: (*a*) although it was limited to outpatient care, it did not distinguish whether soldier-patients were kept at duty during their treatment; (*b*) no data were collected that addressed the presence, if not the relative value, of other treatment elements; and especially important, (c) no attempt was made to monitor the effects of these medications on duty performance, especially performance in combat. It is possible that combat performance was enhanced (Exhibit 7-4). It is also possible that combat performance was diminished through slowed reaction times, reduced concentration, or interference with marksmanship.

The Palinkas and Coben Study Correlating Psychiatric Hospitalization and Wounding Among Marines

Regarding the possibility that some psychoactive medications may have reduced combat performance in Vietnam, the postwar study conducted by Palinkas and Coben is intriguing because it suggested that psychiatric treatment, at least hospital treatment there, could have compromised combat performance for some diagnoses. Although the study involved US Marines, it could have implications for Army troops because of their similar missions.

Palinkas and Coben explored the association between hospitalization rates for injury or wounding in action (N = 78,756) and hospitalization rates for psychiatric reasons (N = 8,835) among Marines deployed over the course of the war (1965–1972). Among those who were wounded in action, 2,369 (3%) also had a record of psychiatric hospitalization; furthermore, psychiatric hospitalization was significantly associated with an increased risk of becoming wounded. The wounding incident most often followed the psychiatric hospitalization and tended to occur within the subsequent 4 months. The sole demographic/service characteristic that distinguished those hospitalized for psychiatric reasons from other wounded Marines was that a greater proportion came from the lowest military ranks. Among the psychiatric hospitalization group, the increased risk for wounding was primarily among those diagnosed with social maladjustment, psychosomatic conditions, "nervous and debility," transient situational disturbance, and acute situational maladjustment.

In contrast, the risk of becoming wounded was lower for those with diagnoses of schizophrenia, anxiety neurosis, and depressive neurosis, but this was explained as the consequence of the policy of evacuating patients with these diagnoses to other treatment facilities out of the combat zone. Notably, risk for becoming wounded after psychiatric hospitalization was also lower for the

243 Marines who received the specific diagnosis of combat fatigue, despite the fact that they typically were returned to their units and combat duty. However, the reduced risk among this subset may have reflected a tendency for Navy psychiatrists to strictly reserve the combat fatigue diagnosis for those without evident predisposing personality deficits.[52,53,54(Table 4-3)]

Hypothesizing a Link Between the Forward Treatment Doctrine, Psychotropic Medications, and Reduced Combat Performance

Taken together these two studies suggest an important question: Is it possible that some treatments received by soldiers with combat-related psychiatric symptoms in Vietnam may have negatively affected subsequent combat performance? More specifically, are there grounds to speculate on a link between the findings of liberal psychopharmacotherapy of Army combat soldiers and the overrepresentation among the wounded of some classes of psychiatrically hospitalized Marines who were returned to duty? (Some publications by Navy physicians indicated that their treatment approach coincided with the Army doctrine, including the extensive use of modern psychotropic medications.[53,54]) If so, it could prompt reconsideration of earlier assumptions as to the salutary effects of symptom suppression among combat troops, especially if it includes prescribing psychotropic medications (at least when there is not a critical military necessity for recovering psychiatric patients to be utilized as replacements). On the other hand, Datel and Johnson's failure to indicate if the soldier-patients continued to be exposed to combat or inquire about drug effects on combat performance, and Palinkas and Coben's omission of the specific elements included in the hospital treatment received by the Marines, render such a conclusion highly speculative.

Current Army doctrine permits the prescribing of psychotropic medications during combat operations if it is to return psychiatrically ill soldiers to their premorbid level of functioning rather than to *enhance* (emphasis added) baseline performance. In a recent review of the subject it was noted that the medications now available in the field are dramatically superior to those available in Vietnam, especially in having significantly lower side effects. However, there was no mention made of the possibility of long-term effects from symptom suppression.[61]

TABLE 7-3. Combat Psychiatrist Participants Reporting Clinical Experience With Combat Stress Reaction Cases, By Symptom Duration Levels (N = 47)

Combat Stress Reaction (CSR) Symptom Duration Level	Number of Psychiatrists	Percentage
Experience with acute CSR cases only (symptoms present < 2 days)	4	8.5%
Experience with extended CSR cases only (symptoms present 2–5 days)	5	10.6%
Experience with persistent CSR cases only (symptoms present > 5 days)	5	10.6%
Experience with both acute and extended CSR cases	11	23.4%
Experience with both extended and persistent CSR cases	11	23.4%
Experience with acute, extended and persistent CSR cases	11	23.4%
TOTAL	47	100.0%

WALTER REED ARMY INSTITUTE OF RESEARCH PSYCHIATRIST SURVEY FINDINGS: TREATMENT OF COMBAT STRESS REACTIONS IN VIETNAM

The following material extends the presentation that was begun in Chapter 5 of findings from the 1982 WRAIR postwar survey of psychiatrists who served with the Army in Vietnam. To explore their recollections of what was done in the theater for combat stress-affected troops, survey participants were asked a series of questions about the treatment of CSR cases in general as well as about treatment of specific symptoms. The responses presented in this section are limited to the roughly two-thirds of survey participants who acknowledged having some experience treating combat stress reaction cases. Subgroup analyses to test for effects of primary differences between respondent psychiatrists pertaining to war era, site of psychiatric training (civilian or military), or combat unit assignment in Vietnam (vs with a hospital) were precluded by small sample sizes. For this section only, respondents will be referred to as combat psychiatrists to distinguish them from the larger group of survey respondents.

Two Dimensions of Combat Stress Reactions Pertaining to Treatment: Severity of Symptoms and Duration of Symptoms

Severity of Combat Stress Reaction Symptoms

As a general reference, combat psychiatrist participants were provided an operational definition of the CSR adapted from Bartimier et al from World War II (refer back to Table 6-1). In this schema, symptoms associated with "normal fear" are listed, followed by those for combat stress reaction according to stages of severity: "incipient," "partial," and "complete" disorganization/dysfunction. Some survey questions utilized this symptom severity-based definition.

Duration of Combat Stress Reaction Symptoms

Some questions in the survey regarding CSR severity were crosscut by others concerning symptom duration, that is, the length of the soldier's disability. These questions utilized a schedule of three symptom duration levels adapted from observations of Albert J Glass in the Korean theater: (1) acute (symptoms less than 2 days), (2) extended (symptoms lasting between 2 to 5 days), and (3) persistent (symptoms lasting more than 5 days).[62] These distinctions also roughly coincide with the medical/psychiatric care echelon system. CSR symptom duration is obviously partly a function of severity, but it also may vary because of differences between individual soldiers or as a function of the treatments provided.

Breadth of Psychiatrists' Experiences With Combat Stress Reaction Cases by Symptom Duration Level

The WRAIR combat psychiatrist participants were asked if they treated combat stress reaction cases, or supervised their treatment, according to the three symptom duration levels, regardless of the setting where this treatment took place. According to their responses, the combat psychiatrist participants fell into one of six possible categories.

TABLE 7-4. Congruence of Combat Stress Reaction Symptom Duration Levels and Army Medical Care Echelons: Means of Combat Psychiatrist Participants Frequency of Experience With Combat Stress Reaction Cases, By Echelon of Care and By Combat Stress Reaction Symptom Duration Level (N = 47)

Medical Care Echelon	Combat Stress Reaction (CSR) Symptom Duration Level		
	Acute CSR (symptoms < 2 days) n = 26	Extended CSR (symptoms = 2–5 days) n = 38	Persistent CSR (symptoms > 5 days) n = 27
1st echelon care setting (battalion aid stations) n = 15		1.67*	1.67*
2nd echelon care setting (division clearing stations) n = 30	2.77		2.21
3rd echelon care setting (hospitals or psych detachments) n = 30	2.48	3.08	

Combat psychiatrist participants were asked about frequency of treatment of combat stress reaction cases in each echelon in which they had experience: Extent of agreement along a 1-to-5 point scale from 1 = very seldom to 5 = very frequent. Empty cells denote where full congruence between echelon care setting and symptom duration was assumed.
*Participants were asked simultaneously about frequency of treating both extended and persistent cases at the 1st echelon care setting.

As Table 7-3 indicates, 47 combat psychiatrist participants reported a wide range of experience in treating combat stress reaction cases in Vietnam. Interestingly, only a quarter of them (11) reported treating cases representing all three symptom-duration levels despite the policy of rotating psychiatrists from field assignments (ie, division psychiatrist) to those with the hospitals. The finding that all did not have such experiences could be a function of the lower incidence of combat stress reaction cases in Vietnam. In addition, it could be a consequence of the previously noted limitations in psychiatrist assignment types through the course of the war (ie, at most, only two-thirds of psychiatrists in a given year could be rotated between combat and hospital assignments, and, as it turned out, even fewer were).

Perceived Effectiveness in Treating Combat Reaction Cases by Echelon of Medical/Psychiatric Care

Combat psychiatrist participants were asked to rate the overall success in the treatment of combat reaction cases for each of the three echelons of medical/psychiatric care based on their knowledge or experience. More specifically they were asked how frequently soldiers referred for combat-related symptoms were successfully treated and returned to combat duty within the timeframe associated with a particular treatment echelon (extent of agreement along a 1-to-5 point scale from 1 = very seldom to 5 = very frequent). Response means were as follows: 1st echelon care, that is, in the battalion aid stations = 3.76 (N = 26); 2nd echelon care, that is, in the division clearing stations = 3.92 (N = 38); and 3rd echelon care, that is, in the psychiatric specialty detachments = 3.35 (N = 27). Overall the trends represented in these findings are in the favorable direction, that is they suggest more success than non-success, because all means are > 3. Although it is consistent with the anecdotal data for treatment success for 1st and 2nd echelon care to be more frequent than that for 3rd echelon care, the prospect that treatment efficacy was more frequent for 2nd echelon care over 1st echelon care is not. The likely explanation is that respondents were not as familiar with the scope of outcomes at the 1st echelon level because they did not typically work at that level of care; they only supervised some of the social work/psychology technicians who did.

Congruence of Combat Stress Reaction Symptom Duration Levels and Army Medical Care Echelons

According to the doctrine of Army medical care in Vietnam, the level of pathology and the echelon of care should have generally coincided, that is, 1st echelon care (within the unit or at the battalion aid station) should treat mostly "acute" CSR cases; 2nd echelon care (in the

FIGURE 7-3. Means of combat psychiatrist participants' estimates of frequency of usefulness of treatments for combat stress reaction (CSR) according to major treatment categories, by symptom duration level (N = 32) [combat psychiatrist participants were asked extent of agreement along a 1-to-5 point scale from seldom useful to often useful].

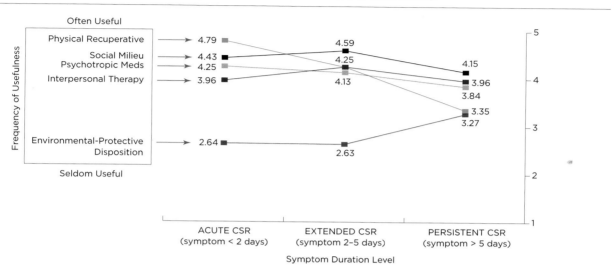

Interpersonal: counseling, catharsis, individual or group therapy, narcosynthesis
Social: ward milieu, military environment, staff expectancy of return to duty, contact with unit or home
Physical recuperative: safety, sleep, nourishment, hydration, rest, recreation, treatment for wounds or disease
Environmental-protective disposition: return to duty in noncombat position or to less stressful unit, evacuation out of the area of risk or out of Vietnam
Psychotropic meds: anxiolytics, neuroleptics, antidepressants, sedatives

division clearing station at the brigade or division base) should treat mostly "extended" CSR cases; and 3rd echelon care (in evacuation or field hospitals in Vietnam, especially those with psychiatric specialty detachments) should treat mostly "persistent" CSR cases. In order to explore the congruence between the echelon of medical care where CSR cases were treated and the symptom duration levels of the soldiers treated there, combat psychiatrist participants were asked a series of questions regarding their recollections of divergence from this schema. Table 7-4 presents a summary of their responses to these questions.

The following is an interpretation of the responses to this series of questions:

- *1st echelon care* (the battalion aid station): 15 combat psychiatrist participants reported having direct clinical contact with acute CSR cases at the battalion aid stations or were involved with technical supervision of the treatment of cases there. These psychiatrists confirmed that most soldier-patients usually remained there only 1 to 2 days. Those who did not recover sufficiently to be returned to duty by that time (ie, extended and persistent cases) were very seldom held longer and were evacuated to the next echelon of care.

- *2nd echelon care* (the brigade/division clearing station): 30 combat psychiatrist participants reported having some experience at the division clearing stations and confirmed that the CSR referrals seen there were usually extended cases (symptoms 2–5 days). Although their treatment of acute cases was in the range of seldom (ie, seldom bypassed the battalion aid stations), it approached intermediate. On the other hand, they seldom kept patients longer than 5 days (ie, persistent cases) as opposed to evacuating them beyond the division to a 3rd echelon, hospital/psychiatric specialty detachment.

- *3rd echelon care* (hospitals with psychiatric specialty detachments): 27 combat psychiatrist participants reported some experience in this setting and confirmed that most CSR cases treated there were persistent cases (symptoms > 5 days). They

FIGURE 7-4. Means of combat psychiatrist participants' estimates of perceived frequency of usefulness of interpersonal treatment elements for combat stress reaction (CSR), by symptom duration level (N = 31) [combat psychiatrist participants were asked extent of agreement along a 1-to-5 point scale from seldom useful to often useful].

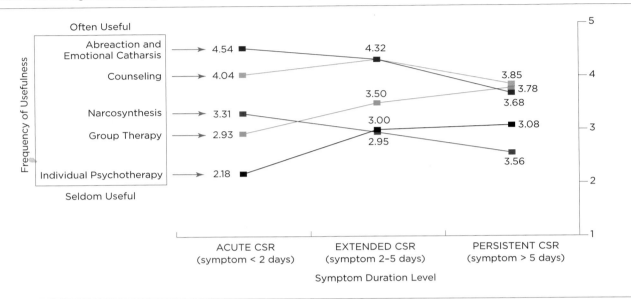

Abreaction and emotional catharsis: therapist mostly listens and offers sympathy and support
Counseling: above plus reassurance, encouragement, information, inspiration, exhortation
Individual psychotherapy: both of the above, but includes interpretation of psychological conflicts
Group psychotherapy
Narcosynthesis: use of short-acting barbiturate to facilitate recall, abreaction, and reintegration

also reported that they seldom treated acute CSR cases (ie, those evacuated directly from the field), but that they frequently treated extended CSR cases (ie, those who bypassed the division clearing station after receiving some nonspecialized care at a battalion aid station/1st echelon care setting).

Although these responses support a conclusion of overall congruence of treatment echelon and CSR symptom duration, they also suggest a more fluid situation than would be anticipated from a strict implementation of the Army medical treatment and evacuation doctrine in Vietnam. In other words, these responses suggest that in practice there was some reduction in the "proximity" management principle for combat reactions in Vietnam. This was undoubtedly the consequence of the growing utilization of air ambulance and "dustoff" helicopters for medical evacuation, which facilitated casualties of all types, bypassing battalion aid stations and even division medical facilities to reach the surgical, field, and evacuation hospitals.[48,63] Deviation

from the anticipated CSR symptom duration/treatment echelon match could also be partly accounted for by the fact that the four independent brigades operating in Vietnam did not have dedicated psychiatrist positions.

Perceived Value of Major Treatment Categories for Combat Stress Reactions

Combat psychiatrist participants were asked to rate the perceived value of five major treatment categories for each of the three combat stress reaction (CSR) symptom duration levels. The results are presented in Figure 7-3. Major treatment categories included:

- physical recuperative (safety, sleep, nourishment, hydration, rest, recreation, treatment for wounds or disease);
- pharmacologic (anxiolytics, neuroleptics, antidepressants, sedatives);
- social (ward milieu, military environment, staff expectancy of return to duty, contact with unit or home);

TABLE 7-5. Means of Combat Psychiatrist Participants' Estimates of Effectiveness in Providing Direct Interpersonal Treatment for Combat Stress Reaction Symptoms by Provider Type [N = 29–40]

Personnel Type	Perceived effectiveness
1. Psychiatrist	4.33
2. Enlisted psychology/social work specialist (91-G)	4.08
3. Social work officer	3.89
4. Enlisted inpatient corpsman (91-F)	3.8
5. Psychiatric nurse	3.47
6. Buddy	3.41
7. General medical officer	3.35
8. Line medic (91-B, C)	3.35
9. Psychologist	3.11
10. Leader (officer, NCO, squad leader, etc.)	3.10

Combat psychiatrist participants were asked extent of agreement along a 1-to-5 point scale from "seldom effective" to "often effective."
NCO: noncommissioned officer

- interpersonal therapy (counseling, catharsis, individual or group therapy, narcosynthesis); and
- environmental-protective disposition (return to noncombat duty position or to less stressful unit, evacuation out of area of risk or out of Vietnam).

The trends in the responses to this set of questions regarding efficacy of major treatment categories for combat stress reaction cases by symptom level suggest that:

- with little to distinguish them from each other, interpersonal treatment, pharmacotherapy, and therapeutic social milieu, which included maintenance of a military context and staff "expectancy" of rapid return to duty, were highly valued for all symptom duration levels;
- physically recuperative measures were valued most for acute cases and progressively less so as symptoms prolonged; and
- environmental-protective dispositions, such as reassignment of the soldier to a noncombat position or evacuation out of the combat area, were seen as the least useful until the stage of persistent cases, but even then they lagged behind most of the other types of interventions in value.

Apart from the unprecedented high value for pharmacotherapy compared to earlier wars, these responses appear to be generally consistent with the principles that comprised the pre-Vietnam doctrine. The high value for pharmacotherapy, however, does mean that mode of intervention was no longer limited in use because of presumed high risk, but was one that was perceived as synergistic with interpersonal and therapeutic social milieu treatments. Thus, in practice in Vietnam there was a substantial alteration of the "simplicity" doctrine principle.

Perceived Value of Interpersonal Treatments for Combat Stress Reaction

Combat psychiatrist participants were asked to rate the perceived value of five subcategories of therapist-provided treatments for the three CSR symptom duration levels. The results are presented in Figure 7-4. Therapist-provided treatments included:

- abreaction and emotional catharsis (therapist mostly listens and offers sympathy and support);
- counseling (above plus reassurance, encouragement, information, inspiration, exhortation);
- individual psychotherapy (both of the above, but includes interpretation of psychological conflicts);
- group psychotherapy; and
- narcosynthesis (use of short-acting barbiturate to facilitate recall, abreaction, and reintegration).

FIGURE 7-5. Prescription patterns for neuroleptic tranquilizing medications—Stelazine, Mellaril, oral Thorazine—and parenteral Thorazine (principally intramuscular, or IM)—in the treatment of combat stress reactions: Percent of combat psychiatrist participants who endorsed use ("commonly prescribed"), by symptom severity stages (N = 47). [The slopes for each drug represent averages across the three symptom duration levels.]

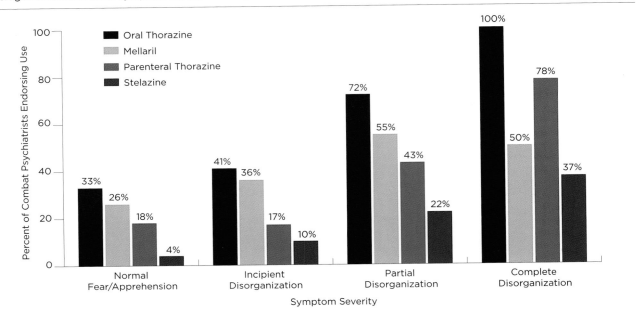

For acute cases, counseling, as well as guided abreaction/emotional catharsis (ie, facilitating the soldier's remembering and ventilating feelings surrounding the disturbing combat events), are the two interventions valued highest; and these are followed by narcosynthesis. Collectively their high rating is consistent with the belief that the acute combat stress reaction is a reversible bio\psycho\social crisis that responds favorably to a guided, supported, psychoemotional decompression. As symptoms prolong, these treatment categories become somewhat less valued (especially narcosynthesis), whereas deeper, more challenging treatments rise in value (ie, group and individual therapy, but somewhat more so with group therapy). This shift is consistent with the assumption that the more prolonged symptomatology includes a greater degree of pre-Vietnam personality susceptibility.

Perceived Differences Between Types of Therapists in Treatment Effectiveness With Soldiers With Combat Stress Reactions

Combat psychiatrist participants were asked to rate the perceived value of 10 types of "therapists" for soldiers experiencing combat stress symptoms regardless of setting. The results are presented in Table 7-5. Although it may not be surprising that survey participants rated themselves as the most effective, it is notable that they acknowledged the high value of the social work/psychology (91G) technicians and the in-patient (91F) technicians—enlisted corpsmen with specialized training who served a direct and vital role in supporting the recovery of soldiers in Vietnam. Also rated very high are the social work officers, which serves to validate their extremely important and generally unsung contribution to the provision of mental healthcare in Vietnam as well. Apart from the psychologists, it is generally understandable that the groups ranked in the top half of the results (1–5) were those with specialized psychiatric training before Vietnam. As for psychologists, they were invariably ranked low because at most only two were assigned in Vietnam per year (with the KO teams), and they usually had other professional responsibilities such as psychological testing. Most of the survey psychiatrists would not have worked with a psychologist in Vietnam. Meanings for the results pertaining to the other groups are subject to speculation.

FIGURE 7-6. Prescription patterns for anxiolytic tranquilizing medications (Valium and Librium) in the treatment of combat stress reactions. Percent of combat psychiatrist participants who endorsed use ("commonly prescribed"), by symptom severity stages (N = 47). [The slopes for each drug represent averages across the three symptom duration levels.]

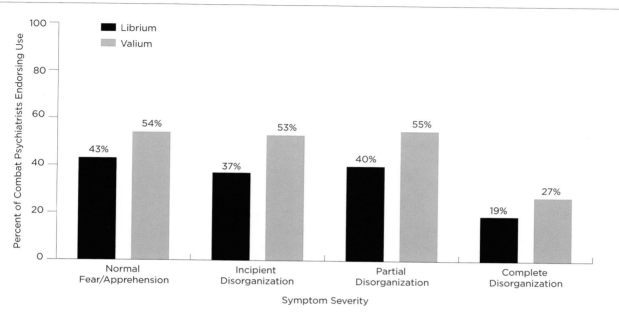

FIGURE 7-7. Prescription patterns for the sedative chloral hydrate, and the tricyclic antidepressant Tofranil in the treatment of combat stress reactions: Percent of combat psychiatrist participants who endorse use ("commonly prescribed"), by symptom severity stages (N = 47) [The slopes for each drug represent averages across the three symptom duration levels.]

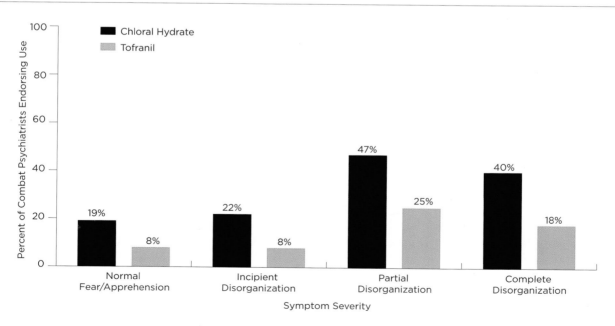

FIGURE 7-8. Recollections of patterns for psychotropic medications "routinely prescribed" for soldiers returned to duty following treatment for combat stress reactions (CSR): Percent of combat psychiatrist participants endorsing use, by symptom duration level (N = 47).

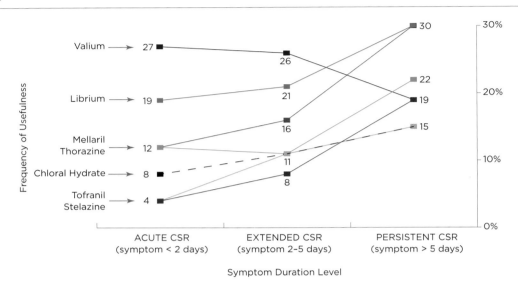

Perceived Use of Pharmacotherapy for Combat Stress Reactions

Figures 7-5, 7-6, and 7-7 summarize findings from survey questions regarding the use of psychotropic medications for soldiers with combat stress reactions by symptom severity and by symptom duration level. Although the combat psychiatrist participants were provided a list of 21 medications that were known to have been available at various times during the war, most acknowledged use of only 12, with seven representing the overwhelming majority. To simplify the presentation, findings for the seven drugs are grouped into three sets: (1) neuroleptics, (2) anxiolytics, and (3) "other," which are set against symptom severity levels. Results by symptom duration were very similar; therefore they were averaged to determine the slopes for each drug. A few participants also made scattered references to prescribing Nembutal, phenobarbital, and amytal. Questions regarding dosages did not produce useable patterns. None of the respondents indicated they prescribed stimulant medications. (Some respondents may have been affected by shortages or unavailability of specific medications, but for lack of data no attempt was made to account for this variable.)

Overall, results presented in Figures 7-5, 7-6, and 7-7 again substantiate that the combat psychiatrist participants highly valued psychotropic medications, especially the neuroleptics and anxiolytics, in the treatment of soldiers with normal fear/apprehension and with combat stress reactions of all stages. Some of the salient findings are as follows:

- In general, the combat psychiatrist participants endorsed increasing use of neuroleptic tranquilizers —Mellaril, Stelazine, and especially Thorazine—as levels of soldier symptoms exceeded normal fear/ apprehension and incipient disorganization.
- For normal fear/apprehension, anxiolytic medications—Valium and Librium—in that order, were preferred.
- For incipient disorganization, there is some overlap in preference for anxiolytic and neuroleptic medications, but Valium was the leader.
- Use of the tricyclic antidepressant Tofranil and the sedative/hypnotic chloral hydrate, obviously targeting different symptoms, were not highly endorsed for normal fear/apprehension and incipient disorganization, increased some as symptoms levels progressed into partial disorganization, but lost favor to Thorazine and Mellaril once the level of complete disorganization was reached.

FIGURE 7-9. Combat stress reaction (CSR) case recovery with return to duty, and relapse after return to duty: Means of combat psychiatrist participants' estimates, by symptom duration level (N = 23–37). [Combat psychiatrist participants were asked to indicate frequency regarding: (a) recovery and return to duty within symptom duration level time limits; and (b) relapse after return to duty, using a 1-to-5 point scale from 1 = very seldom to 5 = very frequent].

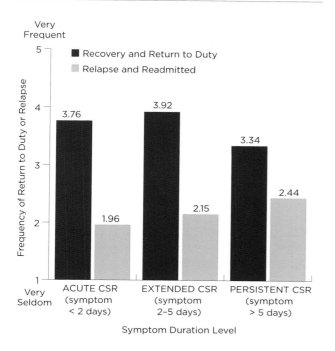

- At the level of complete disorganization, the top five medications were endorsed in the following order: oral Thorazine (100%), parenteral Thorazine—the only neuroleptic available in Vietnam in injectable form (78%), Mellaril (50%), chloral hydrate (40%), and Stelazine (37%).

Perceived Value of Maintenance Pharmacotherapy Following Treatment for Combat Stress Reaction and Return to Duty

Combat psychiatrist participants were asked whether soldiers treated for combat stress reaction were prescribed psychotropic drugs as maintenance medications upon being returned to combat duty. Specifically, they were provided a list of commonly available psychotropic medications and asked to "Indicate with a checkmark or dosage range/schedule those *maintenance* medications that were routinely

prescribed for the soldier who completed treatment and was returning to combat duty." Results are presented in Figure 7-8. Additional questions were asked as to whether there were any perceived influences on combat effectiveness from these medications; however, the responses were too variable for patterning.

Considering the inherent dangers and performance requirements for a combat soldier, it is quite striking that these medications were endorsed as maintenance medications to the extent suggested by Figure 7-8. Regarding acute CSR cases, the two anxiolytics were preferred over the other medications; however, inexplicably, these similarly acting drugs switched rankings as symptoms became more prolonged. Valium began as the leading medication (at 27%) but lost ground to Librium, with Librium ultimately ranked substantially higher for the persistent cases (at 30%, which equaled that of the neuroleptic Mellaril). Mellaril deserves special note as it was positioned relatively low for the acute CSR cases (at 12%, the same as Thorazine), but became the preferred neuroleptic for the persistent cases. The ranking for Thorazine rose in parallel with Mellaril for the extended cases, as did Stelazine, but both dropped below Mellaril, with Thorazine exceeding Stelazine. It can be speculated that, as previously noted, Mellaril was preferred for outpatients over the other neuroleptic drugs because it was thought to be less sedating than Thorazine and less activating than Stelazine. The nontranquilizer medications, the sedative chloral hydrate and the antidepressant Tofranil, also increased for the persistent cases, but they were ranked lowest (at 15%). Regarding the latter, low use of the antidepressant is consistent with the more general finding of Datel and Johnson that depression was not a common psychiatric complaint requiring treatment in Vietnam.

Combat Stress Reaction Treatment Effectiveness

Combat psychiatrist participants were asked a set of questions regarding recollections of frequency of return to duty, and of frequency of relapse after return to duty, for combat stress reaction cases from the standpoint of the three symptom duration levels: acute, extended, and persistent (regardless of treatment echelon where treatment was provided). Figure 7-9 presents the results.

The combat psychiatrist participants' responses regarding combat stress reaction treatment effectiveness presented in Figure 7-9 generally suggest an overall favorable outcome, but with a decline associated with the prolongation of symptoms. Recovery/return to duty

TABLE 7-6. Combat Psychiatrist Participants' Recollections of the Perceived Incidence of Specific Psychiatric Symptoms and Effective Psychotropic Medications

Symptoms Among Combat-Exposed Troops			Prescribing Patterns	
	Mean Incidence	N	n	% indicating use of specific drug or drug family*
5 = VERY COMMON				
"Short-timers" syndrome†	4.33	45	21	66% = Anxiolytic
4 = COMMON				
Threatened assault	3.66	47	24	45.8% = Neuroleptic 25% = Anxiolytic
Insomnia	3.64	44	22	27.3% = Barbiturate 22.7% = Anxiolytic
Anxiety dreams	3.53	45	23	43.5% = Anxiolytic 13% = Neuroleptic 13% = Sedative
Tension headaches	3.36	45	21	47.6% = Anxiolytic 28.6% = Analgesic
Musculoskeletal complaints	3.29	45	18	44.5% = Anxiolytic
Startle reactions	3.07	43	21	57.1% = Anxiolytic
3 = INTERMEDIATE				
Sleepwalking or talking	2.49	45	30	33.4% = Barbiturate 3.3% = Anxiolytic
Nausea, vomiting, diarrhea	2.36	44	15	33.4% = Anxiolytic 13.3% = Lomotil 13.3% = Compazine
Falling asleep on guard	2.34	44	4	No specifics
2 = UNCOMMON				
Hysterical amnesia	1.93	45	9	30% = Amytal interview 20% = Neuroleptic 20% = Anxiolytic
Hysterical deafness, aphonia	1.78	45	12	33% = Amytal (interview)
Narcolepsy	1.68	44	5	No specifics
Hysterical seizures	1.64	44	6	20% = Anxiolytic 16.7% = Anticonvulsant
Nocturnal enuresis	1.64	45	15	60% = Antidepressant
Hysterical stuttering	1.61	44	8	No specifics
Hysterical blurred vision	1.53	43	4	No specifics

The data presume absence of a primary physical cause. Regarding incidence, participants were asked to use a 1-to-5 point scale with:

1 = "very uncommon" to 5 = "very common." Regarding commonly prescribed medications for these conditions, an open-ended question was used. N = numbers of respondents who endorsed psychoactive medications in general for the condition or symptom.

* = Percentages listed are for the endorsement of specific drugs or drug families; the remaining prescribing respondents were vague or noncommittal

† = A low-grade form of disability often exhibited in combat soldiers within 4 to 6 weeks of their DEROS. Symptoms commonly consist of reduced combat tolerance and efficiency; preoccupation with fears about being killed; and sullen, irritable, or withdrawn behavior.

DEROS: date expected return overseas

was endorsed more frequently than not for all three symptom duration levels, that is, all means > 3, although the score decreased for persistent cases. Likewise, for those returned to duty, relapse was not frequently endorsed (ie, all means < 3), but again, it increased as symptom duration levels increased, especially for the persistent group.

Perceived Incidence of Specific Symptoms Among Combat-Exposed Troops and Perceived Value of Psychoactive Medications for Treatment

Combat psychiatrist participants were provided a list of 17 symptoms commonly seen among combat troops either in Vietnam or in wars preceding Vietnam and were asked to indicate their perceived incidence in Vietnam. They were also asked an open-ended question as to medications found useful in their treatment. The results are presented in Table 7-6. For presentation purposes, specific drugs were combined into drug families.

The trends presented in Table 7-6 indicate that the symptoms the combat psychiatrist participants recalled treating among combat-exposed troops were more often milder and less dramatic than those reported in earlier wars. This suggests that the stress levels sustained by US ground troops were lower (for reasons already discussed; see Chapter 6, Figure 6-4, and interpretation), which is consistent with strain trauma as opposed to shock trauma. These findings coincide with the impression that the lack of sustained fighting in Vietnam produced lowered acute stress levels and less overt psychiatric debility; however, social and cultural influences cannot be ruled out as also influencing the forms of symptomatic expression seen.

These results also reinforce the previously noted findings indicating the high prevalence of use of the new psychotropic medications in the treatment of psychiatric symptoms of all types in Vietnam. The most notable finding in Table 7-6 was that anxiolytic medications were preferred for the more common symptoms presenting among combat-exposed troops. The exception pertains to "threatened assault." By these results, this was a high-incidence behavior problem— and, of course, potentially dangerous—where the neuroleptics were preferred by almost 2:1.

SUMMARY AND CONCLUSIONS

The basic assumptions underlying the traditional combat psychiatry forward treatment doctrine can be summarized as:

- combat-related stress casualties have a common biologic\psychologic\social dynamic despite their often variable presentations—one that results from soldiers having sustained unique hardships, challenges, and personal assaults associated with putting ones life on the line to accomplish the military objective;
- they typically represent a temporary, if extreme, natural reaction to overwhelming combat stress and fatigue; and
- they can be clinically addressed in a unitary fashion.

Based on these assumptions, when the United States entered the war in Vietnam, Army psychiatry advocated an empirically derived set of management and treatment principles intended to quickly restore soldiers to their premorbid state of function (PIES). These included (presented in their logical order as opposed to the acronym sequence): elemental treatments, such as safety, rest, replenishment, assisted anamnesis, reassurance, encouragement, and the conservative use of psychotropic medications ("simplicity"); applied as rapidly as possible ("immediacy"); as close to the soldier's unit and the fighting as the tactical situation permitted ("proximity"); and surrounded by a collective expectation that the soldier should quickly recover, resume his military job, and perform his duty ("expectancy").

This chapter reviewed the available psychiatric and related documentation from the war, as well as selected responses from the WRAIR survey of veteran Army psychiatrists, to characterize the treatment that was provided in the theater for soldiers who developed these conditions. Although the incidence of frank combat stress reactions in Vietnam was perhaps only a quarter or less of that found in earlier, high-intensity wars, nonetheless the medical and psychiatric personnel there were often clinically challenged by these and related conditions. Impressions derived from this review are summarized as follows:

- **Because of the relatively low numbers of soldiers disabled with classical combat reaction and other** combat stress-generated psychiatric conditions compared to earlier wars, there was apparently little concern by the Army that this medical/psychiatric problem could compromise its combat capability. There is no greater proof for this than the observation that the only published summary of the US Army medical experience in Vietnam did not include statistics for combat exhaustion or even mention combat-generated psychopathology in any context. This meant that the medical requirement for limiting psychiatric attrition among combat units to "conserve the fighting strength" did not dominate clinical decision making there.

- **The treatment approaches of the psychiatrists and allied medical and mental health personnel who provided care for the troops with combat stress symptoms roughly coincided with the traditional treatment doctrine; there appears to be ample documentation of favorable treatment results.** This is despite inconsistencies in the dissemination of a protocol for the combat psychiatry forward treatment doctrine to the assigned primary care physicians and psychiatrists and growing stateside opposition to the war and psychiatric cooperation with the US military. Although satisfaction in this record must be tempered by the inadequate documentation of the care provided in the last third of the war, findings from the WRAIR survey help to offset the omission and further validate these impressions.

- **In providing treatment for soldiers with combat stress symptoms, adapting to the circumstances in Vietnam meant that the doctrine's principles of "immediacy" and "expectancy" were generally upheld, but "proximity" was substantially reduced by the ubiquity of heliborne medevacuation, and "simplicity" was dramatically altered by the use of the new tranquilizing medications.**

  - Regarding proximity—the ease of helicopter medical transport apparently meant that a somewhat greater proportion of acute combat exhaustion cases were treated at 2nd echelon/division psychiatry facilities (compared with Korea). Similarly, a greater proportion of acute and extended combat exhaustion cases were treated at the 3rd echelon/psychiatric specialty detachments. However, there is no evidence that soldiers who were treated geographically more remote from their units had a more difficult or protracted clinical course than in the past, perhaps also because of the availability of helicopter transport (ie, units could more easily maintain ties with hospitalized soldiers).

  - Regarding simplicity—from the outset, modern psychotropic tranquilizers were widely used by battalion surgeons and most of the psychiatrists for the treatment of classic combat reactions as well as less disabling combat stress symptoms. But there was no clear evidence that pharmacotherapy was antagonistic to military treatment objectives, as was the case with the sedative/hypnotics used in earlier wars. Among the salient findings from the WRAIR psychiatrist survey:

    — Neuroleptic medications were favored for more severe or more prolonged symptomatology. The most popular was Thorazine.
    — Anxiolytic medications were favored for less severe symptomatology. The most popular was Valium.
    — Commonly treated symptoms were (in descending order): short-timer's syndrome, threatened assault, insomnia, anxiety dreams, tension headache, (functional) musculoskeletal complaints, and startle reaction. Anxiolytics were preferred for most of these symptoms, but neuroleptics were strongly preferred for threatened assault, and barbiturates were preferred for insomnia.
    — Anxiolytic medications were also favored by the psychiatrists for stress-related gastrointestinal disturbances, whereas the neuroleptic Compazine was preferred by primary care physicians.

- **Maintenance psychotropic medicines were also commonly prescribed for soldiers operating in the field.** This was more likely for soldiers whose recovery had been somewhat prolonged. Two observations of note:

- The WRAIR survey participants favored the anxiolytics for soldiers recovering from acute combat reactions, but the neuroleptic Mellaril was especially popular (as was Librium) for soldiers who were recovering from more protracted combat reactions.
- These medications were prescribed despite the fact that the physicians had no information as to effects on combat performance or long-term effects.

- **The record from Vietnam is especially strong regarding the value of the enlisted social work/ psychology and psychiatric inpatient specialists in the treatment of combat stress conditions and symptoms.** Not only did they prove to be extremely capable, but they also supported the extension of psychiatric expertise within the divisions (so-called decentralization of care) and in the therapeutic milieu of the inpatient programs.

- **There is little in the record from Vietnam to indicate that the psychiatrists provided primary prevention intervention, that is, program consultation with command cadre, by offering advice for minimizing stress on combat troops and reducing the incidence of combat stress-generated psychiatric conditions.** The available professional literature from Vietnam, both from the psychiatrists assigned to the combat divisions and those serving at the hospitals and with the psychiatric specialty detachments, contained mostly accounts of secondary and tertiary preventive activities and did not document primary prevention activities. Furthermore, the WRAIR psychiatrist survey results suggested that the deployed psychiatrists were not especially knowledgeable as to the wide array of psychosocial stresses bearing on combat troops in Vietnam.

- **There is little to document specific psychiatric involvement in the management and treatment of specific behavior and discipline problems that may have been expressive of especially stressed combat troops (ie, combat avoidance or refusal, excessive combat aggression, neglected hygiene or care of weapons and equipment, violent incidents toward other US troops, etc).**

REFERENCES

1. Salmon TW. The care and treatment of mental diseases and war neuroses ("shell shock") in the British Army. *Ment Hyg.* 1917;1:519–547.
2. President Lyndon Johnson's message to Congress, 5 August 1964. In: US Department of State. *Why We Fight In Viet-Nam.* Washington, DC: Department of State, Office of Media Services; June 1967. Viet-Nam Information Notes (#6).
3. US Department of the Army. *Military Psychiatry.* Washington, DC: HQDA; August 1957. Technical Manual 8-244.
4. Bartemeier LH, Kubie LS, Menninger KA, Romano J, Whitehorn JC. Combat exhaustion. *J Nerv Ment Dis.* 1946;104:358–389.
5. Camp NM. The Vietnam War and the ethics of combat psychiatry. *Am J Psychiatry.* 1993;150(7):1000–1010.
6. Glass AJ. Psychotherapy in the combat zone. *Am J Psychiatry.* 1954;110:725–731.
7. Artiss KL. Human behavior under stress— From combat to social psychiatry. *Mil Med.* 1963;128:1011–1015.
8. Hausman W, Rioch DMcK. Military psychiatry. A prototype of social and preventive psychiatry in the United States. *Arch Gen Psych.* 1967;16(6):727–739.
9. Manning FJ. Morale and cohesion in military psychiatry. In: Jones FD, Sparacino LR, Wilcox VL, Rothberg JM, eds. *Military Psychiatry: Preparing in Peace for War.* In: Zajtchuk R, Bellamy RF, eds. *Textbooks of Military Medicine.* Washington, DC: Department of the Army, Office of The Surgeon General, Borden Institute; 1994: 1–18.
10. Kormos HR. The nature of combat stress. In: Figley CR, ed. *Stress Disorders Among Vietnam Veterans: Theory, Research and Treatment.* New York, NY: Bruner/Mazel; 1978: 3–22.
11. Noy S. Combat psychiatry: the American and Israeli experience. In: Belenky G, ed. *Contemporary Studies in Combat Psychiatry.* Westport, Conn: Greenwood Press; 1987: 70–86.

MK, *The Textbooks of Military Medicine*. Washington, DC: Department of the Army, Office of The Surgeon General, Borden Institute; 2011: 151–162.

62. Glass AJ. Psychiatry in the Korean Campaign: a historical review, 1. *US Armed Forces Med J*. 1953;4(10):1387–1401.

63. Parrish MD. The megahospital during the Tet offensive. *US Army Vietnam Med Bull*. 1968;May/June:81–82.

CHAPTER 8

Deployment Stress, Inverted Morale, and Psychiatric Attrition: "We Are the Unwilling, Led by the Unqualified, Doing the Unnecessary, for the Ungrateful"

. . . [T]he need for clear and meaningful group missions . . . is simply another way in which good leaders can demonstrate to their units that they care—by seeing that their efforts and the risks (and losses) they incur are for something undeniably worthwhile. Certainly the discipline problems, wholesale drug abuse, and fraggings of the US Army in Vietnam came primarily in the latter years of the war, when it was clear that America had made the judgment that their task was not worth pursuing. Interpersonal bonding at the small unit level could not overcome the quite rational desire not to be the last one killed in an effort without glory or thanks.[1(pp1–2)]

Frederick J Manning, PhD
Military Social Psychologist

Graffiti left by "short" soldier. In this 1969 photograph, a soldier who had very little time left to serve in Vietnam, hence "short," taunted other soldiers who had more time than he. It illustrates a pernicious tension among troops that arose from the policy of individualized, annualized troop rotations in and out of Vietnam. Because of high turnover and staggered replacements, unit cohesion and commitment to the mission were weakened. Photograph courtesy of Richard D Cameron, Major General, US Army (Retired).

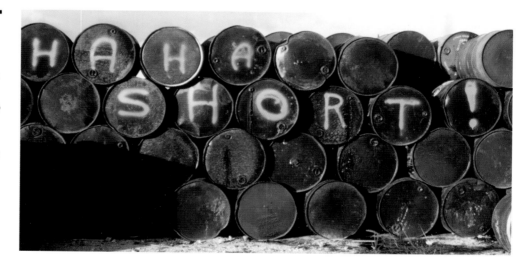

Combat-generated psychiatric conditions have traditionally been the most critical of the problems that military psychiatrists have faced; and, although a broad collection of stress-related factors have been determined to affect how well the soldier can withstand his combat ordeal, the predominant pathogenic one has obviously been its violent nature. However, there are additional challenges—deployment stress—that affect all who are sent to a theater of war, the majority of whom will not face combat directly. In fact history has shown that in a combat theater, commanders, medical personnel, and mental health specialists, as well as those in law enforcement and military administration, must be prepared to respond to large numbers of psychiatrically and behaviorally dysfunctional soldiers who are not combat troops *per se*. Whereas the emergent difficulties may not be attributable to combat stress, nor for that matter always stem from predeployment personality defects, they are invariably linked to the unique stresses and sacrifices associated with assignment in a combat zone, which indirectly includes the primacy of the combat mission.

With respect to the US Army in Vietnam, the flood of combat exhaustion cases that was anticipated never materialized. Also, at least initially, rates for other types of psychiatric conditions and conduct problems were low. However, as already noted, the war passed the midpoint and combat intensity dropped, but soldier dysfunction and attrition nonetheless rose to unprecedented proportions and in unanticipated forms—racial conflicts, heroin use, soldier dissent, and attacks on officers and noncommissioned officers (NCOs)—behaviors that indicated that morale and allegiance to the military mission in the theater were at crisis levels and aligned with the broader antiestablishment spirit of young adults and the antiwar movement. This unraveling of morale and discipline was apparently more common among noncombat personnel,[2] but combat troops were not exempt. Some of this was predictable as a consequence of drawdown; however, the unacceptably high rates and provocative forms that emerged suggested that there were additional circumstances associated with the late Vietnam War and theater that served not just to lower morale but to actually invert it. The "commitment and cohesion" required of even a marginally functional military unit had fragmented to be replaced by loyalties to alternative affinity groups that rallied around opposition to military authority, disabling drug use, and other forms of misconduct and defiance.

Chapter 6 and Chapter 7 focused on combat stress-related psychiatric conditions and their management and treatment in Vietnam. This chapter will build on the overviews presented in Chapter 1 (historical, political, cultural, and military context) and Chapter 2 (accelerating rates for psychiatric conditions and behavior problems in Vietnam) and draw from the available professional literature to address more specifically the broad array of psychological and psychosocial disorders that affected the deployed troops more generally, especially during the second half of the war. It also will include selected clinical examples

and relevant findings from the Walter Reed Army Institute of Research (WRAIR) survey of Vietnam veteran Army psychiatrists. Chapter 9 will review the drug and alcohol problems in Vietnam. Chapter 10 will explore the interactions of mental health personnel with commanders in primary and secondary prevention activities (command consultation).

BACKGROUND

History of (Combat Theater) Deployment Stress Reactions

It should be evident that the high levels and layered nature of the stressors that affect all individuals assigned in a combat zone will result in an increase in psychiatric conditions and behavior problems; but apparently this can be overlooked.[3] The following quotation from Brigadier General William C Menninger, the Army Surgeon General's Chief of the Neuropsychiatry Branch during most of World War II, is illustrative:

> Until [the war] was half over, we as psychiatrists, failed grossly in not appreciating the tremendous importance of distinguishing between emotional illness and faulty attitudes. We did not, until late, adequately grasp the relationship of mental health to group attitudes and pressure, nor did we understand how these could be molded, supported, and changed through leadership, orientation, and information. Too often did we discharge soldiers solely on the basis of the symptoms they presented, rather than consider how environmental support could counteract the cause of these symptoms.[4(pp40–41)]

In his own unique fashion, a senior military psychiatrist, Albert J Glass, offered a similar perspective from the Korean theater: "A majority of those cases are not [neuropsychiatric] conditions because medical officers wish to make patients out of them, but because the line officers have been unable to make soldiers of them."[5(p755)]

In fact, the deployment of troops in sufficient numbers to fight a major war in a remote and inhospitable setting halfway around the world, as proved to be the case in Southeast Asia, is an enormous logistical enterprise. In conjunction, sustaining the requisite morale and commitment to win under such circumstances is equally challenging. From a psychiatric standpoint, in addition to the so-called classic combat stress reaction common in high-intensity warfare (eg, anxiety and psychological fatigue, progressing to gross disturbances in mood, thinking, and behavior), more insidious forms of dysfunction will predictably affect soldiers fighting in low-intensity combat situations as well as those serving in noncombat roles and rear echelon assignments. Similarly susceptible are standing armies in situations involving relative hardship and uncertainty as to justification for continued sacrifices and isolation from home and loved ones. The consequence is a lowering of morale and an increase in psychiatric conditions and dysfunctional behaviors—disorders that can become widespread and undermine combat readiness.[2]

Historically these have taken the form of elevated rates for alcohol and drug abuse, venereal disease, desertion, and disciplinary infractions; but they can be quite variable depending on a broad array of situational, group, and interpersonal influences, which in turn interact with predeployment personality characteristics.[6] Terms like guerrilla neurosis, garrison casualties, and disorders of loneliness or nostalgia have been used, with each label having a somewhat different etiologic emphasis. As an example, it has been estimated that there were approximately three cases of "nostalgia" (disabling homesickness) per 1,000 troops per year among Union soldiers during the US Civil War. Following the Civil War, alcoholism, venereal diseases, and disciplinary infractions continued to be problems for units fighting in the Indian Wars, the Spanish-American War, and the Philippine Insurrection, but these were not considered to be morale and mental health problems until World War I.[3] Data from World War II[7] and Korea[8] documented the rise in psychiatric and behavior difficulties among the large numbers of noncombat soldiers who were stationed far from home, living in confined and isolated groups, and serving primarily in service/support roles. Similar problems have been observed among constabulary forces and those in the process of demobilization in an overseas setting who resented being asked to sustain further sacrifices beyond the conclusion of hostilities.[2,9] Even a dramatic increase in the use of narcotics by US soldiers was seen at the close of the Korean War, which was attributed to drawdown service in an Asian theater.[10] As noted in Chapter 2, current Army doctrine refers to these conditions as misconduct stress behaviors. This author believes that it makes more sense to label them (combat theater) deployment stress reactions to draw attention to the ordeal of assignment in a combat zone as its own center of stress.

Special Role Requirements of Military Psychiatrists in Maintaining the Force

The Army Psychiatrist and Social Psychiatry

The US Army is a huge institution with a strict rank and authority hierarchy. As far as its personnel and culture, the central organizing principle is the subordination of individual values to those of the organization—presumably for the benefit of the larger society. The requirement that the soldier conform to the performance expectations of the Army becomes even more rigorous when the nation is committed to war; and, for obvious reasons, this is even more so when the soldier is assigned in the theater of combat operations. Psychiatry is one among the many Army functions concerned with manpower maintenance. As a consequence, Army psychiatrists are tasked with promoting soldier adaptation to the military's ways and means and, when deployed in a combat theater, to those serving combat objectives in particular. In other words, the military psychiatrist must not only seek to reduce the incidence and morbidity of conventional psychiatric conditions (symptom disorders), as in a civilian setting, but also support the prevention of, or to evaluate and make recommendations regarding rehabilitation of, or facilitate the discharge from the service of, those who would develop aberrant behavior. In this context, aberrant behavior refers to deviations from the military's performance expectations, that is, disciplinary problems—clashes between the soldier and military authority—as well as other behaviors that negatively affect individual and unit performance. In effect, the somewhat unique mission of the military psychiatrist is the reduction of unsatisfactory duty performance that may be due to psychological reasons and that may present in a wide variety of forms.[6] In fulfilling this mission he must not only seek to understand the soldier-patient as an individual, but he must also take into account the soldier's social/military context, which may even include a dysfunctional unit and leadership.

The Evaluating, Sorting, Certifying, and Clearing Functions of Military Psychiatry

During the Vietnam War newly commissioned physicians underwent an accelerated basic training at the Army's Medical Field Service School (MFSS) in which they received instruction regarding the Army's triage model for psychiatric referrals.[11] This was necessary both from the standpoint of their providing clinical care and because they could be required to screen underperforming soldiers who were being processed for discharge from the Army—so-called "noneffectives"—under Army Regulation 635-212.[12] (A similar protocol would apply to officers,[13] but they were far fewer in number.) The triage model involved the following algorithm:

1. Is there evidence a soldier is undergoing a *personal crisis*? Many soldiers develop psychiatric symptoms and maladaptive behaviors in reaction to their individual circumstance and may warrant a psychiatric diagnosis such as a transient situational disorder [in today's nomenclature, they may fall within DSM-IV [*Diagnostic and Statistical Manual of the Mental Disorders*, 4th edition]: adjustment disorder[14,15]]. They may be treatable through counseling, medication, or rehabilitative transfer— as long as the objective is preservation of military function and not symptom elimination. The goal is "effectiveness, not happiness." The practicality of this option rests on unit mission requirements as well as the availability of mental health personnel. The premium is placed on early detection and treatment of the symptomatic soldier so as to avoid removing him from duty status for treatment. The decision whether to treat or not falls to the mental health specialist.

2. Do the soldier's symptoms and behaviors stem from a *disqualifying psychiatric condition*? Some soldiers develop more serious psychiatric conditions that warrant discharge from the Army based on medical and psychiatric fitness requirements for continued service.[16] If the soldier has (*a*) a diagnosable psychiatric condition [which by today's standards would roughly fall within DSM-IV: Axis I set[14,15]], and he has (*b*) substantial and untreatable functional impairment, he should be processed through medical channels for discharge from the Army. The final decision rests with a higher medical authority, that is, the Medical Board.

3. If the soldier's symptoms and behaviors don't conform to (1) or (2), are they expressive of a *character and behavior disorder* (or personality disorder[17])? In instances when an intractable pattern of poor performance or misconduct arises, and

the soldier is not interested in, nor amenable to, corrective measures, a psychiatric opinion must be rendered as to whether the soldier's "faulty attitude"[11] is "characterologic" in nature. If he presents with sustained and untreatable functional impairment and if a pattern of dysfunction is in his preservice background, and if he receives a diagnosis of character and behavior disorder [which by today's standards would fall within DSM-IV: Axis II set], he would receive a psychiatric "certificate" and could be separated from the Army as *unsuitable* [Table 8-1]. The final disposition, however, would be at the discretion of the soldier's commander; but, if utilized, the character and behavior disorder diagnosis and "unsuitable" administrative separation would reduce the soldier's chances of being court-martialed and result in a less punitive type of discharge from the service. It also would allow the commander to bypass a lengthy process of counseling and rehabilitation so as to expedite his discharge from the Army.

If the answers to the questions above are all negative, by the parlance of the time the soldier is "cleared" by psychiatry, and it is presumed that he has the capacity to obey orders but is opposed. He then faces the possibility of judicial punishment or nonjudicial punishment and administrative elimination from the Army as *unfit*.

MOUNTING CHALLENGES IN THE VIETNAM ERA

Incidence of Psychiatric Conditions and Behavior Problems in Vietnam: Containment in the First Half of the War and Hemorrhage in the Second Half

In general, the complex array of psychosocial challenges for the soldiers sent to Vietnam, noncombat troops as well as combat troops, was expected. Technical Manual (TM) 8-244: *Military Psychiatry* provided an excellent depiction of these risks:

The general problem confronting psychiatry in combat is related to the adjustment of the soldier to a life situation which is often unpleasant, and seemingly intolerable. The soldier finds himself deprived in many spheres, away from home, family and friends, in danger, fatigued, in a strange

TABLE 8-1. Schedule for Administrative Elimination of Noneffective Enlisted Soldiers Under Army Regulation 635-212

CATEGORY	UNFIT	UNSUITABLE
Characteristics	Failure to pay debts Drug addiction Discreditable incidents Shirking Sexual perversion Failure to support dependents Homosexual[†]	Inaptitude Character and behavior disorders Apathy Alcoholism Homosexual (class III)
Governing authority	General Court Martial	Special Court Martial
Dispositions*	Retain in the Army Separate as unsuitable Separate as unfit	Retain in the Army Separate as unsuitable
Type of discharge	Undesirable (Honorable or General in special cases)	Honorable General

Note: With the exception of "Homosexual" under Unfit, this is the schedule that was distributed to newly commissioned Army physicians July 1967.[1]
*Individuals could waive a board hearing. If not, they were provided counsel and could testify on their own behalf and call witnesses.
[†]Until March 1970, Army Regulation (AR) 635-212, *Personnel Separations, Discharge: Unfitness and Unsuitability*, included some selected cases of individuals with homosexual tendencies, desires, or interest but without homosexual acts during military service—Class III (latent[2]); individuals not so excluded, as well as individuals who engaged in homosexual acts during military service, were subject to administrative discharge from the Army as unfit under AR 635-89. In March 1970, the elements in AR 635-89 were included in AR 635-212.

References: (1) Elimination of Noneffectives: AR 635-212. San Antonio, Tex: Medical Field Service School Department of Administration; (distributed July 1967). Training Document M 17-450-850-460; (2) Elimination of Noneffectives. San Antonio, Tex: Medical Field Service School Department of Administration; (distributed July 1967). Training Document M 13-360-120-1.

milieu, torn by conflicting interests and desires, subject to military discipline, and emotionally supported principally by the small group with whom he lives and fights. The range of behavior of individuals in such a setting varies from cowardly shirking to heroic, selfless action. The use of the more primitive mental mechanisms in an effort to resolve the situation is a common solution, with the production of both classical and new constellations of symptoms as a result. Certain mechanisms aid in the performance of duty; others seem designed to produce incapacity; and the symptom complex produced by the latter generally takes a form locally likely to lead to evacuation.[18(p63)]

What was not anticipated was the additional strain on the sequential cohorts of replacement troops assigned in Vietnam consequent to the enemy's resolve and tenacity, the prolongation of the war, and the reversal of America's moral sanction for fighting there.

Early in the war, Army psychiatry leaders were impressed by the limited losses from the theater for all psychiatric causes. They surmised that adequate psychiatric resources had been deployed and that the lessons learned from earlier wars were being successfully implemented. For example, William S Allerton, by then the Psychiatric Consultant to the Army Surgeon General, reported that the psychiatric evacuation rate was two to three cases per 1,000 troops per year for the period, from mid 1967 to 1968, which matched the Army-wide rate for psychotic disorders for the preceding 50 years. He deduced that only psychotic individuals were being evacuated from Vietnam for psychiatric reasons, despite it being a theater of combat operations.[19] In other words, it was assumed that the etiology for these cases was endogenous as opposed to situational. Arnold W Johnson Jr, the second US Army Republic of Vietnam (USARV) Psychiatry Consultant, expressed his satisfaction regarding the "relative unimportance of the psychiatric inpatient population

FIGURE 8-1. US Army Vietnam rates (per 1,000 soldiers/year) for wounded in action (WIA), psychiatric hospitalizations, psychiatric outpatient visits, psychiatric out-of-country evacuations, courts martial, and nonjudicial punishments. [Note: These measures were confounded by rising soldier drug use, especially heroin, beginning in 1970.]

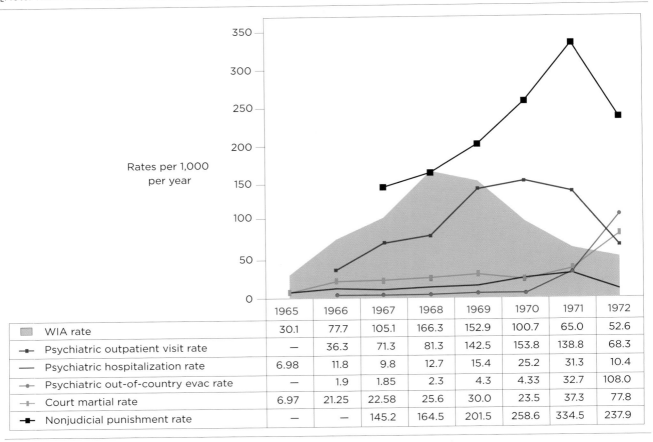

	1965	1966	1967	1968	1969	1970	1971	1972
WIA rate	30.1	77.7	105.1	166.3	152.9	100.7	65.0	52.6
Psychiatric outpatient visit rate	—	36.3	71.3	81.3	142.5	153.8	138.8	68.3
Psychiatric hospitalization rate	6.98	11.8	9.8	12.7	15.4	25.2	31.3	10.4
Psychiatric out-of-country evac rate	—	1.9	1.85	2.3	4.3	4.33	32.7	108.0
Court martial rate	6.97	21.25	22.58	25.6	30.0	23.5	37.3	77.8
Nonjudicial punishment rate	—	—	145.2	164.5	201.5	258.6	334.5	237.9

Sources: US Army Vietnam WIA rates (see Chapter 6, Table 6-3); Army psychiatric hospitalization rates (see Chapter 2, Figure 2-2); Army psychiatric outpatient visit and out-of-country evacuation rates from: Jones FD, Johnson AW Jr. Medical and psychiatric treatment policy and practice in Vietnam. *J Soc Issues.* 1975;31(4):49–65, Figures 3 and 2; and Army disciplinary actions—courts martial and nonjudicial punishment (Article 15)—rates from Prugh GS. *Law at War: Vietnam 1964–1973.* Washington, DC: GPO; 1975: Appendix K.

as far as numbers are concerned."[20(p305)] He also acknowledged that there were "strong efforts made to restrict psychiatric evacuations from Vietnam to those who are disabled with psychosis."[20(p305)]

However, despite this apparently commendable beginning, Army mental health and military discipline in Vietnam became severely compromised after the midpoint in the war. This can be demonstrated using the following gross epidemiologic trends:

- The psychiatric hospitalization rate began to increase throughout the theater beginning in 1968 and accelerated over the 4 years that followed (Figure 2-2 in Chapter2 and Figure 8-1).

- There was a parallel increase for the psychiatric evacuation rate from the theater (Figure 8-1).
- The psychiatric outpatient visit rate (a mix of evaluation and treatment) accelerated after 1966 to plateau in the years 1969 through 1971 at roughly four times the 1966 rate. In 1972, as the last of the troops were being pulled out, it dropped back to two times the 1966 rate (Figure 8-1). (The 1972 metric is undoubtedly misleading, as by then a policy shift had allowed drug dependent soldiers to be medically evacuated out of Vietnam, resulting in an out-of-country psychiatric evacuation rate of 129.8 per 1,000 troops per year or one out of every eight soldiers.)

- There was a parallel and equally dramatic trajectory for an array of discipline problems as measured by judicial and, especially, nonjudicial punishments (Figure 8-1).

- The increases in these indices were inversely correlated with the drop in combat intensity, which began after 1968 (measured both by the Army battle death rate (Figure 2-2) and the Army wounded-in-action (WIA) rate (Figure 8-1).

- Although the rate for psychiatric disorders during the period after 1967 also increased in the Army worldwide, the increase in Vietnam was significantly greater.[21](Figure 18)

Army Psychiatrists as Specialized Human Resources Managers

As the war lengthened, Army psychiatrists of the Vietnam era and their professional and paraprofessional (enlisted specialists) colleagues were required to evaluate, sort, certify, or clear increasing numbers of command-referred soldiers, with and without psychiatric symptoms, who were failing to perform by military standards.[21](Figure 8) (See Appendix II: Format for Psychiatric Reports for Administrative-Type Separation in Appendix 2, USARV Regulation 40-34, to this volume.) In the United States such referrals would spike locally in anticipation of a deployment alert[22]; but the greater problem arose in Vietnam as suggested by the rapidly rising rates for psychiatric outpatient visits and nonjudicial punishments (Figure 8-1).

For the Army overall, these psychiatric determinations assumed great importance in matters of military personnel management and enforcement of discipline. For example, about 7% (72,000) of all enlisted men released from military service in 1971 left with less than an honorable discharge, 40% of whom were diagnosed with character and behavior disorders.[23] Yet as the war became more unpopular, a growing dispute arose among psychiatrists regarding how the character and behavior disorder cases should be defined and managed.[24,25] Some argued that when the military psychiatrist renders a character and behavior disorder diagnosis while being naïve as to causative or aggravating circumstances within the soldier's unit, he serves not as a clinician but as both expert witness and judge in deciding the administrative, or even judicial, fate of the soldier—that the label implied that the soldier had moral defects, not medical/psychiatric difficulties.[23,26] Others felt the psychiatrist was

overlooking true psychiatric conditions that warranted treatment instead.[27] In sharp contrast, the perspective of the Army was that soldiers labeled with a character and behavior disorder were simply being "fired" for failing to perform and that this outcome was without prejudice (see the letter from Hal Jennings Jr, Deputy Surgeon General, to Congressman Ogden Reid in Appendix 15 to this volume).

Functional Impediments to Diagnostic Specificity in Vietnam

With regard to the Army psychiatrists serving in Vietnam, especially those trained in civilian settings (roughly two-thirds), most were unprepared to manage these sorts of referrals for the following reasons:

1. Some of the disciplinary infractions and other offenses for which the soldier was referred for psychiatric screening would have scant civilian equivalency (ie, absent without leave [AWOL], desertion, and insubordination).
2. Some of the behavioral disturbances in question would not generally have been the focus of the psychiatrists' training (ie, racial incidents, violent outbursts, and group pathology, to include organizational dysfunction).
3. The task would be even more problematic for psychiatrists without a military background because the soldier-patient would typically present for the evaluation removed from the context of his specific military situation.
4. Finally, there were no operationally defined criteria established in the theater for the diagnosis of character and behavior disorder that would take into account the performance requirements peculiar to military service, especially in a theater of combat operations (similar to the deficit described in Chapter 6 regarding the lack of uniform diagnostic criteria for combat stress reactions).

Regarding the latter (ambiguous diagnostic criteria) for the most part the Army physicians assigned in Vietnam, including psychiatrists, had not been trained by the Army to reasonably distinguish the soldier with a true character and behavior disorder from the many referrals who were simply antagonistic to military service. For instance, in the summer of 1967, newly commissioned physicians in basic training at MFSS received a training document titled "Management of

TABLE 8-2. Hospitalized Army Neuropsychiatric Cases in Vietnam by Diagnostic Groupings

	USARV/Neel* (mid-1965 to mid-1970)[1]	Colbach and Parrish† (mid-1965 to mid-1970)[2]	Bourne (1966)[3]
Psychotic	16.2%	20%	20.9%
Neurotic	16.6%	15%	19.6%
Character or behavior disorder	29.1%	30%	38.4%
Combat exhaustion		7%	6.0%
NP observation; no psych diagnosis		28%	15.0%
Other psychiatric conditions	38%		
Total	100%	100%	100%

Shaded cells means no category was represented in the data set.

*Derived from Table 2-2, Army Incidence Rate for Psychiatric Hospitalizations in Vietnam [and in Europe] in cases /1,000 troops/year, in Chapter 2 in this volume.

†Colbach and Parrish did not collect data in Vietnam. Like Neel's data, the source would have been from raw data collected by USARV Medical Command; nonetheless what they published diverged from Neel's.

NP: neuropsychiatric
USARV: US Army Republic of Vietnam

Data sources: (1) Neel SH. *Medical Support of the US Army in Vietnam*, 1965–1970. Washington, DC: GPO; 1973; (2) Colbach EM, Parrish MD. Army mental health activities in Vietnam: 1965–1970. *Bull Menninger Clin*. 1970;34(6):333–342; (3) Bourne PG, Nguyen DS. A comparative study of neuropsychiatric casualties in the United States Army and the Army of the Republic of Vietnam. *Mil Med*. 1967;132(11):904–909.

the Noneffective Soldier."[28] It indicated that they may be required to render a medical opinion as to whether a soldier's failure to perform stemmed from preservice personality defects, immaturity, or an inherent lack of capacity to adjust (he "lacks pride," "is selfish," and "unwilling"); but it did not explicitly address character and behavior disorders as a diagnostic entity.[28] These physicians would have been better prepared had they received a copy of the Joint Armed Forces Psychiatric Nomenclature (in Special Regulations 40-1025-2[29]). It indicated that character and behavior disorders demonstrate "developmental defects or pathological trends in personality structure, with minimal subjective anxiety and little or no sense of distress"; that the disorder is typically manifested by a lifelong pattern of action or behavior ("acting out") rather than by mental or emotional symptoms; and that pathological personality types include those with borderline adjustment states, immature and regressive reactions to severe stress, and fixations of certain [adverse] character patterns. However, this publication was not widely distributed. (These stipulations for

character and behavior disorder were consistent with the brief definition included in the American Psychiatric Association's 1952 taxonomy, DSM-I, and its 1968 taxonomy, DSM-II.)

As a consequence, diagnosing and labeling of soldiers may well have been subjectively influenced by the clinician, or through the soldier's military circumstance, rather than by clinical precision. As the war prolonged, polarized attitudes (even among doctors) about the war colored reactions to soldiers who expressed dissent. Furthermore, although it was common knowledge that commanders had final say as to whether the psychiatric diagnosis of a character and behavior disorder would be honored, it was not evident how influential the psychiatric opinion actually was. A study conducted in 1967 and 1968 at Walter Reed General Hospital revealed that not only did 92% of the soldiers diagnosed as character and behavior disorder receive a less than honorable discharge from the Army, but the psychiatrist prediction of performance failure if the soldier was not discharged was accurate only 40% of the time.[25]

Belatedly, at the very end of the war, an Army technical bulletin devoted to drug abuse (authored by Stewart L Baker Jr, a senior Army psychiatrist,) was published that included the following list of common features of the soldier with a character and behavior disorder[30]:

- [The character and behavior disordered individual exhibits] a combination of low self-esteem, limited coping skills, and high susceptibility to peer pressure.
- His history often reveals intellectual and social deprivation secondary to indifferent parenting, environmental circumstances, or both.
- Interpersonal relations with family and peers have frequently been strained, and in some cases military duty was seen as preferable to dealing with a family or judicial problem.
- Not surprisingly, military authority frequently becomes a new focus of conflict for this individual, which he sees as the source of all his difficulty. As a result, his allegiance to a given unit may be tenuous.
- Delinquent behavior, including illicit drug use, usually coexists with poor school and/or job performance.
- Peer relations may be confined primarily to an isolated subgroup within the unit (eg, other drug users).
- His previous military record often reveals a number of minor offenses (late for work, AWOL, uniform violations).
- Typically his immediate commander or supervisor is not eager to have him returned to the unit.

Some relief in the pressure on Army mental health clinics to evaluate, sort, certify, or clear huge volumes of underperforming soldiers came in the Vietnam theater in October 1970 when the USARV Supplement to AR 635-212[31] was revised to allow general medical officers to complete the mental evaluation portion of the medical evaluation when a psychiatrist was not readily available. On 12 April 1971 this became policy throughout the Army. Thereafter, a psychiatrist's evaluation was only required when it was requested by the soldier's commanding officer, the medical officer conducting the separation physical, the board of officers considering the case, or by the soldier. (See item 2-f in Appendix 14, "Bowen's End of Tour Report," to this volume.)

THE PSYCHIATRIC LITERATURE FROM VIETNAM: OBSERVATIONS AND INTERPRETATIONS

Epidemiology of Major Psychiatric Diagnostic Groups: Information Gaps and Overconfidence

During the early buildup years the field research in Vietnam by Peter G Bourne and the WRAIR Neuropsychiatry Research Team proved quite productive (as noted in Chapter 2 and described in Chapter 6). Among his projects he collected data regarding major diagnostic groups for Army troops hospitalized for psychiatric causes during the first 6 months of 1966 that served as an epidemiologic baseline for what was to follow (Table 8-2, column 3).

Bourne paid special attention to the large subset of soldiers diagnosed as character and behavior disorders (almost two of every five psychiatric hospitalizations). According to Bourne, their patterns of symptoms—dysfunction of attitude and behavior—had an uncertain relation to combat stress. They were described as emotionally unstable or immature personalities whose primary difficulty was that they were unable to function apart from their families, and they had become disciplinary problems, apparently as a means of manipulating a transfer out of Vietnam. To further expand the point, in 1966 Borne and Nguyen compared American with South Vietnamese military neuropsychiatric cases in the theater and speculated that the lower proportion of psychosis among the American soldiers (20.9% of psychiatrically hospitalized American soldiers vs 50.0% for Army of the Republic of Vietnam) and the higher rates for character and behavior disorders (38.4% of psychiatrically hospitalized American soldiers vs 13.8% for Army of the Republic of Vietnam) demonstrated how social/cultural and military policy features shaped the dysfunctional patterns of each group's clinical presentations, especially regarding their "manipulative" goals, that is, in pursuit of a socially permissible means for opting out of combat risk.[32] In other words, American soldiers who were hospitalized in Vietnam with character and behavior diagnosis were disabled by the interaction of endogenous influences (premilitary personality deficits) and exogenous ones (risk and privation, institutional requirements, and social dynamics).

In October 1970, Bourne summarized his research in Vietnam in a special section in the *American Journal of Psychiatry* heralding military psychiatry. Like others,

Bourne expressed satisfaction at the unusually low incidence of psychiatric conditions overall, and he attributed this in part to the exceptionally high morale in Vietnam. (He defined morale as "the general sense of well-being enjoyed by the group . . . a reflection of confidence in their ability to successfully survive environmental stress, faith in the quality of their leadership, and an overall sense of cooperation and cohesiveness among its members."[33(p482)]) Bourne concluded his review with confidence and optimism. "The Vietnam experience has shown that we have now successfully identified most of the major correlates of psychiatric attrition in the combat zone, [and] psychiatric casualties need never again become a major cause of attrition in the United States military in a combat zone."[33(p487)]

Remarkably, by the time Bourne made his way home from what in all respects should be considered a successful field research experience in Vietnam and submitted his findings and opinions to American psychiatry's most prestigious journal, little remained of the excellent morale and esprit that he and his colleagues observed. It is not just ironic that the year his piece was published, 1970, was also the year in which the most disturbing expressions of soldier demoralization and revolt in Vietnam made their appearance, specifically, the heroin epidemic and soldier assassinations of officers and NCOs; but it also was the year the American Psychiatric Association eliminated the military psychiatry section of its annual meeting in protest of the war.[34] (It should be noted that in the war's aftermath, Bourne reversed his perspective. After having become impressed with the magnitude of the adjustment problems among Vietnam veterans, he posited that, overall, troops in Vietnam had only appeared to be doing well because they had suppressed their psychological disturbances knowing that their obligation was limited to 1 year.[35])

From the standpoint of epidemiologic observation and interpretation, Edward M Colbach and Matthew D Parrish picked up where Bourne left off.[36] Their summary of mental health activities in Vietnam through mid-1970, mentioned in Chapter 2, included the first official acknowledgement of the rising psychiatric attrition following the enemy's surprise Tet offensives in 1968—the turning point in the war for the United States and the American public. Whereas Colbach and Parrish felt that morale in the theater was holding despite the growing antiwar movement in the United

States, they noted the rising racial tensions and the decline in perception of military purpose within soldiers. They also mentioned increasing marijuana use among enlisted troops and expressed concern that some heavy users developed a transient toxic psychosis with paranoid features. Use of French barbiturate and amphetamine preparations were also seen, but use of hard narcotics was rare.

Nonetheless, the authors concluded that drug use had not seriously affected the overall military mission. Although older career soldiers tended to avoid illegal drugs—"the abuse of drugs has been considered a prerogative of the young soldiers . . ."[36(pp337–338)]—some resorted to alcohol to reduce their stress. Colbach and Parrish also mentioned that poor leadership was contributing to some declining morale and increases in specific psychiatric and related problems. However, they believed that these emergent problems were more likely the consequence of "boredom, loneliness and interpersonal conflicts, [which were] intensified due to the stresses of living a regimented group life in a hot foreign land where there has been a constant threat of bodily harm."[36(p337)]

Finally, in 1973, a year following the withdrawal of Army combat troops, Major General Spurgeon Neel's official synopsis of Army medical activities in Vietnam was released.[37] Unfortunately, this review fell far short of providing a proper overview of psychiatric problems in the theater for several important reasons: (a) like the summary provided by Colbach and Parrish, the data did not include the time period after mid-1970, effectively ignoring almost a third of the war (3 of 8 years); (b) the report included a limited taxonomy for hospitalized psychiatric conditions; (c) as previously noted, combat stress-related conditions received no specific mention; and (d) outpatient psychiatric data were not included. (As somewhat of a remedy, the Jones and Johnson overview, which was published in 1975, included quarterly incidence rates for psychosis and psychiatric inpatients, outpatient visits, and psychiatric medical evacuations throughout the war; however, it did not distinguish between diagnostic groups apart from psychotic disorders.[38])

Table 2-2 in Chapter 2 presented Neel's gross incidence rates for psychiatric hospitalizations of Army troops per year in Vietnam through mid-1970 distributed according to three broad diagnostic groupings (psychosis, psychoneurosis, and character and behavior disorders) as well as "Other Psychiatric

Conditions." As demonstrated, rates stayed low from mid-1965, when American ground troops were first deployed in Vietnam, until mid-1968. Thereafter there was a marked, steady increase in all of the psychiatric diagnostic groups. From Neel's data it is possible to average percentages of psychiatric hospitalized cases within these basic diagnostic groupings over the first 5 (of 8) years and compare them with similar data reported by Colbach and Parrish and that by Bourne for 1966 (Table 8-2).

It is uncertain what meanings to attribute to the differences in the sets of data presented in Table 8-2. In particular there were important discrepancies regarding the composition of some categories that make it difficult to reconcile Neel's data set with the other two. For example, Neel reported 38% of cases as "other psychiatric conditions," but he did not include the category of "NP [Neuropsychiatric] observation, no psych diagnosis." Bourne, as well as Colbach and Parrish, included large percentages of cases as "NP observation" (15% and 28%, respectively), but they did not include "other psychiatric conditions." However, "NP observation, no psych diagnosis" is clearly not synonymous with "other psychiatric conditions." USARV's taxonomy for the collection of morbidity statistics from Army hospitals in Vietnam included the former but not the latter (see USARV Regulation 40-34 in Appendix 2 to this volume). Evidently Neel created "other psychiatric conditions" to encompass two diagnostic groups initially represented in the hospital morbidity report data: (1) stress reactions and (2) combat exhaustion. For example, his 38% for "other psychiatric conditions" approximated the sum of Colbach and Parrish's "combat exhaustion" (7%) and "NP observation" (28%).

Because a category for drug abuse was not created before 1970,[36] for most of the war drug cases would likely have been represented in either the character and behavior disorder or "NP observation" groupings (or Neel's "other psychiatric conditions"). Even more uncertain was the fate of alcoholism and other alcohol-generated conditions. USARV Regulation 40-34 did not designate where they should be counted in the medical treatment facility morbidity reports for psychiatric cases, yet these problems were quite prevalent. Finally, as has already been noted, there were no widely distributed operational definitions for diagnostic groupings so that the categorization of any particular soldier-patient may have been influenced as much by

bias of the clinician, or of the referring command, as by clinical determinants. Douglas R Bey, the 1st Infantry Division (ID) division psychiatrist, offered the following caveat after his return to the United States:

[T]o follow the [DSM] rigidly might also force us to try to fit our observations into diagnostic categories that have questionable application to the [Vietnam] combat setting. This type of decision was always necessary when reporting our monthly [statistics to USARV Headquarters]. At the time we questioned whether some of the syndromes we were seeing were adequately described by the diagnostic categories we were asked to use. For example, was an individual who was unable to adjust to the military in Vietnam and who was given an administrative discharge really suffering from a personality disorder? . . . In many instances he had the same difficulties with teachers, employers and others in the past and probably did have some longstanding characterological problems. However, in some instances he could not tolerate the conditions peculiar to the combat assignment in Vietnam or his unit could not tolerate him and a decision was made…that he should be sent home [via psychiatric and medical evacuation or character and behavior disorder certificate and administrative discharge].

. . . Investigators must be wary of reported statistics as to the number of cases of various diagnostic categories seen by military psychiatrists. In general, those diagnosed as "psychotic" are probably accurate figures. . . . In other instances it might be necessary to diagnose a man in a way that would assure his evacuation rather than by the most technically accurate diagnosis.[39(ChapVIII,pp1–3)]

Frank W Hays, a senior US Air Force psychiatrist who reported on aeromedical evacuations, including Army patients, from Vietnam through Travis Air Force Base, California (1 January 1967–30 June 1967) during the buildup period, illustrated the problem of taxonomic ambiguity. According to Hays, by regulation Air Force and Army psychiatrists recognized two distinct types of emotional and mental disturbances: (1) mental disorders (psychosis, neurosis, impairment of brain tissue function, and psychophysiological autonomic and visceral disorders) and (2) character and behavior disorders. Yet for statistical purposes he and his colleagues lumped soldiers with the diagnosis of combat exhaustion (one case), alcoholism, and adult situational disorder under character and behavior disorders. In his estimation this was warranted because it was common to see military personnel with these diagnoses who had been medically evacuated from throughout the Pacific Theater no longer demonstrate the symptoms that originally brought them to psychiatric attention. Instead they "[manifested] primarily personality trait disturbances, usually of the passive dependent or passive aggressive hue."[40(p659)]

The Navy psychiatrists who took care of Navy and Marine psychiatric casualties in Vietnam used the same limited taxonomy and ended up with a contradiction with regard to some combat stress cases. As noted in Chapter 6, Robert E Strange vigorously reserved the diagnosis of classic combat fatigue (vs "pseudocombat fatigue") for Marines lacking in premorbid personality or psychoneurotic disorders.[41,42] Yet when he and Ransom J Arthur grouped all cases hospitalized on the USS *Repose* (according to psychotic disorder, psychoneurotic disorder, and character and behavior disorder), combat fatigue cases, along with situational reaction, were lumped under character and behavior disorder (actually, personality disorder).[43]

By way of conclusion, collectively the three Army data sets (Neel, Colbach and Parrish, and Bourne) are especially misleading in failing to capture data from the more psychiatrically difficult period in the war—the 2 years following mid-1970. Otherwise, of the three data sets, that provided by Colbach and Parrish appears to be more complete because it spanned the first two-thirds of the war (vs Bourne) and because it retained the original "combat exhaustion" and "NP observation" categories (vs Neel). However, if so, that would suggest that some-where near 50% of Army psychiatric inpatients in Vietnam were not hospitalized for psychiatric "illness." Colbach and Parrish indicated that roughly a quarter of hospitalized psychiatric cases were ultimately deemed to not have psychiatric conditions ("observation neuro-psychiatry—no psychiatric diagnosis"), and another 30% were inappropriately hospitalized (character and behavior disorder), at least according to the regulation. USARV Regulation 40-34 stipulated that:

> Hospitalization is to be avoided except where patients are potentially dangerous to themselves or others, and then only because of mental illness. It is not to be used when personnel, who for

administrative reasons or convenience, need only to remain overnight or await some administrative action. With rare exceptions sociopathic soldiers [*sic*] (character and behavior disorders) are not to be admitted to hospitals. [Hospitals] will not serve as substitutes for administrative action. . . .[44(¶4(a),p2)]

An alternative conclusion might be that diagnostic precision was not a priority—that many soldiers initially presented with disabling stress-generated symptoms but recovered rapidly under a generic treatment regimen (ie, brief hospitalization, observation, milieu treatment, expectancy of rapid return to duty, and tapered psychotropic medications). It was concluded that these individuals had undergone an adjustment disorder, even if facilitated by drug or alcohol use, and they were counted under one of these two headings: (1) "observation neuropsychiatry—no psychiatric diagnosis" or (2) "character and behavior disorder." To make the point, Gary L Tischler, with the 67th Evacuation Hospital, utilized two additional categories: (1) "transient situational disorder" (18%) and "other" (10.5%).[45] Bey, with the 1st ID, added "acute situational reaction" (20%),[46] and H Spencer Bloch, with the 935th Psychiatric Detachment, did likewise (17.5%) as well as added a category for alcohol and drug problems (6.8%).[47]

The Psychotic Disorders

The psychiatric literature from the war indicated that despite induction standards intended to screen out disqualifying psychiatric conditions,[16] the deployed mental health personnel in Vietnam treated a variety of psychotic disorders. This was no surprise to Army psychiatry leaders, like Allerton, because over 5 decades, the Army-wide incidence rate for psychotic conditions was 2% to 3% of troops per year, regardless of the conditions of war or peace.[19] Those Army psychiatrists in Vietnam who provided data indicated that psychotic conditions represented a modest proportion of their referrals. This included three division psychiatrists: (1) Franklin Del Jones ("a few individuals"), (2) Harold SR Byrdy (2.4%), and (3) Bey (5%). Tischler, who also provided 2nd echelon treatment as a solo psychiatrist in an evacuation hospital, reported 3%. Although John A Bowman, the first 935th Psychiatric Detachment commander in Vietnam (3rd echelon care), reported less than 5% of referrals as psychosis, because it was at an early point in the war and he and his team provided care for many combat units, they could be considered as functioning like a division psychiatry unit (providing 1st and 2nd echelon care).

Regarding hospitalized cases, Colbach and Parrish reported that approximately 20% of psychiatric inpatients in Vietnam through the years of mid-1965 through mid-1970 were psychotic disorders (Table 8-2). Consistent with that figure, cases of psychosis (schizophrenia and affective psychosis) were estimated to be 18.8% of the caseloads of the psychiatrist participants in the WRAIR survey (Table 5-3 in Chapter 5). The two reports from the psychiatric specialty units indicated a much higher proportion. Early in the war Louis R Conte, at the 98th Psychiatric Detachment, reported between 40% and 50% of their inpatients were schizophrenic. Later, Bloch, at the 935th Psychiatric Detachment, reported 44% as psychosis. Both of these are double Colbach and Parrish's reported theater-wide percentage for psychosis, but that would be expected because they were the definitive treatment sites in the theater for the more intractable cases.

But some ambiguity also arises because Conte appears to have used schizophrenia interchangeably with psychosis, although they are not synonymous. The soldier who presents with an acute disorganized or disoriented state may be undergoing a schizophrenic decompensation; but alternative possibilities include that of an acute, reactive psychotic episode, such as combat exhaustion, as well as brain trauma or toxic/metabolic conditions. In Vietnam, alcohol abuse and the increasing use of recreational drugs added to the diagnostic complexity. Bey mentioned seeing one intoxicated soldier who had sustained a skull fracture and subdural hematoma. He saw another who had severe hypoglycemia secondary to a pancreatic tumor. He also saw cases of delirium caused by cerebral malaria, heat stroke, alcoholic paranoia and hallucinosis (a mental state characterized by frequent hallucinations).[48]

With respect to drug use other than alcohol, making an accurate diagnosis could also be difficult because possession was a criminal offense, and a history of drug use could be withheld. The early identification and treatment of psychotic conditions was also challenging because soldiers had ready access to weapons. For example, Bey described a tragic incident in September 1969 when a 1st ID soldier walked into a bunker at a fire support base and, without provocation and without knowing his victims, shot all six occupants, killing two.

The sanity board found him to be psychotic at the time. Upon review, his conduct had been quite bizarre for several days before the shooting.[48]

None of the reports by individual psychiatrists provided details pertaining to subcategories of psychoses and numbers seen. They seemed to take these cases in stride and appeared confident in treating them uniformly, primarily in inpatient settings, using milieu therapy and psychotropic medications. (See Case 8-1, PFC Yankee below and Case 8-5, PVT Easy, later in the chapter.) As previously indicated, division psychiatrists were more or less limited to 3 to 5 days of hospital-like care and evacuated unresponsive cases to the psychiatric specialty detachments for additional treatment. Solo psychiatrists at evacuation and field hospitals also were limited in the scope of their treatment and resorted to the psychiatric specialty detachments. In turn, the psychiatric specialty detachments provided more extensive and prolonged treatment but were limited to 30 days before evacuating intractable cases out of Vietnam. However, as already mentioned, the policy was to medically evacuate soldiers with unresponsive psychotic conditions out of Vietnam as soon as possible. Otherwise, psychiatric treatment within the various medical treatment facilities was consistent with the military psychiatry forward treatment doctrine reviewed in Chapter 7.[38]

In general, there was no system established that would inform the psychiatrists in Vietnam regarding the treatment provided and clinical course of their patients at the receiving hospitals out of the country and whether their clinical judgment was confirmed. However, two published reports shed some light on the fate of psychiatric patients evacuated out of Vietnam. Dave M Davis, an Army psychiatrist, noted that of 155 cases sent to his backup hospital in Japan over a 15-month period in 1966–1967, 66 (43%) received a schizophrenic diagnosis (73% of whom displayed prominent paranoid symptoms). Only five of these had a previous history of psychiatric hospitalizations, and the onset of disabling symptoms was not statistically related to any phase of the 1-year Vietnam tour.

The average hospitalization in Japan was 46 days for the schizophrenic patients, and they were returned to duty elsewhere in Asia.[49] The report by Elliot M Heiman, an Army psychiatrist in the United States, provided an intriguing contrast. He indicated that 10 of 12 patients evacuated from Vietnam to the treatment center at Fort Gordon, Georgia, for schizophrenia

Immersion Shock and Adjustment to Vietnam

Army psychiatrists who served during the first year of the war indicated that susceptibility to psychiatric disturbance was highest among recent arrivals. Byrdy, with the 1st Cavalry Division, commented that he often saw new troops during their second week in Vietnam. ("It must take a while before the novelty of the place wore off, before he finally became familiar with the routine of his unit and learned its expectations of him, and before compulsive mechanisms of adjustment were strained by the realization of a year of sad separation from home, tedious days of work and anxious nights."[70]) Bowman, with the 935th Psychiatric Detachment, indicated that the highest incidence of referrals to their mental hygiene clinic was between the 1st and 2nd months[71] (see Appendix 11, "Recent Experiences in Combat Psychiatry in Vietnam"). And Blank, at the 3rd Field Hospital in Saigon, reported a minor peak in referrals at around 4 weeks after a soldier's arrival, but a much larger one after 5 months in-country (Figure 8-3). (A similar diphasic pattern was reported by LE Morris, an Air Force psychiatrist, among 225 Air Force patients hospitalized in 1966 at the 483rd US Air Force Hospital at Cam Ranh Bay. Of the airmen who were hospitalized for adjustment reactions in the first 6 weeks of their tour, 29% were diagnosed with dependent personalities. In contrast, 39% were hospitalized with variations of depression and irritability between their 4th and 6th months and had rigid and overly conscientious personalities.[72])

The following year, three Army psychiatrists—Jones, Jerome J Dowling, and Tischler—provided additional insights into the challenges faced by newly arriving troops. Jones, when he served with the 3rd Field Hospital in Saigon (September 1966–January 1967), reported high numbers of referrals among soldiers in their first weeks in Vietnam and highlighted the unsettling effect of culture shock on the incoming soldiers who were suddenly faced with Vietnam's "poverty, prostitution and pestilence." Being stationed near Tan Son Nhut airfield, the entry point for new arrivals, Jones would treat many of the fresh casualties. Symptoms were fainting or agitation on first arrival, and later, sleepwalking, bedwetting, nightmares, and anxiety. Jones interpreted some of this as serving environmental manipulation, that is, to avoid the hazards of combat. He also noted that after the initial period of adjustment, most adapted and became productive.[38]

Dowling (Figure 8-4) described soldier patterns of adjustment with the 1st Cavalry Division through the course of the 1-year tour. He based his impressions on casual experiences and clinical observations. He especially noted the "trauma" sustained by the arriving soldiers as they encountered:

the naked joy of the out-going troops, hearing their hair-raising stories, plus the sound of artillery, plus the mess halls, the latrines; why everyone doesn't turn around and go home still puzzles me. Death is suddenly very real. In one battalion a newly assigned PFC has a 50-50 chance of surviving.[73(pp45–46)]

According to Dowling, soldiers susceptible to psychosis and those with character and behavior disorders were most likely to require psychiatric attention in the first few months of the tour as a consequence of their inability to adapt to the challenges in this new and highly stressful environment. (Case 7-4, PVT X-ray, in Chapter 7 is an example.) Accommodation to the dangers, deprivations, long working hours, and incessant demands required most military personnel to adopt a mindset of "resignation," which lasted roughly until the last month of their tour. By this he meant a chronic, subclinical depression with interrupted sleep because of the heat and artillery, erratic appetite, and overreliance on alcohol.[73]

Tischler explored more systematically the epidemiology of psychiatric and behavior problems seen among the large collection of support units at Qui Nhon. He correlated demographic and diagnostic features of 200 enlisted soldier referrals to the 67th Evacuation Hospital with the phase of each patient's 12-month tour. Tischler was graphic in his portrayal of the new soldier's anxiety-provoking encounter with the exotic, dangerous, and ambiguous Vietnam. Those who successfully coped drew feelings of security from new group affiliations and subordination to authority; but all were somewhat psychologically depleted by being "exposed to death at first hand" and forced to surrender much of their autonomy to the military.

Nonetheless, the majority of troops were able to distract themselves by becoming absorbed in their military tasks and immediate life space and relationships. This commonly involved redirecting their attention from home and the past to that of seeking maximum pleasure through materialism, scrounging,

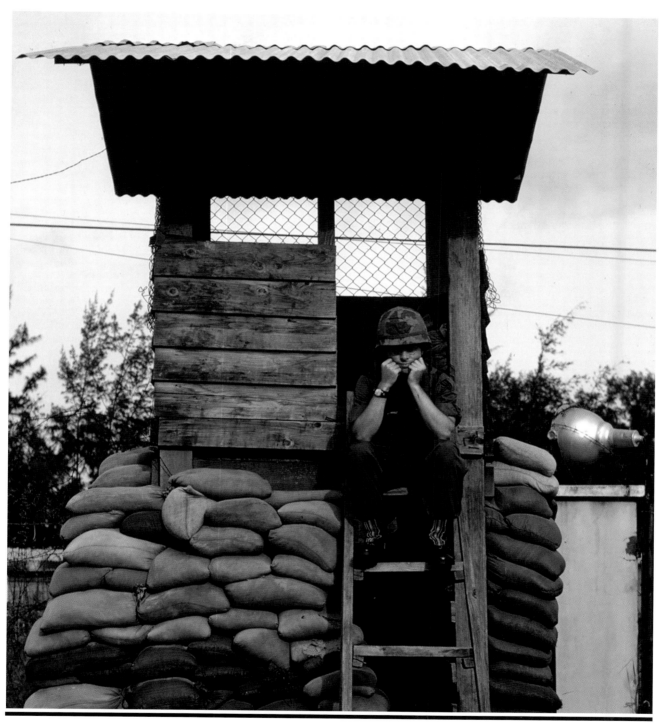

FIGURE 8-3A. Downcast soldier near the gate of the 8th Field Hospital in Nha Trang. The subject in this 1970 photograph appears to be either bored or homesick, or even depressed. The image is consistent with the deepening discontent and despair among replacement troops assigned in Vietnam during the second half of the war. Even though combat risks were gradually declining, the fighting continued and soldiers still had to contend with a year of military restrictions and sad separation from home, tedious days of work, and anxious nights. These factors, combined with the gradual repudiation of the war by fellow Americans and growing disaffection within the military, strained everyone to some degree and certainly contributed to increasing numbers of psychiatric and behavior problems in Vietnam. Photograph courtesy of Richard D Cameron, Major General, US Army (Retired).

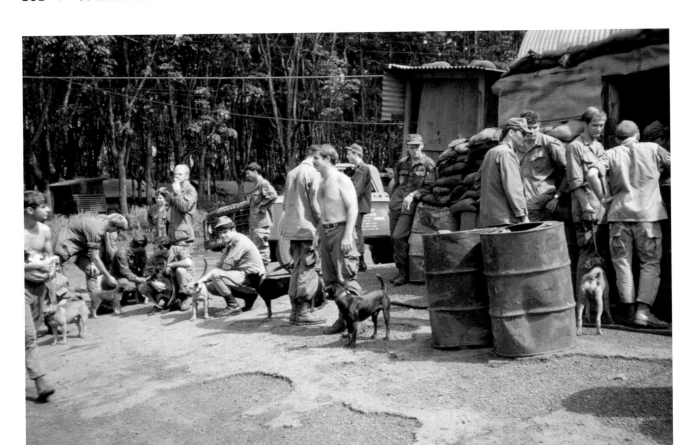

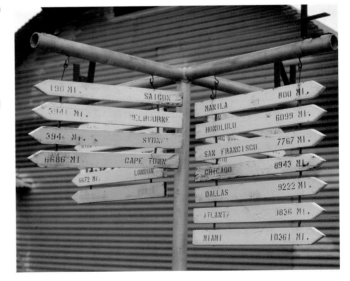

FIGURE 8-3B. (Top) 1st Cavalry Division troops with pet dogs. This is a 1970 photograph of soldiers of the 1st Cavalry Division who have gathered at the 15th Medical Battalion medical clearing station so that dogs they had adopted in Vietnam could be immunized against rabies. This suggests that for some troops relief from deployment malaise and other stresses could be had by taking care of a pet (some adopted monkeys). Photograph courtesy of Richard D Cameron, Major General, US Army (Retired).

FIGURE 8-3C. (Bottom) Mileage marker somewhere on a US military post in South Vietnam. This 1969 photograph gives vivid testimony to the strong sense of physical dislocation and yearning for home that deeply affects troops assigned to fight a war halfway around the world and far from loved ones and the familiar. Any consideration of stress reactions occurring among soldiers deployed in Vietnam had to begin with measuring the weight of this risk factor. Photograph courtesy of Richard D Cameron, Major General, US Army (Retired).

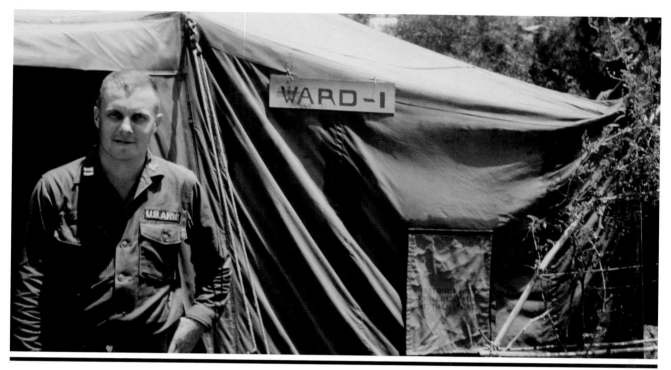

FIGURE 8-4. Captain Jerome J Dowling, Medical Corps, Division Psychiatrist with the 1st Cavalry Division. Dowling was a civilian-trained psychiatrist who served with the 1st Cavalry Division between June 1966 and March 1967, early in the war. He completed the remainder of his tour with the 17th Field Hospital in Saigon. He was the first psychiatrist assigned in Vietnam to describe the psycho-social stressors that commonly affected troops serving in a combat division, as well as patterns of maladjustment and dysfunction, that were coincident with phases of the 1-year tour. Photograph courtesy of Jerome J Dowling.

bartering, R & R (rest and recuperation leave), and frequenting the nearby bars and brothels (a "hedonistic pseudocommunity"). Especially challenging for the new soldier was "anomic anxiety," which was generated by his shock in realizing that preservice assumptions regarding the patterns of events and transactions were no longer predictable—an identity-threatening discovery that brought about intense longing for home and the familiar.

Tischler reported that almost half of his referrals came within the first 3 months of their tour, and that there was a progressively declining incidence over the remaining months until their DEROS (date expected return overseas). His overall impression was that, despite the variations in the forms of psychiatric problems seen, the common pathogenic model involved a mismatch between the soldier's specific personal resource require-ments in Vietnam and his predeployment capacity for stress tolerance. He found that, although time eroded the capacity of the deployed troops to withstand the hazards and privations there in general, the more susceptible

soldier's "neurotic predisposition" also affected the equation.[45]

Somewhat surprisingly, Tischler found that patients who required treatment during their first quarter in Vietnam had been successful in role tasks before Vietnam (both civilian as well as military) but were apparently unprepared for those associated with transition to serving in the combat zone. In contrast were the lower numbers of soldiers seen during the second and third quarters of their tour who were mostly referred by their commanders pending disciplinary actions. These soldiers had functioned relatively ade-quately in their civilian roles but had conflicts with military authority after entering the Army; then, over time in Vietnam they failed to withstand the emotionally depleting circumstances and developed behavior problems.[45]

Bloch, who served in Vietnam the following year, provided further insights into the psychosocial challenges faced by new arrivals based on his casual experiences and clinical observations at the 935th

Psychiatric Detachment. By that point in the war, the combat had intensified and circumstances in the theater had become even more stressful for the new replacement. According to Bloch, the result was a universal variation of depression (persistent loneliness, disgruntlement, moroseness, inertia and lethargy, hypersomnia, and frustration at not being able to alter one's situation)—an observation that seemingly contradicts the impression noted earlier that overall anxiety symptoms predominated over depressive ones, at least in clinical populations. For most everyone, excessive drinking and eating, preoccupation with material acquisitions, compulsive work activity, and maintaining correspondence with those outside Vietnam, were relatively adaptive modes of obtaining relief and distraction. For some, discharge of their personal dysphoria also involved an upsurge of licentiousness, or disabling inhibition, which, according to Bloch, was motivated by the activation of aggressive impulses.

Bloch provided a specific explanation for the strain associated with being sent to war in Vietnam, that is, that it produced an anomalous developmental crisis (ie, a psychological "foreign body"). By that he meant that the typical young soldier had to make radical personal and interpersonal adjustments because of the unnatural combination of: (*a*) the lengthy separation from family and loved ones, which provoked anxieties about separation and abandonment; (*b*) disruptions in expectable stateside life patterns, which aggravated these anxieties; and (*c*) the protracted exposure to the possibility of death and disfigurement. He, like Tischler, also noted that under optimal circumstances, healthy coping required intense bonding with the immediate group and partaking of its morale, which in many respects rested on the caliber of its leadership.

According to Bloch, troops with direct exposure to combat required additional psychological defenses of denial and magical belief in one's luck and indestructibility. Overall, clinical populations, which included combat troops and noncombat troops, were composed of individuals who failed in these adaptive tasks. They commonly presented with free-floating anxiety or psychosomatic conditions and preoccupations. He furthermore speculated on the likelihood that the policy of fixed, 1-year tour limits interfered with the commitment of soldiers to their combat groups and development of esprit de corps, thereby opposing adaptation and positive mental health.[74] (See Appendix 12, "Some Interesting Reaction Types Encountered in a War Zone." It provides a sophisticated analysis of several case examples on a spectrum of soldier maladaptation.)

Bey, who was division psychiatrist with the 1st ID (1969–1970) during the midpoint in the war, was explicit regarding the stress incurred by replacement troops. He reported that they were at high risk to develop symptoms if they resisted transitioning to the new life in Vietnam from their predeployment life at home. According to Bey,

. . . Those individuals who could not develop the counterphobic defenses encouraged by their new units, were unable to give up their hold on "the world," or could not identify with the language and habits of their new peer group, developed symptoms and often didn't make it in Vietnam.[48(p141)]

As a preventive effort, Bey implemented a command consultation model aimed at reducing the incidence of failed integration of solitary green troops into seasoned combat units, which included inserting new unit members by pairs.[75]

To conclude, these reports by psychiatrists who served in the field in Vietnam were consistent in identifying a collection of stressors that challenged all troops there, especially new replacements who arrived in country on staggered schedules. However, because these reviews were limited to the buildup and transition years, they omitted the late war phenomenon of new arrivals being indoctrinated by disgruntled troops who had already established various affinity groups that were bonded through their antagonism to military authority (in defiance of the "green machine"[76(p98),77(p21)]) and devotion to use of illegal drugs.

Support Troops and "The Rear"

Chapter 2 provided some observations regarding the life and circumstances affecting the thousands of military personnel who served in noncombat roles in Vietnam. As noted in Chapter 1, these individuals constituted roughly two-thirds to three-fourths of Army troops in South Vietnam. They lived and worked throughout the country in an array of outposts, semipermanent operation bases (eg, An Khe and An Hoa), corps and division headquarters bases (eg, Phu Bai and Bien Hoa), vast logistics and support complexes (eg, Long Binh and Cam Ranh Bay), and the larger cities

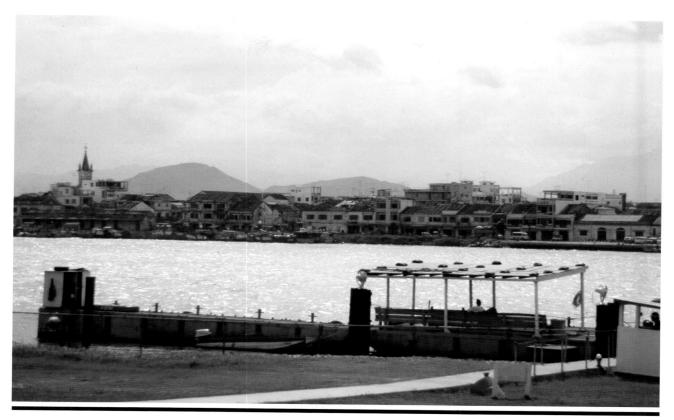

FIGURE 8-5. City of Da Nang from across the Han River. In this 1970 photograph, Da Nang, South Vietnam's second largest city, is seen from 24th Corps Headquarters. Da Nang was located north along the coast of South Vietnam and was surrounded by US military installations. Although there was a US operated pedestrian ferry that crossed the river here, for most military personnel the city was off-limits. Consequently, whereas US troops assigned in the region could find themselves fighting for South Vietnam's freedom, the circumstances meant that they remained mostly remote from the people and their culture. Photograph courtesy of Norman M Camp, Colonel, US Army (Retired).

(eg, Saigon and Da Nang). Within the divisions, they served primarily in headquarters/administration or in the logistical elements.

Although assignment in a noncombat role was not invariably tantamount to serving in a safer and more comfortable circumstance, more often than not it was. Obviously, a conspicuous exception would be the combat medic. (Bey made note of the heightened stresses faced by soldiers who served in certain support jobs: corpsmen, who were prone to reactive depression; military police road guards, because of the long periods of isolation and vulnerability; and engineers, who were not allowed to fight back when attacked.) Of course, reiterating a point made previously, the designation of "the rear" was relative in Vietnam because the combat was very fluid and there was little territory that was completely safe. Michael Herr, the correspondent, described it in compelling fashion:

. . . You could be in the most protected space in Vietnam and still know that your safety was provisional, that early death, blindness, loss of legs, arms or balls, major and lasting disfigurement—the whole rotten deal—could come in on the freaky-fluky as easily as in the so-called expected ways. . . . The roads were mined, the trails booby-trapped, satchel charges and grenades blew up jeeps and movie theaters, the VC [Viet Cong] got work inside all the camps as shoeshine boys and laundresses and honey dippers; they'd starch your fatigues and burn your shit and then go home and mortar your area.[78(pp13–14)]

However, noncombat troops and those living and operating in the rear had one expectable downside—they were treated with total disdain by combat troops who faced greater risk and hardship. Not only were they

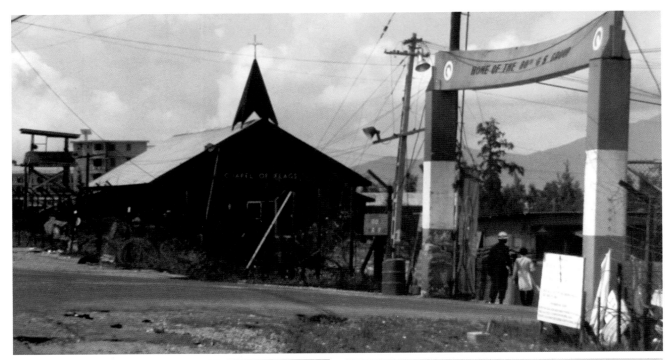

FIGURE 8-6A. (Top) Entrance to the 80th Combat Support Group in Da Nang, 1970. Located on this compound was a very large and diverse collection of support units. The record suggests that rates for psychiatric disorders and behavior problems in Vietnam were generally higher among noncombat troops such as these. Part of the explanation comes from the fact that, outside of the larger installations, such as Long Binh and Cam Ranh Bay, support troops worked and lived in small, isolated, and heavily guarded compounds with few opportunities for escape. Also, compared to combat troops, they were more likely to suffer from the lack of a sense of purpose that could justify their restrictions and privations. For many troops these features combined to aggravate interpersonal conflicts with fellow soldiers and heighten tensions with military authorities. As an aside, although the Chapel of the Flags is prominent in the picture, it is noteworthy that spiritual or religious matters are not mentioned in the psychiatric literature from the theater. Photograph courtesy of Norman M Camp, Colonel, US Army (Retired).

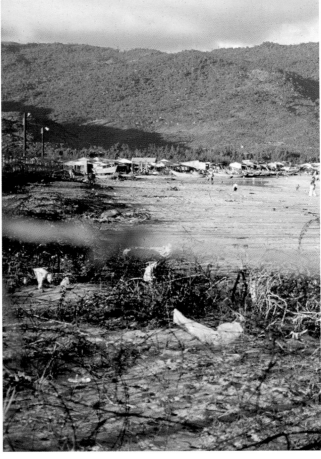

FIGURE 8-6B. (Bottom) Fishing village seen through concertina wire. This is a 1970 photograph of a Vietnamese fishing village taken through the heavily guarded perimeter of the 95th Evacuation Hospital near the city of Da Nang on the coast of the South China Sea. It illustrates the view that the majority of nondivisional, support troops had of the Vietnamese people and their culture apart from incidental contact with Vietnamese day laborers on their compound or while hastily traveling on the roads with an armed escort. Photograph courtesy of Norman M Camp, Colonel, US Army (Retired).

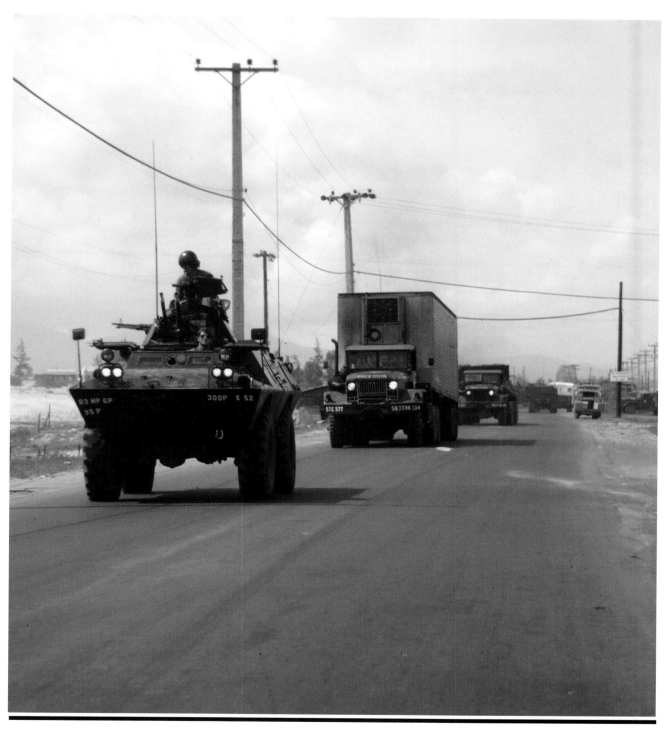

FIGURE 8-6C. US military convoy with armed escort near Da Nang, 1970. Because of the dangerous conditions throughout most of South Vietnam, areas outside of military compounds and bases were designated off-limits to American military personnel except during combat maneuvers. This meant that, whereas the troops assigned to the larger, better equipped installations, such as Long Binh and Cam Ranh Bay, had off-duty access to recreational facilities, the majority of soldiers in Vietnam were more restricted in opportunities to escape the embrace of their immediate military setting and authority because of the need to travel in an armed escort or aircraft. Photograph courtesy of Norman M Camp, Colonel, US Army (Retired).

resented for their life of safety and ease (relative), but they were also often suspected of unfairly appropriating the best of the equipment and benefits for themselves. Support and service troops were aware of how they were regarded by "real" combat troops and invariably felt varying degrees of guilt in their presence.[79] Bey provided the following observations regarding the tension between combat troops and noncombat troops.

> . . . [T]here was the REMF [rear echelon mother f--ker] social order. This term was used to refer to anyone in a more desirable, comfortable, or safer assignment than your own. The men in the combat units with the most dangerous duties such as Rangers who were LRRPs (long-range reconnaissance patrol), were at one end of the continuum. Military personnel serving in the United States were at the other end. In between, the general hierarchy went from the men at the fire support bases, those at base camps, and those assigned to large support areas such as Long Binh or Saigon. I was as far forward as a psychiatrist could be assigned, but I was a REMF to the combat troops who fought the enemy out in the paddies. Similarly, Dau Tieng and Lai Khe received rocket and mortar attacks more frequently than Di An; therefore the men stationed at those bases regarded the men stationed at Di An as REMFs.
>
> There was a kind of one-upmanship that took place when forward- and rear-assigned individuals interacted.
>
> . . . Sometimes the anger toward REMFs produced explosive violence, especially when aggravated by factors such as the communication gap between white, inexperienced officers and black enlisted men from inner city environments.[48(pp158–159)]

To maintain morale, the US government went to great expense to supply the troops in Vietnam with material comforts and recreation/entertainment opportunities (Figure 8-7). According to Spector, a military historian:

> In general, the larger the base or headquarters, the greater were the amenities. As a minimum, however, troops at the major installations enjoyed beds with sheets, hot food, electricity, hot showers, a club, athletic facilities, movies, and plenty of beer. Barracks and hootches often had Vietnamese maids

and laundresses. Many clubs were air-conditioned, and the larger ones featured dining rooms where hamburgers, French fries, fried chicken, or steak were always available.[79(p263)]

Still, large numbers of soldiers, especially support and service-support, were assigned to small, isolated compounds that weren't so well equipped. For most of them, the confines of their day-to-day life felt like being in a prison camp (Figure 8-5 and Figure 8-6).

Troops serving in the rear in general found themselves battling boredom and loneliness for home as opposed to fighting the enemy. For them, the stress-mitigating spirit of unit commitment and group cohesion characteristic of a combat unit was missing, and disputes and fights between soldiers were common; as the war progressed, these became increasingly racially centered and facilitated by drug use. (Indeed, according to Spector, racial problems, and then serious morale problems more generally, first appeared in the combat support and service support units in 1968.[79])

From his vantage point as a research psychiatrist in Vietnam during the first couple of years of the war, Bourne remarked that the bulk of psychiatric cases came from support units. Two years later, in 1969–1970, Bey, a division psychiatrist, made the same observation, that support units had a higher incidence of some problems, especially drug and alcohol problems and racial tensions, and he believed this was because they were not involved in the combat and had to contend with the routine and monotony of daily life and boredom.[46] However, reports by Blank[80] and by William F Kenny,[81] which centered mostly on the psychiatric problems of the thousands of support and service-support personnel who lived and worked in the Saigon area, suggest a more complex pathogenesis. They observed that most referrals were dependent and passive-aggressive individuals and felt their adjustment problems stemmed especially from heightened dependency needs, underlying separation anxiety, and primitive defense mechanisms; in other words, preservice personality susceptibility was a critical risk factor.

But even within the combat units, apparently the lulls could be as corrosive to the spirit as was the marginality borne by support troops. According to Dowling, a division psychiatrist, greater stress came from daily base camp routines than combat itself—often accompanied with preoccupations with problems back home.[73] Bowman, with the 935th Psychiatric

Detachment in 1966, was specific that although combat-centered stress was diffusely debilitating in the cases they treated, it was compounded by the more general stress of combat zone deployment.[71]

The only attempt to systematically compare combat and support troops among psychiatric patients came from Jones,[82] who collected diagnostic and demographic data regarding 120 consecutive enlisted referrals to the 3rd Field Hospital in the Saigon area in late 1966, the second year of the war. The median rank for these patients was E-4 (corporal), and they were only distinguishable by age (23 for combat troops vs 29 for support troops) and marital status (35% for combat troops vs 51% for support troops). Among the 98 support troops, the leading "symptom or behavior" was alcoholism (20%), followed by character and behavior disorder (18%), and anxiety (16%). Among the 22 combat troops (25% of referrals, compared to the 15% reported by Blank who preceded him), the leading "symptom or behavior" was character and behavior disorder (32%), followed by conversion symptoms (23%), and anxiety (18%).

Although Jones did not include denominator data that would permit establishment of incidence rates, he did offer the following summary of his findings: "the [combat support troop] casualty stands out as being very much more likely to be alcoholic, homosexual, or psychotic."[82(p14)] Jones felt that the type of psychological conflict borne by these men could only be determined with some degree of certainty in 47 cases (39%) (20 combat troops, 27 support troops). Still, thirteen of the 22 combat troops (59%) had a primary conflict over being in a combat zone versus only five of the 98 support troops (5%); but the two groups were otherwise similar regarding marital or family problems as a primary conflict (23% and 21%, respectively)[82] (see Appendix 16, "Vietnam Study: Reactions to Stress Comparing Combat and Support Troops").

Renner, a Navy psychiatrist who served aboard the hospital ship USS *Repose*, provided some general observations regarding the higher rates of disciplinary infractions among Marine support troops in 1969. According to Renner, despite the overall lower morale in Vietnam by that point in the war, members of the small combat unit were able to justify their dangers, hardships, and self-discipline based on a shared "primitive struggle for survival." By extension, as long as they were in the field, unit identity remained intact ("superficial closeness"), whereas military identity

more generally was mostly irrelevant. However, once these Marines were rotated out of combat, conflicts between group members, or opposition toward military authority, erupted. "The reduced degree of external danger in the rear permitted these men to express dissent more openly . . . and reduces their need for conformity."[27(p177)]

Soldiers, Sex, and Romance

The inevitable sexual tensions generated among the several hundred thousand bored, lonely, and frustrated men serving in Vietnam was an important matter affecting morale and duty performance. Evidently from the first months of the war military personnel had access to local prostitutes based on combat circumstances, the unit's location, and the unit's culture. Byrdy, the Army psychiatrist who served with the 1st Cavalry when it was inserted into Vietnam in 1965, reported that "Vietnamese camp followers quickly moved into the area in a very well organized fashion and, depending on the attitudes of command, the troops variably had access to them."[70(p10)] (See Appendix 8, "Division Psychiatry in Vietnam," to this volume for a further discussion.) According to Spector, a Marine historian, sex inevitably became a major preoccupation for the deployed troops in Vietnam. "In practice, sex was relatively easy to obtain in the shanty towns surrounding many of the large bases."[79(p268)] Whereas these were almost always designated as off-limits, with threats of fines, demotions, and so forth, the venereal disease rate was high, which indicated that the troops found ways around these restrictions. Many units set up clubs on post, "recreational areas," ostensibly to showcase entertainers, but they typically also served as a venue for prostitution ("semiofficial brothels"). The advantage was that the women could be monitored by military medical personnel. In the field, soldiers could make a deal for quick sex using a C-Ration meal. Although military policy sought to restrict troop access to Saigon and the other big cities, this proved impossible, and sex, as well as drugs and black marketeering, became "growth industries."[79(pp268–269),83]

Gary K Neller, an Army psychiatrist, provided this description from his experience as a Special Forces medic in Vietnam in 1967:

> In many of the units that were away from populated areas and were heavily engaged, drinking and prostitution were even encouraged by [military

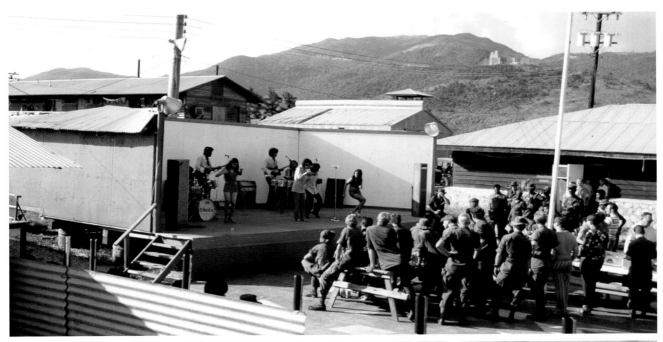

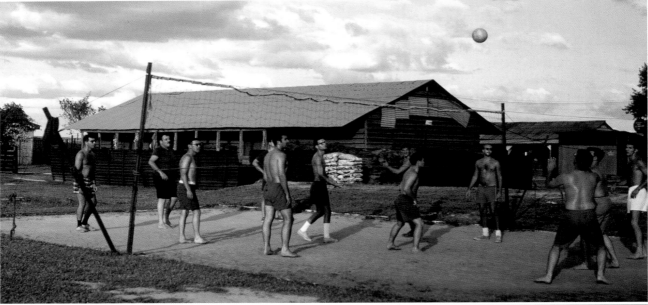

FIGURE 8-7A. (Top) Unit party at the 95th Evacuation Hospital (1971). Such activities were greatly prized as a means of stress mitigation by troops who had access. Furthermore, alcohol was openly available at functions like these and otherwise readily available to the troops through the system of post exchanges (PX) and noncommissioned officers' (NCO) and officers' clubs. Even in units whose commanders did not permit alcohol sales to lower ranks, there were manifold ways to bypass this restriction. Photograph courtesy of Norman M Camp, Colonel, US Army (Retired).

FIGURE 8-7B. (Bottom) Volleyball at the 15th Medical Battalion, 1st Cavalry Division base at Phouc Vinh. Sports and recreation were highly valued by troops as an antidote to stress and boredom. In general, the larger the compound or base, the greater the likelihood that there were facilities available for these activities. However, this predictably led to high tension between the combat troops who served in the more primitive forward positions and the noncombat, support troops who worked and lived in the better equipped and relatively safer bases such as this one. Photograph courtesy of Richard D Cameron, Major General, US Army (Retired).

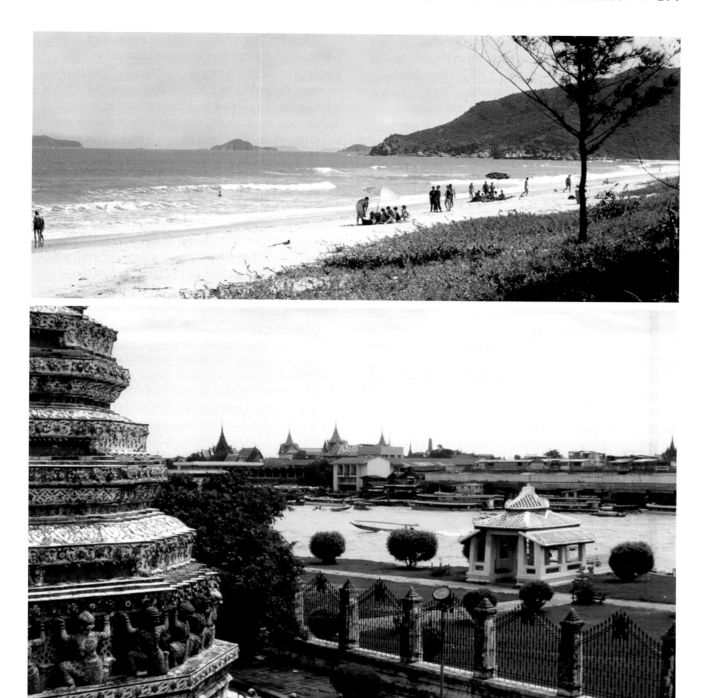

FIGURE 8-7C. (Top) American beach at Vung Tau on the coast of the South China Sea east of Saigon. Many troops were lucky enough to be assigned near one of the American-controlled beaches and were periodically allowed to spend time there to relax and recreate. This had obvious morale-boosting effects. Photograph courtesy of Norman M Camp, Colonel, US Army (Retired).

FIGURE 8-7B. (Bottom) View from The Grand Palace in Bangkok, Thailand. The US military R & R (rest and recuperation) leave program, in which all personnel serving in Vietnam were permitted a week away from their unit and transportation to remote settings such as Australia, Hong Kong, Bangkok, and Hawaii, was very efficient and successful over the course of the war. Overall it served as a highly prized form of psychological release from the war. Photograph courtesy of Norman M Camp, Colonel, US Army (Retired).

referred refused to cooperate and were administratively discharged from the Army.[92] One explanation for the minimal references to homosexual referrals in Vietnam is that at that point in time the Army's concerns for identifying and eliminating homosexual soldiers were at a low ebb,[93] perhaps in conjunction with the necessity for maximizing troop strength.

Staggered 1-Year Tours and the Short-Timer's Effect

The overlapping psychosocial risk consequent to the staggered troop replacement policies and the fixed 1-year tours were explored in Chapter 6 with regard to combat troops, but their effects in Vietnam were far more widespread. The individual rotation and replacement policy that was utilized was an adaptation of a term-limitation policy initiated in Korea after the first year there. It was intended to counteract the excessive psychiatric attrition seen in World War II among soldiers who were deployed "for the duration" (an expression indicating that troops were committed until the end of hostilities). However, in contrast to tours with a predetermined length, as in Vietnam, in Korea soldiers were assigned for 9 to 12 months and rotated out based on a point system of exposure to risk. In fact, Stewart L Baker Jr credited the *earned* rotation system in Korea, along with the forward placement of mental health professionals and helicopter evacuation capability of the wounded, for greatly reducing the psychiatric percentage of medical evacuations within that theater.[94]

Observers in the field during the first couple of years in Vietnam, like Bourne (a psychiatric researcher), Moskos (a military sociologist), and Byrdy (a division psychiatrist with the 1st Cavalry Division), touted the benefits of the fixed, 1-year tour as stress reducing because of the soldier's sense of limitation of the hardship and risk. However, as the war progressed, the individual fixed tour developed offsetting negative effects because: (*a*) soldiers became preoccupied with the passage of their year as opposed to performance measures (according to Jones, "Everything [in Vietnam] occurred in the context of time-awareness"[38]); and (*b*) various causes of attrition within units (combat casualties, sickness, etc) meant that the troop replacements became increasingly randomly distributed.

Thus after the first couple of cohorts of troops had rotated back to the United States and their replacements began to arrive on a staggered basis, the fixed, 1-year tour meant that there was invariably a large measure of interpersonal dysynchrony because the timing for everyone's cycle in-country was different. As a result, these two force management policies (ie, the 1-year fixed tour and individual rotations) greatly impeded the maintenance of unit cohesion and commitment. This was truer for support troops because it was not necessary that they bond for the sake of combat efficiency, as was the case for combat troops. However, this effect was otherwise very evident throughout the theater as, with every new encounter, sooner or later a comparison was made as to how much time each party had remaining in their tour.

As a corollary, a soldier's self-esteem rested to some degree on how "short" he was, that is, how much time he had left in his tour in Vietnam. Soldiers ritualistically marked their personal DEROS calendars, and they adopted a variety of expressions serving to gloat over someone who was not as short (ie, a "two-digit, midget!" boast meant that one had fewer than 100 days remaining). Although the soldier's status increased with every passing day because new arrivals began at day 365, he was still vulnerable to feeling pangs of envy when he encountered another soldier who had less time remaining in his tour. In effect, these rotation policies meant that too much importance became attached to the differences between individuals as opposed to their interdependent needs as soldiers fighting to win a war. Unfortunately, apparently the Army never systematically studied the policy's negative effects on unit morale and performance.

Also problematic, earlier in the war, Bourne had argued that traditional unit cohesion was not as necessary in Vietnam because of the ease with which the soldier could stay in contact with home during his assignment (speedy mail, tapes, periodic phone calls, and a stateside R & R leave). This may have been true as long as family and loved ones supported the war. However, when their attitude reversed as the war became increasingly despised, the opposite outcome arose: those on the home front fostered tremendous resentment within the soldier who felt forced to face unjustified risks, hardship, and losses.

The problems faced by commanders regarding soldiers who were nearing their DEROS and who were becoming progressively ineffective, or even combat averse—the so-called short-timer's syndrome—was mentioned in Chapter 2 and further elaborated in Chapter 6 (illustrated with Case 6-9, SP4 Kilo). To reiterate, the short-timer's syndrome consisted of a low-grade form of emotional and behavior disability commonly seen in soldiers nearing the end of their tour and manifested by sullen, irritable, or withdrawn behavior; a preoccupation with fears of being killed or injured; and a general resistance to duty.

With regard to combat units, Dowling, who was with the 1st Cavalry Division, observed clinically that soldiers were commonly affected by mounting apprehension during the weeks leading up to DEROS; and that this could lead to a syndrome of emotional distress in which irritability alternated with euphoria, and obsessions about "returning intact" took such forms as anxious requests for X-rays, VDRL testing (Venereal Disease Research Laboratory test for syphilis), and the removal of genital warts.[73] Jones, who was with the 25th ID, suggested that the combat soldier became symptomatic when approaching his DEROS because, in emotionally withdrawing and turning his attention to life after Vietnam, he was relinquishing a critical psychological defense based on combat group identification because he could no longer share in the group's illusion of immortality.[38] Jones also said that, whereas the short-timer's syndrome was worse among combat troops, it rarely required psychiatric attention.[22] Bloch, who saw both combat and support troops at the 935th Psychiatric Detachment, speculated that variations on the short-timer's syndrome were best understood as ways that soldiers "buttress themselves against the waves of strong internal reactions to external stresses . . . ,"[74(p625)] which were character-specific for them.

Tischler, who was with the 67th Evacuation Hospital, also reported from his study mentioned earlier that during the last few months of the soldier's tour, emotional withdrawal from both the environment and the group was inevitable, and that the dominant challenge he faced was that of psychosocial disengagement. Even among support units, soldiers became especially cautious and fewer were willing to leave the safety of the compound. According to Tischler, combat troops increasingly suffered from "[a] feeling of resentment that approaches loathing and hatred . . . when combat missions are called for."[45(p39)] Although the last quarter of the tour brought the fewest psychiatric referrals, in part because of each soldier's tendency to draw strength from an idealized future, some troops required psychiatric attention because they had difficulty separating from their "exquisitely interdependent" group of combat buddies.

Tischler found that soldiers seen in the last quarter were individuals from disrupted families with poor educational and service records who struggled with the process of reorienting to a post-Vietnam future (home, family, friends, and things forgotten). Although there were more married soldiers in this group than those seen in the previous three quarters, more than half (57%) of these cases had not been receiving letters from home. According to Tischler, overall these cases could be regarded as "role failures," and many experienced "apathetic disenchantment" because they assumed that they would continue to fail after they returned to the United States.[45]

The preceding observations have centered on the problematic effect on the soldiers because they rotated in and out of units on a 1-year tour basis; however, greatly aggravating this policy's potential to impair unit morale and bonding, as well as unit combat effectiveness, was that leadership elements—officers and NCOs—were also entering and leaving the theater on a random basis.[79,95] Remarkably, the resultant churning and depletion of experienced Army officers consequent to their serving 1-year tours was doubled by the theater policy of rotating officers from command to staff positions after 6 months to increase opportunities to command.[96] Bey, to his credit, discovered that a rise in some indices of unit dysfunction in the 1st ID correlated with leadership turnover, and he instituted a preventive, command consultation project aimed at reducing the associated stress on unit members.[97]

LATE WAR PROBLEMS IN VIETNAM: PLUMETTING MORALE, DISCIPLINE, AND MENTAL HEALTH

The second half of the war brought with it a dramatic rise in soldier dissent with widespread behavior problems that seriously compromised military order and discipline. Although primarily representing challenges to Army leadership, four of the emergent problem areas overlapped with the mission of Army psychiatry, certainly that pertaining to social and community psychiatry: (1) racial tension and conflicts; (2) suicides; (3) soldier violence, especially the targeting of military leaders; and (4) use of dangerous drugs, primarily heroin. This section will summarize the available professional information regarding items

(1) through (3), and Chapter 9 will address the available information regarding drug use in the theater.

Racial Tension and Conflicts

Despite its prior successes in desegregation, the Army was not exempt from racially based tension and strife as new recruits entered the military from an increasingly polarized American society. The combination of the burgeoning black-pride/civil rights movement in the United States and the general disaffection among enlisted soldiers corrupted the morale and military allegiance of many black soldiers in Vietnam during the second half of the war. Aggravating the problem, 40% of the 320,000 men brought into the service under the previously described Project 100,000 program, with its lowered intelligence and educational standards, were nonwhite. Furthermore, a disproportionate number (37%) of Project soldiers served in combat roles (vs 14% for non-Project soldiers).[66]

By way of backdrop, The National Advisory Commission on Civil Disorders, known as the Kerner Commission, was established in July 1967 by President Lyndon Johnson to investigate the causes of the recent upsurge in race riots in the black neighborhoods of major US cities. After 7 months of proceedings, the Commission's final report was released. Among its conclusions, which generally underscored the economic and social hardship borne by African Americans, was that racial tensions and polarization in the United States had increased to unprecedented levels, and, if unaddressed, would ultimately lead to "the destruction of basic democratic values."[98] On 4 April 1968, 1 month after the release of the Kerner Report, the inspirational civil rights leader Martin Luther King Jr was assassinated. This provoked an upsurge of racial violence, prompting riots in 169 cities and resulting in $130 million in property damage, 24,000 arrests, and 43 deaths.[99(p102)]

The riot in the Long Binh Jail the following August was emblematic of the incendiary level of black–white tensions in Vietnam. The rebellion, which ultimately destroyed the facility, started when a group of black inmates attacked the guards, ostensibly over unacceptable living conditions. However, clearly indicating its racial roots, bands of black prisoners roamed through the compound, beating white prisoners and setting fire to their tents. One white inmate was killed.[100]

In 1970, Colbach and Parrish's semiofficial summary of mental health activities in Vietnam to that point in the war acknowledged that "the racial problem" in the United States had extended to Vietnam:

> Black power feelings have become quite strong at times, and such things as Afro haircuts, extreme clannishness, and black power signs have become commonplace. There have been some outbreaks of black-white violence, and everyone has become increasingly edgy about the situation. . . . [A]ny incident involving black and white soldiers has been considered to be of racial origins. The whole situation has had an adverse effect on morale.[36(p338)]

That same year Wallace Terry, a war correspondent, surveyed soldiers in Vietnam regarding racial perceptions and attitudes. His findings made it clear how much race relations had deteriorated there compared to a survey conducted 3 years earlier. He found a "very deep layer of bitterness" among black soldiers. In particular (*a*) they were averse to fighting in a war they considered to be the white man's war; (*b*) their anger was fueled by the racial prejudice in America; (*c*) they believed their fight was really in the United States against repression and racism; (*d*) they were "schooled in the violent art of guerrilla warfare"[101(p222)]; and (*e*) many declared their intention to align themselves with radical groups upon return home, join riots, and take up arms in the United States to achieve rights and opportunities previously denied them.[101]

Results of a similar survey administered by Fiman, Borus, and Stanton to 126 black and 359 white enlisted soldiers returning from Vietnam between 1968 and 1971 generally confirmed Terry's findings. Black soldiers, primarily the younger ones, held a more negative view of race relations than did whites. Interestingly, black–white relationships were perceived as better in Vietnam than in the United States, especially among soldiers who served in combat.[102] Borus also interviewed 64 Vietnam returnees who served there between June 1969 and December 1970 and concluded that, when compared with combat units where the goal of survival necessitated a spirit of trust and cooperation, racial relations were far more strained among those serving in the rear echelons. This took the form of racially segregated groupings, discrimination, tension, and open interracial conflicts.[103]

Regarding serious crimes in Vietnam, Kroll, an Army psychiatrist, conducted an in-depth study at the Fort Leavenworth Disciplinary Barracks (also known as the United States Disciplinary Barracks [USDB]) of soldiers transferred there from Vietnam between February 1968 and November 1969, that compared white soldier-prisoners (n = 149) with black soldier-prisoners (n = 127).[100] (The USDB was the only confinement facility for soldiers and airmen convicted by court-martial and required to serve more than a 6-month sentence.) Kroll's methodology included clinical interviews, psychological testing, extensive background reviews, and longitudinal observations. The two groups were indistinguishable regarding age (mean = 22.3), educational level (mean = 10.6 years), and GT (General Technical; roughly equivalent to IQ) scores (mean = 99.5), but the average time in service was greater for the white prisoners (3.3 years vs 2.2 years for black prisoners).

However, overall rates for incarceration of black prisoners significantly exceeded those for white prisoners. Black prisoners were twice as likely to be convicted for AWOL, 10 times as likely to be convicted for combat refusal, and 7.5 times as likely to be convicted for violence against a US soldier, that is, assault or murder. Rates for violence against Vietnamese nationals were roughly equal.[100(Table 4)] Kroll offered no conclusions as to individual psychiatric or personality factors that would explain how these men were different from the other soldiers who served in Vietnam without incident. However, he provided other impressions along the lines of social determinants:

- Although Kroll sought to remain neutral regarding their guilt or innocence for specific crimes, he argued for the underlying innocence of these black soldier-prisoners because of their being victims of the extremely stressful social influences and circumstantial pressures in Vietnam at that time.
- Regarding the higher rates for most crimes among black prisoners, this was explained in part by "[t]he emergence of a strong anti-military attitude among the present draft-eligible generation, combined with…a black identity movement that ridicules obedience to a white system [like the military] . . . and a war that seems vicious, pointless, and endless."[100(p59)]
- Regarding those convicted of murder, the finding that over 50% of the murder victims were buddies or friends and that the murders occurred in the rear was combination of the inherently ambivalent nature of combat buddy relationships and the regression-inducing nature of combat. "This raises the problem of whether men who become [black/white] buddies of necessity in the combat field can safely remain buddies in base camp, where the factors pushing each away from the other [in this instance, racial polarization] may be stronger than the ties pulling them together."[100(p59)]

It should be underscored that Kroll reported there was only one case of leader assassination among the cohort he studied (1968–1969). This will be contrasted with a later study conducted at the USDB by Gillooly and Bond of 24 such cases.

In 1971, following a worldwide increase in inter-racial conflicts on American military installations, the Secretary of Defense and Secretary of the Army declared that improving race relations was of the highest priority.[104] As a result educational courses in race relations were piloted throughout the chain of command. Small group discussion seminars ("rap sessions") were introduced at several posts. In November the first Department of the Army Race Relations Conference was held to implement Army-wide planning of programs to deal with racial tensions. Nonetheless throughout the remaining years of the war the programs remained inconsistent, partly because they were dependent on local initiative and support. At a number of posts these were impeded by commanders who either vehemently denied existence of any racial difficulties in their units, or the opposite—feared that introduction of race relations programs would cause bloodshed between black and white soldiers.[104]

In the Vietnam theater, the low morale and growing racial tensions affecting the military forces prompted the Military Assistance Command, Vietnam (MACV) to establish a Human Relations Branch. In turn, USARV created its Human Relations Branch, which was under the direction of Chaplain (Lieutenant Colonel) Benjamin E Smith, and required that each company-level Army unit in Vietnam establish a human relations council. By October 1971, there were 725 such councils meeting at least monthly—typically in unstructured discussions—in an attempt to improve relationships within the unit between blacks and whites as well as between enlisted men, NCOs, and officers. Commanders were responsible for facilitating the exchanges and obligated to act upon legitimate complaints. In addition, at least six major subordinate commands appointed officers or

NCOs to serve as full-time human relations specialists. Unfortunately, the stability of the councils was often undermined by the rapid turnover in personnel brought about by the contracting force structure.[105]

From the perspective of the psychiatrists in Vietnam, references to racial tensions or incidents do not appear during the first 3 years of the war. Later, Colbach, who served as a solo psychiatrist at the 67th Evacuation Hospital (November 1968–November 1969) acknowledged feeling ill-equipped to defuse racial tensions.[106] The following year, Bey (1969–1970) alluded to problems within the 1st ID, which were primarily seen among units in base camp:

> . . . Most of the black men in Vietnam were high school dropouts from ghetto neighborhoods. The officers, on the other hand, were mostly white, college-educated, newly trained lieutenants who had little or no experience at commanding troops or dealing with inner-city blacks. . . . Some company commanders and cadre tended to respond to their fears by bearing down on the black soldiers. They would issue orders prohibiting symbols of black identity, such as music, clothing, and power salutes. This led to further anger and resentment on the part of the blacks, who viewed such acts as provocations.
>
> Combat units did not have many racial problems when in the field. . . . When the soldiers were faced with a common enemy who was trying to kill them all, racial differences were mostly ignored. The problems arose when units left the field for stand down at base camps.[48(p80)]

Although having to improvise, Bey appeared to have some measure of success in intervening through the mental hygiene unit's program of primary and secondary psychiatric prevention activities. In so doing, he had a distinct advantage over Colbach as he was organizationally connected to the units within his division and had a social work officer and enlisted specialists to help. According to Bey:

> Reducing racial tensions was not officially part of the psychiatric unit's mission, but since many psychological issues were linked to racial problems, we did what we could to improve the situation in the division. I had no formal training in race relations, and I am white. A black psychiatrist

trained to deal with race relations and capable of making policy changes would likely have been more helpful to the division than I was able to be. However, there was little time to work with the black inner-city troops and the white suburban lieutenants who led them. Had there been more time and resources, we could have done more to help them reach a better understanding and working relationship. Nonetheless, we did what we could and succeeded some of the time.[48(pp80–81)]

Bey also noted that

> We only tried it (organizational case study) on a few units, but the feedback, i.e., about the racial tensions in the unit, did seem to have some positive results in terms of command loosening up about allowing black music in the enlisted men's area, tolerating their symbols of black solidarity, taking down the confederate flags, etc. I think we were able to achieve a little better understanding by both parties. Some of the techs were more knowledgeable and helpful.[107]

(See descriptions of primary prevention activities in Chapters 3 and 10; Chapter 3 includes a summary of a publication by Bey and Smith[108] that describes combined primary and secondary prevention activities surrounding racial tensions.)

In the remaining years of the war it became clear that racial tensions had become even more divisive, as well as dangerous.[109] Although the antagonism to military authority in the theater was widespread among soldiers of both races, some data suggested disproportionate numbers of black soldiers targeted their military leaders (all white) for assassination.[110,111] Under these conditions, it is not surprising that for some psychiatric cases, symptoms centered on racial differences and suspicions. (See Bloch's "Some Interesting Reaction Types Encountered in a War Zone" in Appendix 12.) The following case of paranoid schizophrenia is illustrative.

CASE 8-5: Private With Paranoid Schizophrenia and Racist Genocidal Preoccupations

Identifying Information: PVT Easy was a 19-year-old single black male with 12 months of active duty service and 7 months in Vietnam (noncombat, supply). He was treated in a succession of four medical treatment facilities. He was initially hospitalized at the 71st Evacuation Hospital in Vietnam in early 1968. He was next transferred to 8th Field Hospital, then to the 249th General Hospital, Japan, and finally to Walter Reed General Hospital (WRGH) in Washington, DC. He was discharged from WRGH 6 weeks after his initial hospitalization.

History of present illness: PVT Easy was initially hospitalized because of homicidal thoughts and grandiose delusions. ("I heard God.") At that time he related that he had been chosen "to lead my people" and that his mission was to "kill all the whites in Vietnam." These symptoms arose after he had been in Vietnam for 3 months, apparently during a period of considerable racial tension in his unit. Two days prior to admission he was reduced in rank following an incident of insubordination toward an officer (he alleged that the officer had addressed a black sergeant as "boy"). Complicating the diagnosis was that, since his arrival in Vietnam, PVT Easy frequently used marijuana. His emotional problems apparently began while he was on leave in anticipation to being assigned in Vietnam and were precipitated by the breakup with a girlfriend and the murder of his cousin by a white man. He became depressed and made several suicide attempts. He finally deduced that, since he could not be killed, God had a greater purpose for his life.

Past history: The patient was raised in the South as the youngest of four siblings. His father left the family when he was a year old and his mother worked as a secretary to raise the family. He denied significant childhood adjustment difficulties, however, in his teens he was involved in delinquent behaviors (fights, muggings, and breaking and entering). He also acknowledged deep resentment of his father for abandoning the family. His military performance history was marginal. He had received a summary Court Martial for being AWOL and an Article 15 in Vietnam for the length of his mustache.

Examination: When PVT Easy was admitted to the field hospital in Vietnam, he was observed to be euphoric, irritable, and hostile. He was grandiose in speech and manner, disoriented as to date, and had delusions of a militant, genocidal nature. Upon his transfer to WRGH and after a month of hospitalized treatment he was described as a large, muscular, mustachioed black male who appeared drowsy and without evident anxiety. He was mildly suspicious and distant, but his thinking was mostly clear, coherent, and rational. His thoughts centered on explaining how his delusions had led to his hospitalization. He was eager to minimize his earlier symptoms, prove his normalcy, and return to duty.

Clinical course: At the 8th Field Hospital he was mostly observed for a few days before his transfer to Japan. In Japan he was treated with phenothiazines, milieu therapy, and psychotherapy, resulting in abatement of his symptoms. A brief exacerbation occurred consonant with the news of the assassination of Martin Luther King Jr and the rioting in the United States. He was evacuated to WRGH on 150 mg of Thorazine and 5mg of Stelazine per day. At WRGH his hospital course was unremarkable.

Final diagnosis: Schizophrenia, paranoid type, acute, severe. Stress: moderate, recent personal losses plus duty in Vietnam. Predisposition: moderate, chaotic family background. Impairment: none, in complete remission.

Disposition: Returned to duty (in the United States) with temporary profile; to continue his medications and be reevaluated in 30 days.

Source: Narrative Summary, Walter Reed General Hospital.

Suicide

The DoD's most comprehensive records for military personnel assigned in Southeast Asia, the Combat Area Casualties Current File (CACCF), list the total number of casualties within South Vietnam for all service branches as 58,193, with 10,787 (18.5%) recorded as not being the direct result of hostilities.[112] Among the 10,787 nonhostile deaths, 382 records (3.5%) are designated as suicides. It can be reasonably assumed that this number significantly underrepresents the suicides in the theater because the CACCF also lists counts for accidental self-destruction (842); vehicle loss, crash (1,187); drowned, suffocated (1,207); misadventure (1,326); and "other accident" (1,371)—categories of death for which lowered morale and other types of psychological difficulties and psychiatric conditions may have directly or indirectly been contributory.

However, there is little in the documentation from the war in Vietnam to indicate that Army psychiatrists were utilized to conduct a psychological autopsy on any of the suicides or otherwise suspicious deaths. (Byrdy mentioned without details that once he was asked to conduct a postsuicide investigation; and Bey reported that he was asked by the division surgeon to look into the unexpected death of a 19-year-old E-4 cook. Bey's conclusion was that he died after accidentally ingesting twice the recommended dose of malaria prophylaxis, chloroquine/primaquine, while intoxicated.[48(p124)]) Such reviews might have led to the conclusion that some among the almost 6,000 nonsuicide, noncombat, violent deaths were unwitting suicides or suicides that were purposefully disguised to avoid consequences such as stigma, religious guilt, or adverse financial consequences. Illustrative of the latter is the following material that was provided in correspondence to the author many years after the war by Phillip W Cushman, who served as division psychiatrist for the 25th ID in the fall of 1970:

> One of my first experiences with the 25th Infantry Division was a young 18-year-old man whose unit had brought onto the base a prostitute to service the men. He was unable to get an erection and/ or did not want to participate. His fellow soldiers pursued him relentlessly with every derogatory name imaginable. This had gone on a week or so prior to my arrival in the division and the corpsmen at the Mental Hygiene Clinic would put the soldier up in the infirmary when his anxiety level became intolerable. I approached his Captain and told him the young man had to be transferred to a different unit where his history would hopefully not follow him. The Captain was appalled that a soldier would be so rewarded for being unable to function sexually like other "normal" males and absolutely refused my recommendation. The next evening while the soldiers were at mess the young man put his M16 in his mouth and blew out his brains. I suspect his Officer felt justice had prevailed and I suspect his family was never told the nature of his death.

The possibility of undercounting aside, according to an analysis of an earlier version of the CACCF data, the suicide rate among the US military personnel assigned in Vietnam was 0.16 per 1,000 troops (based on a total of 378 suicides), which the authors indicated was approximately double that for the general population.

Surprisingly, whereas Army troops accounted for 65.7% of the total deaths in Vietnam, 92.6% of the suicides were Army soldiers—a rate that was 7 times that for the other branches combined. In contrast, the Marines accounted for 25.5% of the total deaths in Vietnam but only 6.1% of the suicides. A multivariate analysis revealed the best predictor for suicide compared to all other deaths was being single, older, serving more time in Vietnam, not having been drafted, service in Vietnam in 1968 or later, and serving in the Army.[113] Regarding the latter, Figure 8-8 illustrates the rising suicide incidence rate among Army troops in Vietnam.

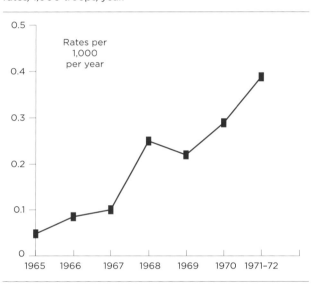

FIGURE 8-8. Estimated US Army Vietnam suicide incidence rates/1,000 troops/year.

Data sources: Numerator data for rate calculations are derived from Adams DP, Barton C, Mitchell GL, Moore AL, Einagel V. Hearts and minds: suicide among United States combat troops in Vietnam, 1957-1973. *Soc Sci Med*. 1998;47:1687–1694 (Tables 3 and 4). Denominator data are from Department of Defense, OASD (Comptroller). Directorate for Information Operations. US Military Personnel in South Vietnam 1960–1972;15 March 1974;60.

There is no published record of official concern among Army leaders, including psychiatric leaders, for this rising suicide incidence rate. From the field, Bey provided a II Field Force, Vietnam, Talking Paper that included the following: "During a 4½ month span (5 July 68 through 13 Nov 69) there were thirty-one II Field Force, Vietnam (FFORCEV II) soldiers who committed suicide—a serious problem. Gunshot (24); drug overdose (5); grenade (1); stabbed self = (1)."[39(ChapVIII,pp49–50)] (According to Bey, the number of troops represented in II Field Force's area of operations, III Corps Tactical Zone [later renamed Military Region 3], at that time was 140,000 troops.[48(p193)] If these figures are correct, the 31 suicides represented an incident rate of 6.1 suicides/1,000 troops/year.)

From the perspective of the psychiatrists who served with the Army hospitals in Vietnam, Huffman (May 1965–1966) indicated that 6.1% (37) of his patients had suicide attempts or gestures, and that there was one completed suicide in a 49-year-old master sergeant who had a depression complicated by alcoholism.[114] Blank also reported one completed suicide of a chronically depressed alcoholic sergeant.[80] During the same timeframe, Strange reported that 8% of the Navy/ Marine psychiatric caseload aboard the USS *Repose* (February and August, 1966) included suicide attempts and threats as symptoms, but that overall, "the externalization of aggression in combat is important in decreasing the comparative frequency of self-directed violence."[42(p87)]

In the combat divisions, Bey reported a few referrals for suicidal behavior in the 1st ID, and one did result in a completed suicide. In that instance it was again an alcoholic sergeant.[48] Byrdy indicated that there were no suicides among his patients at the 1st Cav, but that he knew of three "offhand."[115] He also commented:

No systematic effort was made in chronicling suicidal gestures. In fact, there were very few suicide gesturers that were directly referred [in] to me. Some soldiers with self-inflicted wounds were sent for evaluation after they had healed and were ready to return to duty. Completed suicides were the province of the military police. Only once was an effort made to involve me in a post-suicide investigation.[70]

Tischler, with the 67th Evacuation Hospital, alluded to the frequency of alcoholic intoxication in conjunction with suicidal and assaultive behavior, but he did not indicate that he was aware of any completed suicides. The case of E-4 Fox below is a summary of some illustrative material Tischler provided; however, he did not include follow-up information on the treatment.

CASE 8-6: Suicide Attempt in a Recent Arrival

Identifying Information: E-4 Fox was a 20-year-old, married, white soldier with 9 months of Army service and 3 weeks in Vietnam. He was assigned to a transportation unit.

History of present illness: Patient was hospitalized following an incident in which he drank a bottle of whisky and then slashed his wrists in his tent.

Past history: Patient had a good military record. Since his arrival in Vietnam he had not received mail from his pregnant wife. She was living with his parents and most of his pay went to her. He was working 15 hours/ day. Soon his sleep became erratic and his appetite fell off. He became obsessed that something was wrong with her and desperate to get home. His company commander was sympathetic but reminded him that everyone was in the same boat. The Red Cross and Chaplain's office personnel told him the same thing.

Examination: Patient shuffled into the appointment; his eyes were downcast and his face was a "mask of despair." He burst into tears and said, "I can't do it. Without her, I'm nothing. Since I've been here I've never felt so all alone, so cut off." All indications were that he was highly interdependent with his wife.

Clinical course: No record.

Diagnosis: No record of a formal diagnosis. Informally— "He failed to master the psychosocial task of transition associated with being newly assigned in Vietnam."

Final disposition: No record.

Source: Adapted with permission from Tischler GL. Patterns of psychiatric attrition and of behavior in a combat zone. In: Bourne PG, ed. *The Psychology and Physiology of Stress: With Reference to Special Studies of the Viet Nam War.* New York, NY: Academic Press; 1969: 34.

It seems reasonable to conclude that soldier complaints of suicidal urges and ideation were common enough among the referrals to the mental health services that they were taken seriously as clinical matters but not tracked statistically. More reportable would be the instances when the act was completed, but because those individuals were no longer in need of psychiatric care, the mental health personnel may have remained unaware of the fatal outcome.

Gartner, a political science professor, recently utilized a statistical analysis of the rising suicide rate among US troops in Vietnam, which he noted to be a historically unique phenomenon, and found it strongly correlated with the shift in US strategy to that of Vietnamization of the fighting and the growing unpopularity of the war. He argued that when combat success measures became defensive in Vietnam, that is, to avoid casualties, that, along with public disapproval of the war, created a motivational contradiction within solders (ie, challenged the individual and the collective "warrior" identity); soldiers, in turn, reverted to a psychological "learned helplessness" (a condition associated with higher rates of depression and suicide[116]). According to Gartner, "It is not [simply] the fear of dying that drives dysfunctional behavior [ie, suicide]. I expect factors driving dysfunction stem from the fear of failure, the inability to do a job successfully, and the fear of dying and killing in an unpopular war."[117(p18)] In other words, Gartner theorized that a set of highly disturbing late war factors produced sufficient strain among solders that some would have succumbed to an urge to kill themselves as if to control the means of permanently eliminating their dysphoria. As a corollary, Gartner is also critical of the US military for its persisting belief that soldier suicide during wartime is a problem of individual psychology rather than a function of the political and strategic environment.[117]

Soldier Violence and the Targeting of Military Leaders

Early War Baseline

It is evident from material presented earlier that Army psychiatrists assigned in Vietnam in the second half of the war were more likely than their predecessors to be required to assess and manage soldiers exhibiting a broad array of conduct and behavior problems, including violent, antimilitary threats and behavior. Aggressive, antagonistic soldiers were encountered during the first half of the war, but violence was not usually directed at leadership personnel. But there were exceptions. As early as 1966 Bowman, with the 935th Psychiatric Detachment, noted that his team managed a large group of soldiers referred for behavioral problems such as indiscriminate firing of weapons, insubordination, assaults, and threats of violence against their officers and NCOs, which were typically associated with heavy drinking.[71,118] Mentioned earlier, Blank, also from the first year of the war (at the 3rd Field Hospital in Saigon), reported that 17% of his patients were command-referred soldiers who were being administratively separated from the service because of repeated incidents of either verbal abuse or physical assault on superiors, usually while armed and often intoxicated.[80] And Jones told of a "gung ho" major in the Medical Service Corps who received death threats (finding bullets with his name on them) because he was felt to be too "STRAC"[2(p76)] (1960s era US military acronym, meaning "strategic, tough, and ready around the clock"). Finally, Langner, a Navy psychiatrist who served aboard the hospital ship USS *Sanctuary* (1967–1968), described often having to evaluate the individual who "came in or was sent to me with the fear or threat of killing one of his superior officers who he felt had harassed him or treated him unfairly."[119]

Two years later Bey, with Zecchinelli, studied 43 soldiers (July 1969–December 1969) who were responsible for explosive violence toward other soldiers in the 1st ID. The composite picture was that of a young, immature, action-oriented soldier with a history of limited or punitive upbringing, marginal intellect or education, and deficient social skills. Early in his Vietnam tour this soldier remained remote from his peers, or worse, was the object of scapegoating, and failed to identify with his unit and its mission. He ultimately resorted to using the available weaponry and his heightened combat reactions to vent accumulated frustrations, which were worsened by the hot, hostile, and deprived environment. He reached a flashpoint because of his exaggerated passivity and the reduced availability of alternative release behaviors such as AWOL or sick call attendance. The authors also acknowledged the compounding influence of the combat group culture in which violent behaviors commonly served to defuse group tensions (including derivatives of latent homosexuality aroused by the intense closeness of peer groups). However, a confounding variable was that African American soldiers were overrepresented among the violence-prone soldiers in the study (25%), which raises the specter of racially based grievances as well.[69] Regarding the role of intoxication, Bey provided the following:

> In our division it appeared that acts of violence were more often associated with alcohol abuse than with drug abuse. However, it was noted that men were more likely to admit to alcohol abuse than to drug usage because during that period in Vietnam a reduction in sentence could be obtained

if the man could demonstrate that the extent of his intoxication precluded his being able to premeditate the crime of which he was accused. In comparison, drug abuse did not result in mitigation of sentence and was more likely to result in additional punishment and certainly no sympathy from the military court.[39(ChapVII,p10)]

Quite notably, although Bey and Zecchinelli provided a case example of a soldier who shot to death a supply sergeant, even by 1969 there was no trend toward soldiers attacking superiors. The plausible explanation is that the study took place the year before fraggings (leader assassinations and threats) became common in Vietnam. It also may reflect that their study was conducted with combat troops who may have had somewhat lower rates of boredom and feelings of purposelessness (as noted earlier), which served to reduce resentment of military leaders compared to troops serving in support units.

During roughly the same time frame, Pasternack, a Navy psychiatrist, studied 22 Marines who were evacuated from Vietnam to a Navy hospital in the United States (late 1969–early 1970) following acts of violence, or threats to commit them, against fellow Marines. Although indicating there was considerable diversity, Pasternack noted that common trends among the subjects were the presence of psychotic or near-psychotic mental states and severe and brittle underlying character pathology. Family backgrounds included extensive chaos with parental alcoholism, mental illness, criminality, or brutality toward the patient. These patients had been poor students, socially inept, and rigidly defended with projection, denial, and reaction formation; they sought combat service to prove their masculinity. Furthermore, like Bey and Zecchinelli's study, no reports of attacks on military leaders were reported.[120]

Late War Enmity

After early 1970, the deteriorating morale and esprit in Vietnam was accompanied by rapidly rising levels of discipline problems, racial conflicts, drug use (especially heroin), and threats or attacks on officers and NCOs specifically. Linden's alarming description of the "class war" he saw as a journalist in late 1971, mentioned in Chapter 2, warrants elaboration. Linden reported that fraggings (assault using an explosive device) and threats of violence were commonly used as a means of controlling officers and NCOs through intimidating the intended victim and his peers—

primarily by enlisted soldiers who opposed performance expectations, black activists who claimed racial prejudice, and drug users who wished to pursue their heroin use without interference. According to Linden, troops serving in the rear were "acutely aware of the authoritarian nature of the system and the privileges and luxuries enjoyed by officers; yet they saw little justification . . . because both officers and enlisted men are doing essentially nothing."[109(p13)] He surmised that for most military personnel, fighting the war in its latter stages was so meaningless and bewildering that it took on a dreamlike quality—an unreality that paved the way for acts like fraggings and using heroin—behavior that would otherwise be unacceptable in other environments.[109]

There is very little in the professional literature from Vietnam to document the involvement of mental health personnel with the late-war antagonism toward military authority by lower-ranking enlisted soldiers. It was certainly evident from Linden's description that this was a big and very disruptive problem for the 101st Airborne Division and a challenge for Robert Landeen, a psychiatrist who served with the division. Contemporaneously, David J Kruzich, a social work officer who served with the 1st Cavalry Division (Airmobile) far to the south, provided a similar depiction:

> Usually superiors had advance notification that their lives were in danger. Units with which I was familiar, the usual "warning" procedures were: (1) One or more gassings of the person's living quarters with a tear gas grenade; (2) Placing a fragmentation grenade, with the detonation pin intact, under the person's pillow or in some other area where it would be readily discovered and unmistakably interpreted as a serious warning; (3) If the initial measures failed to result in the desired response, then one evening a frag would be lobbed at the individual or slipped into his sleeping bag or living area.[121(p8)]

Kruzich reported that the soldiers who resorted to fragging tended to be "antisocial." These were individuals "with little stake in either the Army or society. They were often societal rejects who had joined (or been coerced into joining by legal authorities) the Army after a succession of failures in adjusting to life as a civilian."[121(p9)] However, he gave no indication of the response by the mental hygiene staff of the 1st Cavalry Division to these problem soldiers.[121(p9)] Finally, Fisher indicated that 22 Marines among his 960 consecutive referrals in 1970–1971 were seen "in association with the charge of murder." Unfortunately, his description was not specific regarding assassination attempts on military leaders, although he included the following, "Fraggings of authorities seemed to occur in commands intimidated by threats or who were ambivalently permissive and tacitly encouraging hostile behavior in their troops."[55(p1166)]

Although official figures for fraggings were never released by the military services, it was reported that Senator Mike Mansfield (D-MT) was able to get the Pentagon to disclose that fraggings in Vietnam totaled 209 during 1970, which more than doubled those in 1969.[76(p101)] Officially, the following numbers are included in the CACCF data for the war: intentional homicide (234) and accidental homicide (944).[122] These are not broken out by year or branch of service, but some estimation can be made as to the numbers of Army soldiers affected because Army troops represented roughly two-thirds of the deployed force. Unofficial data collected by Gabriel and Savage identified a total of 1,016 incidents among all branches for the years 1969–1972 ("actual assaults" combined with incidents where "intent to kill, do bodily harm, or to intimidate" was suspected).[123(Table3)] However, there is no indication as to the proportion of these incidents that were in fact directed at officers and NCOs. Assassinations of unpopular officers and NCOs had been seen in earlier wars, typically during combat; but in Vietnam, not only was the incidence of fragging exceptionally high, but these attacks mostly arose in the phase of the war after the combat intensity had declined. They were also more common in rear areas and with the tacit approval of peers.[110] Also alarming, it is estimated that only 10% of fraggings ever came to trial because of the extreme difficulty in identifying the perpetrators.[76]

Charles Moskos, a military sociologist, provided the following impressions of the dominant patterns of late-war fragging incidents. According to Moskos, roughly 20% were "personal vendetta" fraggings in which a solitary soldier acted on his resentment of the military system by targeting a representative. Such an individual was psychologically impaired at the time and seemed to act on impulse, usually with his own weapon. Furthermore, he made no effort to hide his identity. However, the majority of fraggings, which he referred to

as group-engendered, resulted from small-group process and were the result of soldier groups believing that their integrity had been violated in some way. Within this type, he identified three varieties: (1) racially inspired fraggings—usually by black soldiers against a white superior who was regarded as racist; (2) "dope hassle" fraggings—by drug using soldiers who were reacting to a superior who was seeking to enforce antidrug regulations; and (3) fraggings by combat soldiers who regarded a superior as having excessive combat enthusiasm, which in turn exposed them to unwarranted danger. The character of these incidents differed from those based on personal vendetta in that the assault was group sanctioned, often included an escalation of threat (in order to intimidate the targeted authority figure into conforming to the group's will), and the actual perpetrator was less easily identifiable. Unfortunately Moskos' data was limited to anecdotal accounts of veterans.[124]

One study did address the perpetrators of fragging incidents in Vietnam. Gillooly and Bond examined 24 soldiers confined at the USDB regarding the circumstances and attitudes surrounding their assaults on superiors with an explosive weapon.[110] (Gillooly and Bond did not indicate when these incidents occurred, however, the authors were at the USDB about 2 years after Kroll, and their findings present a striking contrast with his earlier study that included only one case of leader assassination among soldiers confined over a 10-month span for crimes committed in Vietnam.) Most of the attacks occurred at a base camp, in darkness, and with unauthorized weapons. Among the offenders, 87.5% acknowledged being intoxicated and 90% had direct confrontational interactions with the victims up to 3 days prior; 67% had made no effort to avoid getting caught. They reported feeling scapegoated by the targeted leader, who was perceived as insensitive to the frustrations of his troops. Quite striking, as noted above, was the evidence that these assassinations were often associated with concurrence, or even collaboration, with fellow enlisted soldiers. The authors found that 62.5% of offenders reported that other soldiers knew of their plans for the attack, and 46% indicated they acted with cohorts serving as accessories.

The authors reported that according to their interviews with the offenders, racial tensions were of minor importance in the incidents. However, they also noted that nonwhite soldiers (four) only targeted white officers or NCOs. Otherwise, perhaps the most alarming finding of all was that "very few felt remorse and still did not at the time of the study."[110(p701)] Later Bond published additional analysis of the personality features of these men and gave more detail on contributory social dynamics. He described how the restive lower-ranking soldiers in Vietnam commonly held open discussions about fragging, collected cash bounties on various targets, and participated in a macabre ritual of anonymously warning potential victims so as to control them through intimidation. Apparently captains and sergeants were more common targets than lieutenants because they were more responsible for discipline or implementing the punishments.

Common background and personality features were found that indicated these soldiers had defective character formation. These included family histories of deprivation and/or brutality, poor self-image, chronic feelings of insecurity or vulnerability, poor object relations, lack of critical self-observation, excessive use of the defense mechanism of externalization, and poor impulse control. In Vietnam their drug use joined with these and other factors pertaining to their local "predicament" to create a lethal combination in which they perpetrated an assault on a leader they perceived as powerful and threatening. Still, Bond felt his sample was not necessarily typical of the lower-ranking soldiers in Vietnam, especially because two-thirds of these individuals had made almost no effort to avoid being caught. He also reiterated that racial tension and political activism were not primary factors in their motivation. What did seem especially relevant was their expectation that, by eliminating the authority figure, they would gain greater self-esteem and acceptance among their peers.[111]

WALTER REED ARMY INSTITUTE OF RESEARCH PSYCHIATRIST SURVEY FINDINGS: THE NONCOMBAT PSYCHIATRIC CHALLENGES IN VIETNAM

The following material extends the presentation begun in Chapter 5 of findings from the WRAIR post-war survey (1982) of Army psychiatrists who served in Vietnam that pertains to the overall psychiatric challenges in Vietnam, that is, ones not specifically tied to combat exposure. In particular this section explores the respondents' recollections of the prevalence of behavior problems that required their professional attention, impressions of troop morale, and factors they perceived as lowering morale.

Estimates of Professional Involvement with Behavior Problems

As was presented in Table 5-3 in Chapter 5, WRAIR survey respondents estimated that diagnosable behavior problems—specifically personality disorders and drug and alcohol dependence syndromes—accounted for over half of their patients; and that of those, only drug dependence syndromes rose significantly in the second half of the war. To further clarify the picture of psychiatric challenge in Vietnam, survey respondents were also asked to indicate how common it was for them to be involved in the evaluation and diagnosis of soldiers manifesting problematic behaviors in 17 categories. Results are presented in Table 8-4.

These results have particular utility in making comparisons across the two halves of the war and between psychiatrists who provided care mostly for combat troops and those who provided mostly for noncombat troops. Visual inspection reveals that the five most common behavior problems encountered—(1) characterological maladaptation; (2) excessive use of alcohol; (3) violent, antisocial behavior; (4) excessive use of marijuana; and (5) nonviolent, antimilitary behavior—are not specific for a combat theater, and a high incidence could be found among garrisoned troops almost no matter where they were located. The mean for individual combat avoidance behaviors—obviously only a problem in a combat theater—ranked 6th, slightly below nonviolent, antimilitary behavior, and subgroup analyses revealed it to be the only behavior problem that appeared significantly greater among psychiatrists who served *only* in a combat assignment compared to their colleagues who served *only* in the hospital setting.

However, more notable is the collection of behavior problems that rose significantly after the war passed the midpoint (violent, antisocial behavior; violent, antimilitary behavior; use of addictive, illegal drugs; and racial conflicts). These findings are consistent with the theater-wide metrics indicating accelerating morale and discipline problems after 1968 and the emergence of novel forms of opposition to military authority (Figure 8-1). Furthermore, with respect to the means for these 6 items among the psychiatrists who served in the second half of the war, there were no significant differences

TABLE 8-4. Survey Psychiatrist's Estimates of Their Professional Involvement With Behavior Problems in Vietnam

Behavior Problem	Overall mean N = 65	"Early" assignment mean (n = 35)	"Late" assignment mean (n = 30)
4 = COMMON			
Characterological maladaptation	3.55		
Excessive use of alcohol	3.36		
Antisocial behavior (violent)	3.02*	2.67	3.31
3 = INTERMEDIATE			
Excessive use of marijuana	2.97		
Antimilitary behavior (nonviolent), eg, insubordination, combat refusal, etc.	2.89		
Individual combat avoidance, eg, malingering, self-inflicted wound, etc.	2.83‡		
Antisocial behavior (nonviolent), eg, theft, corruption, etc.	2.41		
Use of heroin via smoking	2.27†	1.57	2.83
Use of Binoctal or other barbiturate	2.20†	1.62	2.69
Other drug use, eg, LSD, amphetamines, etc.	2.11*	1.76	2.42
Use of heroin via IV or inhalation	2.08†	1.48	2.59
Antimilitary behavior (violent), eg, attack NCO; fragging, etc.	2.00*	1.68	2.26
2 = UNCOMMON			
Group racial conflict	1.95*	1.55	2.29
Excessive combat aggression, eg, to civilians, prisoners; souvenirs of the dead	1.76		
Neglect hygiene, eg, venereal disease, antimalarial, footcare, etc.	1.74		
Group combat refusal	1.28		
Antiwar demonstrations and tensions	1.25		

Means of survey participants' estimates as to their involvement (evaluation and diagnosis) with 17 behavior problems in Vietnam ranked along a 5-point scale where 1 = very uncommon and 5 = very common (N = 65). Adapted with permission from Camp NM, Carney CM. US Army psychiatry in Vietnam: preliminary findings of a survey, II: Results and discussion. *Bull Menninger Clin.* 1987; 51(1):19–37.

*Statistically significant difference comparing war stage difference ("early" and "late" refer to those who served before or after mid-1968) with p < .05.

†Statistically significant difference comparing war stage difference with p < .005.

‡ Statistically significant difference comparing psychiatrists by assignment type with p < .05. The mean value for the 14 psychiatrists who served only with combat units was 3.36 versus a mean value of 2.49 for the 36 psychiatrists who served only with the hospitals.

IV: intravenous

LSD: Lysergic acid diethylamide

NCO: noncommissioned officer

TABLE 8-5. Perceived Causes of Soldier Demoralization

Factor Loadings	Soldier Demoralizing Influences	Mean value
	4 = HIGH EFFECT	
0.49 (B)	Vagueness of military objectives or lack of apparent success	3.85
	Vulnerable feelings associated with enemy guerrilla tactics	3.48
0.73 (A)	Antiwar attitudes	3.38
0.74 (B)	Soldiers perceive they have meaningless jobs	3.36
0.36 (A)	Soldier heroin use	3.33
	Soldier marijuana use	3.31
	Leader alcohol use	3.28
0.32 (C)	Isolation from home and loved ones	3.26
	Individualized rotation schedules diminish bonding with unit members	3.26
0.61 (A)	The media overstated the war's destructiveness	3.25
0.65 (B)	Perceive inequality of hardship and risk (resent "REMF"s)	3.09
0.57 (C)	Individualized rotation schedules weaken belief in military objectives	3.03
0.78 (B)	Too strict enforcement of rules and regulations	3.01
	3 = INTERMEDIATE EFFECT	
0.79 (A)	Soldier antiestablishment, antimilitary attitudes	2.96
0.60 (A)	Racial polarity and tension	2.96
	Officers' 6-month rotation in/out of the field reduced unit cohesion	2.92
0.80 (A)	Soldier repudiation of traditional, conservative American values	2.88
0.57 (A)	Soldier belief that the war was immoral and exploitive	2.85
	South Vietnamese perceived as ungrateful and exploitive	2.80
	Combat operations within an alien culture and setting	2.79
0.69 (C)	Soldiers too restricted; Vietnam beyond perimeter was off-limits	2.79
0.65 (A)	"Generation gap" polarization and animosities	2.75
0.68 (B)	Leaders seen as uncommitted to the troops, incompetent, or unethical	2.74
0.70 (C)	Limited recreational opportunities	2.70
0.63 (A)	Media represent soldiers as destructive villains	2.61
0.58 (C)	Too easy contact with home (tapes, calls, leave) promotes homesickness	2.54
	Too lax enforcement of rules and regulations	2.51
0.60 (A)	Class polarization and reciprocal resentment	2.50
0.44 (C)	Severe living and working conditions	2.49
	2 = LOW EFFECT	

The WRAIR Psychiatrist Survey contained 29 items ranked by means of survey participants' perception as to the negative effect on the average soldier's morale using a 1-to-5 scale where 1 = very low effect and 5 = very high effect. [N = 74–82] Also presented are three factors formed from factor analysis of responses (21 items) interpreted and named as: Factor A: perception of societal blame; Factor B: alienation from the Army; and Factor C: isolation and loneliness.

REMF: "rear echelon mother f--ker"

FIGURE 8-11. Multiple regression results for Factor B: Low morale as a function of alienation from the Army by interaction of war phase and psychiatrist assignment type (p < .004). Low score means psychiatrists reported soldiers as more alienated from the Army.

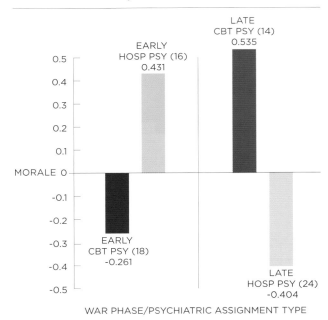

EARLY CBT PSY: psychiatrist arrived before mid-1968 and served with any combat unit in Vietnam

EARLY HOSP PSY: psychiatrist arrived before mid-1968 and served only with a hospital or psychiatric detachment in Vietnam

LATE CBT PSY: psychiatrist arrived after mid-1968 and served with any combat unit in Vietnam

LATE HOSP PSY: psychiatrist arrived after mid-1968 and served only with a hospital or psychiatric detachment in Vietnam

Factor A: Low Morale as a Function of Perceived Societal Blame

For the first morale factor—low morale as a function of perceived blame from American society—low score means soldiers believed they were forced to fight in an immoral war yet felt blamed by American society and the media for being destructive killers, with many soldiers reacting through passionate dissent and polarization along such natural cleavage lines of racial, class, value, and generational differences as well as the use of heroin. Figure 8-10 depicts the statistically significant main effect of psychiatrist phase of the war, with morale perceived as dropping among troops throughout the theater during the second half of the war based on this factor. It also may be especially

noteworthy that "soldier heroin use" is a component only of Factor A.

Factor B: Low Morale as a Function of Alienation From the Army

With respect to the second morale factor—low morale as a function of alienation from the Army—low score means soldiers were distressed by vague and unsuccessful military activity, meaningless and redundant tasks, apparent inequalities of hardship and risk, excessive rules and enforcement, and disinterested or self-serving leaders. Figure 8-11 depicts the statistically significant interaction between the phase of the war and the type of psychiatrist assignment. For those Army psychiatrists with combat unit assignments, low troop morale attributable to alienation from the Army appears to have improved from the early to the late half of the war. Conversely, for Army psychiatrists with a hospital assignment, morale attributable to alienation from the Army appears to worsen as the war progressed. These results suggest a strong shift in soldier alienation from the Army among combat units during the first half of the war when combat intensity was high, to support units after the war passed the midpoint and the combat intensity dropped.

Factor C: Low Morale as a Function of Isolation and Loneliness

Regarding the third morale factor—low morale as a function of isolation and loneliness—low score means soldiers are beset with homesickness and loneliness for family and loved ones, sequestered in scattered and austere compounds, restricted in such outlets as recreation, and uncommitted to the military mission because of the individualized rotation schedules. Figure 8-12A depicts a statistically significant interaction between phase of the war and respondents' psychiatry residency type. Civilian- and military-trained psychiatrists alike report relatively little degradation of morale during the early phase of the war secondary to soldier isolation and loneliness; and although both groups report increased degradation of morale during the second half of the war, the increase for these reasons is much more noticeable for the military-trained psychiatrists. Figure 8-12B also depicts a trend associated with psychiatrist assignment type. Regardless of phase of the war, the psychiatrists who served in the hospitals were more likely to note the morale to be degraded by the factor of soldier isolation

FIGURE 8-12A. Multiple regression results for Factor C: Low morale as a function of isolation and loneliness by interaction between war phase and psychiatry residency training (p < .05). Low score means psychiatrists reported soldiers as more demoralized by isolation and loneliness.

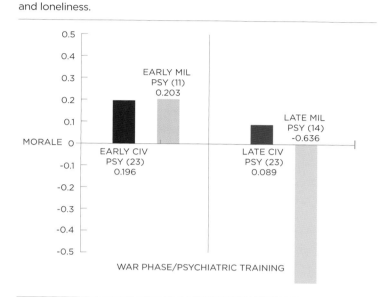

FIGURE 8-12B. Multiple regression results for Factor C: Low morale as a function of isolation and loneliness by psychiatrist assignment type (p < .10). Low score means psychiatrists reported soldiers as more demoralized by isolation and loneliness.

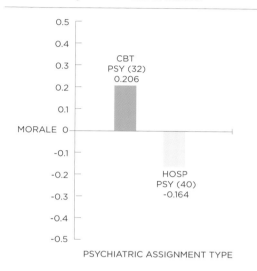

EARLY CIV PSY: psychiatrist arrived before mid-1968 and received psychiatry training in a civilian program

EARLY MIL PSY: psychiatrist arrived before mid-1968 and received psychiatry training in a military program

LATE CIV PSY: psychiatrist arrived after mid-1968 and received psychiatry training in a civilian program

LATE MIL PSY: psychiatrist arrived after mid-1968 and received psychiatry training in a military program

CBT PSY: psychiatrist served with any combat unit in Vietnam

HOSP PSY: psychiatrist served only with a hospital or psychiatric detachment in Vietnam

and loneliness. Taken together these results suggest that degradation of morale secondary to isolation and loneliness increased in the second half of the war, but it was more noticeable to the psychiatrists with military training and by the hospital psychiatrists who saw more soldiers assigned to support units.

In conclusion, these questions regarding morale were intended to transcend psychopathology affecting the individual soldier to focus on circumstances influencing his group. Although the results are invariably impressionistic, they may still be useful as they permit the reader to see this dimension through the eyes of those especially qualified to report on it—the behavior science specialists operating in the field. Furthermore, they provide an especially useful longitudinal perspective by comparing and contrasting the perceptions of psychiatrists who served at the

beginning of the conflict with their counterparts who served later. The results of the multiple regression suggest that morale took a severe downward course after the midpoint in the war; that all those deployed in the second half of the war had their morale depleted by the sense of public blame; that the propensity for the soldiers to fault the military was greater among those serving in support units as combat intensity waned and earlier military objectives became doubtful; and that psychiatrists with military training were more likely to perceive that the isolation from home and restricted living conditions in Vietnam had a seriously negative impact on troops in the second half of the war. (Unfortunately it cannot be ruled out that lowered morale among some survey psychiatrist participants influenced their responses to these items.)

SUMMARY AND CONCLUSIONS

Chapter 6 and Chapter 7 centered on combat exhaustion and related psychiatric and behavior conditions apparently generated by the stress of combat. This chapter reviewed the overlapping stresses that affected the soldiers serving in Vietnam more generally (combat as well as noncombat troops), the emergent patterns of psychiatric conditions and behavior problems that were not directly associated with combat exposure, and the responses of Army psychiatry and Army leaders. Sources were the available psychiatric/behavior science and military documentation from the war; however, the skew favoring the first half of the war was a major impediment in drawing conclusions. This was somewhat offset with results from the WRAIR survey of veteran Army psychiatrists, but that study had its limitations.

The only official synopsis of Army medical care in Vietnam, *Medical Support of the US Army in Vietnam 1965–1970*, is critically misleading regarding psychiatric care because it omits the last 3 years of the war (mid-1970–1973). It also is unrepresentative because it does not include rates for combat exhaustion or certain other important diagnostic groups, that is, stress reactions (adjustment disorders), alcohol-related disorders, and drug dependency—conditions whose collective incidence probably averaged 25% to 35% of hospitalized cases and far overshadowed that for combat stress casualties. As it turned out, psychiatric and behavior conditions that were mostly unrelated to combat exposure, especially the upsurge in soldier heroin use, became the most challenging medical problems that the Army faced in the last years of the war.

Reiterating from earlier chapters, the Army psychiatric inpatient rate, which hovered between 10 and 12 per 1,000 troops per year until 1968, quadrupled by July 1971, before dropping sharply after new policies were instituted that allowed soldiers with heroin dependency to be medically evacuated back to the United States. Concordantly, the Army psychiatric evacuation rate remained under four per 1,000 troops per year until July 1969; less than five per 1,000 troops per year from then through April 1971; and then skyrocketed to 129.8 per 1,000 troops per year by April 1972. The absence of epidemiologic information pertaining to soldier attrition from alcohol-related conditions is also problematic. The WRAIR survey psychiatrists indicated that these represented

about 10% of their overall caseload and caused as much dysfunction and disability throughout the war as did heroin dependency late in the war. (Drug and alcohol problems will be addressed in Chapter 9.) Impressions derived from this review are as follows:

- **Soldier attrition for diagnosable psychiatric conditions (hospitalized or confined to quarters) for the first 5 years in Vietnam, mid-1965 through mid-1970, assumed roughly these proportions: one-third as psychosis and neurosis, one-third as character and behavior disorders, and the remaining one-third as stress reactions, including combat exhaustion and drug and alcohol-related conditions. After mid-1970 heroin dependency predominated.** Confidence in these figures is reduced by the lack of psychiatrist reports from the second half of the war, variability in the diagnostic criteria utilized by the psychiatrists, and lack of clarity in some instances as to whether reported patient counts were limited to hospitalized soldiers.

- **Army psychiatric personnel appeared confident in the diagnosis and treatment of symptom disorders such as psychosis, neurosis (anxiety, depression, and conversion reaction), acute stress reactions, and brain syndromes secondary to drugs and alcohol because these clinical challenges were aligned with their professional training—training that centered on biological and psychological disturbances within the individual patient.** In general, the treatment provided for the noncombat psychiatric cases followed the traditional principles of the Army doctrine for the care of acute combat stress casualties. This was augmented with the judicious use of psychotropic medications and appeared to produce favorable results.

- **The available clinical data from Vietnam, including that pertaining to combat stress casualties, emphasized anxiety as the primary dysphoric affect experienced by symptomatic soldiers as opposed to depressive affect.** Despite a rising Army suicide rate in Vietnam, the available psychiatrist reports, which are primarily from the first half of the war, said little about the treatment of depression or suicidality. Of course, as suggested in the Prologue as well as the WRAIR survey findings regarding late war demoralization, the rising rates for behavior disorders can be interpreted as actions serving a defensive function against depressive affect.

- **Regarding behavior disorders:**
  - The psychiatrists' reports from the first half of the war indicate a steady and sizable stream of command-referred soldiers for evaluation for misconduct and maladjustment. Whereas the mental health personnel evidently undertook the psychiatric "clearing function" required by the regulations, no data indicate that any particular treatments were successful with these soldiers.
  - Although there are few reports from those who served in the second half of the war, it can be inferred from the results of the WRAIR survey, the documented rise in Army rates for outpatient psychiatric visits generally and for drug use more specifically, and the dramatic increase in administrative discharges from military service worldwide, that the Army psychiatrists in Vietnam were increasingly challenged by referrals for misconduct and maladjustment as the war lengthened, especially in new forms: defiance and dissent; racial conflicts; violent, antimilitary behaviors; and drug dependency and addiction. There are no data indicating that any particular treatments were successful with these soldiers either. In this vein the wholesale medical evacuation of soldiers with heroin dependency out of Vietnam in the last 2 years of the war served as a remedy if not a treatment, per se. Some considered these soldiers to be "evacuation syndromes," that is, they were seeking to manipulate the system to get relief from their assignment.

- The psychiatric literature and related documentation from Vietnam centered around a series of overlapping risk factors that predicted soldier maladjustment and the emergence of psychiatric and behavior problems:
  - The enemy's strategy of guerrilla/terrorism warfare.
  - Soldier immaturity. The typical first-term enlisted soldier in Vietnam was 19 to 21 years of age.
  - Preinduction personality deficits.
  - Lowered induction standards for intelligence and education.

- The staggered, individual, 1-year, replacement policy for enlisted troops. Throughout the war force management policies exempted Reserve and National Guard units and relied heavily on young, conscripted troops who were randomly rotated into the theater for 12-month tours. The Army psychiatrists who served in Vietnam believed these policies proved to be enormously corrosive to the cohesion of military units and the adaptation of individual soldiers, including promoting the development of widespread, if subclinical, "short-timer's" dysfunction. It seems obvious in retrospect that if group membership and identification serve as a critical stress-mitigating factor for soldiers, it must be assumed that this would especially apply to troops serving in a theater of combat operations, especially replacement troops.
- The staggered, individual, 1-year, replacement policy for officers and NCOs. The harmfulness of this policy was compounded by rotating officers out of the field after 6 months.
- The African American soldier. Because of increasing racial discord in the United States, antimilitary attitudes and behaviors found their fullest expression among the large numbers of black troops in Vietnam—mostly young, first-enlistment soldiers from lower socioeconomic backgrounds. As the war prolonged and the force became increasingly demoralized, disruptive, sometimes violent, behaviors by frustrated, angry young African Americans became increasingly common.
- Serving in a support role. The reports suggested there was a higher incidence of psychiatric casualties among noncombat soldiers, and this impression was reinforced by the WRAIR survey data. This evidently occurred because of the lack of clearly defined (safe) rear areas in Vietnam and because these troops could not utilize the stress-mitigating bond, that is, survival-necessitated commitment and cohesion, that was available to soldiers in small combat units.
- Service after Tet '68. Even before the troop withdrawal gained momentum following the political and military events in 1968 and 1969, the morale of the troops in Vietnam began to decline; but after 1969 the replacement soldiers

found themselves in a steadily deteriorating circumstance compared with their counterparts who served earlier. By 1970, enthusiasm in America for the war had dissolved, and a growing opposition to military authority by the troops in Vietnam resonated with the virulent antiwar feelings of those at home. Along with needing to adapt to assignment in the theater and the stress of combat, the second half of the war brought successive cohorts of soldiers to Vietnam to face an additional, and what proved to be more insidious, collection of stressors that were mostly unrelated to combat. These troops were quite far from home, part of a large retrograding Army of resentful conscripts and disillusioned career soldiers—some of whom were on their second or third tour—fully armed but mostly serving in a defensive role, impatiently waiting for their year to pass while feeling vulnerable to attack from communist forces or even hostile South Vietnamese who were apprehensive about being abandoned by the Americans. For the diminishing numbers of troops who were still required to face combat, they were surrounded by a military culture that had become preoccupied with the attainment of individual safety, status, and comfort. Although combat refusal incidents were not reported officially, most accounts of the late-war morale problems include references to their rising numbers. Less confrontational were the "search and avoid (or evade)" missions carried out by troops. Especially important, soldiers who served during the drawdown were bombarded by the media and loved ones in the United States that their mission in Vietnam was dishonorable. The result was sagging morale and a severe unraveling of military order and discipline. This is demonstrated not only by unprecedented rates of psychiatric disorders and misconduct, but also by their extreme nature, that is, violent threats on military leaders and widespread heroin use. As the Prologue attested, late-war soldiers had become an embittered and desperate aggregate of young men who deeply resented being asked to take risks and make sacrifices in order to salvage America's lost cause there while being surrounded by the

moral outrage of the American public. In response they bonded around their anger at feeling exploited, abandoned, and blamed and took refuge in alternative affinity groups, which were based on race or drug of choice and fueled by subversive attitudes toward military authority and enmity toward rival enlisted men groups. A senior Army research psychiatrist, Holloway, referred to the turn of events in late-Vietnam as a "human tragedy."[125] Jones and Johnson opined that these psychosocial casualties and the associated rock-bottom morale jeopardized combat readiness in Vietnam as much as the high incidence of combat stress casualties in earlier wars.[38]

- **Pathodynamic consideration regarding the deterioration of morale and mental health of the drawdown Army in Vietnam requires approaches at both the level of the affected soldier and that of his primary group (buddies).**
  - **At the level of the individual soldier.** Many of the soldier-patients who received mental health attention in Vietnam can be understood as manifesting a situation-specific stress response pattern, that is, a failure of adaptation arising in previously functional men who evidently sustained an intolerable interaction of personal circumstance and disturbing biological (often including drug- and alcohol-induced), psychological, and social stressors (in Vietnam, as well as from home)—stressors that became more onerous for sequential cohorts of replacement soldiers as the war wound to its disheartening conclusion. In effect, they underwent a (combat theater) deployment stress reaction.
  - **At the level of the military group.** Although many of the conspicuously misbehaving soldiers in Vietnam brought preservice personality susceptibility to the theater that facilitated their acting out their frustrations, the unprecedented rise in the incidence of psychiatric disorders and nonpsychiatric behavioral problems during the drawdown phase of the war suggests these soldiers were only the tip of an iceberg of discontent and resentment shared by the majority of first-term troops there. In other words, a social stress

reaction resulted—a failure of adaptation at the level of the collective.

Some have assumed that the disgruntled, disintegrating Army in Vietnam was a predictable consequence of government promises of withdrawal and the perception of demobilization. This review suggests a more complex bio\psycho\social model of deployment stress and dysfunction that includes service in a combat zone as a specific and critical variable—a model that psychiatrists who'd not been there could not fully appreciate.

On the social level, Rose, a sociologist, proposed that during the final years in Vietnam the Army experienced a collective "macromutiny," which represented a collapse of the requisite mutual allegiance and cooperation between military leaders and soldiers, and the ascendance of individual self-interests. In other words, the deteriorating morale and military order and discipline exceeded the tipping point, with troops expressing by various means their antagonism toward military authority and an unwillingness to make further sacrifices—the inversion of morale[126]—clearly an unacceptable and dangerous situation.

REFERENCES

1. Manning FJ. Morale and cohesion in military psychiatry. In: Jones FD, Sparacino LR, Wilcox VL, Rothberg JM, eds. *Military Psychiatry: Preparing in Peace for War.* In: Zajtchuk R, Bellamy RF, eds. *Textbooks of Military Medicine.* Washington, DC: Department of the Army, Office of The Surgeon General, Borden Institute; 1994: 1–18.

2. Jones FD. Disorders of frustration and loneliness. In: Jones FD, Sparacino LR, Wilcox VL, Rothberg JM, Stokes JW, eds. *War Psychiatry.* In: Zajtchuk R, Bellamy RF, eds. *Textbooks of Military Medicine.* Washington, DC: Department of the Army, Office of The Surgeon General, Borden Institute; 1995: 63–83.

3. Jones FD. Psychiatric lessons of war. In: Jones FD, Sparacino LR, Wilcox VL, Rothberg JM, Stokes JW, eds. *War Psychiatry.* In: Zajtchuk R, Bellamy RF, eds. *Textbooks of Military Medicine.* Washington, DC: Department of the Army, Office of The Surgeon General, Borden Institute; 1995: 1–33.

4. Menninger WC. *Psychiatry in a Troubled World: Yesterday's War and Today's Challenge.* New York, NY: Macmillan; 1948.

5. Glass AJ. Lessons learned. In: Mullens WS, Glass AJ, eds, *Neuropsychiatry in World War II.* Vol 2. *Overseas Theaters.* Washington, DC: Medical Department, United States Army; 1973: 732–737.

6. Glass AJ, Artiss KL, Gibbs JJ, Sweeney VC. The current status of Army psychiatry. *Am J Psychiatry.* 1961;117:673–683.

7. Tureen LL, Stein M. The base section psychiatric hospital. In: Hanson FR, ed. *Combat Psychiatry.* Washington, DC: US Government Printing Office; 1949: 105–134.

8. Harris FG. Some comments on the differential diagnosis and treatment of psychiatric breakdowns in Korea. *Proceedings of Course on Recent Advances in Medicine and Surgery.* Army Medical Service Graduate School. Washington, DC: Walter Reed Army Medical Center; 30 April 1954: 390–402.

9. Lee RA. The army "mutiny" of 1946. *J Am History.* 1966;53(3):555–571.

10. Froede RC, Stahl CJ. Fatal narcotism in military personnel. *J Forensic Sci.* 1971;16(2):199–218.

11. Medical Field Service School. *Philosophy of Military Psychiatry.* Fort Sam Houston, Tex: Department of Neuropsychiatry, Medical Field Service School; distributed July 1967. Training Document GR 51-400-006, 045.

12. US Department of the Army. *Personnel Separations, Discharge: Unfitness and Unsuitability.* Washington, DC: DA; July 1966. Army Regulation 635-212.

13. US Department of the Army. *Personnel Separations, Officer Personnel.* Washington, DC: DA; February 1969. Army Regulation 635-105.

14. American Psychiatric Association. *Diagnostic and Statistical Manual of Mental Disorders.* 4th ed (DSM-IV). Washington, DC: APA; 1994.

15. American Psychiatric Association. *Diagnostic and Statistical Manual of Mental Disorders.* 4th ed, text rev (DSM-IV-TR). Washington, DC: APA; 2000.

66. Starr P. *The Discarded Army: Veterans After Vietnam*. New York, NY: Charterhouse; 1973.

67. Dougan C, Lipsman S, Doyle E, and the editors of Boston Publishing Co. *The Vietnam Experience: A Nation Divided*. Boston, Mass: Boston Publishing Co; 1984.

68. Crowe RR, Colbach EM. A psychiatric experience with Project 100,000. *Mil Med*. 1971;136(3):271–273.

69. Bey DR, Zecchinelli VA. GI's against themselves. Factors resulting in explosive violence in Vietnam. *Psychiatry*. 1974;37(3):221–228.

70. Byrdy HSR. Division psychiatry in Vietnam (unpublished); 1967. [Full text available as Appendix 8 to this volume.]

71. Bowman JA. Recent experiences in combat psychiatry in Viet Nam (unpublished); 1967. [Full text available as Appendix 11 to this volume.]

72. Morris LE. "Over the hump" in Vietnam. Adjustment patterns in a time-limited stress situation. *Bull Menninger Clin*. 1970;34(6):352–362.

73. Dowling JJ. Psychological aspects of the year in Vietnam. *US Army Vietnam Med Bull*. 1967;May/June:45–48.

74. Bloch HS. The psychological adjustment of normal people during a year's tour in Vietnam. *Psychiatric Q*. 1970;44(4):613–626.

75. Bey DR. Group dynamics and the "F.N.G." in Vietnam: a potential focus of stress. *Int J Group Psychother*. 1972;22(1):22–30.

76. Lipsman S, Doyle E, and the editors of Boston Publishing Co. *The Vietnam Experience: Fighting for Time*. Boston, Mass: Boston Publishing Co; 1983

77. Ratner RA. Drugs and despair in Vietnam. *U Chicago Magazine*. 1972;64:15–23.

78. Herr M. *Dispatches*. New York, NY: Avon Books; 1980.

79. Spector RH. *After Tet: The Bloodiest Year in Vietnam*. New York, NY: The Free Press; 1993.

80. Blank AS Jr. In: Johnson AW Jr, Bowman JA, Byrdy HS, Blank AS Jr. Panel discussion: Army psychiatry in Vietnam. In: Jones FD, ed. *Proceedings: Social and Preventive Psychiatry Course, 1967*. Washington, DC: GPO; 1968: 41–76. [Available at: Alexandria, Va: Defense Technical Information Center. Document No. AD A950058.] [Full text available as Appendix 10 to this volume.]

81. Kenny WF. Psychiatric disorders among support personnel. *US Army Vietnam Med Bull*. 1967;January/February:34–37.

82. Jones FD. Reactions to stress comparing combat and support troops. Presentation to: World Psychiatric Association; 29 August 1977; Honolulu, Hawaii.

83. Doyle E, Weiss S, and the editors of Boston Publishing Co. *The Vietnam Experience: A Collision of Cultures*. Boston, Mass: Boston Publishing Co; 1984.

84. Neller G, Stevens V, Chung R, Devaris D. Psychological Warfare and Its Effects on Mental Health: Lessons Learned From Vietnam (unpublished); 1985.

85. Bey DR. In: Forrest DV with commentary by Bey DR, Bourne PG. The American soldier and Vietnamese women. *Sex Behav*. 1972;2:8–15.

86. Menard DL. The social work specialist in a combat division. *US Army Vietnam Med Bull*. 1968;March/April:48–57.

87. Bey DR Jr, Smith WE. Organizational consultation in a combat unit. *Am J Psychiatry*. 1971;128(4):401–406.

88. Forrest DV, with commentary by Bey DR, Bourne PG. The American soldier and Vietnamese women. *Sex Behav*. 1972;2:8–15.

89. US Department of the Army. *Personnel Separations, Homosexuality*. Washington, DC: DA; July 1966. Army Regulation 635-89.

90. Dynes WR, Donaldson S, eds. *Homosexuality and Government, Politics and Prisons*. New York, NY: Garland Publishing; 1992.

91. Baker WL. Division psychiatry in the 9th Infantry Division. *US Army Vietnam Med Bull*. 1967;November/December:5–9.

92. Druss RG. Cases of suspected homosexuality seen at an Army Mental Hygiene Consultation Service. *Psychiatr Q*. 1967;41(1):62–70.

93. Shilts R. *Conduct Unbecoming: Gays and Lesbians in the US Military: Vietnam to the Persian Gulf*. New York, NY: Ballantine Books; 1993.

94. Baker SL Jr. Traumatic war disorders. In: Kaplan HI, Freedman AM, Sadock BJ, eds.

Comprehensive Textbook of Psychiatry. 3rd ed. Baltimore, Md: Williams & Wilkins; 1980: 1829–1842.

95. Sorley L. *A Better War: The Unexamined Victories and Final Tragedy of America's Last Years in Vietnam*. New York, NY: Harcourt Books; 1999.

96. Fulghum D, Maitland T, and the editors of Boston Publishing Co. *The Vietnam Experience: South Vietnam on Trial, Mid-1970 to 1972*. Boston, Mass: Boston Publishing Co; 1984.

97. Bey DR. Change of command in combat: a locus of stress. *Am J Psychiatry*. 1972;129(6):698–702.

98. Kerner O, Lindsay JV, Harris FR. *Report of the National Advisory Commission on Civil Disorders*. Washington, DC: GPO; 1968: Abstract. Available at: http://www.eisenhowerfoundation.org/docs/kerner.pdf. Accessed 28 May 2013.

99. Dougan C, Weiss S, and the editors of Boston Publishing Co. *The Vietnam Experience: Nineteen Sixty-Eight*. Boston, Mass: Boston Publishing Co; 1983.

100. Kroll J. Racial patterns of military crimes in Vietnam. *Psychiatry*. 1976;39(1):51–64.

101. Terry W. The angry blacks in the army. In: Horowitz D and the editors of Ramparts, eds. *Two, Three . . . Many Vietnams: A Radical Reader on the Wars in Southeast Asia and the Conflicts at Home*. San Francisco, Calif: Canfield Press; 1971: 222–231

102. Fiman BG, Borus JF, Stanton MD. Black-white American-Vietnamese relations among soldiers in Vietnam. *J Soc Issues*. 1975;31(4):39–48.

103. Borus JF. Reentry, I: Adjustment issues facing the Vietnam returnee. *Arch Gen Psychiatry*. 1973;28(4):501–506.

104. Borus JF, Stanton MD, Fiman BG, Dowd AF. Racial perceptions in the Army: an approach. *Am J Psychiatry*. 1972;128(11):1369–1374.

105. Williamson E. From both sides now. *Army Reporter*. 25 October 1971:5.

106. Colbach EM. Ethical Issues in combat psychiatry. *Mil Med*. 1985;150(5):256–265.

107. Bey DR. Personal communication, 23 March 2010.

108. Bey DR, Smith WE. Mental health technicians in Vietnam. *Bull Menninger Clin*. 1970;34(6):363–371.

109. Linden E. The demoralization of an army: fragging and other withdrawal symptoms. *Saturday Review*, 8 January 1972:12–17, 55.

110. Gillooly DH, Bond TC. Assaults with explosive devices on superiors: a synopsis of reports from confined offenders at the US Disciplinary Barracks. *Mil Med*. 1976;141(10):700–702.

111. Bond TC. The why of fragging. *Am J Psychiatry*. 1976;133(11):1328–1331.

112. National Archive Records Administration (NARA). Statistical information about casualties of the Vietnam War: [Southeast Asia] Combat Area Casualties Current File (CACCF), 2007.

113. Adams DP, Barton C, Mitchell GL, Moore AL, Einagel V. Hearts and minds: suicide among United States combat troops in Vietnam, 1957–1973. *Soc Sci Med*. 1998;47(11):1687–1694.

114. Huffman RE. Which soldiers break down. A survey of 610 psychiatric patients in Vietnam. *Bull Menninger Clinic*. 1970;34(6):343–351.

115. Byrdy HSR. In: Johnson AW Jr, Bowman JA, Byrdy HSR, Blank AS Jr. Panel discussion: Army psychiatry in Vietnam. In: Jones FD, ed. *Proceedings: Social and Preventive Psychiatry Course, 1967*. Washington, DC: GPO; 1968: 41–76. [Available at: Alexandria, Va: Defense Technical Information Center. Document No. AD A950058.]

116. Klein DC, Fencil-Morse E, Seligman ME. Learned helplessness, depression, and the attribution of failure. *J Pers Soc Psychol*. 1976;33(5):508–516.

117. Gartner SS. Strategic and political factors affecting suicidality in the armed forces. Paper presented at: American Political Science Association; September 2010; Washington, DC.

118. Bowman JA. In: Johnson AW Jr, Bowman JA, Byrdy HS, Blank AS Jr. Panel discussion: Army psychiatry in Vietnam. In: Jones FD, ed. *Proceedings: Social and Preventive Psychiatry Course, 1967*. Washington, DC: GPO; 1968: 41–76. [Available at: Alexandria, Va: Defense Technical Information Center. Document No. AD A950058.]

119. Langner HP. The making of a murderer. *Am J Psychiatry*. 1971;127(7):950–953.

120. Pasternack SA. Evaluation of dangerous behavior of active duty servicemen. *Mil Med.* 1971;136(2):110–113.

121. Kruzich DJ. *Army Drug Use in Vietnam: Origins of the Problem and Official Response* (unpublished manuscript). University of Minnesota, School of Public Health; May 1979.

122. National Archive Records Administration (NARA). Statistical information about casualties of the Vietnam War: [Southeast Asia] Combat Area Casualties Current File (CACCF), 1998.

123. Gabriel RA, Savage PL. *Crisis in Command: Mismanagement in the Army*. New York, NY: Hill and Wang; 1978: Table 3.

124. Moskos CC Jr. Surviving the war in Vietnam. In: Figley CR, Leventman S, eds. *Strangers at Home: Vietnam Veterans Since the War*. New York: Praeger; 1980:71–85

125. Holloway HC. Vietnam military psychiatry revisited. Presentation to: American Psychiatric Association Annual Meeting; 19 May 1982; Toronto, On.

126. Rose E. The anatomy of a mutiny. *Armed Forces Soc.* 1982;8(4):561–574.

CHAPTER 9

Substance Abuse in the Theater: The Big Story

. . . [O]ne young warrant officer who was described by his flight surgeon as "one of the better all around pilots in our unit" . . . was discovered to be smoking marijuana 10 to 15 times per day while flying combat missions. . . . [When confronted, he replied,] "It didn't bother me being shot at for . . . every time I was stoned on marijuana. It was beautiful to me. The tracers were even pretty. I got to where I could fly pretty good on marijuana, but sometimes when I landed I could hardly walk."[1(p57)]

Lieutenant Colonel Norman Evans
Army Psychiatrist and Flight Surgeon
98th Psychiatric Detachment
August 1967–August 1968

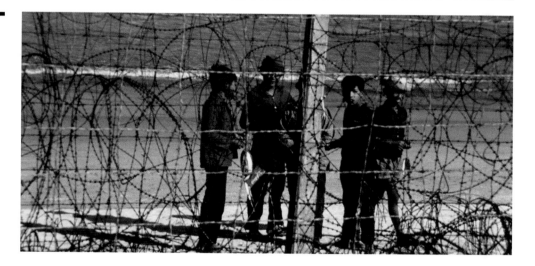

Heroin dealers at the 95th Evacuation Hospital compound fence. In this 1971 photograph, Vietnamese boys wait at the hospital's perimeter to trade heroin with US soldiers for prized goods, such as cigarettes. By mid-1970, 5 years into the war, earlier concerns by command in South Vietnam regarding soldier use of marijuana and other drugs had been eclipsed by threats to the health, morale and discipline, and combat readiness of the force stemming from the rapid spread of heroin use and addiction. Photograph courtesy of Norman M Camp, Colonel, US Army (Retired).

Alcohol abuse and marijuana use were persistent but mostly manageable problems for the US military during the first 2 years after ground troops were inserted in Vietnam in spring of 1965. As the US forces numbers grew and the war entered its middle phase (1968–1969), accelerating use of illegal drugs by soldiers—especially marijuana but also barbiturates and amphetamines—prompted command to increase suppressive efforts. Still, although many soldiers became psychologically dependent, and some developed disabling medical and psychiatric reactions, the scope of problems associated with drug use was limited and not perceived as a serious detraction to accomplishing the mission.

In early 1970, a new and far more pernicious problem arose following the emergence of a very efficient Vietnamese heroin marketing system and the enthusiastic embrace of heroin by the lower-ranking troops in Vietnam. Within a short span of time, concerns about rapidly accelerating heroin-related arrests, medical problems, and overdose deaths greatly overshadowed earlier ones regarding marijuana use.[2] This epidemic of self-inflicted soldier disability fell especially on Army units, and all levels of command were hard-pressed to effectively respond. Furthermore, because its causes, effects, and attempted remedies were at the intersection of physical fitness, mental health, morale and discipline, and combat preparedness, Army psychiatry faced its biggest challenge of the war. Unfortunately, vigorous efforts by command and medical/psychiatric elements in Vietnam to address the new heroin problem through education and other suppressive means, detection, and treatment and rehabilitation had little effect. By 1972 the Army in Vietnam shifted to an unprecedented hybrid medical/law enforcement model: soldiers with positive urines were "quarantined" for observation, detoxified as needed, and returned to the United States as patients. This peaked in July with an annualized rate of one out of every eight soldiers medically evacuated back to the United States for this reason. Although that figure may be somewhat inflated because the Army was in the final stages of drawdown, it is nonetheless evident that rampant heroin use in Vietnam and the military's inability to find solutions proved to be one of crowning blows to America in its failed war in South Vietnam.

Chapter 1 made the case for the dramatic rise in drug use by young Americans over the course of the war. Chapter 2 described how this trend influenced the soldiers assigned to the Vietnam theater, including medical and psychiatric effects. This chapter provides the fuller story of drug use and abuse among Army troops in Vietnam, especially the heroin epidemic, and the collective efforts of Army psychiatry and other medical elements to provide humanitarian care while supporting Army leadership in the accomplishment of the military mission.

ALCOHOL ABUSE AND ADDICTION IN VIETNAM: A SERIOUS BUT OVERLOOKED PROBLEM

Pre-Vietnam

In the years leading up to the Vietnam War, the "substance" that generated the greatest ongoing concern for the US military was alcohol.[3] Across wars and between wars, alcohol abuse (drunkenness) and physical and psychological dependence (alcoholism), as well as related medical conditions and misconduct, were recurrent problems with serious consequences, as seen in reduced military performance, ruined military careers, and the consumption of military healthcare resources. However, in that the scope of these problems remained modest among troops deployed overseas (compared to other nonbattle conditions such as malaria, hepatitis, tuberculosis, and sexually transmitted diseases), and because alcohol possession for off-duty use was legal (compared with illegal drugs, as in Vietnam), at the time the United States went to war in Southeast Asia military leaders had not been inclined to address alcohol problems in wider, public health/epidemiologic terms (as command, medical, or law enforcement issues); for the most part, their definition as a problem remained centered on each affected individual.

From the historical standpoint, the prevalence of alcohol problems in the US Army can be appreciated from the following rates, which interestingly, steadily declined. During the Civil War, besides desertion, the primary psychiatric/behavior problem affecting US Army soldiers was alcoholism.[4] In the decade preceding America entering World War I, US Army admissions for alcohol problems were 16 per 1,000 troops per year. During the years of Prohibition (1920–1933), the admission rate was 7–8 per 1,000 troops per year. In the period following the Prohibition years and the repeal of the Volstead Act in 1933, the rate gradually dropped to 3.3 per 1,000 troops per year, apparently because of higher selection criteria for service in the Army, which was consequent to the Great Depression and high unemployment. Through World War II the alcohol admission rate was an even lower 1.7 per 1,000 troops per year, and the drug addiction rate was only 0.1 per 1,000 troops per year. Together they accounted for only 4.7% of all psychiatric diagnoses; and these rates held steady until the buildup in Vietnam.[5]

One important feature should be underscored: until 1970, Army regulations and policies distinguished alcohol problems (as well as the use of illegal drugs) from other psychiatric disorders. Alcohol dependency/alcoholism was regarded as the consequence of willful misconduct, along with "shirking," failure to pay debts, "inaptitude," homosexuality, enuresis, and character and behavior disorders—with the insinuation that they were the product of a character or moral defect.[5] This was true through most of the Vietnam War period despite alcoholism's inclusion in both the American Psychiatric Association's classification system of mental disorders[6] and the *Armed Forces Medical Diagnosis Nomenclature and Statistical Classification System* (Army Regulation [AR] 40-401 dated 15 June 1963).[7] As a consequence, with limited exceptions the Army did not provide treatment/rehabilitation programs for alcohol (and drug) dependency for those on active duty. Treatment was provided for medical complications such as delirium tremens and liver cirrhosis, but personnel with sustained alcohol (and drug problems) were typically administratively eliminated from the Army as unsuitable under the provisions of either AR 635-212 for enlisted ranks or AR 635-105 for officers.[8] These regulations and policies were partially nullified during the last 2 years of the war as the result of federal legislation that included the stipulation that alcohol dependence be treated before an individual was released from the armed services (The Comprehensive Alcohol Abuse and Alcoholism Prevention, Treatment, and Rehabilitation Act, PL 91-616, 1970). However, in that Vietnam was a combat theater, this had little relevance there.

Finally, it should be noted that because of inconsistency of terms, confusion is somewhat inevitable when attempting to compare patterns of alcohol use with those for drug use within military populations. Whereas one can speak of "alcohol use" versus "alcohol abuse" (excessive or problematic use), any use of illegal drugs is commonly referred to as "drug abuse" simply because use is against the law and military regulations under all circumstances.

Vietnam

Prevalence of Alcohol Use

It is not surprising that there are few records that addressed the prevalence of alcohol use in Vietnam. It was a legal "drug" that was widely distributed and sold in Vietnam by the US government throughout the war. Ethyl alcohol in its many forms was available in the Post Exchange (PX) facilities and noncommissioned officers' (NCO) and officers' clubs (although those under 18 were prohibited from buying distilled beverages [hard liquor]), and it was openly served at unit functions (Figure 8-7A). Evidently, it was assumed by military planners that, apart from the predictable but acceptably small numbers of individuals who would manifest problems, alcohol would aid the troops in decompressing from the ordeals of combat and the stress of deployment.

For example, according to Harold SR Byrdy, a division psychiatrist with the 1st Cavalry, "[i]n the very early days of the division, the mail and the daily allotment of

two cans of beer, usually warm, were crucial issues which were quickly perceived by command."[9(p9)] In Chapter 1 of this volume, Dennis L Menard, an enlisted social work specialist with the 1st Infantry Division (ID), described a beer ration in the field of two or three cans per day.[10] Herein is Douglas R Bey's postwar recollection from his experience as division psychiatrist with the 1st ID (April 1969–April 1970):

> For officers and NCOs, the drug of choice was alcohol. It was inexpensive and readily available. Every "Hail and Farewell" celebration, every T.G.I.F. [thank god it's Friday], every change of command was associated with alcohol. We had regular parties with steaks and booze. The medical officers had an officer's club and bartender. . . . The military encouraged drinking—to a point. However, if drinking led to problems with performance or discipline, the Army would come down hard, punish the drinker, and end his career.[11(p124)]

More broadly, the following is a description by Ronald H Spector, a military historian, of the place of alcohol within the military culture in Vietnam:

> As in all wars, soldiers [in Vietnam] turned to alcohol as a temporary escape from loneliness, boredom, and fear. "I was drinking two quarts of Old Grand Dad, 100 proof, every day," a soldier who served four tours in Vietnam recalled. "You drank it and you'd just sweat it out. You needed it to keep going, I guess. I got tired, real tired. You saw so much happening." In Vietnam the clubs and PXs made access to booze cheap and convenient, almost effortless in the rear areas. "You could go to the PX and buy . . . a whole fifth for a dollar," recalled one [soldier], "and some of the high-grade alcohol, even J&B scotch, only three dollars." Some commanders prohibited the sale of hard liquor to men below the rank of E-5 [sergeant]. Yet those men could easily obtain what they desired through purchases from other GIs [soldiers] not so restricted, and in any case had access to virtually unrestricted quantities of beer.
> Senior officers and career NCOs expected that soldiers far from home and in a war zone would do a good deal of drinking. Drunkenness was not exactly encouraged, but drinking was widely viewed as an acceptable outlet for the stress, fatigue, and tension of military life. So long as a man indulged himself while

off duty and kept his behavior within certain broad bounds, heavy drinking was tolerated or ignored. Indeed, the tough, experienced soldier was almost expected to be a hard-drinking man as well.

The generals recognized that there was a price to be paid in accidents, fights, and even occasional homicides, yet this price was understood and accepted, while the traditional apparatus of military control ranging from the tough old sarge who knew how to handle drunks to the Military Police to unit punishment to the military justice system was expected to keep a lid on things.[12(pp272–273)]

Apparently alcohol remained the preferred drug for off-duty use for the majority of assigned personnel in Vietnam, especially the NCOs and officers, despite the easy availability of marijuana throughout the war and heroin during the last third. (Although, in their summary of mental health activities in Vietnam [mid-1965–mid-1970], Colbach and Parrish declared that the young soldiers "generally avoided alcohol," which was replaced with illegal drug use.[13]) The majority of the drug use surveys conducted in Vietnam (reviewed later in this chapter) did not inquire about alcohol. One exception was the survey of lower-ranking enlisted soldiers departing Vietnam by Roffman and Sapol in 1967 (N= 484). Among their respondents, almost 95% acknowledged some alcohol use in Vietnam, with almost 55% indicating alcohol use "fairly often" or "a great deal."[14]

Incidence of Alcohol Problems: Abuse and Psychological/Physical Dependency

Overview. Because of the lack of available data, it remains difficult to ascertain the full extent to which alcohol abuse and dependency were problems for the Army in Vietnam. In his summary of Army psychiatric experience through the first third of war, William S Allerton, Chief, Psychiatry and Neurology Consultant Branch, Office of The Surgeon General (OTSG), declared that "[p]roblems with alcoholism, though present, do not seem to be in any way out of proportion to the problems observed elsewhere in the Armed forces."[15] Unfortunately Major General Spurgeon Neel's official overview of US Army medical experience in Vietnam through two-thirds of the war made no specific mention of alcohol-related problems, even though he did mention the emerging drug problems.[16] This did not mean that alcohol problems were insignificant, just

not documented. Official counts for alcohol-related problems were evidently not compiled because alcohol-related statistics were not collected as such from Army medical units for analysis (see Appendix IV: USARV [US Army Republic of Vietnam] Psychiatry and Neurology Morbidity Report in Appendix 2, "USARV Regulation No. 40-34" to this volume). Spector suggested that military leaders might have been willing to overlook such matters to facilitate the troops using alcohol to blow off steam from combat stress and the various privations of deployment. This is consistent with the argument by Joseph R Rothberg, a Walter Reed Army Institute of Research (WRAIR) biomathematician, that, in general, there is good statistical evidence to suspect a long-standing tendency toward underreporting of alcohol problems within the Army throughout this time frame.[17] One measure of alcohol's clinical impact during the buildup period came from Hays, who indicated that out-of-country evacuees with the diagnosis of alcoholism, which he lumped with character and behavior disorders, constituted only 2.2% of all Army psychiatric evacuees from Vietnam between January 1967 and June 1967 (the same percentage as that for Air Force, but less than the 2.9% for the Navy).[18] Yet Jones and Johnson's postwar review of Army psychiatric problems over the entire span of the war referred to the "high rate of alcoholic incidents" and a "high frequency" of alcoholism—but unfortunately without metrics.[19]

The Datel and Johnson psychotropic prescription survey, although limited to mid-1967 and to outpatient care, did provide a partial measure of the clinical challenge of "alcohol abuse" in the theater.[20] Of the 233 Army primary care physicians assigned in Vietnam, which included battalion surgeons, 92 (84% of respondents) indicated that 2.6% of their cases warranted the diagnosis of alcohol abuse. In contrast, the six Army and two Navy (attached to the Marines) respondent prescribing psychiatrists (100% of respondents) reported treating alcohol abuse over four times as often (11.8% of their caseloads); however, these results are less certain because the study did not distinguish between inpatient care and outpatient care as it did with the primary care physicians. The Datel and Johnson findings received some confirmation from the 1982 WRAIR survey of veteran Army psychiatrists who served in Vietnam. Survey participants reported a mean of 10.4% for alcoholic dependence syndrome among their caseloads (see Chapter 5, Table 5-3). Furthermore, when asked about frequency of professional involvement with a list of behavior problems in Vietnam, they estimated "excessive use of alcohol" as the second most frequent problem, somewhat less than characterological maladaptation but greater than problems secondary to use of marijuana, heroin, or other illegal drugs— estimates that held steady over both halves of the war (see Chapter 8, Table 8-4).

Reports From the Field. Evidently, the deployed medical and psychiatric specialists in Vietnam were often required to manage and treat soldiers with acute and chronic alcohol problems and associated medical conditions. From the beginning, most of the Army psychiatrists who published accounts from Vietnam indicated that alcohol problems were a prominent part of their workload. Robert E Huffman, the first Army psychiatrist assigned in Vietnam after the commitment of American ground troops in May 1965, reported that 18.5% (113) of the patients he treated, both combat and noncombat troops, had severe problems related to alcohol intoxication. "Men drank to excess in Vietnam so commonly that unless they engaged in extremely bizarre behavior, they were not usually referred."[21] Also in the first year, Byrdy, with the 1st Cavalry, indicated that of the 116 soldiers he hospitalized, 27 (23%) were either acutely or chronically alcoholic. However, unless these men were repeatedly hospitalized or were being considered for disciplinary or administrative action by their unit, they were "dried out" and returned to duty.[9] John A Bowman, with the 935th Psychiatric Detachment (December 1965–October 1966), referred to excessive drinking as a common form of regressive behavior, which resulted in punitive consequences or psychiatric attention in conjunction with administrative actions by commanders.[22] William F Kenny reported from the 17th Field Hospital in Saigon (May 1966–December 1966) that many of his cases, especially the characterologically dependent/emotionally unstable ones, were seen in their emergency room acutely agitated and under the influence of alcohol. He noted that, in general, it was common for soldiers who were poorly managing stresses of separation from home, marital discord, and frustrations with their jobs, to suffer with mixed anxiety and depression and resort to increasing alcohol intake.[23] Finally, Franklin Del Jones provided more detailed information. Besides his description of the numerous instances of "berserk" 25th ID troops (drunk and frenzied soldiers who threatened fellow soldiers with their weapons) mentioned in Chapter 3 in this volume, his study of Army patients at the 3rd Field Hospital in Saigon found alcoholism

to be the primary reason for referral for almost 20% of the support troops and an associated symptom for an additional 7% (compared to 5% and none among his combat troop referrals).[24] (See also Appendix 16, "Vietnam Study: Reactions to Stress Comparing Combat and Support Troops.")

Two years later, in 1968, during the transition phase of the war, John A Talbott, also in the Saigon area, reported that during the fighting in Saigon in conjunction with the Tet offensives, 44 (of 100 consecutive patients) were diagnosed as character and behavior disorders, 26 of whom were alcoholics.[25] Also, Edward M Colbach recalled from the 67th Evacuation Hospital in Qui Nhon that "alcohol caused most of the trouble of a sensational variety [when compared with marijuana],"[26(p206)] and John Imahara, who was assigned to the Long Binh stockade, reported that alcohol was often correlated with violent crimes by soldiers.[27] Surprisingly, that same year, H Spencer Bloch indicated that soldiers with drug or alcohol dependency problems represented only 6.8% of their total caseloads at the 3rd echelon treatment center, the 935th Psychiatric Detachment,[28] suggesting that many of the soldiers who developed significant alcohol problems in Vietnam did not get referred for sustained treatment and rehabilitation.

Some measure of explanation for the latter came from Bey the following year. He served as division psychiatrist in the 1st ID (1969–1970) and indicated that, despite widespread use of marijuana by troops, alcohol continued to be the major problem drug, and that violent incidents occurred most often while the soldier was under the influence of alcohol. However, for the most part, soldiers with chronic problems eluded clinically effective treatment. ("Psychiatric consultation . . . may harm an individual's chance for promotion, may jeopardize his security clearance and diminish his acceptability by his superiors."[29(ChapVII,p5)]) According to Bey, the alcoholic sergeant was a common problem. In fact, many alcoholics volunteered for Vietnam duty as a way to escape from rehabilitation pressures and an impatient company commander in the United States. In Vietnam he anticipated cheap liquor and social acceptance of high alcohol use, avoidance of family responsibilities, and decreased scrutiny by command. On the other hand, some men were sent to Vietnam by their commanders in the United States as a punishment for their drinking. As far as the consequences, Bey provided these observations:

Nearly every type of acute and chronic problem associated with alcohol abuse was seen in the division. Cases of simple drunkenness, DT's [delirium tremors], pathological intoxication, Korsakoff's psychosis, acute hallucinosis, alcoholic paranoia and alcoholic deterioration were seen in our division.

. . . It often appeared to us that the Army tolerated, supported and even encouraged the use of alcohol to a point, but once a man lost control of his dependence on alcohol he became a threat to the organization's security. [The commander's] first response to this confrontation was one of denial, by getting the individual out of sight through unit transfer. Where this was not possible, command urged increased controls on the part of the individual, and when this failed the alcoholic was often the scapegoat and punished.[29(ChapVII,pp7–8)]

Bey later noted that, "the vast majority of individuals who had problems with alcohol did not come to our attention."[11(p126)]

By the drawdown phase of the war, alcohol was apparently still an endemic problem, but it was so overshadowed by heroin use that it was hardly noticed as such by clinicians or the Army. Still, according to Richard Ratner, an Army psychiatrist with the 935th Psychiatric Detachment (1970–1971), "Drinking, when it occurs in excess, is at least as potent a cause of ineffectiveness among the troops as heroin . . . and marijuana [as a cause of ineffectiveness], is so rare it is reportable."[30] Contemporaneously, Howard W Fisher, a Navy psychiatrist who served with the 1st Marine Division, found that of 1,000 consecutive Marine referrals, 590 were presumed to be involved with illegal drugs, and "[a]lcoholism was an overwhelming problem in 130 men, but many more abused it."[31(p1166)]

Risk Factors for Alcohol Problems

Documentation regarding risk factors for alcohol problems in Vietnam is also sparse. Because alcohol problems tend to have a bimodal distribution, with problems of abuse and psychological dependency grouping in the late teens and twenties, and problems of physical dependency grouping a decade or more later, considerations for the younger soldiers are often separable from those of the older soldier.

Younger Enlisted Soldiers. Some measure of baseline for alcohol problems within the stateside Army during the war period can be derived from a study conducted by Cahalan et al in 1972 that found a third of the sample of young enlisted men (EM) were heavy drinkers and another third had drinking problems (vs civilian counterparts with 21% heavy drinkers and 9% with drinking problems[32]). The investigators concluded that enlisted soldiers drink more and get in more trouble than their civilian counterparts.[33]

However, the Army psychiatrists in the field in Vietnam had almost nothing to say bearing on risk factors for alcohol abuse, especially those specific for Vietnam. After the war, Jones and Johnson opined that the alcohol-related problems seen in Vietnam were attributable to "disorders of loneliness," too much leisure time, and the lack of potable ice, which led to drinking of canned beverages, especially beer.[19]

More definitive findings regarding the prevalence of alcohol use/abuse in Vietnam and associated risk factors among the young, enlisted soldiers, came from the large, government-sponsored study of drug use in Vietnam by Robins and her colleagues in 1972 (described later in this chapter). As part of their study, 451 randomly selected Army enlisted men who left Vietnam in September 1971 were interviewed 8 to 12 months after their return to the United States regarding their patterns of alcohol use. The percent acknowledging regular, nonproblem alcohol use before, during, and after Vietnam was 16%, 23%, and 16%, respectively, indicating a significant increase among that group while in Vietnam but a return to pre-Vietnam levels afterward. On the other hand, the percent acknowledging problem alcohol use (symptomatic or alcoholic) before, during, and after Vietnam was 26%, 15%, and 38%, respectively, indicating a large reduction of problem alcohol use in Vietnam, followed by problem-use levels back in the United States that were significantly higher than pre-Vietnam levels. Reciprocal patterns were found among the percent acknowledging (*any*) opiate use before, during, and after Vietnam (10%, 48%, and 10%, respectively), barbiturate use (11%, 24%, and 12%, respectively), and amphetamine use (22%, 27%, and 21%, respectively). Whereas, while in Vietnam, drinking levels declined among the subgroup that acknowledged pre-Vietnam drinking problems, use of illegal drugs (not including marijuana) there rose sharply, evidently as preferred alternatives to alcohol (almost one-half tried opiates, and 20% became opiate-dependent). Upon their return to the United States, use of these drugs declined dramatically (less than 2% were opiate dependent), while the percent of those acknowledging problem drinking greatly exceeded pre-Vietnam levels (from 26% to 38%). Furthermore, among a set of demographic variables tested, the highest scores for preservice predictors of alcoholism were early age of drinking, school troubles, and parental alcoholism. The authors concluded that this general sample of lower-ranking soldiers indicated that alcohol was a more serious pre-Vietnam problem than were other drugs.[34] Unfortunately, it is difficult to generalize from their study. Not only was the sample gathered from those who served in the later, more tumultuous phase of the war, but the increased heroin accessibility there—a phenomenon that was limited to Vietnam and to the last couple of years—is a feature the authors acknowledged as having been quite influential.[35]

Career Soldiers. A whole different set of problems surround the older soldier who is more likely a careerist and who may develop a serious physical and psychological alcohol-dependency problem (alcoholism). Interestingly, the aforementioned stateside survey by Cahalan et al in 1972 also compared officers (n = 4,331) and enlisted soldiers (n = 5,579) and found that despite reported attitudes toward imbibing alcohol that were similar to the younger enlisted soldiers (37% of enlisted soldiers and 36% of officers endorsed the statement, "Getting drunk occasionally is a good way to blow off steam"), officers were half as likely to manifest problems associated with drinking, and half again as likely to develop health problems secondary to drinking, and half again as likely to require hospitalized treatment for alcohol-related problems.[33,36] Nonetheless, it seems reasonable to suspect from the anecdotal psychiatrist reports that many officers and NCOs in Vietnam did use alcohol to such an extent that their duty functions were affected and that the circumstances there discouraged them from seeking help. This refers to the likelihood that their superiors were reluctant to identify them as problem drinkers because of the previously mentioned Army policies and regulations that classified alcohol problems as misconduct, which meant that a career soldier with a recurring drinking problem faced the possibility of a career-ending administrative discharge from the Army.[5]

Treatment of Alcohol Problems in Vietnam

The foregoing material indicates that acute alcohol-generated problems among personnel assigned in

Vietnam were a steady and significant issue for military leaders and medical personnel, including psychiatrists. However, there are no reports in the professional literature that documented the application of specific treatments for these cases. It seems likely that clinical reports did not emerge because referrals were expected and manageable in number, and the approaches for acute conditions were well established. The 1967 Datel and Johnson survey sheds some light on medications found useful in the treatment of "alcohol abuse" in Vietnam.[20] In particular, the majority of both the prescribing primary care physicians (91%) and the prescribing psychiatrist respondents (68%) favored neuroleptics (usually Thorazine) over the next most commonly used anxiolytics (usually Librium) and sedative/hypnotics. (See Chapter 6, Case 6-9, SP4 November as an example of a soldier with alcohol abuse requiring a brief hospitalization.)

Treatment of alcohol dependency was more difficult. Jones and Johnson mentioned that "[c]hronic alcoholism usually showed up as job inefficiency in a man who had a history of alcohol excesses in the past. Treatment by total abstinence was impossible in most cases and administrative handling usually resulted."[19(p55)] In their review of Army psychiatry in Vietnam through two-thirds of the war, Colbach and Parrish reported that two psychiatric specialty detachments sponsored Alcoholics Anonymous meetings; however, none of the anecdotal psychiatrist reports provided substantiation.[13] (In contrast, see Appendix 17, "Mental Hygiene Bulletin No. 1: Suggestions in the Management of Alcoholism.") There also is no indication in the record of the use of Antabuse (a medication that produces an immediate and severe negative reaction to the subsequent intake of alcohol) as a disincentive to drink. In general, Antabuse, or disulfiram, has proved very useful in restraining alcohol use among abuse-prone service members because the military's structured environment includes mechanisms to ensure compliance. Bey described its effective use with alcoholic service members when he served in the United States[11]; but, inexplicitly, he apparently did not use it in Vietnam. Case 9-1 below, the case of Lieutenant Colonel George, is an example of the emergence of depression and disabling alcohol dependency in a career soldier under the circumstances accompanying his assignment in Vietnam—symptoms that receded to subclinical status after he was returned to the United States and reunited with his family. It is notable that his medevacuation out of Vietnam was command directed rather than a medical decision. This was likely also the disposition for numerous, uncounted individuals with higher ranks who manifested recurrent difficulties with alcohol in Vietnam.

CASE 9-1: Career Officer With Performance Failure Secondary to Repeated Alcohol Abuse

Identifying Information: Lieutenant Colonel (LTC) George is a 45-year-old, married, white, Medical Service Corps officer with over 20 years of Army service. After serving in Vietnam for 2 months, he underwent two hospitalizations at a field hospital in Vietnam for alcohol abuse before being medevacuated to Walter Reed General Hospital (WRGH) in Washington, DC, for alcoholism.

History of present illness: The patient describes increasing difficulty handling a series of jobs in Vietnam as well as a strained relationship with his wife in the States. He recalled mounting tension and despair; insomnia, anorexia, malaise, and work inefficiency after arriving in Vietnam; which lowered his self-confidence and contributed to disagreements with his superiors; and which led to attempts to relieve these feelings with alcohol. A series of transfers and reductions in responsibility only aggravated his condition. His first hospitalization revealed him to be objectively and subjectively depressed. After 10 days he was discharged with a diagnosis of "reactive depression manifested by acute mental syndrome due to alcohol intoxication," placed on the antidepressant Tofranil (100 mg/day), and instructed to not drink any alcohol. Although somewhat improved initially, further disagreements with superiors and episodic alcohol abuse occurred. He was again hospitalized after an incident of drunk and disorderly behavior. His commander directed his medical evacuation to the United States and recommended he be separated from the Army.

Past history: LTC George was the oldest of three sons. His father died of heart problems when he was 22. His mother is now 72 and also has heart disease. Neither parent had a drinking history. The patient completed high school and received several college credits. His childhood and adolescence were referred to as happy. He and his wife of 21 years raised two children; however, their relation had recently become strained. Both he and his wife were moderately heavy social drinkers. LTC George was drafted into the Army in 1943 and served as an enlisted soldier for 3 years before being commissioned. The character of his service was distinguished. He received the Bronze Star for performance in combat as an enlisted soldier in World War II (artillery). Since he married, he had never been required to be apart from his wife.

Examination: At Walter Reed General Hospital (WRGH) he was noted to be obese, pleasant, alert, and cooperative. He showed only minimal signs of anxiety and none of depression. His thoughts centered on arguing, with vehemence, that the record of his failure to meet his responsibilities in Vietnam and the contention of his misuse of alcohol was a distortion of the facts. More generally, there was no evidence of disordered thinking or intellectual impairment. Judgment and insight were also unimpaired. Physical exam was unremarkable and without signs of chronic alcoholism or dietary deficiency.

Clinical course: Unremarkable. He quickly adapted to the ward milieu at WRGH. There was no evidence of a thought or mood disorder or a significant personality disorder. He was discharged after a month of observation and milieu treatment.

Final diagnosis: (1) Transfer diagnosis: Alcoholism, chronic, not concurred in ["Not concurred in" was evidently a commonly used term to mean that the final diagnosis did not agree with the transfer diagnosis.] (2) Observation, neuropsychiatric; no disease.

Disposition: Returned to duty in the United States.

Source: Narrative Summary, Walter Reed General Hospital.

On 17 June 1971, President Richard Nixon, in a special message to Congress on drug abuse prevention and control, referred to drug abuse as "America's public enemy number one" and, among other provisions, directed the Secretary of Defense to establish a program to eliminate drug abuse in the military, especially in Vietnam.[37] This led to great interest in soldier use of illegal drugs in Vietnam, but concerns for alcohol abuse and dependency continued to be overlooked there from the epidemiologic perspective.

In conclusion, the available documentation suggests that alcohol-related problems were widespread among Army troops in Vietnam and may have consumed roughly 10% to 20% or more of the clinical resources of the psychiatric specialists, especially in the evaluation and treatment of alcohol toxicity and acute alcohol dependence syndrome. This was evidently true across both halves of the war and included both combat and support troops. Acute alcohol problems were managed routinely on a case-by-case basis and did not exceed the threshold for professional reportability (ie, because the deployed psychiatrists found these to be neither qualitatively nor quantitatively exceptional). On the other hand, there was little or no provision for a sustained or systematic treatment of individuals with chronic or recurrent alcohol dependence syndromes in Vietnam, even though the anecdotal series of suicidal NCOs mentioned by several of the psychiatrists (see Chapter 8 of this volume) is consistent with the prospect of a sizable mental health problem regarding this subset of alcohol-related problems.

DRUG ABUSE IN VIETNAM AND THE SABOTAGE OF THE "GREEN MACHINE"

Problems associated with soldiers using drugs other than alcohol had been seen during foreign deployments preceding Vietnam, and most often these were attributed to boredom and ended as the troops were withdrawn. Marijuana use by American soldiers first aroused concerns in Panama in the 1920s and early 1930s, and several investigative boards were held, and one study of hospitalized marijuana users was undertaken. The conclusion was that "the effects upon military efficiency and discipline were practically negligible."[14] When US troops were first deployed in Southeast Asia, most medical authorities considered marijuana to be a dangerous drug and a rising public health problem.[38] However, as young adults in the United States were increasing their use of illegal drugs, especially marijuana, doubts were being raised by some civilian psychiatrists as to its deleterious effects. A prominent example is that of Joel Fort, public health specialist and former Consultant on Drug Abuse for the World Health Organization, who weighed in on the side of decriminalization.[38]

As for the much more serious matter of soldier use of narcotics, the end of the Civil War brought with it a sizable problem of opiate addiction among veterans, the then-called "Army Disease," in part because of the invention of the hypodermic syringe. Around the turn of the 20th century concerns arose regarding US troops smoking opium during the Philippines occupation. Within the civilian sector, narcotic use became a serious endemic problem with illicit features following the discovery of the opium derivative, heroin, in 1898, and the enactment of the Harrison Narcotic Act in the United States in 1914—a law whose strict control measures provided an opportunity for underworld exploitation. The typical addict of those times was white, female, rural, lower to lower-middle class, and middle-aged.[39] Use of narcotics does not appear to have been a problem for the US military in World War I. In fact, drug addiction was not an absolute disqualifying condition for service during the mobilization. In 1939 drug addiction became recognized as a public health problem in America, and in August 1940, the US Army removed drug addiction from conditions acceptable for special and limited service. According to Perkins, a psychiatric historian, although drug addiction represented 0.1% of all overseas psychiatric admissions through the course of World War II, there is no record of psychiatric attention in the literature.[40] When all cases of fatal narcotism in American military personnel between 1918 and mid-1970 filed with the Armed Forces Institute of Pathology were reviewed (N = 174), it was noted that the majority of deaths occurred in the Asian theaters in nonwhite males aged 18 to 25 and in the three lowest pay grades; most resulted from drug overdose or hypersensitivity rather than from the medical complications of narcotic addiction; rates before and during the mobilization years of World War II were insignificant, followed by a slight rise in the closing phases of the war; and between 1951 and 1953, an extraordinary increase in deaths occurred, primarily among troops assigned in Korea.[41]

As morale and commitment sagged during the Vietnam era and antimilitary sentiment grew among the lower-ranking EM, officers and NCOs came to be derided by many enlisted men as "juicers." This alluded to the presumption that they were abusing alcohol, just as the enlisted men were abusing other drugs. It was also meant to suggest there was hypocrisy in command's efforts to suppress soldier drug use, which in turn served as rationalization for troops not respecting military order and discipline, especially that regarding their own drug use. In fact, the historically validated distinction between those more inclined toward simple drunkenness (ie, the younger soldiers) and those who developed alcohol dependency problems (ie, the older, career NCO or officer), took a new form: young, first-term soldiers often found their drug of choice to be an illegal one. This was corroborated by Rock, who found soldiers admitted to Tripler Army Medical Center (Hawaii) for chronic alcoholism in 1967–1970 were, on average, 39 years old, had 15 years of service, and held a rank of E-6; and soldiers also admitted for chronic alcoholism at Army hospitals in Europe between January 1972 and March 1972, were 35 years old, had 11.6 years of service, and held a rank of E-6; but soldiers admitted for drug abuse in Europe between January 1972 and March 1972 were in their early 20s, were on their first enlistment, and were lower-ranking EM.[42]

A particularly cogent explanation for the upsurge in preference for illegal drugs by lower-ranking enlisted soldiers of the Vietnam era was provided by Manning, an Army social psychologist. In past generations, sanctioned, alcohol-centered events had been a military custom because, by creating memorable episodes, the formation of small unit morale and cohesion could be accelerated. By contrast, as the younger, noncareer, Vietnam-era soldiers shifted to illegal drugs, they were pointedly seeking to form their own cohesive group that repudiated the military command structure and its values—that is, they sought a horizontal cohesion, unhinged from vertical (hierarchical) cohesion to their leaders and military priorities (what they referred to disdainfully as the "green machine."[43(p21),44(p98)])[45]

The material that follows will review, chronologically, the growing problem of drug use in Vietnam along with the various efforts by military leaders and the mental health component to counteract these trends. Interspersed are excerpts from Major General (MG) George S Prugh's summary of the military law enforcement activities in response to illegal drug use in the theater.[46(pp106–108)] MG Prugh served as Staff Judge Advocate at the US Military Assistance Command in Vietnam through July 1966 and later as the Army Judge Advocate General in the early 1970s. This review is set against the backdrop of the dominant social, political, and military events at the time (see Chapter 1) as well as the associated challenges to Army psychiatry in Vietnam (see Chapter 2).

THE BUILDUP PHASE (1965–1967): MARIJUANA, HASHISH, AND OTHER DRUGS (PRE-HEROIN)

1965–1966

Following the insertion of US ground troops in Vietnam in May 1965, and once the buildup phase was underway, military personnel in Vietnam, especially those in the lower ranks, not only eagerly consumed alcohol,[14,21] but in addition, smoked marijuana. Some soldiers also smoked opium-soaked marijuana (the "OJ"—the opium joint).[47] (The references to marijuana that follow will also include hashish, a much more concentrated extract. Both are preparations from the plant Cannabis Sativa, [although Army psychiatrist Frank D Master, who served at the 67th Evacuation Hospital, said it was Cannabis Indica[48]] and the primary active ingredient is delta-9-tetrahydrocannabinol [THC].)

> MG Prugh:
>
> In September 1966 the U.S. Military Assistance Command made a survey of the availability of drugs in the greater Saigon area. The survey showed that there were twenty-nine fixed outlets in this area, and that drugs were readily available from cycle and pedicab drivers, bar girls, shopkeepers, hotel clerks, and others who dealt with the public. The Vietnamese drug laws were ill-defined. No central Vietnamese narcotic enforcement agency existed, and enforcement of existing laws was lax. There was no government control over marihuana and only a little over opium. The U.S. Embassy was informed of the results of the survey, and on 12 November 1966 General Westmoreland asked the embassy for action on the matter; none had been taken by the year's end. Of the 100 drug cases investigated in the U.S. command in Vietnam from 1 July 1965 to 30 June 1966, 96 involved marihuana.[46(p106)]

Numerous Vietnam veterans have published personal accounts of marijuana use in Vietnam. One written by John Steinbeck IV[49] received notoriety in the late 1960s. He served as an Army enlisted radio/television specialist early in the war and was stationed at Qui Nhon, the large logistical base midway up the coast of South Vietnam. Steinbeck noted the easy interpenetration of GIs and civilian Vietnamese and

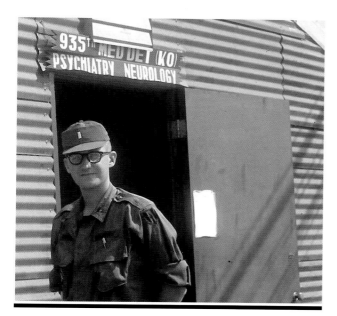

FIGURE 9-1. First Lieutenant Roger A Roffman, Medical Service Corps, Social Work Officer with the 935th Psychiatric Detachment. Roffman conducted the first study of patterns of soldier drug use, especially marijuana, in Vietnam. In June 1967 he surveyed confinees of the Army stockade at Long Binh. This was followed by a similar survey (with Army Psychologist Ely Sapol) of troops leaving Vietnam. The results, along with findings from similar studies by others who followed them, ultimately permitted command to monitor the problem of growing drug use in Vietnam, a phenomenon that steadily undermined military morale and discipline and paralleled the rise in drug use among civilian peers in the United States Photograph courtesy of Roger A Roffman.

described the central role of marijuana for both sides in the war. "There is no central market for it in Vietnam. It is simply a way of life."[49(p34)] He also commented on the relatively tolerant attitude by American command structure for soldier use of marijuana and emphasized its ubiquitous availability and extremely low cost. Steinbeck was clearly in favor of soldiers using marijuana and had no reservations about impairment ("you can learn to function normally with marijuana"[49(p33)]), but with a rather critical proviso regarding combat troops ("[being stoned] is not the best condition to be in when confronted with an ambush, terror attack, or some like activity"[49(p33)]). He speculated that 75% of his fellow soldiers used it regularly. He provided the following interpretation as to why: "Everyone was taking the release from the war. Perhaps to many GIs [marijuana] was the only and last relief that Vietnam had to offer."[49(p35)] He observed that marijuana induced

"a calm, perceiving detachment . . . [during which] a wonderful change in war starts to occur. Instead of the grim order of terror, explosions modulate musically; death takes on a new approachable symbolism that is not so horrible."[49(p35)]

Regarding the prevalence of psychiatric problems associated with use of so-called recreational drugs, like marijuana, the little available clinical data from this early point in the war suggested that drug abuse was not seen as a serious problem. Huffman reported that among his caseload (N = 573 American military personnel), patients with alcohol-associated psychiatric problems (18.5%) far overshadowed those associated with drug use (0.82%). Huffman was not specific about the drugs used in his cases, but he did note that "[t]he use of marijuana among American troops was known to be occurring, but among physicians seeing patients in Vietnam it was seldom mentioned as a recognized problem."[21] Also, among 22 combat soldiers treated by Jones at the 3rd Field Hospital in Saigon, there were no cases of drug abuse reported. However, among his 98 patients who were support troops, 5% had drug abuse as either a primary reason for referral or as an associated symptom. Jones also did not indicate which drugs were being used, but it was presumably marijuana.[24]

1967

Rising Prevalence of Drug Use

As troop strength in Vietnam increased, so did the prevalence of drug use especially marijuana and hashish, but including opiates to a limited degree among the soldiers assigned in Vietnam. This coincided with the increasing popularity of illegal drugs among the generation of young Americans in the mid-to-late 1960s. Although many soldiers felt that marijuana was simply an alternative intoxicant (comparable to alcohol), because its possession was illegal, it presented a new problem for the military.

MG Prugh:
By 1967 marihuana cigarettes were selling for 20¢ each in Saigon and $1.00 each in Da Nang. Opium was $1.00 per injection, and morphine $5.00 per vial. Heroin had not appeared on the market. There were 1,391 US military investigations, involving 1,688 persons, for use of marihuana in 1967. This monthly rate of .25 per 1,000 troops was still lower than the Army-wide average of .30 per

1,000 troops. There were 29 hard narcotics investigations, involving 25 persons, for illegal possession, use, or sale of opium and morphine. There were 427 courts-martial for marihuana and hard narcotics abuse in Vietnam in 1967.[46(pp106–107)]

Three additional features prompted the Army's growing concern about the expanding use of marijuana by soldiers in Vietnam: (1) evidence suggested that marijuana was being used in the field,[12(p275),47,50,51] which could affect combat performance; (2) clinical reports indicated that it was negatively impacting the health of some troops in the form of neuropsychiatric conditions; and (3) the native-grown marijuana was more potent than that sold in the United States (estimates ranged from 2[52] to 5–10 times[51] as potent) and was inexpensive and ubiquitously marketed by the Vietnamese. With regard to marketing, Roger A Roffman (Figure 9-1), an Army social work officer assigned to the 935th Psychiatric Detachment, provided the following observation:

> Marijuana had become widely available in Vietnam, and its packaging was quite ingenious. The cellophane wrapping on American commercial brand cigarette packages was carefully unsealed by the Vietnamese marijuana distributors, and the twenty tobacco cigarettes were removed and replaced by nineteen rolled joints. The cellophane was then resealed and the package looked untouched.[53(Chap2,p7)]

In June 1967, Roffman surveyed 96 confinees (excluding those convicted for marijuana possession) in the Army stockade at Long Binh regarding marijuana use. He found that 63% acknowledged use at least once in their lives and 45% since they arrived in Vietnam.[54] This was followed closely by a similar survey by Roffman (with Ely Sapol, an Army psychologist) of 584 lower-ranking (E-6 and below) enlisted soldiers leaving Vietnam. Of the 32% who had ever smoked marijuana, 61% began in Vietnam, but only one-quarter of all users were classified as heavy users (defined as greater than 20 times while serving in Vietnam). The heavy marijuana user was unique in being younger, of lower rank, and more likely to have marijuana-using friends. He also was more likely to have used marijuana before coming to Vietnam, used it earlier in his tour, used other drugs, and had a history of at least one minor disciplinary action.

Overall, reported marijuana use was higher among soldiers exposed to combat, tended to be a communal activity, and users overestimated prevalence among peers. The investigators also found that not only was alcohol use more prevalent among marijuana users, but 41.8% of the soldiers who described using alcohol "a great deal" were marijuana smokers compared to only 19.4% of those who indicated no alcohol use. In other words, among these soldiers, marijuana use did not replace alcohol use but was additive.[14]

Clinical Observations on Effects of Marijuana

Several clinical reports on the effects of marijuana were generated from the 935th Psychiatric Detachment near Saigon in 1967. Raymond A Fidaleo, an Army psychiatrist, described the effects of marijuana on soldiers and distinguished the "high" from the "trip." The high followed two-to-four long, air-filled inhalations of marijuana and consisted of a dreamlike state with feelings of well-being, exhilaration, and contentment. Imagination and perception were increased and pleasant experiences were reported. In contrast, when two to 10 cigarettes were smoked, a trip, similar to that experienced with LSD, could occur. This consisted of feelings of estrangement and depersonalization; perceptual illusions; distortions of time, space, and place; along with a euphoric feeling. Fidaleo noted that some combat soldiers on operations in the field maintained a high with marijuana to keep anxiety down. On the other hand, support troops were more likely to use it in greater amounts so as to obtain a trip, not just a high. However, in some instances this resulted in a "bad trip," which might include: nystagmus, ataxia, tremor, headache, dry mouth, flushed faces, dilated pupils, nausea and vomiting, diarrhea, and the typical red-eyed hangover state, as well as depression and hostile-aggression, apprehension and acute anxiety, paranoid delusions, and hallucinatory states. Fidaleo reported that they treated approximately two admissions per month (5% of admissions) for paranoid psychosis in combination with acute organic brain syndrome in soldiers with patterns of heavy marijuana use, and that these cases responded in 1 to 4 days to conservative management and Thorazine (300 mg–600 mg/day).[47(p58)]

John A Talbott, Fidaleo's colleague at the 935th Psychiatric Detachment, described treating a continuum of inpatients that had psychiatric complications from marijuana use ("pot reactions"). These ranged from a relatively benign intoxicating high to a frank schizophrenic-like psychosis. He also noted that the diagnosis could be complicated because soldiers feared punishment and would not acknowledge their marijuana use. In general, the more typical reactions to marijuana requiring hospitalized care included: tachycardia and shortness of breath; anxiety and fearfulness; depression and tearfulness; confusion, disorientation, dissociation and depersonalization; and paranoia, delusions, and auditory hallucinations. Talbott commented that although those who developed such reactions may have had pre-Vietnam character defects, the etiological importance of susceptibility was difficult to judge because the locally grown marijuana was highly potent.[55] (See also Case #3 in Bloch's paper, "Some Interesting Reaction Types Encountered in a War Zone" [in Appendix 12 of this volume] for a more challenging clinical example of a soldier with a pattern of marijuana use who presented with bizarre and aggressive psychotic symptoms.)

Subsequently, he and Teague described 12 cases of "marijuana psychosis" (an acute toxic psychosis with paranoid features) treated at the 935th Psychiatric Detachment. They were noted to have acute attacks of disorganizing combinations of organic brain dysfunction and anxiety, with 10 cases showing paranoid symptoms. All were successfully treated and returned to duty within a week, typically without use of psychotropic medications. Notably these episodes often followed the soldier's first attempt to smoke marijuana, and in only two cases was a premorbid personality disorder diagnosed (the case of PFC King, below, serves as illustration). The authors posited that the primary etiologic agent for these cases was the Cannabis; however, they also mentioned that 50% of marijuana contraband seized in Vietnam contained opiates. They further speculated that because they were working in a tertiary treatment setting (the 935th), they were seeing only the tip of an iceberg of toxic reactions to marijuana that other soldiers were successfully managing by other means.[52]

CASE 9-2: Toxic Psychosis in a New Marijuana User

Identifying information: Private First Class (PFC) King is a 24-year-old, black soldier (MOS [military occupational specialty] and unit indeterminate) who was transferred to the 935th Psychiatric Detachment for additional specialized psychiatric treatment after 2 days of treatment at another Army hospital in Vietnam.

History of present illness: The patient was initially admitted after he had smoked a pipe full of "strange-tasting tobacco," which caused him to feel light-headed and "funny." He subsequently had feelings of depersonalization and derealization, and he thought his mind was split into two parts—good and evil. He expressed the morbid preoccupation that he was dead, admitted to unusual illusions or hallucinations (clouds pulling him in, bright lights coming out of the clouds toward him), and expressed frightening fears that he would kill someone or be killed. He was disoriented, confused, and forgetful. He was treated with Thorazine with some improvement before his transfer to the 935th.

Past history: The record regarding PFC King's history only included that he grew up without his father at home, he had aggressive outbursts in late adolescence, and he later manifested excessive drinking and difficulty keeping a job. The character of his military service was not recorded.

Examination: At the 935th he was noted to be apprehensive, worried, and preoccupied with fears, sensations, and impulses. His restlessness, tremulousness, agitation, and rapid speech alternated with staring, mutism, and inability to complete his thoughts. He continued to express the belief that his mind was split but denied hallucinations, delusions, or other unusual sensations. He seemed adequately oriented, and he denied prior exposure to marijuana.

Clinical course: The patient was treated with Librium and his anxiety rapidly abated. He was active in group therapy and presented no problems in ward management. He was discharged after 5 days with no residual symptoms.

Discharge diagnosis: Acute toxic psychosis associated with Cannabis intoxication in an individual with an aggressive premorbid personality.

Disposition: Returned to full duty.

Source: Adapted with permission from Talbott JA, Teague JW. Marihuana psychosis. Acute toxic psychosis associated with the use of Cannabis derivatives. *JAMA*. 1969;210(2):301.

To conclude, during the buildup phase the rise in the prevalence of drug use (especially marijuana and hashish) was substantial, but only a small percentage of users required treatment, primarily for toxic brain syndromes. The psychiatrists at the 935th Psychiatric Detachment described these as brief and self-limited (if marijuana use was discontinued), and they advocated that these soldiers be rehabilitated and returned to duty in Vietnam. However, as noted in Chapter 8 of this volume, Elliot M Heiman, an Army psychiatrist who received psychiatric patients at Fort Gordon, Georgia, who had been medically evacuated from Vietnam, suggested that the clinical course for some heavy marijuana users was not as benign as those at the 935th presumed. Heiman speculated that many acute psychoses seen in Vietnam who appeared to have a functionally based condition (eg, schizophrenia), may instead have chronic or excessive marijuana use as a critical, if ultimately reversible, etiologic factor.[56]

THE TRANSITION PHASE (1968–1969): A GROWING POLYDRUG PROBLEM (PRE-HEROIN)

1968

Because the raison d'être of the US Army is preservation of America's security through the maintenance of an effective fighting force, it would seem that prohibiting soldier use of illicit, mind-altering drugs requires no further explanation. Yet in 1968, in response to the growing drug problem in the US military, the Department of Defense reiterated that

Drug abuse has a particularly important consequence for the Armed Forces. Unlike civilians, those in military service have a special dependency on each other. The lives of all those on a Navy ship may depend on the alertness of one man assigned to close certain watertight doors. Each member of a Marine Corps fire team is dependent on his buddies for survival in a combat situation. There are no 'passengers' in fighter aircraft or bombers, or in the Army's tanks. No commander can trust the fate of his unit, ship, or plane to a man who may be under the influence of drugs.[57(p9)]

Nonetheless, illegal drug use by the US troops became increasingly popular in Vietnam and alarming to military leaders.

MG Prugh:

In October 1968 the Vietnamese government publicly condemned the use of or trafficking in marihuana and opium and issued instructions to province chiefs to forbid the growing of marihuana. The recently established Vietnamese Narcotics Bureau was expanded, and the U.S. government sent an agent from the Bureau of Narcotics and Dangerous Drugs to Saigon to provide professional assistance to the Vietnamese. A program of using aircraft to discover marihuana crops and sending in Vietnamese troops to destroy the crops was instituted. In June 1968 the marihuana use rate among U.S. troops, based on reported incidents, had risen to 1.3 per 1,000 (194 cases); by December it had climbed to 4.5 per 1,000 (523 cases). The opium rate rose from .003 per 1,000 in June to .068 by December.[46(p107)]

Prevalence of Marijuana Use

In early 1968, Wildred B Postel, the division psychiatrist assigned to the 4th ID in Pleiku, conducted the first survey regarding marijuana use with infantry units. Fifty psychiatry clinic patients and 76 surgical inpatients participated, all of them first-term enlisted soldiers. Fifty-six percent of psychiatry clinic patients and 46% of surgical inpatients acknowledged marijuana use overall, with 30% of the former and 21% of the latter qualifying as habituated (defined as having smoked marijuana five times or more). Compared to the surgical habituated, psychiatry clinic patients who were habitual users tended to have started marijuana before entering the service and experimented more with other drugs. All marijuana groups indicated that marijuana use tended to be a social group activity and was commonly used in the field, usually to calm down after a battle; however, one soldier acknowledged going into battle while under its influence.[50]

Edmund Casper, the division psychiatrist with the 23rd ID (Americal), along with Hugh Martinell Jr, an enlisted social work/psychology specialist, and James Janacek, a psychiatrist with the 98th Psychiatric Detachment, surveyed a cross section of 771 soldiers with the 23rd ID regarding marijuana use at Chu Lai. They reported that among the general population at least

20% had tried marijuana but only a few had become chronic users. Those who did not continue use said they found it either unrewarding or unpleasant. Furthermore, the investigators had the general impression that the chronic users had been users before joining the Army. A comparison of psychiatric clinic patients to general medical patients showed marijuana use rates of 52% and 33%, respectively (close to Postel's findings with the 4th ID). The authors also found a higher percentage of soldiers arriving in Vietnam who reported marijuana use (27%) than those leaving (20.6%) and hypothesized a more rapid rise in use among civilian peers.[58]

Clinical Effects of Marijuana Use

From the 67th Evacuation Hospital, which served the Qui Nhon catchment area of 45,000 mostly support troops, Colbach, an Army psychiatrist, and Raymond R Crowe, an Air Force psychiatrist, reported on their clinical experiences with a series of marijuana psychosis cases. Among the 40 to 50 soldiers hospitalized per month at the 67th Evacuation Hospital over a 10-month period beginning in late 1968, approximately five per month presented with a schizophrenia-like psychosis with paranoid features secondary to heavy marijuana use. These cases were similar to those described by Talbott and Teague the year before, but Colbach and Crowe indicated that in some cases the symptoms did not remit despite hospitalization for 1 to 2 weeks, phenothiazine treatment, and supportive psychotherapy. They also credited the much more potent marijuana in Vietnam, but they furthermore reported that the more prolonged treatment course was required by individuals with personality disorders. Colbach and Crowe provided the following case example of Private Love. Also of note, these investigators were the first to speculate on contributory antimilitary attitudes among the more serious cases.[59]

CASE 9-3: Toxic Psychosis in a Chronic Marijuana User

Identifying information: Private (PVT) Love is a 19-year-old combat soldier with 6 months service in Vietnam who was hospitalized at the 67th Evacuation Hospital for psychotic behavior.

History of present illness: At the time of his admission, he claimed he was smoking 20 marijuana cigarettes per day. Upon returning from the field, he began

preaching about a new religion he was founding that would bring peace to all mankind. He swore at his commanding officer, calling him an instrument of the devil.

Past history: PVT Love came from a broken home and described his father as an alcoholic. He was a high school dropout who thought of running to Canada rather than coming into the Army because he was against the war. In the Army he had been a chronic disciplinary problem and had once tried to organize an antiwar protest.

Examination: On admission he was noted to be quite grandiose and hyperactive, and he immediately set about trying to convert other patients on the ward to his new religion. Otherwise he was oriented but had some recent memory loss, was very concrete in proverb interpretation, and had flight of ideas.

Clinical course: After 10 days and heavy Thorazine medication, he improved considerably. He was discharged to duty although he was still somewhat [sic] delusional.

Discharge diagnosis: Psychosis associated with marijuana use and personality disorder.

Disposition: He was released to the custody of his commanding officer, who kept him under strict surveillance in the unit orderly room to prevent him from using marijuana. After 2 weeks he was evaluated for administrative separation from the Army. At that time he was hostile and guarded, felt others were always picking on him, and related a long history of mistrust of others. He had no memory defect, and his proverb interpretation had markedly improved.

Source: Adapted with permission from Colbach EM, Crowe RR. Marihuana associated psychosis in Vietnam. *Mil Med.* 1970;135(7):572.

Clinical Effects of Other Drugs

Also in 1968, psychiatrists' reports were beginning to refer to clinical complications from soldier use of drugs other than marijuana. Colbach, with Scott M Wilson, a social work/psychology technician, described increasing barbiturate use, and in some cases, addiction, among American troops in the Qui Nhon area after November 1968. Typically, this involved the use of a French preparation, Binoctal, a combination of amobarbital (50 mg) and secobarbital (70 mg), which American troops could purchase from Vietnamese pharmacies. A study of 100 randomly selected nonpsychiatric admissions to the 67th Evacuation Hospital over a 3-month period revealed 7% of patients had used Binoctal, with two acknowledging use more than five times. Among 100 randomly selected psychiatric inpatients, 16% were admitted for Binoctal use, and 15% of randomly selected psychiatric outpatients acknowledged significant use. The authors described the typical user of Binoctal as having been raised in a chaotic home of low socioeconomic status, became an anxious person with a long antisocial history, and had severe authority conflicts. He had been a marginal soldier and used marijuana before discovering Binoctal. He reported using drugs in Vietnam as an escape from the stress of military life there, and, whereas he had no goals for the future, he had no wish to stop his drug use. The authors underscored the additional clinical requirements associated with assessing the extent of barbiturate addiction while treating the acute intoxication. In cases of substantiated addiction it was necessary to avoid an abrupt withdrawal crisis using a 10-day barbiturate-tapering program and oral pentobarbital.[60]

David V Forrest, an Army psychiatrist who closely followed Talbott and the others at the 935th Psychiatric Detachment, reported that he and his colleagues were seeing regular marijuana users "almost always" also using Binoctal; Obesitol, a liquid amphetamine preparation; intravenous (IV) methedrine; and opium- or heroin-dipped marijuana. He also reported that some soldiers had requested hospital-level support for withdrawing from opiates, but he did not provide further details regarding their clinical course.[61]

1969

Prevalence of Use of Marijuana and Other Drugs

MG Prugh:

> [t]here was continued rise in the drug use rate in 1969, with 8,440 apprehensions.[46(p107)]

In the fall of 1969, M Duncan Stanton, an Army psychologist with the 98th Psychiatric Detachment, surveyed soldiers of all ranks entering or departing Vietnam regarding drug use (N = 2,547). When compared with the Roffman and Sapol survey 2 years earlier, sizable increases were noted in the reported use of marijuana among those who were leaving Vietnam (28.9% vs 50.1% respectively). However, most of the increase was accounted for by a comparable increase reported by soldiers entering Vietnam. Among Stanton's outgoing group, 21.5% used marijuana for the first time in Vietnam, which was only slightly higher than the 19.4% found by Roffman and Sapol. However, Stanton did find a shift toward heavier use among his sample of departing EM (only 7.4% of the Roffman and Sapol study group were heavy or habitual users vs 29.6% in Stanton's). Otherwise, when comparing his entering and departing groups Stanton found no sizable increases in reported use of amphetamines, barbiturates, or heroin/morphine during the Vietnam tour; however, the incidence of opium use in the form of the "OJ"— marijuana dipped in opium—carried a threefold increase (6.3% to 17.4%). Reported use of drugs was negligible among the officer and noncommissioned officer groups. Stanton also found a slight positive relationship between frequency of marijuana use and amount of exposure to enemy fire. Finally, he opined that much of the drug use in Vietnam served as a substitute for the alcohol of past wars, and he speculated that marijuana and some other drugs could actually allow certain types of individuals to function under the stresses of a combat deployment.[62]

The 4th Infantry Division Pilot Drug Amnesty/ Rehabilitation Program

In the 4th ID, a drug "amnesty"/rehabilitation program was established in 1969. This was limited to soldiers who presented themselves as drug users to their commander, chaplain, or unit surgeon and who had not previously come to the attention of command for drug use. It provided rapid medical assessment, counseling including group therapy, and the assignment of a "buddy" to provide positive reinforcement in the soldier's effort to give up drugs. Otherwise, participants were expected to perform full military duties.[2] It is not clear, however, from the surviving information to what extent the division's psychiatric personnel were involved in the inception or operation of the 4th Infantry Division drug amnesty/rehabilitation program. Still, it was apparently successful enough that 2 years later it was adapted for Army-wide implementation as Army Regulation 600-32, *Drug Abuse Prevention and Control* (December 1970).[16]

Experience in the 1st Infantry Division

Bey's postwar account of his tour in Vietnam was quite illuminating regarding marijuana use in the 1st ID at the time. Bey noted that soldiers could buy a 6-pound bag full of very pure marijuana for $50, and a joint for $0.50. He estimated that 25% of soldiers in Vietnam used marijuana, including combat troops in the field who wished to reduce their anxiety. He described the 8 December 1969 publication of 1st ID Regulation 190-3, *On the Detection and Suppression of Marijuana and Illegal Drugs*, and he noted the Army's increased emphasis on apprehending and punishing drug users. Each division had a drug education team, but Bey recalled his satisfaction in being "kicked off" the team for his opposition to their "scare" approach to drug prevention. ("My assignment was to explain [to the troops] that drugs made you crazy."[11(p121)]) By his standards, "If a person used either [drugs or alcohol] in moderation and it didn't impair their functioning on the job, we [in mental hygiene] didn't see it as a problem."[11(p122)] (A perspective that was consistent with Stanton's.) He also noted that all but one of his social work/psychology techs used marijuana. "They functioned well in their jobs, and there was never a reason to bring the subject up. They knew that I drank booze with the officers."[11(p123)]

However, Bey was clear regarding his concerns about the soldiers for whom marijuana use was part of a pattern of maladaptation. "Our approach shifted from [scare tactics] to one . . . indicating that anyone using drugs or alcohol to excess . . . advertised his incontinence . . . [and] was probably having serious problems and needed help."[29(ChapVII,p18)] As examples, Bey and Zecchinelli, his social work/psychology technician, presented demographic and clinical data collected from 20 consecutive 1st ID soldiers treated for acute psychotic reactions associated with marijuana use. These reactions were successfully treated over 1 to 3 days using the *dauerschlaft* protocol described in Chapter 7, that is, 100 mg chlorpromazine taken hourly while awake to maintain sleep for 24 hours, with dosage being progressively decreased as the acute symptoms subsided. Subsequent examination revealed all the affected soldiers to have borderline personality features ("core problems of identity diffusion, ego weakness, low self-esteem, and inability to form close interpersonal relationships"[63(p450)]) and to be marginally adjusting to their Vietnam circumstance. In the authors' opinion, "[M]arijuana served directly and indirectly to assist patients [with predisposing personality defects] in achieving a costly homeostasis. . . ."[63(p450)] Besides the tranquilizing effects and the oral gratification attained through smoking the drug, they concluded that many appeared to also be using marijuana to reduce anxiety through developing a "head" group identity and membership in a clique whose affiliation centered on shared defense mechanisms of splitting and projection—that is, blaming the Army.[63]

Bey also mentioned that he learned at a drug and alcohol conference about the initial success of the 4th ID's drug amnesty/rehabilitation program for soldiers not currently under investigation and that this model was being adapted for use by most of the combat divisions in Vietnam. However, he indicated that following its implementation in the 1st ID, few soldiers volunteered for the program.[29]

Experience at the 67th Evacuation Hospital

Frank D Master, an Army psychiatrist, followed on the heels of Colbach at the 67th Evacuation Hospital and summarized his experience with the burgeoning drug problem during his year there. Of 58 psychotic patients treated by Master during his tour, 55 reported marijuana use, half of whom used it in conjunction with other drugs. In general, Master became convinced that "a very real organic brain syndrome regularly developed among chronic cannabis users (those who would smoke 5–10 marijuana cigarettes per day over a 3–6 month period)."[48(p195)] He also commented on the strong social pressure exerted by cannabis users on nonusers to join them. Barbiturate compounds, Binoctal, Iminoctal, and Ansional, which are central nervous system depressants, commonly accounted for addiction (two cases) or accidental overdose (20 cases). Equally available and popular were amphetamine mixtures, Obesitol and Maxitone Forte, which produced 80 cases of toxic psychoses. Master's approach for such cases was to advise the soldier's unit to provide 48-hour observation; then, if he failed to recover (as did 10 cases [12.5%]), he was hospitalized by Master and treated with up to 800 mg of Thorazine per day. Nonetheless, eight of the 10 maintained a schizophrenic-like course and required medical evacuation out of Vietnam. Narcotic use, typically in the form of smoking raw opium mixed with marijuana, was not a serious clinical problem at the time. However, Master noted that when he left Vietnam (October 1970), reports of heroin snorting were emerging.[48]

Experience at the 95th Evacuation Hospital/ 98th Psychiatric Detachment

As mentioned in Chapter 4 of this volume, Joel H Kaplan, the commanding officer of the 98th Psychiatric Detachment at that time, later reported his impressions from his tour in Vietnam that mostly centered on the growing drug abuse problem. Kaplan and his staff estimated that 50% to 80% of soldiers in Vietnam were using marijuana, at least as "experimenters." He also indicated that, during the year, 70% of 4,000 outpatients and 50% of roughly 500 inpatients they saw were drug abusers (defined as "using drugs heavily day in and day out"). Most of the drug use was marijuana, but soldiers commonly added barbiturates and opium (the latter was either smoked with marijuana or administered intravenously). Also popular with troops were amphetamines (Methadrine), lysergic acid diethylamide (LSD), glue, alcohol, and the dextropropoxyphene (a weak opioid) pellet out of the Darvon with aspirin capsule. Kaplan also noted that underlying personality disorders were typically found among the drug-abusing soldiers who required psychiatric care. Combat and noncombat troops were evenly represented, and the more extreme marijuana-associated reactions were not only shaped by personality defects but also by the social/environmental context. Whereas his case examples of combat soldiers suggested they were more prone to marijuana-associated violent episodes—"[the combat soldier may develop] paranoid feelings, become frightened and more angry and vengeful"[64(p264)]—amotivational syndromes were apparently more common among some marijuana-using support troops—"passive behavior, irresponsibility, lack of ambition, obstinacy, procrastination, irritability, poor concentration, and withdrawal from activities."[64(p264)] As for treatment efforts, the 98th Psychiatric Detachment's group therapy program (6 nights/week) became highly popular among soldier volunteers who attended because they were eager to "kick the habit" before rotating back to the United States. However, other than that, there were no easy answers to the growing "subculture of drugs" throughout Vietnam, according to Kaplan.[64]

In conclusion, by the transition years, (1968–1969), drug problems had begun to seriously erode military health and discipline in Vietnam. With respect to clinical challenges, psychiatrists in the field were not only able to measure increasing marijuana use prevalence and heavier use among their referrals, including combat troops, but the cases they described appeared to have more severe neuropsychiatric symptoms and required more prolonged recovery than earlier. There was also evidence of greater use of other illegal drugs, especially among support troops. The most clinically challenging cases involved barbiturate overdose or addiction and toxic psychoses secondary to heavy use of stimulants. Finally, reports from the field were starting to include evidence of troop disaffection as a motivating factor in increasing drug use. Nonetheless, despite evidence of mounting drug problems, in his summary of Army psychiatric experience in Vietnam up through 1969. Allerton, the senior psychiatrist in the Office of The Surgeon General, provided the following reassurance—similar to his assertion regarding low levels of alcoholism in Vietnam mentioned earlier:

> [T]here does not appear to be any significant statistical information which would lead one to believe that problems with marijuana, the opium alkaloids, or hallucinogens have any higher incidence among troops in Viet Nam than might be the case for the same age group in metropolitan centers in the [United States].[15(p10)]

THE DRAWDOWN PHASE (1970–1972): THE SHIFT TO HEROIN

1970

Waning Concern for Marijuana and Barbiturate Use

Through the first half of 1970, marijuana (or hashish) was still the most common drug used by soldiers in Vietnam, the sizable clinical challenges associated with its use continued unabated, and the Army still had not implemented a reliable system for monitoring soldier morbidity stemming from its use or that of other drugs.[2] The last drug-use survey in Vietnam that featured marijuana was conducted in the 173rd Airborne Brigade in early 1970 by JJ Treanor, a brigade surgeon, and JN Skripol, an Army social work officer. They surveyed all ranks (N = 1,064) and found that 31% acknowledged regular marijuana use, 37% admitted to an isolated incidence of experimentation, and 32% denied ever using an illegal drug. Of special note, 35% of soldiers with combat duty assignments reported regular use, and 48% of all subjects felt marijuana use should be allowed on fire support bases. There is no mention of heroin in

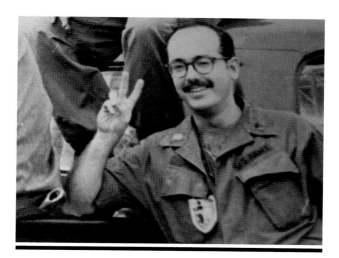

FIGURE 9-2. Major Richard A Ratner, Medical Corps, 935th Psychiatric Detachment. Ratner, a civilian-trained psychiatrist, served with the 935th between August 1970 and July 1971. Among his duties, he worked in the KO team's newly created "Crossroads" drug detoxification and rehabilitation program, which was attached to the 24th Evacuation Hospital on the Long Binh post. Ultimately, Ratner provided many unique and cogent observations regarding the heroin-dependent soldiers who were residents of the program. Photograph courtesy of Richard A Ratner.

their report, but opium users represented 6% of those surveyed. Increased marijuana use correlated positively with lower rank, age, military experience, and formal education level. It also correlated with higher incidents of civilian and military legal entanglements, low job satisfaction, and incidents suggestive of disaffection with the military such as absent without leave (AWOL) and insubordination. The authors concluded that marijuana users were primarily incapable, frustrated, and poorly educated soldiers with passive-aggressive personalities, that is, they were psychologically predisposed as opposed to expressing low morale and psychosocial anomie.[65]

From the psychiatric specialty detachments, Anthony Pietropinto, an Army psychiatrist who served with the 98th Psychiatric Detachment, estimated from the cross section of cases seen there that the incidence of marijuana use among the troops was "very high—nearly two-thirds have experimented with it and at least half are using it frequently."[66(p106)] A similar observation came from Ratner (Figure 9-2), with the 935th Psychiatric Detachment: "eighty percent or more of the men in Vietnam below the rank of E-5 use marijuana on a fairly regular basis."[30] However, in contrast to Treanor and Skripol, he believed that the high rates of drug

use, including alcohol, also represented a passive-resistant means for soldiers to survive their discontent and opposition to the oppressive embrace by military authority. He quoted one soldier: "When I'm turned on, I don't get excited; I might feel like belting the First Sergeant for something, but when I'm high, I just close my eyes, and it doesn't bother me."[30] Ratner commented that most unit commanders denied their unit's drug problems, and he quoted a battalion surgeon as saying, "Most commanders have accepted that, so long as personnel don't get caught using drugs, or mess up while on duty, they should let sleeping dogs lie."[30]

More broadly, Colonel Thomas B Hauschild, a senior Army psychiatrist, polled the 22 Army psychiatrists in Vietnam and found that all had treated cases of acute marijuana intoxication or acute brain syndrome secondary to marijuana use. He also reported that 70% of psychiatric evacuees from Vietnam to the US Army hospitals in Japan had histories of drug abuse, especially marijuana. For some, their toxic states rapidly cleared, and they were diagnosed as acute brain syndrome; others did not and were believed to have had psychotic reactions that were precipitated by the disorganizing effect of these drugs.[38] Also, to offset the growing numbers of medical professionals in the United States who were minimizing the risks of marijuana use, Hauschild reminded his audience that, besides being a euphoriant, it:

- is a powerful intoxicant;
- distorts time, space, body image, and thought processes;
- has psychotomimetic properties (ie, can imitate psychotic states);
- produces a drug dependence syndrome that is very habit-forming (if not as addicting as morphine derivatives);
- can produce lethargy, apathy, and debilitation in chronic users; and
- can precipitate mental illness in predisposed individuals.[38(p108)]

Finally, the winter of 1970 saw testimony before the US Senate Subcommittee to Investigate Juvenile Delinquency, Senate Judiciary Committee, by Kaplan, a former Army psychiatrist and commander of the 98th Psychiatric Detachment (November 1968–November 1969). Kaplan felt that the Army was failing to recognize the enormity of the drug abuse problem in Vietnam (at that time, primarily marijuana and barbiturates) and urged Congress to take action on their behalf.[67] Also testifying before the same subcommittee (August 1970) was Roffman, who presented findings from the aforementioned survey of lower-ranking enlisted soldiers departing Vietnam that he and Sapol conducted in 1967. His testimony included that: (1) in 1967 the enlisted soldier in Vietnam was no more likely to use marijuana, or to heavily use it, than his stateside peers; (2) the Army had sought to suppress his survey findings to avoid negative publicity; and (3) there was little evidence to substantiate that marijuana use in Vietnam accounted for combat atrocities as some had suggested.

The Heroin Epidemic and the Scramble for Containment and Countermeasures

By mid-1970, earlier concerns by command regarding soldier use of marijuana and other drugs were greatly eclipsed after it became apparent that heroin use by lower-ranking soldiers was spreading rapidly throughout South Vietnam. The tipping point between a manageable level of drug abuse and that which seriously jeopardized the health, morale and discipline, and combat readiness of the deployed forces corresponded to an upsurge in heroin trafficking by indigenous South Vietnamese.[68] Now, soldiers could easily acquire extremely pure (95%[69]) and extremely inexpensive heroin, and were becoming avid consumers. A carton of cigarettes costing $2.00 at the PX could be traded for a 250 mg vial of heroin that would have been worth hundreds of dollars in the United States. Because heroin was so cheap, pure, and accessible, soldiers in Vietnam used it recreationally, most commonly mixed with tobacco and smoked in ordinary-looking cigarettes. In fact, soldiers bragged that they could smoke it on duty without fear of being detected because it did not give off a characteristic odor like marijuana and did not typically cause conspicuous functional impairment.[70] Many soldiers preferred instead to snort heroin (insufflation), and a minority injected it intravenously.[69]

Some illustration of the growing problem came from Ratner's journal:

> We had a visit from a division battalion surgeon today, quite unexpectedly. His responsibility is an Aviation battalion (Phu Loi), just a few minutes from Long Binh Post by helicopter. He dropped by because he has begun to feel overwhelmed by the magnitude of the hard drug problem in his area. At

the moment, no less than 15 men were withdrawing from heroin overdoses. He reminded us that these men manned helicopters, and the dangers are obvious. Happily, no pilots seemed to be involved; the crew chiefs and door gunners were, however. The battalion surgeon confessed dolefully that, if he were to ground all the heroin users he knew about, not a single helicopter would get off its pad. It is, of course, impossible that the unit not complete its mission; therefore, the helicopters go up, and the unit "does not have a drug problem."[30]

Besides the rising rates for drug-related hospitalization and arrests for drug possession and distribution in late 1970, the first of many heroin overdose deaths also came to the attention of USARV Command. In August, the 483rd Air Force Hospital reported the first heroin overdose death of a soldier that was proven by autopsy. In fact, by October, the 483rd Air Force Hospital was receiving the largest number of Army personnel with drug problems among all medical facilities in the theater because of the very large concentration of Army support units in the Cam Ranh Bay area (see Bowen's End of Tour Report in Appendix 14).

Epidemiologic Measures

Two studies conducted by Army medical personnel sought to measure heroin use but produced widely divergent results. One survey administered by Cookson to 1,125 enlisted soldiers in 19 randomly selected companies yielded modest self-reported prevalence rates. Acknowledged drug use by respondents was as follows: (1) marijuana use by 30% (10.8% daily); (2) heroin use by 7% (2.3% daily), while 5% acknowledged infrequent opium use; (3) amphetamine use by 7%; and (4) barbiturate, hallucinogen, and sedative use combined was 4%.[71] Unfortunately, information as to the details of the Cookson's survey method and instrument or the types of units surveyed are not available.

A more alarming picture of the heroin problem in the field came from a survey conducted by Jerome Char, the division psychiatrist with the 101st Airborne Division. Char explored drug use patterns within his division utilizing three cohorts of lower-ranking enlisted soldiers: those departing after a year-long tour (n = 568), new arrivals (n = 111), and psychiatric outpatients (n = 467). Among those departing, 41% admitted use of some drug during their tours. Roughly one-third of the drug users (36%) acknowledged use of heroin or other "hard" drugs, whereas the remainder limited their drug use to marijuana. The departing soldiers' overall drug use rate was roughly twice that for the soldiers arriving from the United States (21%). A drug use history was acknowledged by 71% of the psychiatric patient group. Of the men using drugs in all three groups, 58% reported they began as civilians.[72]

The Overlapping Challenge for Military and Government Leaders, Law Enforcement, and Medical Personnel

MG Prugh:

. . . During 1970 there were 11,058 arrests of which 1,146 involved hard narcotics.

In August 1970 the Drug Abuse Task Force was formed to seek new solutions to the drug problem and make recommendations to General Westmoreland. The task force included representatives from most of the U.S. staff agencies, major subordinate commands of the MACV, the embassy, the U.S. Agency for International Development, customs, and the Bureau of Narcotics and Dangerous Drugs. The task force worked through September to complete a report, the conclusions of which were embodied in MACV Directive 190-4 of December 1970. The objectives of this directive were to eradicate the sources of drugs, to strengthen customs and postal procedures, to improve detection facilities, to co-ordinate the various drug abuse programs, to integrate law enforcement programs, to improve statistical reporting, and to rehabilitate drug abusers.

The campaign against drug abuse was waged on many fronts. Commanders incorporated drug abuse talks as part of the command information program; drug abuse councils were established in commands throughout Vietnam; chaplains, physicians, and judge advocate officers worked to impress on the troops the dangers of drug abuse; amnesty programs were established and detoxification/counseling centers were opened; law enforcement agencies intensified their efforts. . . .[46(p107)]

As indicated by MG Prugh, responding to the Army's burgeoning drug problem in Vietnam required integration of the activities of command (mission, performance, morale, discipline), medicine/psychiatry (health, fitness, prevention, detection, treatment), and law enforcement. However, cooperation between these elements was sometimes complicated due to differences in perspective. Before heroin entered the picture, marijuana use, because of its relatively benign effects and because it was an illegal substance, was mostly regarded as misconduct. Also, although some soldiers became heavy users and psychologically dependent, evidence suggested that their compulsion to use it coincided with a personality disorder. However, heroin use and the use of other drugs, especially barbiturates, were associated with a powerfully complicating factor in the form of their addictive potential—a physically driven compulsion/dependence that carried with it the threat of a medical crisis under circumstances of abrupt withdrawal. (Recent research has established a significant, but substantially lower addictive potential in the case of marijuana—more on a par with tobacco.[73]) In other words, heroin use as widespread misconduct was also heroin use as medical epidemic.

Because of heroin's well-established reputation for causing physical dependence—that is, addiction—military leaders and physicians assumed this would be the case for most soldier-users as well. However, establishing a system for case identification and monitored detoxification in a medically supportive environment proved to be quite difficult for the following reasons:

- In general, symptoms of narcotic withdrawal are quite suggestive. Confirmation of the presence and extent of withdrawal requires monitoring of objective signs or laboratory measures.[74,75]
- Medical facilities in Vietnam had no reliable laboratory means for ensuring drug abstinence in soldiers undergoing withdrawal until roughly 1 year after the epidemic began.
- Inpatient facilities could not be kept free of illegal drugs.[76]
- Soldiers in Vietnam defended their drug use as being justified by the circumstances (service in Vietnam), or as generally not problematic; thus, their motivation for abstinence was very low.
- Medical observers noted that the withdrawal syndromes for many soldiers could be mild and managed through dispensary-level care.
- Despite these features, soldiers claimed that the likelihood of unbearable withdrawal symptoms necessitated their continued use. And, if pressed, especially when they were threatened with prosecution for drug possession, they demanded

TABLE 9-1. US Military Deaths in Vietnam Attributed to Heroin

	1970	1971	1972
January		9	1
February		10	1
March		2	
April		3	
May		4	
June		1	
July		2	
August	8	3	
September	7	0	
October	9	0	
November	15	5	
December	10	2	

Source: DoD Information Guidance Series. *Drug Abuse In the Military—A Status Report (Part II)*. Office of Information for the Armed Forces; 1972, August (No 5A-18):1-3.

hospitalization (for both detoxification and isolation from drug suppliers).

- By this time soldiers were so antagonistic to military authority and opposed to serving in Vietnam that identified heroin users welcomed removal from military duties as a medical diversion; thus heroin use alone served as an "evacuation syndrome."[4(p70)]
- The incidence of heroin use became so high that if inpatient hospital-level service was provided for all users, that is, without identifying those in need of 24-hour monitoring and care, the hospitals could be overtaxed, which meant that the care of other patients could be compromised.

Colonel Clotilde D Bowen, Psychiatry Consultant to the Commanding General/USARV Surgeon at that time, reported that as early as September 1970, all combat divisions were setting aside six to 25 hospital beds for the treatment of heroin-using soldiers. As for the even more numerous nondivisional troops scattered across South Vietnam, between September and December, heroin abusers were being admitted to the psychiatric services of field and evacuation hospitals in rapidly increasing numbers. After December, the various amnesty/

rehabilitation programs took over the coordination of these inpatient functions. Also, after September, all Army psychiatric activities in Vietnam were to include in their monthly morbidity reports a list of drug-using soldiers by name, rank, unit, drugs used, and amount. (However, as late as June 1971, the system of patient classification and reporting, including for alcohol and drug hospitalizations, was still confused; see Bowen's End of Tour Report in Appendix 14 for further detail.)

Unfortunately, throughout this period there were problems in reaching consensus among the medical personnel in Vietnam as to operational definitions of problematic levels of use, psychological dependence, and addiction. As a result, some inpatient programs were more liberal in their admission policies, became swamped as a result, and in many respects found themselves mostly relegated to providing custodial services for antagonistic soldiers.[43] The following description by John Ives, an Army psychiatrist, most of which was written shortly after he returned to the United States, is illustrative:

I was loaned to the 483rd USAF [US Air Force] Hospital [in August 1970] at Cam Rahn Bay as the Air Force had complained to the Army about all the Army troops burdening their case load. . . . Some [of the patients] had even re-enlisted to come back to Vietnam as they hated garrison duty in the states . . . [then] were enraged to find that by September 1970, Vietnam involved garrison duty as well, with little or no "action.". . . For them (as for me) Vietnam was more prison than combat. . . . Heroin withdrawal at the 483rd was a factory operation. We accepted all who were sent to us "for the amnesty." The withdrawals didn't seem severe. We used only Valium. . . . We then sent them back where they came from, and there was little or no communication with their unit.[77]

Other programs sought to limit admission to soldiers requiring inpatient-level detoxification support. By way of example, the psychiatrists at the 98th Psychiatric Detachment in Da Nang utilized the narcotic antagonist N-allynormorphine [Nalline] to screen for physical dependency[78] (see Appendix 1, Camp's Report of Activities of the 98th Psychiatric Detachment). In their experience, among the many soldiers who claimed to be physically dependent to heroin, only roughly one in ten tested positive.[79]

To illustrate the resultant confusion, one Army psychiatrist recalled to this author [Camp] many years after the war,

One case I remember was a soldier withdrawing after having been in lock-up (the Army stockade). He was sweating and shaking. I did not admit him for gradual withdrawal as he wanted, but I gave him—I am embarrassed to say—Thorazine, I think. He was found dead of a heroin overdose the next day. This outcome haunts me today.[80]

Table 9-1 presents numbers of drug overdose deaths in Vietnam (proven by autopsy) for all services during the last 2 years of the war. Whereas this figure suggests rapidly declining levels after February 1971, this is misleading because the progressive reduction in troop strength is not taken into account. When the numbers for the last 5 months in 1970 (ie, the months following the emergence of the heroin market) are annualized, the rates for narcotic overdose deaths show only a modest decline, from 0.34 per 1,000 in 1970 to 0.30 per 1,000 in 1971. (Some of these figures in Table 9-1 are lower than those provided by Colonel Stewart L Baker Jr, a senior Army psychiatrist.[2] He indicated that in 1970, there were 75 confirmed or suspected incidents between August 1 and October 18, only 11 of which were confirmed by autopsy. He also said there were 14 before August 1970, and 11 in 1969 [all confirmed by autopsy]. However, it must be concluded that those before mid-1970 involved drugs other than heroin, such as barbiturates, because heroin was not being marketed. Recall from earlier that Bowen indicated that the first heroin overdose death of a soldier in Vietnam proven by autopsy was in August 1970.)

To some degree, overdose deaths were predicted. Froede and Stahl were impressed by the marked elevation of fatal drug overdose cases in the Vietnam in 1969 and 1970 (pre-heroin) and noted the parallel with the extraordinary increase in narcotic-related deaths between 1951 and 1953 within the US military, primarily among soldiers assigned in Korea. They projected that the high prevalence of narcotic use would continue among the troops serving in Vietnam through the end of the war.[41]

1971–1972

MG Prugh:

Despite the concerted efforts of the command, there was an alarming increase in the use of hard narcotics in 1971, when the number of offenders involved with hard drugs, mostly heroin, increased sevenfold, to 7,026. This trend was particularly disturbing in view of the continually decreasing troop strength in Vietnam.[46(p107)]

Challenges in Implementing the Army Drug Abuse Prevention and Control ("Amnesty") Program in Vietnam

According to MG Spurgeon Neel, the former MACV Surgeon, "Growing awareness of the nature and extent of the drug problem in Vietnam led to a search for a flexible, non-punitive response. . . ."[16(p48)] In response to the growing Army-wide drug problem, especially in Vietnam, in December 1970 the Department of the Army published AR 600-32, *Drug Abuse Prevention and Control*, to provide "limited rehabilitation for restorable drug abusers, when appropriate, and consistent with the sensitivity of the mission. . . ." As noted, the program outline presented in this regulation was an adaptation of an "amnesty"/rehabilitation program implemented in the 4th ID in 1968.[16,76] The regulation defined the Army drug use prevention strategy and procedures for processing drug abusers, including conditions that would allow a commander to grant a soldier a one-time-only exemption from legal jeopardy if he voluntarily requested medical and rehabilitative help (but not for other acts associated with drug abuse).

The creation of this uncharacteristically lenient program by the Department of the Army meant that it believed it was up against a serious and urgent problem within its ranks. As previously noted, at the time the Army went to war in Vietnam, the management of soldiers using illegal drugs or misusing alcohol was straightforward—their behavior was treated as misconduct, which resulted in judicial and administrative consequences, often including discharge from the service. Associated medical conditions received in-service medical treatment, but the condition retained the final designation of "Line of duty, no, due to own misconduct," and the Army held the soldier financially responsible for costs of treatment and nonduty time.

The new regulation, AR 600-32, resembled policies stemming from the challenge of venereal disease in earlier conflicts. The Army had learned that associated medical and morale issues could not be mitigated as long as detection carried with it the consequence of punishment. However, in the case of drug abuse, a critical miscalculation may have followed the fact that, whereas soldiers are most usually eager to be treated for venereal diseases, this same attitude was not the case for soldiers using illegal drugs in Vietnam.

Although AR 600-32 addressed command responsibilities in situations where a soldier voluntarily asked for amnesty and rehabilitation, and it listed the agencies (eg, local medical personnel, chaplains, and legal officers) that were to support the commander in rehabilitating the soldier, there was no specific program defined by this regulation. On 29 December 1970, USARV Headquarters distributed the "Drug Rehabilitation/Amnesty Program" (nicknamed "the amnesty program") as a Vietnam theater adaptation of Army Regulation 600-32. It outlined procedures and conditions regarding "amnesty" as well as stipulated the elements that were to comprise a unit's rehabilitation program:

1. Direct the drug-using soldier to the nearest medical facility for any acute care that medical personnel determined was necessary.
2. Upon return to his unit, command was to assess the soldier's potential for successful return to previous duties and responsibilities and inform the soldier's supervisor of his ". . . key role in the rehabilitation of the soldier."
3. Pair him up with a (nonusing) "buddy"—a peer who could "act as a positive influence, and . . . provide counseling and supportive assistance in the soldier's endeavors to remain free of drugs."
4. "Establish a group therapy program wherein the rehabilitee may receive support from ex-drug abusers; associate with others who are attempting to stop using drugs; and receive professional counseling from the unit surgeon, chaplain or qualified visiting professionals."
5. Destroy all records of the soldier's participation in these programs (ie, amnesty and rehabilitation) when the soldier departed the unit.

However, the program was easier to describe than to implement. Firstly, once the drug-using soldier was identified and apart from ensuring that there were no other Uniform Code of Military Justice (UCMJ) charges pending against him and that he was medically cleared, the commander had to decide whether the soldier was genuinely motivated to discontinue drug use and whether he qualified as a one-time-only volunteer. This clearly represented a challenge because item #5 above meant that the commander had no way to know if this soldier

had already been a participant in another unit's program. But more generally, as will be described, the whole program rested on the Army's capacity to objectively verify abstinence or monitor withdrawal among participants, which was impossible because of the lack of available laboratory screening procedures.

Nonetheless, to comply with the USARV amnesty program, major Army commands hastily improvised treatment/rehabilitation programs and facilities utilizing whatever resources they had at hand. This produced diverse approaches because command attitudes ranged widely with regard to commitment and material support. The result was a collection of unstandardized, semibootleg treatment/rehabilitation programs with colorful, nonmilitary names—Sky House, Highland House, Operation Guts, Head Quarters, Pioneer House, Crossroads, Operation Rebuild, Golden Gate, Freedom House, Reality House, Three-Quarter-Way House, and Black Amnesty.[81] They were typically staffed with individuals with little or no experience in treating substance abuse and counselors who claimed to be former addicts.

Ratner, with the 935th Psychiatric Detachment/Crossroads program illustrated some of the attendant difficulties in establishing such a treatment/rehabilitation program in a 3 January 1971 post in his journal:

> Drug use has become the star of the psychiatric show here in Vietnam. In anticipation of a visit by some Congressman, the 68th Medical Group commander has ordered the 935th [Psychiatric Detachment] to create a drug amnesty [detoxification] and treatment center in nine days, separate from our already existing psychiatric facilities and services. The Colonel emphasized that he did not want it to look like an "opium den" with "psychedelic posters" as decorations. The program calls for a ten-day hospitalization in two wards of the 24th Evacuation Hospital. These facilities previously served as prisoner of war confinement wards, have barbed wire all around, and create a general atmosphere of incarceration. But more ironic, the three men picked from among our enlisted specialist staff to run the program include a regular heroin smoker and another who possesses the largest [drug] habit in the entire barracks. I can see using reformed users in a program like this, but I am dubious about continuing users. More generally, I have gradually become aware of a

rather high degree of drug use among the personnel of the 935th. It seems as if nearly everyone uses "grass" in the unit—the frequency differing with the person, from less than once weekly to more than once daily. But what shocked me was the use of "smack" (heroin) by our young enlisted corpsmen [and Ratner lists the initials of six of them]. These men could in no way be construed as the dropouts of society—in fact, they are often brighter, though I think more troubled, than most EM.[30]

By June 1971, apparently because of these kinds of problems, the Crossroads program was removed from medical authority of the 935th Psychiatric Detachment/24th Evacuation Hospital and transferred to the post commander, and the staff was replaced with nonmedical personnel from other Long Binh Post activities [see Appendix 14, "Bowen's End of Tour Report" and Appendix 18, "The Baker/Holloway Report"].

Public Alarm and Increased Scrutiny

As word of the soldier heroin epidemic reached the United States, the American public became alarmed and further insistent that the troops be brought home immediately. The first of many congressional hearings regarding rising drug abuse in the military had begun with the aforementioned subcommittee hearings by the Senate Judiciary Committee to Investigate Juvenile Delinquency. This was followed by hearings before the Special Subcommittee to Investigate Alleged Drug Abuse in the Armed Services, House Committee on Armed Services.[76] In April 1971, a congressional visit to Vietnam reported an estimated 30,000 to 40,000 troops—10% to 15% of deployed soldiers—were addicted to various drugs, especially heroin, and proposed that high among possible causative factors, along with boredom, group pressure, and experimentation, was the soldier's dilemma of being sent to risk death or injury when the government has elected not to seek to win.[82]

An inspection visit was also made in March 1971 by Colonel Stewart L Baker Jr, the Neuropsychiatry Consultant to the Army Surgeon General. Especially notable, in his official report Baker catalogued the wide diversity of medical approaches to the detoxification of soldiers suspected of being physically dependent on heroin:

- at the 18th Surgical Hospital in the Quang Tri area, they prescribed Valium and Donnatal to support withdrawal as outpatients;
- at the Drug Center of Camp Eagle, Headquarters for the 101st Airborne Division, morphine was used for withdrawal symptoms;
- at the 67th Evacuation Hospital in Qui Nhon, they employed methadone; and
- at the Pioneer House (II Field Force headquarters) they advocated a "cold turkey" approach, but 25% of participants required medical support at the hospital, which utilized thorazine, probanthine, and valium.

Appendix 18, "The Baker/Holloway Report," has a fuller account of Baker's findings.

Two months after Baker's visit, a team from the Army's Medical Research and Development Command led by Colonel Harry C Holloway, a research psychiatrist, toured throughout Southeast Asia, including visits to 30 drug rehabilitation facilities in Vietnam (May–June 1971). Holloway's official report verified the pervasive nature of the problem of soldier use of serious drugs, especially heroin, including within combat units. It also documented the unsystematic nature of the Army's efforts at identification, detoxification, and rehabilitation and the very limited success these programs achieved in keeping enrollees from returning to heroin use.[83] From interviews and surveys of over 1,000 servicemen, Holloway constructed a profile of the typical Army heroin user in Vietnam: 18- to 23-years old, low ranking, and employed in a less-skilled job; might not have completed high school; probably used marijuana, alcohol, or other drugs prior to heroin and preferred smoking or snorting to injection (10:1) in Vietnam.[69] Holloway and his associates concluded that "[t]he heroin abuser is not distinguishable from the average soldier in any practically helpful way."[84(p7)] (See Appendix 18, "Excerpts From the Baker/Holloway Report," for a fuller account of Holloway's findings.)

Reports From the Field by Psychiatrists and Other Medical Personnel

Some accounts from the medically sponsored Army detoxification/rehabilitation programs in Vietnam have survived and testify to the enormous challenges faced by the Army and the deployed medical resources. Regrettably, none included case examples (see Case Prologue-3, PVT Charlie).

From the heroin user's point of view, the following disguised material is from an interview that took place in summer 1971 of a soldier (truck driver) who was recovering at the 67th Evacuation Hospital from wounds sustained when his truck was hit by enemy fire:

For a while, when I first got [to Vietnam], I didn't use any [heroin]. Then, in October and November there was a period when I snorted quite a bit and got strung out. Then, I think about the 10th of December, a couple of friends and I said, "Well, we're going to quit." About the 17th, I got a little Christmas spirit. My aunt sent me a bunch of presents, you know, and I thought, "Wow, what am I doing on dope?" So I quit until around the middle of January. I got off by myself. It was kind of tough the first couple of days, you know? And the only kind of drugs I used to come off was grass now and then. I'd smoke a little grass to help me sleep a little better, you know? You just kind of drift off. And after I got off of it I really felt good. I got my health back again. I wasn't losing weight. And I just felt freer, healthier. And then . . . I don't know what made me go back. I never snorted it again, but I started smoking it. And I even stayed on until I got hit. I don't think I even had anything that morning. I might have . . . I think I did smoke skag [heroin]. But, No, I drove on the road before and I remember I used to take a lot of dope, and I could handle the truck very good because I was used to it, I guess. When I was in the hospital, the doctor asked me what kind of narcotics I was on because I was going through withdrawal, you know? I had cold sweats and cold chills, so I told them I was on heroin. So they gave me some pills and stuff. I didn't wake up until, like about a day and a half. But that's why I'm glad they're sending me home, because I'll never have the temptation to go back to that again, you know? I think I've learned my lesson. Christ, I could go outside the hospital right now and get some, but I just don't want to mess with it no more, you know?[85]

From the psychiatric point of view, Ratner provided the following impressions after he and his colleagues treated over 1,000 drug-dependent soldiers voluntarily admitted to the 935th Psychiatric Detachment/Crossroads program between January and June of 1971:

[The prototypical soldier/patient is a SP4] who has gotten strung out on heroin. The olive drab uniform . . . hangs listlessly [on] a weak, cachectic, sallow and sickly looking young man whose adolescent acne stands in dreary relief to his pasty coloration and sunken cheeks. He has lost thirty pounds; he is unkempt and dirty."[43(p15)]

. . . [However], the withdrawal syndrome, known as "Jonesing" to the troops, was far milder than I had expected when undergone in our Amnesty Center. The "hard" symptoms of cramps, muscle pains, restlessness, vomiting, diarrhea, sweating with running nose and tearing, nausea, and somewhat paranoid ideation almost never took more than five days to clear up. We attributed this to the psychological climate of the center, in which perhaps twenty-five men were simultaneously withdrawing under the supervision of a trained and experienced staff. For one thing, most men were reluctant to suggest that they were less able to withstand pain than their neighbors. . . . But even more important was that nearly everyone was strongly motivated to get off drugs, since a majority of our patients had three months or less to go before returning home.[43(p15)]

However, as described in Chapter 2, Ratner was frank about their program's general lack of success and the resultant professional discouragement he and his psychiatric colleagues there shared. He also speculated that alienation from the military and its mission in Vietnam was chief among the psychosocial variables responsible for heroin use ("a drug traditionally so reviled and feared") and underscored the ubiquitous despair he encountered among program participants.[43(p15)]

Somewhat in contrast is the perspective of Army psychiatrist Ives, over at the 483rd US Air Force Hospital at Cam Rahn Bay. As noted earlier, he seemed cynical as well (withdrawal at the 483rd was a "factory operation"), but he favored predisposition as the primary etiologic factor:

. . . I was struck by the fact that they all seemed to be virtually the same person. I rarely saw a combat soldier or a draftee. Their backgrounds almost invariably included divorce or separation, poor relationships between the addict and his parents, and use of alcohol or tranquilizers by the parents. The addict himself would almost invariably have dropped out of high school, mostly for disciplinary rather than academic problems, and he often had difficulty finding and holding a job. He usually enlisted in order to get away from home or avoid a jail sentence. The addict rarely took any drugs in the states, with the exception of moderate use of alcohol and slight use of marijuana. . . . [In short] he was a disaster that was waiting to happen.[77]

At their program with the 1st Cavalry Division (Airmobile), Frank Ramos, the Army-trained psychiatrist, and David J Kruzich, the division social work officer, favored an etiological mix that combined elements of both perspectives. They initiated a heroin detoxification program in November 1970 within their division using a 20- to 30-bed inpatient service and biweekly group therapy for outpatients. Over five months they hospitalized 236 soldiers under the amnesty program, 40% of whom were listed as combat soldiers. The median age was 20, the median education level was 12 years, and the mean time in Vietnam before hospitalization was 9 months. Besides their drug use histories (72% of participants reported use of illegal drugs prior to joining the Army, but only 14% had used opiates), review of their civilian and military records did not suggest significant delinquent behavior. The combination of availability of drugs, peer group pressure, boredom, frustration, and "unmet dependency needs" best explained the high heroin use rates in Vietnam. ("[T]heir personalities and socioeconomic backgrounds were not greatly dissimilar to those of the average high school graduate."[86(p2)]) Ramos and Kruzich were only able to confirm outcomes for a third of those who completed the program; and, of those, the ratio of success to failures was two to three.

In a separate document, Kruzich estimated that, among the troops of the 1st Cavalry Division, 25% used heroin and over half of those were addicted, and that detoxification only succeeded for soldiers within a week of their DEROS (date expected return overseas). He also noted that, because the heroin sold was of such purity that it could be smoked, it allowed soldiers to avoid the more objectionable injection route, which in turn fostered wider use. In addition, it was a common misconception among soldiers that they were using cocaine, which allowed them to rationalize that what they were smoking was not as addictive.[87]

Further information regarding heroin-using soldiers and treatment approaches came from Samuel J Lloyd and Ralph C Frates, both Army battalion surgeons, with SP4 Douglas C Domer, who summarized their treatment of 81 consecutive heroin soldier-patients at a brigade clearing station with the 101st Airborne Division in Vietnam. These soldiers were program volunteers, and all were of lower enlisted ranks. For 23%, it was not their first attempt at withdrawal under medical supervision. Demographic comparisons with an equal number of controls revealed that the heroin users included a higher proportion of first-enlistment Regular Army soldiers who more often came from disrupted homes. The average daily consumption of heroin was six to eight vials (about 600 mg–800 mg of 97% pure heroin). The majority either smoked or snorted the drug. In the authors' opinion, most of the patients appeared to have begun using heroin as a transitory reaction to the distorted environmental and peer pressure in Vietnam. Physical withdrawal symptoms were typically managed using low doses of Thorazine combined with Librium. Detoxification success was qualified (67%) and was strongly correlated with the soldier's intent to pass DEROS drug screening test.[88]

An interesting contrast came from Brian S Joseph, an Army flight surgeon and partially trained psychiatrist, who described his voluntary 3-week program for heroin users at an Army airfield in the Mekong River Delta. The program could accept 11 residents per week, and its staff included a psychiatric social worker and a chaplain. The program design was that of a "therapeutic community," which began with a 5-day detoxification process. After 6 months of operation, Joseph and his staff concluded that the program was a failure because participants acquired heroin surreptitiously despite being housed in a closed ward. They also surmised that the program failures were soldiers with character disorders who entered the program to evade disciplinary action, and that the more stable users apparently were able to continue to function and escape detection. In Joseph's opinion, heroin use in Vietnam was primarily a social problem rather than one of individual psychopathology.[89]

Also pertinent is the report by Golosow and Childs, two Army psychiatrists assigned in Hawaii. They provided findings from their treatment of 36 soldiers from Vietnam who developed withdrawal symptoms from heroin while temporarily in Hawaii (September 1970–June 1971). Twenty-seven of their subjects were on R & R (rest and recuperation) leave from

Vietnam, and nine were in transit after completing their tour there. Thirty-one subjects manifested abstinence syndromes in three levels: "mild" (nine) included mild myalgias, restlessness, chills, diaphoresis, rhinorrhea, lacrimation, anorexia, and mild insomnia; "moderate" (eight) included moderate distress, severe agitation, insomnia, and severe myalgias; and "severe" (14) included severe distress in addition to the above, cramps, nausea, vomiting, and diarrhea. These were treated with methadone or drugs such as Valium and chloral hydrate. Seventeen of the 36, roughly half, had received treatment and rehabilitation in Vietnam under the amnesty program, and all but one were rehabilitation failures.

Collectively, their subjects resembled lower socio-economic civilian addicts in having histories of broken homes, disturbed family relationships, academic failures, and juvenile delinquency; however, they were also different in their majority-group membership, middle-class origins, presence of paternal figures in the family, and absence of criminal activity. Psychological testing did not reveal a unifying diagnostic pattern, but all received a psychiatric diagnosis in addition to one identifying their substance abuse status; 31 were personality disorders and five were psychotic or neurotic. Nonetheless, the authors concluded that, although these soldiers demonstrated increased premorbid susceptibility, conditions peculiar to Vietnam were necessary for addiction to develop in most (eg, increased drug availability, environmental stressors, peer group pressures).[90]

Initiation of Urine Screening for Drugs

Some realistic containment of the drug epidemic in Vietnam became possible in June 1971, when urine-testing technology was standardized and employed to screen the soldiers who were scheduled to DEROS from Long Binh, Cam Ranh Bay, and Da Nang. Refinement of the existing clinical technology for use as a drug-screening tool was the result of an urgent and ambitious effort by DoD. Once implemented in Vietnam, the military finally had a biochemical means for identifying drug users (opiates, barbiturates, and amphetamines) and could begin to assess the prevalence, at least among those departing Vietnam and unable to free themselves of these drugs, and to monitor detoxification in controlled centers.[91]

As of 21 September 1971, 92,096 soldiers had been tested before leaving Vietnam, and 4,788 (5.2%) positives were detained for detoxification and rehabilitation.[92(p859)] (Also of note, positive urine testing results were lower for officers, women, and members of the Navy and Air Force than for Army enlisted men.) However, these numbers invariably and substantially underrepresented actual use prevalence in Vietnam because, as has already been made clear, soldiers who were preparing to leave were extremely motivated to discontinue their heroin use on their own in order not to delay their departure. It also suggested that the level of addiction was not as high as presumed by military medical authorities.[93] Five months following the establishment of a DEROS urine-screening program, the technology was extended for unannounced screening of units operating throughout South Vietnam (November 1971). Once employed, the rate found for "dirty urines" was also roughly 5%, however the variability between units ranged from 1% to 20%.[94]

MG Prugh:

On 18 June 1971 the Secretary of Defense sent a message to the US services informing them of the presidential directive that the drug problem be given urgent and immediate attention and announcing a program to identify military personnel leaving Vietnam who were on narcotics and to give them the opportunity for drug treatment at facilities in the United States. . . .

As the drug problem intensified . . . , the legal emphasis for dealing with drug offenders gradually shifted from prosecution to administrative action.

It became increasingly clear that trial by court-martial was an awkward, ineffective, and expensive means of attempting to cope with a large-scale problem. Moreover, the public attitude toward individual drug users, particularly young soldiers, was changing; the public began to see these men not as criminals deserving punishment, but as suffering individuals requiring treatment. This attitude was reflected by the government and the armed services. . . . Soldiers whose behavior indicated that they lacked the desire or ability to rehabilitate themselves were eliminated through administrative channels. Soldiers who had unresolved court-martial charges pending against them for drug offenses and who did not wish to remain in the service often were allowed to resign for the good of the service rather than face trial by court-martial, unless the facts pertaining to the charges indicated they were active, commercial pushers of drugs, in which case trial was sought.[46(pp107–108)]

The Investigative Visit by Psychiatrist
Norman E Zinberg

In August and September 1971, Zinberg, a
civilian psychiatrist and addiction specialist, toured
Vietnam at the request of the Department of Defense
to study heroin use patterns and efforts toward the
rehabilitation of users, which resulted in two published
reports.[74,95] Zinberg's principal observation was that
heroin use there was unusual in being a widespread,
social group phenomenon among otherwise healthy
young soldiers who self-administered extremely
inexpensive and available heroin. In general their
behavior was motivated by efforts to get relief from the
stresses of low morale; mistrust of military authority;
insignificant jobs; jail-like restriction to military bases;
and the perception that Americans at home had
discredited those serving in Vietnam. Furthermore,
soldiers considered the military's heroin education
programs neither credible nor effective.

According to Zinberg, heroin users in Vietnam
belonged to three groups: (1) an urban type with a
criminal record; (2) a middle-class individual with
a record of trouble in school; and (3) a small-town
dweller in good physical condition and representing
all ethnic groups. The 16 Army rehabilitation and
treatment programs he visited were of three types: (1)
psychologically oriented programs outside of either
medical or penal authority, managed by former addicts
and minimizing the physical symptoms of withdrawal;
(2) medically oriented programs with reversed priorities;
and (3) involuntary programs emphasizing detoxification
enforced through urine testing.

Still, despite differences in orientation, the results
of these programs were uniformly poor (estimated
at fewer than 10%). Success was mostly limited to
soldiers nearing their DEROS who could sustain the
motivation to discontinue heroin use. Zinberg believed
the unsatisfactory outcomes ("counterproductive")
from these efforts were fostered by three common
programmatic errors:

1. Case selection: There was a failure to separate
   out those with characterologically based drug
   dependence for specialized medical/psychiatric
   attention, from the larger segment of socially [drug]
   habituated soldiers ("Their fury at the Army is
   boundless, and the group reinforcement of this
   bitterness is virtually palpable"), who needed other

rehabilitative or administrative steps.[74(p290)] Zinberg
also noted that, whereas occasional and moderate
users often recovered, heavy, committed users did
not benefit from these programs.

2. Treatment design: Zinberg questioned the
   emphasis on group treatment and indicated that
   this approach had been shown among civilian
   addicts to foster persistence of low motivation and
   strong countermores. More specifically, he was
   puzzled by these programs' "lack of discussion of
   the personal reasons a man uses heroin" (eg, the
   typical line of soldier discussion was impersonal:
   revolt against Army authority and the conditions
   in Vietnam).[74(p282)] In civilian substance abuse
   programs, it is unacceptable to blame one's use on
   outside authority or the social setting.

3. Case disposition: According to Zinberg the post-
   treatment planning for soldier participants was
   especially problematic:

   [T]he soldier returns to his unit immediately
   after detoxification or after a few days in a different
   ward or halfway-house arrangement. His unit
   contains the very group structure that may have
   been a crucial factor in his initial drug use. One
   might imagine that, with the enormous importance
   of peer groups in Vietnam, the pull to rejoin
   one's friends would be very great. The alternative
   of sending him to another unit seems equally
   inadequate.[74(p290)]

Inception of the Drug Confinement Facilities

In August 1971, the Army opened a new, more
restrictive, holding facility on the Long Binh post
near Saigon for acute treatment (detoxification) and
rehabilitation of soldiers who showed positive urine-
testing results. It was officially known as the Drug
Treatment Facility, Long Binh, and participation was
mandatory. The facility had a capacity of up to 150
patients/confinees within 10 wards, two of which
were set up to provide intensive care. Admissions
were searched for drugs and issued hospital pajamas
and slippers to be worn exclusively during their stay
(averaging 5 days). Their baggage was also searched
and secured. They were physically evaluated upon entry
and continually observed by medical officers and other
healthcare staff until they were released either into the
custody of the medical evacuation system (most) or back
to their units if they were not due for reassignment back
to the United States.[96] However, the latter disposition

was extremely unpopular for confinees. The following is Zinberg's description of this facility:

> The nonvoluntary treatment program I visited is a division of a base hospital, but a security fence and locked gates sharply separate it from the rest of the installation. The population varies from about 180 to 250, all housed in barracks. A career Army physician is in charge, with a staff whose size varies according to patient load: there are always at least 2 physicians, 15 to 25 nurses, and 25 to 40 technicians. There is also a detachment of security police for periodic drug and weapons searches. The mood of this installation is ugly. Most of the patients have been picked up by the [urine screening] and are held until they can pass it. Detoxification and a final negative result for urine tests are the grim goals of every man. Average patient stay is 4.2 days. Appetites return on the second day, and patients are so ravenous that snack carts must be protected by technicians. Small doses of methadone hydrochloride (20 to 40 mg) are given on the first and second nights to relax the patients, according to the medical officer in charge, and to make withdrawal a less trying procedure for them and the staff.[95(p488)]

According to Shelby Stanton, a military historian, the military police were soon stretched thin by guarding this and a similar facility established at the 6th Convalescent Center—the Drug Treatment Center at Cam Ranh Bay. The following is his description of the heightened security requirements for the Cam Ranh Bay facility:

> By mid-August the 97th Military Police Battalion had to be reinforced, and finally, the separate 127th Military Police Company was permanently assigned. It was charged with protecting the lives of volunteer patients and medical staff, preventing the entry of drugs and other contraband, stopping unlawful exits prior to detoxification, and maintaining order at the center. Static guard posts had to be manned along all fence lines, and police armaments at gate entrances were increased to shotguns and submachine guns. The company guarded messing areas, occupied patient wards at night, and built a separation ward with one and two-man cells.[97(p358)]

The Final Shift to a Law Enforcement/Custodial Approach

By September 1971, watershed legislation had been passed in Washington, directing the Secretary of Defense "to identify, treat and rehabilitate members of the Armed Forces who are drug or alcohol dependent." Public Law 92-129 required the military to participate in full compliance with the earlier noted Comprehensive Alcohol Abuse and Alcoholism Prevention, Treatment, and Rehabilitation Act of 1970. As a result, detection efforts were no longer aimed at identifying soldiers for the purposes of treatment and rehabilitation within Vietnam; their objective was to keep from sending serviceman home addicted to drugs. The failure of the Army's efforts at treatment and rehabilitation of heroin users in Vietnam was acknowledged, and the US military adopted a law enforcement–custodial approach.

All soldiers found to have morphine breakdown products in their urine were quarantined in one of three detoxification centers (Cam Ranh Bay, Long Binh, and Da Nang) and, when medically cleared, returned to the United States as medevac patients and distributed among 34 Army hospitals for further evaluation and treatment.[81] As a consequence, rates for heroin arrests, hospitalizations, and positive urines dropped rapidly in Vietnam until all combat troops were pulled out in mid-1972 (in May 1972, DEROS screening yielded 1.5% positives). Allowing drug-using soldiers to utilize the medical evacuation system represented an unprecedented relaxation of US Army Medical Department criteria—a modification that was limited to the Vietnam theater. As a side effect, however, the profile of psychiatric evacuation rates during the drawdown phase of the war became materially confounded.[19,98]

In June 1972, Department of the Army (DA) Circular (Cir) 600-85 was published stipulating the Army's Alcohol and Drug Abuse Prevention and Control Program (ADAPCP), which sought to balance humanitarian considerations and mission requirements with respect to drug and alcohol problems.[5] But again, by then the implementation of these changes was meaningless in Vietnam as the drawdown was nearing completion.

To conclude, the drawdown years saw rampant heroin use by first-term enlisted soldiers, including those within combat units, which was associated with addiction in about one in ten users. As a result, in addition to humanitarian costs, the Army faced a significant threat to combat readiness. Furthermore, concerns for marijuana use, or even alcohol abuse, were completely overshadowed. In response command and the medical/psychiatric component hastily expanded treatment facilities, devised a program offering limited amnesty to drug users who expressed a willingness to abstain, and mounted an urgent effort to develop laboratory technology for drug use detection and to support treatment and rehabilitation programs in the theater for the thousands of affected soldiers. However, results were spotty and mostly failed to curb this serious and unprecedented epidemic of self-inflicted soldier disability. Ultimately, public alarm and congressional pressure forced the medical evacuation of many of these soldiers from the theater. In the end, the Army psychiatrist who was the most knowledgeable about the subject, Holloway, could only offer this consolation: "[Despite their failure, these programs] were at least a source of hope to heroin users seeking help and commanders concerned about the welfare of their troops. The effort, creativity, and enthusiasm of the treatment program personnel must be admired."[69(p109)]

COLLATERAL DATA

Other Service Branches in Vietnam

Parallel experiences with identification and treatment/rehabilitation of heroin users by the other armed services in Vietnam, as well as those of Army units serving in Thailand, suggest insights into use patterns among Army troops in Vietnam.

US Marine Corps

As mentioned in Chapter 2, during the drawdown in Vietnam the Marines had their own problems with drug abuse, including heroin. Nonetheless, of the four military services in Vietnam, the US Marine Corps is the only one not to adopt some form of limited amnesty for personnel who could be rehabilitated. Their heroin use prevalence was estimated at 10%, and most identified users were subjected to legal or administrative discharge procedures.[83] Anecdotally, the experience in 1971 by Fisher, a Navy psychiatrist with the 1st Marine Division near Da Nang, is quite remarkable. Although his report did not center primarily on drug abuse, of the 1,000 consecutive Marine referrals he saw, 960 were diagnosed as personality disorders, and more than half (590) were "presumed to be involved with illegal drugs."[31(p1166)]

US Navy

Kolb, Nail, and Gunderson compared demographics of heroin inhalers (those who smoked or snorted heroin) versus injectors among 121 men serving in the Navy on shore in Vietnam. Although inhalers believed that by not injecting they would not become addicted, about two-thirds did become addicted. Inhalers did not differ significantly on demographic characteristics from other nonheroin drug users in Vietnam or from a Navy control sample serving aboard Navy ships off the coast. However, injectors demonstrated lower socioeconomic status (based on father's educational level), decreased family stability, and greater reported tension between the service member and his family, especially as a result of harsh paternal discipline.[99]

US Air Force

Descriptions of two US Air Force heroin rehabilitation programs in Vietnam paint a more favorable picture than do those of the aforementioned Army programs. Johnson and O'Rourke, both physicians in the US Air Force, reported a 73% success rate for their program on the US air base at Phan Rang, South Vietnam, in 1971. The program rested on the US Air Force Limited Privilege Communication (LPC) policy, which was similar to the Army's amnesty program but not as lenient. They described a three-pronged approach—that is, (1) prevention, (2) isolation from the source, and (3) rehabilitation of the heroin user. Treatment and rehabilitation procedures utilized weekly urine testing, psychological testing, and individual and group therapy.

Program candidates were classified as drug addicts ("those with deeper psychological problems") or situational drug abusers ("victims of drug abuse"). The addict group generally had pre-Vietnam histories of heroin involvement, and it was concluded that it was impossible to deal with them within the scope of the program. Apparently, they were administratively separated from the Air Force. Situational drug abusers were relatively open to therapy and, in general, were successfully rehabilitated. Most participants were assigned to the rehabilitation barracks ward, but a small number required initial hospitalization for withdrawal. In general, physical withdrawal lasted 3 to 5 days and left the individual in a weakened state for approximately 2 weeks. After acute withdrawal symptoms abated, participants returned to their jobs but were required to live in the rehabilitation barracks for at least 6 weeks and participate in 10 to 12 hours of group and individual therapy per week.

Johnson and O'Rourke felt that the (relative) success of this program was the consequence of urine-test monitoring, the active involvement of each individual's commander and supervisors, and the US Air Force's high enlistment selection criteria.[39] It also likely benefited from the exclusion of the "drug addict" group.

Similarly successful (relatively) was the US Air Force Drug Abuse Rehabilitation Therapy (DART) program at the Da Nang Airfield in 1971. Dehart and Sorrentino, both US Air Force physicians, noted that the explosion of heroin use by Air Force personnel in the fall of 1970 was similar to that reported by the Army, and they described their experience with detoxification of nearly 100 users stationed there. Like at Phan Rang, several individuals with long-term drug abuse histories were not included in the program but instead were returned to the United States. Dehart and Sorrentino's program was more inpatient-focused than that described by Johnson and O'Rourke, but it included a base-wide program, which was coordinated by a multidisciplinary staff council and had the full support of the base commander. Also like the program at Phan Rang, urine testing was a critical element.

Dehart and Sorrentino found the typical user to be of low motivation with few established goals, low tolerance for frustration, immaturity in dealing with authority figures, and boredom with his job, Vietnam, and life. However, his drug use history was short, and he resembled the situational drug abusers at Phan Rang who had the better prognosis. Of the 35 patients who could be followed for at least 3 months after completing the program and returning to duty, 74% (26) remained drug free, essentially the same outcome as reported at Phan Rang.[100]

US Army in Thailand

Considering the mostly successful outcomes reported by the Air Force programs in Vietnam, and the mostly unsuccessful outcomes of multiple Army programs there that had varying approaches, it is tempting to speculate that a critical variable was combat participation, direct or indirect. Perhaps serving stress mitigation and reducing overall heroin use prevalence, or compulsion to use, was the fact that airmen were not routinely combat participants. An opportunity to test the relation of combat participation (direct or indirect) and heroin use among Army troops arose in Thailand, where large numbers

were assigned near, but not in, the theater of combat operations, and heroin was readily available.

Major Arthur J Siegel, the drug control officer for the Army hospital in Bangkok, provided his general impressions from the treatment of 200 drug abuse cases among Army support troops stationed there in 1971 and 1972.[70] The population at risk had easy access to a wide range of illegal drugs, including highly pure and very inexpensive heroin, and, by Siegel's estimate, the prevalence of drug use in Thailand was identical to that occurring in Vietnam. Whereas the stressors affecting the soldiers assigned in Thailand did not include the combat environment, like the troops in Vietnam they did involve: (a) isolation from home, (b) service in a foreign (Southeast Asian) environment, (c) lack of identification with the military and opposition to its mission, and (d) absence of close military supervision. Of course, these soldiers were also affected by prodrug-use peer influence, and they reported extensive preassignment drug use experience (70%, primarily marijuana). According to Siegel, "Drug taking assumes an even stronger appeal in [Thailand], less for recreation than as a refuge from unpleasant reality."[70(p1259)] Although other drugs were commonly used by soldiers, serious morbidity from drug use as measured by the rates for hospitalization was limited to heroin users. Most heroin users preferred the oral-respiratory route because it removed the fear of needles, hepatitis, overdose, and the stigma of the stateside "junkie." Many users continued to function in their jobs while under its influence and remained inconspicuous— "a population of quasi-competent habituated users developed, quite distinct from the stereotype of the obvious 'smack freak.'"[70(p1260)]

According to Siegel the majority of heroin users suggested major underlying personality deficiencies, histories of adaptive failure, and a poor prognosis. A minority demonstrated personality strengths, and their habituation seemed to be consequent to the special setting where loosened social and legal constraints were reinforced by intense peer-group pressures to use heroin. Detoxification relied on urine monitoring, and abstinence syndromes generally proved to be "strikingly benign" (insomnia, mild agitation, and transient muscle cramps), which were controlled by reassurance or small doses of antianxiety compounds. Although 5% had a more severe flu-like illness, rarely were narcotic replacement medications required. Otherwise, Siegel's report did not include information regarding a treatment program or treatment success rate.

The similarities between the patterns of drug use in Thailand and in Vietnam suggest that being a soldier in the theater of combat operations was a minor risk factor for heroin use. However, contemporaneous with Siegel's observations, Zinberg also visited Army units and rehabilitation programs in Thailand and provided contradictory data. He judged there to be a pattern of lower heroin use among these troops and correlated this with the drastically reduced social and environmental stresses affecting the soldiers compared with those serving in Vietnam. "In Thailand, the men get days off, they can go off base, the Thais are friendly, soldiers can travel freely in the country when they have time off, there is no war anxiety, and the small numbers remaining have jobs which, while often boring, seem to have a function."[74(p268)]

As a postscript, a later report from Thailand by George Kojak Jr, an Army psychiatrist, and John P Canby, the Army hospital commander, is of less certain relevance because it occurred after all ground troops were withdrawn from Vietnam (in other words, for practical purposes the war was over) and because the study participants were a mix of Army and non-Army personnel. Kojak and Canby compared a group of 25 heroin-dependent American servicemen with a matched control group of men not dependent on heroin. The heroin dependent group averaged significantly lower IQ scores, education levels, and work performance records, and many revealed difficulties related to a distant or negative relationship with their fathers. However, overall the authors felt that their population of heroin users did not confirm a relationship between heroin dependence and any particular personality pattern.[101]

RESEARCH AND ANALYSIS: WAS THE RUNAWAY DRUG PROBLEM IN VIETNAM BEST EXPLAINED AS RECREATIONAL, AN ADDICTIVE COMPULSION, SELF-MEDICATION, COUNTERCULTURE "SACRAMENT," OR COLLECTIVE DISSENT?

The preceding review of the reports by the military physicians and psychiatric specialists and the related literature associated with use of drugs in Vietnam indicates that the management of the acute medical and psychiatric conditions there did not present unique clinical challenges. However, with respect to questions regarding epidemiology and obstacles to treatment and rehabilitation, four dimensions of soldier drug use in Vietnam warrant further exploration: (1) prevalence of use; (2) prevalence of addiction; (3) extent of soldier impairment (health and fitness, duty performance, morale, discipline, military commitment, unit cohesion, and combat readiness); and (4) motives for use. Answers to these questions also bear on the question of post-Vietnam effects, especially regarding the widespread use of heroin in Vietnam, because addiction typically carries a poor prognosis for health and general adaptation. Specifically, was use of heroin likely to recur after leaving Vietnam? Did the introduction to heroin in Vietnam initiate a seriously disabling, chronic condition? Or was soldier use of heroin there a transient phenomenon predicated on a unique collection of environmental extremes and sociocultural dynamics?

Prevalence of Use

By the drawdown phase of the war, the Department of Defense estimated that 60% of deployed personnel in Vietnam were using marijuana and 25% to 30% were using heroin[44]—figures that coincide with the unprecedented rates for use of illegal drugs reported from the field and surveys of soldiers departing Vietnam. However, the DEROS urine-identification system implemented in Vietnam after June 1971 found that only 5.2% of departing personnel were positive for morphine breakdown products (the test was not able to identify marijuana users). The likely explanation for this discrepancy is that the urine testing only captured those who were unable to discontinue use of heroin by themselves—either because they were seriously addicted (eg, physically dependent), substantially psychologically dependent, or both. In other words, 5.2% probably significantly underrepresented the prevalence of heroin use in Vietnam at that time.

Studies of Vietnam returnees permit some further clarification of heroin use patterns and prevalence in the theater late in the war. In a survey of over 1,000 returning enlisted soldiers being honorably discharged from the Army at Oakland Army terminal, also in early 1971, 23% acknowledged using heroin or other opiates while in Vietnam, and almost two-thirds of these acknowledged use greater than 10 times during their last month in Vietnam.[102,103] The 23% is somewhat less than the Department of Defense (DoD) estimate, probably because only those receiving honorable discharges were queried;

but it is substantially higher than the 5.2% with positive DEROS urines in Vietnam.

The most thorough research addressing the prevalence of heroin use in Vietnam came from the government-sponsored study of US Army Vietnam returnees conducted by Robins et al mentioned earlier. She and her colleagues interviewed 900 Army enlisted men (accompanied by urine testing) between May and September 1972, 8 to 12 months after their return to the United States. Only 16% were still in the service at that time. "User" subjects (n = 449) were a representative sample of those whose urine was opiate-positive when they left Vietnam; the remaining "general sample" (n = 451) represented all men who returned in September 1971.

These investigators found that of the general sample, 69% reported any use of marijuana, 44% reported having tried any narcotic, and 34% reported any use of heroin, usually through smoking it with tobacco—a rate that is somewhat higher than the DoD estimate. Twenty percent reported using narcotics more than weekly for at least 6 months (which the investigators labeled "addicted"). One-fifth of all heroin users began within the first week of arrival and three-fifths within the first 2 months.

Robins et al also found among the general sample surprisingly large numbers who reported using amphetamines (25%) and barbiturates (23%) in Vietnam. Only 2% of those reporting any heroin use there had used heroin specifically prior to their arrival in Vietnam (whereas 11% reported using "any" narcotic before Vietnam), and only 11% had positive urines detected at the time of their rotation home.[93,104,105] This latter figure appears to substantiate that the numbers of those who screened positive at DEROS significantly underrepresented narcotic use prevalence in Vietnam.

The last attempt to measure drug use in Vietnam was made by Frenkel et al who surveyed noncombat soldiers stationed in three locations in Vietnam (N = 1,007) compared with counterparts assigned to a stateside post (N = 856). The most striking finding—that 13.5% of the Vietnam soldiers and 14.5% of those in the United States reported use of heroin (not a significant difference)—was interpreted by the investigators as contradicting those of Robins and others, who believed that the heroin epidemic in Vietnam was unique to that theater. However, there were important differences in the findings from these studies, including that 32% of the heroin users in Vietnam reported that they started in Vietnam and that the number who used within the previous 72 hours was significantly higher among the

Vietnam participants (69%) than those in the United States (44%). Frenkel et al acknowledged that their data were questionable because the late date of the survey (1972) meant that many changes had already taken place in Vietnam, particularly the implementation of unannounced urine screening of units.[106]

Following the war, M Duncan Stanton reviewed results from the most credible drug use prevalence studies in Vietnam, which were centered on marijuana and narcotic use and were conducted at various points during the war (Figure 9-3). Although the data he included in the review were not collected at regular intervals, Stanton's composite still revealed: (a) steadily rising pre-Vietnam marijuana use among the soldiers deployed there (with some decline after mid-1970); (b) a parallel but less pronounced rise in first use of marijuana in the theater (through 1970); (c) a dramatic rise in first use of narcotics by soldiers in the theater after mid-1969; and (d) a more modest increase in narcotic use before deployment among those serving after the midpoint of the war (late-1968).[94]

Not only do these data portray the rise in use of marijuana in Vietnam through the course of the war and heroin later in the war, but collectively they suggest a trend in which soldiers assigned during the drawdown phase preferentially used marijuana in the United States but switched to narcotics, or added narcotics, to their drug use repertoire in the theater. (Also worth recalling is the survey by Robins et al of EM alcohol use before, during, and after service in Vietnam mentioned in this chapter. Twenty-five percent of their general sample of recent returnees reported drinking problems before Vietnam; but 20% to 50% of those switched to opiate use in the theater, only to revert to alcohol upon returning to the United States.[34]) In conclusion, these studies appear to indicate that EM use of both marijuana and heroin peaked in 1970 and 1971, with roughly two-thirds of EM reporting any use of marijuana and roughly one-third reporting any use of heroin.

Prevalence of Addiction

The medical problems in Vietnam directly linked to soldier use of marijuana were evidently limited, including because of marijuana's far lower potential to be addictive compared to other illegal drugs.[73] The prevalence of narcotic addiction, however, became a critical question from mid-1970 until ground troops were withdrawn in mid-1972. Apart from obvious concerns as to heroin's effect on the health and fitness of the troops, the political

FIGURE 9-3. Trends among Army enlisted personnel in pre-Vietnam use of marijuana and heroin/morphine, and in new use of marijuana and heroin/morphine in Vietnam.

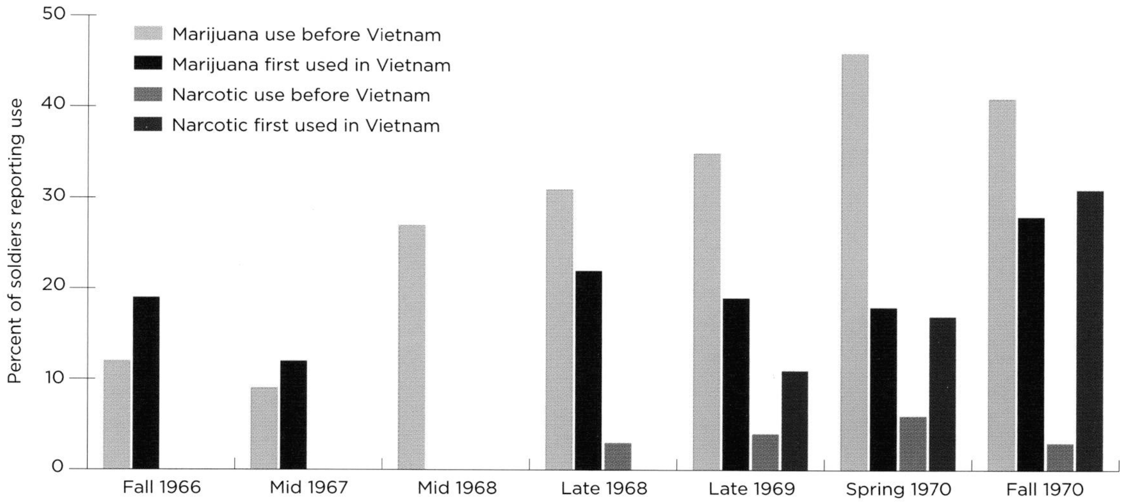

Data source: Stanton MD. Drugs, Vietnam, and the Vietnam veteran: An overview. *Am J Drug Alcohol Abuse.* 1976;3(4):560.

storm at home in response to publicity regarding soldier use and addiction in Vietnam[107] made it incumbent on the Army to distinguish between those who used heroin recreationally (a discipline problem) and those who had become addicted to heroin (a combined medical and discipline problem). Unfortunately, as the reports from the field indicated, making this distinction with confidence was practically impossible until June 1971, when a reliable laboratory method could be implemented for mass urine screening.

Considering heroin's demonstrated high addictive potential among at-risk civilians, the Army naturally assumed that rates of addiction would closely parallel rates of use. Some even considered prescribing methadone as a maintenance narcotic substitute for participants of in-service rehabilitation programs.[70,81] The observations by Zinberg from his Vietnam inspection visit in 1971 were especially revealing. He was impressed by the range of withdrawal-symptom intensity seen between the various detoxification/rehabilitation programs compared to what could be predicted based on civilian experience and concluded these differences arose because of the suggestibility of withdrawal symptoms. From this, he deduced that physiological withdrawal among the soldiers in Vietnam was most likely not as severe as the soldier, or those providing care, had anticipated.[74(p285)]

As it turned out, the apprehension of government and military leaders that the military needed to identify and treat large numbers soldiers for heroin *addiction*—that is, physical dependency—after their return from Vietnam proved to be greatly exaggerated. Although the aforementioned field reports and the DEROS urine-testing results had suggested a "relatively" low addiction rate (the 5.2% positive rate mentioned earlier), corroborative data came from a study by WRAIR. In early 1972, a team from WRAIR under the leadership of Holloway conducted physiological studies of 31 heroin users (with 5 controls) undergoing withdrawal in Vietnam. Both patients and controls were observed and monitored continuously for 5 to 7 days in a specialized ward.

The investigators were impressed by how much these heroin users differed from civilian addicts, especially the soldiers' youth, good general health, and brief exposure to heroin. The pattern of use for most of the study subjects was that of nasopulmonary insufflation ("snorting") of extremely pure heroin (92%–98%). This is a route that was not typical of most heroin users in Vietnam (who smoked it mixed with tobacco), resulting in absorption of heroin of approximately the same magnitude as through intravenous injection. However, the study subjects showed a surprisingly brief and benign withdrawal symptomatology. This was notable considering their tolerance to very large quantities of heroin and despite the fact that morphine metabolite excretion was found as late as 14 days after their last dose. In fact, especially striking was the fact that abstinence syndromes were so mild that it was possible to conduct these withdrawal studies without pharmacologic intervention. Holloway et al concluded that the withdrawal patterns in Vietnam were less severe than anticipated, in particular because of an uncoupling of tolerance and physiological dependence.[68,108–111]

Also strongly confirming a low prevalence of physical dependence to heroin in Vietnam were post-Vietnam adjustment findings from the aforementioned survey by Robins et al of Army enlisted soldiers who left Vietnam in September 1971. As noted, close to half of the general sample (44%) reported having tried one or more narcotic drugs in Vietnam and 20% used narcotics more than weekly for at least 6 months (so labeled, addicted). However, most of those who used narcotics heavily stopped on their own when they left Vietnam and had not begun again 8 to 12 months later; and only about 5% had received some treatment for drugs in the United States—mostly mandated by the military. One percent reported addiction since their return (and 1% had positive urine tests at the time of the study), whereas the percentage reporting addiction before they were assigned in Vietnam was negligible.

Finally, among substance abuse patterns in Vietnam, a preference for heroin snorting or injecting (versus smoking), combined with frequent use of amphetamines or barbiturates and little use of alcohol, was the strongest predictor of continued narcotic use after Vietnam. Robins concluded that "[t]he results of this study indicate that dependence on narcotics is not so permanent as we had once believed. . . . Not only did many of the addicted stop their drug use without any special treatment at the time they left Vietnam but many of those who continued use have not been re-addicted."[93(p63)]

In conclusion, the findings of Robins et al are consistent with the rates for positive urine tests on DEROS testing and the unannounced unit urine testing in Vietnam and suggest that 5% of soldiers is a reasonable figure for narcotic addiction prevalence in Vietnam in 1971, the peak year for heroin use. Furthermore, drawing upon the findings of Robins et al, the DoD settled on the rate of 1.3% for those who had persisting narcotic dependence following return to the United States. Thus, of the 315,500 Army enlisted soldiers who served in Vietnam in

1970–1972, it was projected that 4,075 returnees would need government-sponsored treatment and rehabilitative services.[91]

Extent of Drug-Induced Soldier Impairment

Of course, the greatest concern of Army leaders and the Army Medical Department in Vietnam was regarding the possible negative effects of soldier use of illegal drugs on military discipline, preparedness, and performance. Confusing the picture is that the professional literature surrounding marijuana and heroin use in Vietnam made various references to soldiers using these drugs electively, stably, and without noticeable performance degradation. Some even suggested that these drugs served adaptation to the especially aversive circumstances there (to be discussed below).

Marijuana

Colbach, when he served as Assistant to the Psychiatric Consultant for the Army Surgeon (October 1969–October 1970), summed up the Army's experience with marijuana in Vietnam before it was eclipsed by heroin use. According to Colbach, although marijuana smoking became a significant problem in Vietnam, it was not as serious as the mass media indicated. ("The consensus was that marijuana had thus far not seriously affected the military mission and that there was no real sense of urgency about eliminating it."[26(p206)]) This impression coincided with Bourne's—that marijuana use, at least in the buildup phase, created almost no psychiatric problems in the theater.[112] On the other hand, in recalling his own clinical experiences serving as a psychiatrist at the 67th Evacuation Hospital in Vietnam (November 1968–November 1969), Colbach noted, "[Although] I came across no case in which there was definite evidence that aggression directed toward the self or others could be attributed primarily to marijuana [it] was associated with ineffectiveness, panic states, and psychoses. . . ."[26(p206)] Bey and Zecchinelli were not completely sanguine about marijuana use among the soldiers of the 1st ID in 1969 either. In their opinion, under those circumstances it provided a "costly homeostasis," at least among psychologically susceptible soldiers, because of its potential to generate disabling neuropsychiatric reactions.[63]

Heroin

In Stanton's review of the drug use prevalence studies across the course of the war mentioned earlier, he speculated that both Robins' finding of a remission rate of 95% for heroin-using soldiers once they returned to the United States and the lack of other data indicating that heroin use degraded individual or group performance in Vietnam, suggested that heroin may not have been more deleterious than alcohol use in previous wars.[62,94] Echoing this perspective, that is, that regular heroin use was not broadly disabling, were some findings from Zinberg's inspection visit to Vietnam in 1971. Among various corroborative observations, Zinberg recalled the military judge who indicated that, to his surprise, 80% of the men appearing before him because of heroin use had top efficiency ratings from their commanding officers.[74]

The report from Joseph, an Army flight surgeon, appeared confirmatory as well. He and his rehabilitation program staff felt that they had little impact in part because most of the heroin users in their area had stable habits and did not desire to stop their drug use.[89] Siegel, an Army physician with the Army hospital in Bangkok, was more specific. He indicated there was a large population of habituated soldiers in his area who continued to function in their jobs while they were inconspicuously under the influence of heroin ("quasicompetent").[70]

Finally, there were the observations of Baker from his 1971 inspection visit to Vietnam and the Pioneer House rehabilitation program on the post of II Field Force headquarters:

> Analysis of the most recent 100 graduates of the program revealed a surprising profile of the hard drug user compared [to] that of civilian addicts: his average age was 20 y.o.; 25% of the time he's married; in 90% of the instances both parents are alive, and in 75% of the instances the parents are neither separated nor divorced; 50% of cases had no record of disciplinary actions and another 25% have had only one Article 15. In summary, the profile of the potentially rehabilitatible drug user was described as strung out on heroin, but you don't know it—he's doing his job. [See Appendix 18, "Excerpts From the Holloway/Baker Report."]

Still, it cannot be overlooked that the aforementioned clinical reports from Army psychiatrists and other physicians indicated they were required to treat a sizable subset of soldiers in Vietnam who became disabled by neuropsychiatric conditions, including serious withdrawal syndromes, associated with both marijuana and heroin use. These were individuals who adopted atypical patterns of drug use, for example, heavy use of marijuana and heroin, intravenous use of heroin or use via snorting, and polydrug use, which led to psychological dependency, and, with respect to heroin, physical dependency. They also typically had premilitary histories of personality deficits and other forms of individual psychopathology, including polydrug and narcotic use.

Effects on Combat Performance

Of course, among combat troops, nothing rivals the importance of the effects of drug and alcohol use on the capacity of the soldier to perform in battle. Unfortunately, specific conclusions regarding combat efficiency in Vietnam for drug-using soldiers must remain impressionistic because of the lack of data. With respect to marijuana use, Spector, the military historian, noted that at least through 1968 and 1969 (before heroin was available), few if any soldiers used drugs during combat; however, marijuana was used by some after a battle to help them calm down.[12(p275)] The latter observation was corroborated by the Roffman and Sapol survey of soldiers departing Vietnam in 1967,[14] by Postel with the soldiers of the 4th ID in 1968,[50] and by Treanor and Skripol with soldiers of the 173rd Airborne Brigade in early 1970.[65] As late as fall 1971, senior Air Force psychiatrists Mirin and McKenna inspected a dozen military installations in Southeast Asia and conjectured that marijuana's sedative and tranquilizing properties were beneficial in helping combat troops diminish anxiety and blunt the hyperaroused state frequently seen between periods of combat.[51] Sanders came to a similar conclusion from his interviews with returning veterans between 1967 and 1970: that although few reported use of marijuana while on patrol, they habitually used it to unwind after the intense pressures of combat.[113] However, perhaps as a contradictory finding, Stanton's survey of soldiers departing Vietnam in late 1969 found only a slight positive correlation between frequency of marijuana use and "exposure to enemy fire."[62(p285)] (See also Chapter 7, Exhibit 7-4, "Use of Pharmaceuticals to Bolster Combat Performance.")

Matters are more ominous once widespread heroin use entered the picture in Vietnam. Even if habitual heroin users could meet performance standards, risks of use would invariably become magnified because of the necessity of an accessible supply. In their survey of 1,000 returning enlisted soldiers in 1971, Bentel et al found some who spoke of using drugs to increase sensory awareness. They described soldiers reporting that they carefully titrated the use of marijuana plus heroin while on combat patrols to calm down, enhance alertness, and increase suspicion of enemy activity.[114] During his inspection visit in 1971, Holloway found evidence of prevalent heroin use among combat and combat support units. According to Holloway, "Trips to nearby fire bases verified that heroin was being used in the field and on patrol, but heroin use had infiltrated every level of the brigade structure including the medical battalion."[83(p2)] More broadly, he and his research colleagues ultimately concluded that drug abuse, primarily heroin, among US military forces represented a "significant threat to combat readiness."[68(p1191)]

Risk Factors for Drug Use

In many respects the dominant patterns of soldier use of the most common drugs used in Vietnam— marijuana and heroin—resembled those of alcohol in previous wars, that is, they were casually and spontaneously consumed in off-duty circumstances among socially defined groups for the purposes of emotional numbing, disinhibition, and promoting group solidarity. But understanding the motivation for the skyrocketing rise in the use of these drugs as the war prolonged, especially marijuana and heroin, by lower-ranking EM requires consideration of additional features, including predeployment variables—(a) the youth drug culture; and (b) individual predisposition; and Vietnam theater variables: (c) the ubiquitous drug market; (d) reduced combat activity and military demobilization; (e) social dynamics of enlisted troops there; (f) antiwar, antimilitary authority passions; and (g) drug use as "self-medication."

Predeployment Variables

The Drug Culture. The most conspicuous predeployment influence on drug use among the general population of young EM in Vietnam was that of peer group norms. Chapter 1 made the case for the increasing popularity of illegal drug use among civilian peers, especially marijuana. But it should be remembered that this was more than a peer group fad and an alternate means to increase pleasure; marijuana had also become emblematic for the burgeoning antiestablishment passions shared by young adults in America at the time. The serial drug use surveys in Vietnam reviewed in this chapter substantiated that the sequential cohorts of soldiers brought these drug attitudes and habits into the theater with them. However, as Stanton demonstrated, their civilian counterparts were not as accepting of heroin use as they were of marijuana use,[94] thus the enthusiasm for heroin among the soldiers in Vietnam requires further explanation.

Individual Predisposition. Extent of pre-Vietnam susceptibility is a more complex variable. Soldiers alleged that their heroin use in Vietnam was a reasonable adaptation to the unreasonable situation the Army had thrust them into; that they were not sick or impaired and could stop heroin use when they were released from Vietnam and the Army; or, if not, it was the Army's fault and the Army should provide a painless way to facilitate their discontinuing drug use as well as relieve them of any negative consequences for their drug use such as punishment or an unfavorable discharge from the service. But according to psychiatric researcher Holloway, drug use was more frequent among soldiers with characterological low self-esteem, for example, psychopathology, especially those with pre-Vietnam history of polysubstance use.[69]

The literature from the Army mental health professionals who worked in the field with drug users in Vietnam showed some lack of consensus regarding predisposition, ranging from characterologically susceptible and maladjusted[59,63,65,77] to uncertain,[52,89] at least for the soldiers who presented with symptoms. A corollary question also remained unanswered: how much should be generalized from clinical populations to the majority of drug using soldiers—those who did not require medical attention? Was their use also secondary to character defect? In attempting to answer these questions, professional disagreements surrounded the question of which soldiers were physically dependent, that is, whether a given soldier's continued drug use was an expression of "sickness" or misconduct (as mentioned earlier, it is notoriously difficult to distinguish the extent of physical dependence without objective means). (See also the summary of Cohen's speech to the I Corps Medical Society in Chapter 4.)

A study of the Minnesota Multiphasic Personality Inventory (MMPI) results of 101 Army enlisted soldiers detained for heroin detoxification prior to their return from Vietnam to the United States (September 1971–April 1972) by Hampton and Vogel did not definitively answer the question of predisposition. These investigators found a marked heterogeneity of psychological test types. They concluded that 55% of their sample had abnormal MMPIs, whereas 35% had normal MMPIs. However, when they matched their results against those from civilian addicted groups, they noted that the military group had less psychopathology and a lower incidence of sociopathy.[115]

In their study, Robins et al collected demographic information comparing Vietnam returnees who used heroin in Vietnam with those who used no drugs or only marijuana. They found heroin users to be younger, single, less educated, from larger cities, and more often reared in broken homes. They also were more likely to come to Vietnam with a history of deviant behavior (crime, drug use, or high school dropout). Race was not significantly related to drug use, although blacks were more likely to be detected as opiate-positive at the point of their return to the United States. However, the strongest preservice factor that predicted continuing use after Vietnam was preservice narcotic use. The only pre-Vietnam military indicator was a history of disciplinary action.[104,105]

Especially salient was the finding that neither predisposition nor setting alone predicted narcotic use in Vietnam; they must be considered as an *interaction*. In other words, because Vietnam offered much greater availability of heroin than in the United States, this increased the impact of a predisposition to abuse narcotics ("abuse" is defined broadly). Soldiers with histories of preservice deviant behavior who did not use heroin prior to Vietnam may simply have lacked opportunity, but those who had the opportunity before service and chose not to use narcotics then might be expected to be mostly invulnerable to use in Vietnam (and they added, "perhaps because they were satisfied with alcohol.") It must be noted, however, that in their analysis Robins et al considered high drug accessibility as the principal intratheater, drug use-promoting influence.[35]

Finally, studies of Army returnees from the draw-down phase in Vietnam who exhibited persisting combinations of drug and alcohol problems as well as depression 2 to 3 years following their reentry into the United States strongly pointed to preservice risk factors of early alcohol problems, polydrug use, and antisocial behavior.[116]

Vietnam Variables

The Drug Market. The most prominent intratheater factor that fostered soldier use of illegal drugs was accessibility, especially to marijuana and heroin. These drugs were characterized by their exceptionally high potency (or purity in the case of the heroin), exceedingly low cost (by the standards of the soldiers), and the efficient distribution system throughout the country by indigenous Vietnamese. However, as has been noted, military order and discipline became far more threatened by the widespread use of heroin than marijuana. Many suspected that the marketing of heroin in Vietnam represented a communist strategy to demoralize both the US troops and the American public.

Over time, more convincing data suggested that widespread corruption among South Vietnamese officials, highly efficient criminal syndicates, and opportunity were primarily responsible. Increased demand among US troops in Southeast Asia brought expansion of the Golden Triangle's heroin-refining facilities, almost all of which were owned and protected by pro-American Thai and Laotian forces. Thai, Laotian, and South Vietnamese air forces and the paramilitary charter airline companies, such as Air America and Continental Air, soon dominated the opiate transportation business.[117] This suggested that the soldier demand for drugs fueled the market as opposed to the opposite, that is, that the market fueled the demand. Probably the best guess is that they were mutually reinforcing.

Heroin's High Addictive Potential. Did soldiers who experimented with heroin become physically compelled to extend their use because they needed increasing amounts to experience the same high or to avoid unbearable withdrawal symptoms? The afore-mentioned reports from the field that indicated low levels of addiction, the corroborative findings from the withdrawal study of Holloway et al, and the postdeployment addiction rates measured by Robins et al seem to rule out the likelihood that heroin's high addictive potential explained more than a fraction of the high prevalence of use by the lower-ranking enlisted soldiers in Vietnam (eg, 34% use prevalence vs 5% addiction prevalence). Still, this suggests that one out of every seven soldiers who used heroin became addicted— not an insignificant fraction).

Reduced Combat Activity and Military Demobilization. Because roughly one-third of soldiers, E-4 and below, were using heroin, at least occasionally, and use at this high rate cannot be fully explained by its accessibility or addictive potential, premorbid personality defects, or civilian peer-group norms, its use must, in large measure, be circumstantially determined, as was suggested by Robins et al. And if so, it also must be considered volitional. So, what can be said about the circumstances faced by these drawdown-phase soldiers? A common myth that emerged from the Vietnam era was that heroin use was driven by combat stress; but this is very unlikely because use of heroin was rising as combat risk and numbers of casualties were dropping.

Holloway reported that heroin users told his investigation team they used drugs "to turn the place off" and that this was necessary because of the unique stresses in Vietnam (eg, boredom, being "hassled by lifers," bad living conditions, or combat).[69] Similarly, Stanton reported "boredom, disenchantment with the war, and feelings of victimization"[94(p562)] as soldier justifications.[94] In their study of late-war Vietnam returnees, Robins et al found no statistical correlation between heroin use and assignments, danger, or death of friends. Besides the wish to achieve euphoria, the most common explanations for use by their study participants included intolerance of Army regulations, homesickness, boredom, depression, and fear.[104]

In many respects these were predictable symptoms of a disengaging military force.[98,118–120] Even the use of narcotics by US soldiers was seen at the close of the Korean War, apparently partly attributed to increased drug accessibility.[41] Still, various indicators suggest that the troops during the drawdown in Vietnam were even more restive and antagonistic than those deployed at the close of the earlier conflicts and that the widespread use of narcotics, which was unprecedented in its scope and inconsistent with civilian, peer group norms, was a symptom of, and expressive of, their discontent and impatience.

As attested by Holloway from his drug program inspection trip, soldier survey, and studies of narcotic withdrawal in Vietnam, the process of withdrawing US forces from Vietnam brought significant, morale-depleting stressors for the soldiers deployed in the last years. Not only were combat risks still present, the outcome ambiguous, and public opposition intensifying, but also: (*a*) reduced combat activity was producing role uncertainty (eg, loss of a sense of purpose and justification for personal sacrifices of deployment); and (*b*) attrition and reconfiguration of units were contributing to decreased unit identification and cohesion (eg, reduced sense of commitment to military cohorts and the military mission).[69]

Social Dynamics of Heroin Use Among Enlisted Soldiers. Consideration of the soldier's social relationships is critical in understanding his drug use. Although a full discussion of the social psychology of soldiers is generally beyond the scope of this work, suffice it to say that the establishment of groups (cliques) by soldiers is necessary and predictable. Such groups constitute the alliances the soldier makes with those he feels are most like him and from whom he draws a sense of intimacy, affirmation, and security in the face of the rigors and strictness of military life. As such, they have traditionally allowed soldiers to maintain their psychological balance and resiliency. Group life is centered on maintaining boundaries, common values, and status discriminations within the group and establishing group-sanctioned/required behaviors.

Formation and maintenance of such groups is even more important for lower-ranking enlisted soldiers because they are the least powerful individuals within the larger system (lowest status, fewest assets). As a baseline, group stability and membership would be predictably even more important for the soldiers deployed in a dangerous, austere situation a long way from home—circumstances such as Vietnam. But, as noted previously in this work, the Army's 1-year, individualized rotation/replacement system in Vietnam was especially disruptive to soldiers maintaining unit ties and mission-centered allegiances.

MG Spurgeon Neel, the former MACV Surgeon, noted that there were signs as far back as 1969 and 1970 indicating the growing presence of dissenting soldier subgroups in Vietnam that were more motivated by racial, political, and especially drug culture priorities[16(p48)] (vs those centered on traditional military/combat objectives and respect for military leaders). By 1971, Zinberg understood the heroin-using soldiers in Vietnam as "socially habituated"—vs the psychologically or physically habituated, civilian addicts.[95] Similarly Holloway concluded, "[H]eroin use in Vietnam is best viewed in terms of the social structure that encouraged and maintained usage rather than in terms of personality, demographic, or pathological characteristics of individual users."[68(p1198)]

Exploration of the group dynamics that operated in Vietnam was undertaken by Larry Ingraham, an Army social psychologist. In late 1971, he conducted a stateside study of a cohort of 78 soldiers who had been identified as opiate-positive at the conclusion of their Vietnam assignment. Nearly three-quarters had used at least one illegal substance weekly prior to entering the Army, and at least one-fifth had tried heroin before Vietnam. However, demographic and other descriptors of the study respondents did not clearly identify premilitary service risk factors. Most reported they smoked or "snorted" the heroin while in Vietnam, and, within their "head" society (communal, drug-using lower-ranking enlisted), status discriminations centered on drug choice and usage pattern, with the highest level for the exclusive marijuana users and lowest for those preferring barbiturates and amphetamines.

Although acknowledging that they had become dependent upon heroin in Vietnam, the study participants justified their use as adaptive to the unique stresses of the theater (not typically combat stress), considered their use as on a minor scale because they had not injected drugs, and denied any need for further treatment or rehabilitation because they maintained their habits in Vietnam without losing function or resorting to theft. Their jargon exalted the enlisted "heads," denigrated the "lifer/juicers" (alcohol-consuming career military superiors), and expressed intense anti-Army and antiwar passions. According to Ingraham, the principal dynamic underlying their drug use was that it fostered a bonding with others who shared specific attitudes and values, especially regarding drug use.

Group membership meant the soldier could experience an immediate and intense sense of acceptance and support. Curiously, perhaps because he did not conduct his research in Vietnam, Ingraham alleged the soldiers' antagonism about the Army and the war did not represent a political ideology or a rejection of conventional values. He argued they were repeating enlisted coping styles that had been observed in prior armies in war.[121] Nonetheless, his study made clear that among these heroin-positive soldiers, drug use and counter(military) values were fused and served to define these as "counter(military)-culture" groups.

Heroin Use Expressing Opposition to the War and Military Authority. As described in Chapter 1 and Chapter 2, following the drug-naïve years of the build-up phase in Vietnam, use of marijuana and other drugs began to rise in tandem with dropping soldier morale—a prelude to the heroin epidemic after mid-1970. Over time, the emergence of EM splinter groups, which were commonly centered on surreptitious drug use and antiwar, antimilitary attitudes, became evident to medical and mental health observers in the field. First notice of these motivational influences appearing in the psychiatric literature came in 1968 from observations by Colbach and Crowe working at the 67th Evacuation Hospital with a mix of combat and support troops. Imahara, from his vantage point of stockade psychiatrist in the "Long Binh Jail" (stockade) in 1968 and 1969, warned that there was a growing problem with disruptive, deviant soldiers—men who expressed, including through drug use, intense, essentially collective, hostility toward the military as an oppressive institution. This was especially prominent among black soldiers who viewed the white officers and NCOs as their persecutors.[122(p57)]

Bey, division psychiatrist for the 1st ID, and Zecchinelli, social work/psychology specialist, saw increasing marijuana use among the soldiers of the division in 1969 as expressive of counterauthority sentiments. Recall from earlier his observations regarding the growing trend for soldiers to adopt a "head" identity and primary affiliations with like-minded soldiers.[63] Mirin and McKenna found a similar social dynamic with respect to the patterns of marijuana use during their 1971 drug investigation tour, that is, that use served as a peer group sacrament, binding comrades and defining (alternative) group boundaries.[51] And in his journal, Ratner, serving at the 935th Psychiatric Detachment in 1970 and 1971, emphasized that antimilitary "passive-aggressiveness" was central in the psychodynamics of the heroin user (eg, it was a form of low-risk dissent and protest against the "ghetto" existence the lower-ranking soldiers felt forced to endure in Vietnam). Finally, contemporaneously with Ratner, this author found collective, antimilitary authority passions at least as motivationally influential as the pursuit of euphoria among the drug-using mix of combat and support troops encountered at the 98th Psychiatric Detachment (see Prologue).

Linden's report of his investigative visit in 1971 provided first-person testimony on the critical link between heroin use and the near-the-flashpoint dissidence that was so prevalent among the lowest ranks:

> Contending with heroin use in a mutinous unit with strained race relations is overwhelming to an officer trained only to order and deploy his men. The rear echelon officer stands over a caldron where the soldier's every atavistic impulse is boiled to the surface by the heat of enforced proximity. . . .
>
> At some bases, such as Camp Eagle [101st Airborne Division base], it seems that the commanding officer of every unit leads what in any other war would be singled out as a rare "trouble" unit. . . .
>
> [Heroin] is one device the [soldier] uses to live through a tour in Vietnam without being there.

The drug—or evidence of it—is everywhere. If you look down through the slats of a base bus station anywhere in Vietnam, you will see dozens of the little glass vials that once contained the 96 to 99 per cent pure heroin. . . . Army psychiatrist Dr. [Robert] Landeen, who was with the 101st Airborne . . . found that in several companies as many as 40 per cent of the men used heroin. Peer group pressure only partially explains the rapid spread of use of heroin. Bill Karabaic, a drug counselor with the division, told me that for many [soldiers], fighting a war in Vietnam is so confusing and inassimilable that . . . they feel they are in a dream, that they are not really themselves. Because life there is not real, it becomes acceptable to snort skag [heroin] and frag [assassinate] the sarge. That's what your buddies are doing. When the dream stops and you return safely to the [United] States, you will stop—or so goes the dream. "Vietnam is a bad place to be," said Karabaic, "and most people want to get through as quickly and painlessly as possible. Heroin makes the time fly."[123(p13)]

Drug Use as "Self-Medication." Of course, the flip side for drug use as pathological is the prospect that it could support adaptation. As the preceding section described, an apparently untenable situation arose near the end of the war in Vietnam in which enlisted troops were pitted against their military leaders. By 1970, the first-term soldiers assigned in Vietnam, along with a sympathetic American public, became convinced that the government and the military were making them sick by keeping them there, and they felt blameless in using heroin—as self-medication. Of course, in a colloquial sense the same claim can be made by anyone who electively uses a mind-altering drug—that it is "therapy." On a practical basis, because these substances were illegal to possess in Vietnam, this is a moot point. But as a natural experiment it behooves one to consider that possibility, at least for soldiers not predisposed to misuse. Could marijuana, or heroin, used in the fashion most soldiers did, that is, via smoking, have served a coping, stress-mitigating function? In other words, did it promote adaptation under the particular morale-depleting combat theater circumstances in Vietnam? It certainly appears to have been unwittingly assumed by military leaders that alcohol use would serve this function throughout the war as it might have in earlier conflicts.

It would seem self-evident that the casual use of mind-altering substances is a threat to military discipline and overall combat preparedness but, in fact, many professional commentators, most of whom were not serving in Vietnam, interpreted the accelerating marijuana use and the later heroin epidemic in Vietnam as "self-medication," "therapy," and a "coping device." For example, from their interviews with Vietnam returnees, Bentel et al described the social bonding facilitated among soldiers by the communal use of heroin akin to marijuana use in the United States. They also claimed that many used drugs as therapy for their despair, boredom, and frustration.[114] Stanton served as an Army psychologist in Vietnam in 1969 and conducted a major drug use survey there.[62] Later he explored the drug abuse histories of Vietnam veterans and developed a similar perspective:

> What we had [in Vietnam] was a form of massive *self-medication* [author's emphasis] utilizing substances which, in addition, provided thrills and were amenable to a kind of small group communion experience. Certainly factors such as curiosity, rebellion, escape, and anti-fatigue were also important, along with deterioration in morale/discipline concomitant with mounting disenchantment with the war.[94(pp566–567)]

Sanders came to a similar conclusion from his interviews with returning veterans between 1967 and 1970. According to Sanders, drugs provided soldiers a means for counterauthority and antiwar group affiliation, as well as a personal mechanism for "manipulating time" and withdrawing from the pressures and frustrations of Vietnam—"a realistic and rational attempt at self-medication."[113(p64)] Colbach and Crowe saw motives for marijuana use along two planes: it served simultaneously as a "coping device" for the surrounding stresses and a "means of acting out against military authority. . . ."[59(p572)] Similarly, from their inspection visits to a dozen military installations in Southeast Asia in fall 1971, Mirin and McKenna, both Air Force psychiatrists, opined that the extensive use of marijuana was a means for lowering individual tension and that it represented a mostly adaptive coping strategy. ("Its ready availability and wide peer group acceptance made it the drug of choice among younger enlisted personnel for the self-medication of anxiety, anger, and depression."[51]) In Hawaii, Golosow and Childs concluded that among the 36 soldiers they treated for withdrawal, heroin use in Vietnam had become a "coping device under trying and unusual circumstances in an alien world."[90]

So, given all these references to drug use in Vietnam as self-medication (ie, to blunt feelings of distress and even to quell the temptation to desert, mutiny, or attack a leader), and considering the requirement that the military field an effective fighting force in a theater of war, to what extent should drug use in Vietnam be considered misconduct, or overlooked as adaptive? Applying a medical model for explaining soldier drug use creates a conundrum: if possession of a drug is illegal, its use is "bad" (ie, misconduct), and military leaders are correct to, apart from offering some flexibility (the amnesty program), enforce the laws and regulations against drug use in order to shore up the deteriorating discipline and ensure combat readiness. On the other hand, if there is a growing consensus, including among military medical personnel, that use of these drugs is medicinal, is it not instead "good"? This riddle (adaptive, justifiable vs maladaptive, not justifiable) is conceptually resolvable if the overlapping motives behind soldier heroin use are deconstructed. To paraphrase from this volume's Prologue, through using heroin, soldiers in drawdown Vietnam sought to fulfill the four goals of: (1) temporary psychological "removal" (from place and circumstance); (2) submersion in an affirming affinity group; (3) pharmacological relief of individual tension; and (4) counterauthority behavior, that is, expressing passively and collectively an intent to sabotage the institution and thwart its authorities—a potential that was heightened *because* possession was illegal.

The first three of these motives might reasonably be seen as self-medication (and could refer to the use of alcohol as well), but because "counterauthority behavior" is also included, then the overall set serves as misconduct, at least by military standards. As a corollary, it would seem possible that only those with similar antimilitary sympathies would conclude that a behavior motivated by that objective should be defined simply as coping or (self-) therapy. Thus, by extension, the conundrum only persists if motive (4), which implies self-inflicted disability and sabotage—if not mutiny, or even desertion (psychological), remains unacknowledged. Somewhat in defense of the troops serving in drawdown Vietnam are Holloway's observation that the troops serving late in the war were "carrying out a mission which is less than universally popular,"[69(p112)] Mirin and McKenna's "[soldiers] lack a shared ideologic conviction

about the war,"[51(p483)] and Baker's "[the soldier there] draws little esteem from contributing to an unpopular war effort"[124(p857)]; however, these characterizations dramatically understate the bitterness and resentment borne by these soldiers. More accurate and complete would be to say that the war became universally despised among those assigned there, most of whom were "citizen soldiers"; and that for the majority, pre-Vietnam loyalty to military objectives, means, and authority were consequently replaced by mistrust and antagonism as evidenced by inverted morale. Furthermore, by inference, these passions were among the primary reasons that lower-ranking soldiers elected to use illegal, socially forbidden, mind-altering drugs with such abandon while they were there and not upon their return to the United States.

WALTER REED ARMY INSTITUTE OF RESEARCH PSYCHIATRIST SURVEY FINDINGS: PATTERNS OF DRUG AND ALCOHOL ABUSE IN VIETNAM

The following extends the summary of findings from the WRAIR postwar survey (1982) of Army psychiatrists who served in Vietnam that was begun in Chapter 5. In that chapter, Table 5-3 noted that the Army psychiatrist participants in the WRAIR survey estimated that over the course of the war, alcohol dependence syndromes represented 10.4% of their diagnosable cases. They also indicated that drug dependence syndromes collectively represented 15% of their diagnosable cases, with psychiatrists who served in the second half of the war reporting significantly higher estimates (19%) than those who served in the first half of the war (8.1%). Also, in Chapter 8, Table 8-4 indicated that among a list of 17 behavior problems in Vietnam requiring professional involvement, survey psychiatrists ranked excessive use of alcohol as second and marijuana use as fourth. When the second half of the war was considered separately, heroin use (via smoking) was the sixth problem behavior, barbiturate use was seventh, and use of stimulants or hallucinogens was eighth.

To further explore patterns of use and effects for alcohol, marijuana, and narcotics, survey psychiatrists were provided 12 statements and asked to indicate for each the extent of their agreement on 1-to-5 scale with 1 = strongly disagree to 5 = strongly agree. Results are presented in Figure 9-4 and Table 9-2.

FIGURE 9-4. Means of survey psychiatrists' experience with substance abuse in extent of agreement on 1-to-5 scale with 1 = strongly disagree to 5 = strongly agree (N = 30–69). Responses are arranged in five conceptual groups.

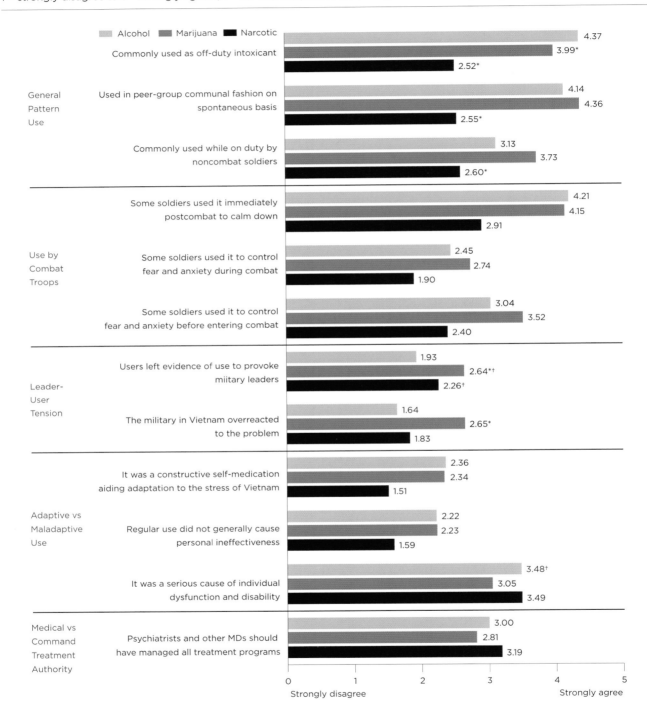

Significant Anovas are indicated as follows:

* Early/late, that is, comparing responses of psychiatrists who served in the first versus second half of the war

† Support/combat, that is, comparing responses of "support" psychiatrists (those who only served with hospitals) and "combat" psychiatrists (those who served any time with a combat unit). [Subgroup values are shown in Chapter 9, Table 9-2].

TABLE 9-2. Statistically Significant Results for Subgroup Values (From Figure 9-4 Using Analysis of Variance)

Item	Drug	Total Sample	"Early" psych (n=33)	"Late" psych (n=38)	p. value	Support psych (n=39)	Combat psych (n=32)
Commonly used as off-duty intoxicant	Marijuana	3.99	3.59	4.30	.026		
	Narcotic	2.52	1.85	3.00	.001		
Used in peer-group communal fashion on spontaneous basis	Narcotic	2.55	1.89	2.94	.011		
Commonly used while on duty by noncombat soldiers	Narcotic	2.60	1.78	3.10	.001		
Users left evidence to provoke military leaders	Marijuana	2.64	2.09	3.03	.009		
					.031	2.96	2.25
	Narcotic	2.26			.034	2.65	1.75
The military in Vietnam overreacted to the problem	Marijuana	2.65	2.04	3.09	.015		
It was a serious cause of dysfunction and disability	Alcohol	3.48			.014	3.81	3.07

Psych: psychiatrist
Early: survey psychiatrists who served in the first half of the war
Late: survey psychiatrists who served in the second half of the war

Support: survey psychiatrists who served at hospitals
Combat: survey psychiatrists who served *anytime* with a combat unit

Several of the survey findings are striking and consistent with the preceding material. The more dramatic findings are high frequency for: extensive off-duty, communal use of marijuana, alcohol, and (late war) narcotics; common use of all three by noncombat troops while on duty; and extensive use of alcohol and marijuana by combat troops postcombat and, to a lesser extent, before entering combat. It is also noteworthy that the survey psychiatrists appear to refute the idea that any of these substances served adaptation in Vietnam. Instead they perceived that not only were all three drugs serious causes of individual dysfunction and disability, but that alcohol was the most deleterious, especially among noncombat troops.

SUMMARY AND CONCLUSIONS

Chapter 8 reviewed the psychiatric record and related literature pertaining to psychiatric and behavior problems for Army troops in general, especially the accelerating rates associated with the collapse of morale and military discipline in Vietnam as the war lengthened. Chief among them were clinical conditions stemming from the use and abuse of mind-altering substances,

primarily alcohol, marijuana, and heroin. This chapter extends that review through a closer examination of the effects of these drugs, which proved to be especially insidious and disabling forms of soldier misconduct and dissent. The following summarizes the most salient observations:

- **It can be concluded from the available psychiatric reports and results of the WRAIR psychiatrist survey that among both enlisted troops and officers, there was a steady and high prevalence of alcohol problems, both as abuse (most) and as addiction (some), over the course of the war. Whereas modest alcohol use may have served traditional military ends in Vietnam by facilitating off-duty psychological numbing of the ordeals inherent in serving there and small group bonding, it also negatively affected the health, fitness, and performance of a sizable subset of susceptible soldiers.**

  - The Army in Vietnam did not collect epidemiologic data on alcohol problems identified as such.

- Psychiatrists' reports from the field suggested that between 10% and 20% of their cases were either primarily alcohol related or that alcohol was an aggravating factor.
- Psychiatrist respondents to the WRAIR survey indicated that alcohol was as serious a cause of soldier dysfunction and disability in Vietnam, as was heroin, especially among support troops.
- Psychotropic drugs (Thorazine was used most frequently, followed by Librium), were reported to be helpful in treating acute alcohol abuse.
- There were no effective treatments utilized for alcohol dependency in the theater. Apparently, for many of the affected soldiers (typically those with higher ranks), intractable or recurrent bouts of alcohol abuse ended their careers through administrative elimination from the service for alcoholism or related ineffectiveness. The anecdotal record suggests that some individuals chose suicide as an alternative. Also, some received medical evacuation out of the theater, even though this would have been contrary to Army policy because their acute condition would have quickly remitted while receiving hospital-level treatment in Vietnam.

- **Illegal drugs—primarily marijuana and hashish, barbiturates, stimulants, and narcotics—were commonly used socially by lower-ranking enlisted soldiers in Vietnam, and their use accelerated as the war prolonged. The Army failed to contain this epidemic or develop successful treatment and rehabilitation programs in the theater. These circumstances presumably jeopardized combat readiness and hastened the American pull out.**

  - During the buildup years, the rising prevalence of drug use, primarily marijuana and hashish, among first-term enlistees was evident, with a small percentage of users requiring inpatient psychiatric treatment for toxic brain syndromes (often with psychotic symptoms). The treating psychiatrists concluded that the locally grown marijuana was primarily responsible because of its especially high potency. After a few days of hospital management under conditions of abstinence, often augmented with use of psychotropic medications, the conditions

remitted and these soldiers could be returned to duty with their units. However, some soldiers, apparently those with greater premorbid susceptibility, had more prolonged disability and required evacuation out of the theater for additional treatment.

- By the transition years, drug problems became more common and complex and suggested eroding military health and discipline in the theater. Psychiatrists' reports and WRAIR psychiatrist survey data indicated higher and heavier marijuana use prevalence (approximately half of younger enlisted reported some use) than earlier, including among combat troops, with an associated rise in the number of soldiers requiring treatment for toxic brain syndromes. Clinical problems resulting from polydrug use also increased, especially among support troops, which involved their use of marijuana mixed with opium, amphetamines, or barbiturates. Some of the reports indicated that emerging troop disaffection appeared to be correlated with increasing drug use.
- The drawdown phase of the war was dominated by an epidemic of heroin use among first-term enlisted soldiers (reported use as about one-third of soldiers), both combat and noncombat troops, accompanied by addiction and withdrawal problems for many (prevalence for addiction, ie, physiological dependence, was estimated to be approximately 5% of troops). The accelerating rates coincided with the widespread antagonism of lower ranks toward military authority and the US mission in Vietnam. Army leadership and medical/ psychiatric personnel strenuously sought to stem this trend and identify and treat/ rehabilitate heroin users, but poor results and public protest led to the medical evacuation of thousands of soldiers from the theater for continuing narcotic use. Although there was ample evidence that the soldiers who were more likely to become heavily involved in drug use were developmentally and characterologically predisposed, the widespread use of heroin indicated that social pathology and associated crisis had trumped individual psychopathology as causation. Moreover, in the end this insoluble medical/morale problem within the

ranks became the Army's Achilles' heel and emblematic of America's failure in Vietnam.

REFERENCES

1. Evans ON. Army aviation psychiatry in Vietnam. *US Army Vietnam Med Bull.* 1968;May/June:54–58.

2. Baker SL Jr. Drug abuse in the United States Army. *Bull N Y Acad Med.* 1971;47(6):541–549.

3. Rock NL, Stokes JW, Koshes RJ, Fagan J, Cline WR, Jones FD. US Army combat psychiatry. In: Jones FD, Sparacino LR, Wilcox VL, Rothberg JM, Stokes JW, eds. *War Psychiatry.* In: Zajtchuk R, Bellamy RF, eds. *Textbooks of Military Medicine.* Washington, DC: Department of the Army, Office of The Surgeon General, Borden Institute; 1995: 149–175.

4. Jones FD. Disorders of frustration and loneliness. In: Jones FD, Sparacino LR, Wilcox VL, Rothberg JM, Stokes JW, eds. *War Psychiatry.* In: Zajtchuk R, Bellamy RF, eds. *Textbooks of Military Medicine.* Washington, DC: Department of the Army, Office of The Surgeon General, Borden Institute; 1995: 63–83.

5. Watanabe HK, Harig PT, Rock, NL, Koshes RJ. Alcohol and drug abuse and dependence. In: Jones FD, Sparacino LR, Wilcox VL, Rothberg JM, eds. *Military Psychiatry: Preparing in Peace for War.* In: Zajtchuk R, Bellamy RF, eds. *Textbooks of Military Medicine.* Washington, DC: Department of the Army, Office of The Surgeon General, Borden Institute; 1994: 61–89.

6. American Psychiatric Association. *Diagnostic and Statistical Manual of Mental Disorders.* 2nd ed (DSM-II). Washington, DC: APA; 1968.

7. US Department of the Army. *Armed Forces Medical Diagnosis Nomenclature and Statistical Classification.* Washington, DC: DA; June 1963. Army Regulation 40-401.

8. US Department of the Army. *Personnel Separations, Officer Personnel.* Washington, DC: DA; July 1968. Army Regulation 635-105.

9. Byrdy HSR. *Division Psychiatry in Vietnam* (unpublished); 1967. [Full text available as Appendix 8 to this volume.]

10. Menard DL. The social work specialist in a combat division. *US Army Vietnam Med Bull.* 1968;March/April:48–57.

11. Bey D. *Wizard 6: A Combat Psychiatrist in Vietnam.* College Station, Tex: Texas A & M University Military History Series, 104; 2006.

12. Spector RH. *After Tet: The Bloodiest Year in Vietnam.* New York, NY: The Free Press; 1993.

13. Colbach EM, Parrish MD. Army mental health activities in Vietnam: 1965–1970. *Bull Menninger Clin.* 1970;34(6):333–342.

14. Roffman RA, Sapol E. Marijuana in Vietnam: a survey of use among Army enlisted men in two southern corps. *Int J Addict.* 1970;5(1):1–42.

15. Allerton WS. Army psychiatry in Vietnam. In: Bourne PG, ed. *The Psychology and Physiology of Stress: With Reference to Special Studies of the Viet Nam War.* New York, NY: Academic Press; 1969: 1-17.

16. Neel SH. *Medical Support of the US Army in Vietnam, 1965–1970.* Washington, DC: GPO; 1973.

17. Rothberg JM. A note on alcoholism: incidence and policy (letter). *NEJM.* 1975;292(21):1137.

18. Hays FW. Military aeromedical evacuation and psychiatric patients during the Viet Nam War. *Am J Psychiatry.* 1969;126(5):658–666.

19. Jones FD, Johnson AW Jr. Medical and psychiatric treatment policy and practice in Vietnam. *J Soc Issues.* 1975;31(4):49–65.

20. Datel WE, Johnson AW Jr. *Psychotropic Prescription Medication in Vietnam.* Alexandria, Va: Defense Technical Information Center; 1981. Document No. AD A097610. Available at: http://handle.dtic.mil/100.2/ADA097610.

21. Huffman RE. Which soldiers break down. A survey of 610 psychiatric patients in Vietnam. *Bull Menninger Clinic.* 1970;34(6):343–351.

22. Bowman JA. *Recent Experiences in Combat Psychiatry in Viet Nam* (unpublished); 1967. [Full text available as Appendix 11 to this volume.]

23. Kenny WF. Psychiatric disorders among support personnel. *US Army Vietnam Med Bull.* 1967;January/February:34–37.

24. Jones FD. Reactions to stress comparing combat and support troops. Presentation to: World Psychiatric Association; 29 August 1977;

Honolulu, Hawaii. [A summary of the principal study underlying this presentation is available as Appendix 16 to this volume.]

25. Talbott JA. The Saigon warriors during Tet. *US Army Vietnam Med Bull.* 1968;March/April:60–61.

26. Colbach EM. Marijuana use by GIs in Viet Nam. *Am J Psychiatry.* 1971;128(2):204–207.

27. Imahara J. In: Colbach EM. Marijuana use by GIs in Viet Nam. *Am J Psychiatry.* 1971;128:204–207.

28. Bloch HS. Army clinical psychiatry in the combat zone: 1967–1968. *Am J Psychiatry.* 1969;126(3):289–298.

29. Bey DR. *Division Psychiatry in Vietnam* (unpublished), copy provided to author.

30. Ratner RA. Unpublished journal, unnumbered pages, copy provided to author.

31. Fisher HW. Vietnam psychiatry. Portrait of anarchy. *Minn Med.* 1972;55(12):1165–1167.

32. Cahalan D, Cisin IH, Crossley HM. *American Drinking Practices: A National Study of Drinking Behavior and Attitudes.* New Brunswick, NJ: Rutgers Center of Alcohol Studies; 1969.

33. Cahalan D, Cisin IH, Gardner GL. *Drinking Practices and Problems in the US Army, 1972.* Washington, DC: GPO; 1972. Report No. 73-6. [Available at: Alexandria, Va: Defense Technical Information Center. Document No. AD A0763851.]

34. Goodwin DW, Davis DH, Robins LN. Drinking amid abundant illicit drugs. The Vietnam case. *Arch Gen Psychiatry.* 1975;32(2):230–233.

35. Robins LN. The interaction of setting and predisposition in explaining novel behavior: drug initiations before, in, and after Vietnam. In: Kandel E, ed. *Longitudinal Research in Drug Use: Empirical Findings and Methodological Issues.* Washington, DC: Hemisphere and Wiley; 1978: 179–196.

36. Rothberg JM. Alcoholism and the US Army (letter). *NEJM.* 1976;294(6):343.

37. Richard Nixon: "Special Message to the Congress on Drug Abuse Prevention and Control," 17 June 1971. Peters G, Woolley JT. *The American Presidency Project.* http://www.presidency.ucsb.edu/ws/?pid=3048. Accessed 30 July 2013.

38. Hauschild TB. Marijuana. *Mil Med.* 1971;136(2):105–109.

39. Johnson A, O'Rourke K. Drug rehabilitation in the combat zone. *Mil Med.* 1974;139(5):362–366.

40. Perkins ME. Opiate addiction and military psychiatry to the end of World War II. *Mil Med.* 1974;139(2):114–116.

41. Froede RC, Stahl CJ. Fatal narcotism in military personnel. *J Forensic Sci.* 1971;16(2):199–218.

42. Rock NL. Treatment program for military personnel with alcohol problems (unpublished). 1973.

43. Ratner RA. Drugs and despair in Vietnam. *U Chicago Magazine.* 1972;64:15–23.

44. Lipsman S, Doyle E, and the editors of Boston Publishing Co. *The Vietnam Experience: Fighting For Time.* Boston, Mass: Boston Publishing Co; 1983.

45. Manning FJ. Morale and cohesion in military psychiatry. In: Jones FD, Sparacino LR, Wilcox VL, Rothberg JM, eds. *Military Psychiatry: Preparing in Peace for War.* In: Zajtchuk R, Bellamy RF, eds. *Textbooks of Military Medicine.* Washington, DC: Department of the Army, Office of The Surgeon General, Borden Institute; 1994: 1–18.

46. Prugh GS. *Law at War: Vietnam 1964–1973.* Washington, DC: GPO; 1975.

47. Fidaleo RA. Marijuana: social and clinical observations. *US Army Vietnam Med Bull.* 1968;March/April:58–59.

48. Master FD. Some clinical observations of drug abuse among GI's in Vietnam. *J Ky Med Assoc.* 1971;69(3):193–195.

49. Steinbeck J IV. The importance of being stoned in Vietnam. *Washingtonian Magazine.* January 1968: 33–35, 56, 58, 60.

50. Postel WB. Marijuana use in Vietnam: a preliminary report. *US Army Vietnam Med Bull.* 1968;September/October:56–59.

51. Mirin SM, McKenna GJ. Combat zone adjustment: the role of MJ [marijuana] use. *Mil Med.* 1975;140(7):482–485.

52. Talbott JA, Teague JW. Marihuana psychosis. Acute toxic psychosis associated with the use of Cannabis derivatives. *JAMA.* 1969;210(2):299–302.

53. Roffman RA. *Vietnam* (unpublished memoir), copy provided to author.

54. Roffman RA. Unpublished material ("Marijuana Use Survey of Confinees in the Army Stockade at Long Binh") discussed in: Roffman RA, Sapol E. Marijuana in Vietnam: a survey of use among Army enlisted men in the two southern Corps. *Int J Addict.* 1970;5(1); 1–42.

55. Talbott JA. Pot reactions. *US Army Vietnam Med Bull.* 1968;January/February:40–41.

56. Heiman EM. Marihuana precipitated psychoses in patients evacuated to CONUS. *US Army Vietnam Med Bull.* 1968;May/June:75–77.

57. Department of Defense. General Order No. 33, 1968. In: Roffman RA, Sapol E. Marijuana in Vietnam: a survey of use among Army enlisted men in the two Southern Corps. *Intl J Addict.* 1970;5:9.

58. Casper E, Janacek J, Martinelli H Jr. Marijuana in Vietnam. *US Army Vietnam Med Bull.* 1968;September/October:60–72.

59. Colbach EM, Crowe RR. Marihuana associated psychosis in Vietnam. *Mil Med.* 1970;135(7):571–573.

60. Colbach EM, Willson SM. The binoctal craze. *US Army Vietnam Med Bull.* 1969;March/April:40–44.

61. Forrest DV. Marijuana to heroin . . . A missing link? [letter]. *Am J Psychiatry.* 1970;127:704–706.

62. Stanton MD. Drug use in Vietnam. A survey among Army personnel in the two northern corps. *Arch Gen Psychiatry.* 1972;26(3):279–286.

63. Bey DR, Zecchinelli VA. Marijuana as a coping device in Vietnam. *Mil Med.* 1971;136(5):448–450.

64. Kaplan JH. Marijuana and drug abuse in Vietnam. *Ann N Y Acad Sci.* 1971;191:261–269.

65. Treanor JJ, Skripol JN. Marijuana in a tactical unit in Vietnam. *US Army Vietnam Med Bull.* 1970;July/August:29–37.

66. Pietropinto A. Quoted in: Hauschild TB. Marijuana. *Mil Med.* 1971;136(2):105–109.

67. GIs called 'pot users' in Vietnam. *US Medicine.* 1 April 1970:7.

68. Holloway HC, Angel CR, Bardill DR and the members of Work Unit 032. Drug abuse in military personnel. In: *Annual Progress Report, 1972.* Washington, DC: Walter Reed Army Institute of Research; 1972: 1185–1201.

69. Holloway HC. Epidemiology of heroin dependency among soldiers in Vietnam. *Mil Med.* 1974;139(2):108–113.

70. Siegel AJ. The heroin crisis among US forces in Southeast Asia. An overview. *JAMA.* 1973;223(11):1258–1261.

71. Cookson P. Unpublished information cited in: Holloway HC. Epidemiology of heroin dependency among soldiers in Vietnam. *Mil Med.* 1974;139:108–113.

72. Char J. Drug abuse in Vietnam. *Am J Psychiatry.* 1972;129(4):463–465.

73. Budney AJ, Roffman R, Stephens RS, Walker D. Marijuana dependence and its treatment. *Addict Sci Clin Pract.* 2007;4(1):4–16.

74. Zinberg NE. Rehabilitation of heroin users in Vietnam. *Contemp Drug Problems.* 1972;1(2):263–294.

75. US Department of the Army. *Drug Abuse (Clinical Recognition and Treatment, Including the Diseases Often Associated).* December 1972. Technical Bulletin No. 280.

76. Westin AV, Shaffer S. *Heroes and Heroin: The Shocking Story of Drug Addiction in the Military—and Its Impact on Society.* New York, NY: Pocket Books; 1972.

77. Ives JO, Army psychiatrist in Vietnam. Personal communication, July 2011.

78. Braumoeller FL, Terry JG. Nalline: an aid in detecting narcotic users. *Calif Med.* 1956;85(5):299–301.

79. Camp NM. Report of activities of the 98th Med Det (KO) for the six months ending 31 Dec 1970. [Full text available as Appendix 1 to this volume.]

80. Anonymous quote to the author, 15 September 2008.

81. Baker SL Jr. US Army heroin abuse identification program in Vietnam: implications for a methadone program. *Am J Public Health.* 1972;62(6):857–860.

82. Murphy M. When 30,000 GIs are using heroin, how can you fight a war? *Drug Forum.* 1971;1:87–98.

83. Holloway HC. CINCPAC Study for Evaluation of PACOM Drug Abuse Treatment/Rehabilitation Programs–Interim Report (1 September, 1971). [Abbreviated text available as Appendix 18 to this volume.]

84. Holloway HC. Profile of the military drug addict. Proceedings of Army World Wide Drug Abuse Conference, Fort McNair, Washington, DC, 27–29 September 1971.

85. Provided by Francis J Mulvihill Jr, MD (formerly assigned to the 67th Evacuation Hospital, Qui Nhon, September 1970–June 1971), 1983.

86. Ramos FE, Kruzich DJ. A survey of heroin users in Vietnam (unpublished); 15 April 1971.

87. Kruzich DJ. Army drug use in Vietnam: origins of the problem and official response (unpublished); May 1979.

88. Lloyd SJ Jr, Frates RC Jr, Domer DC. A clinical evaluation of 81 heroin addicts in Vietnam. *Mil Med*. 1973;138(5):298–300.

89. Joseph BS. Lessons on heroin abuse from treating users in Vietnam. *Hosp Community Psychiatry*. 1974;25(11):742–744.

90. Golosow N, Childs A. The soldier addict: a new battlefield casualty. *Int J Addict*. 1973;8(1):1–12.

91. Wilbur RS. The battle against drug dependency within the military. *J Drug Issues*. 1974;4(1):11–31.

92. Special Action Office for the National Drug Abuse Prevention Program. As reported in: Baker SL. US Army heroin abuse identification program in Vietnam: implications for a methadone program. *Am J Public Health*. 1972;62(6):859.

93. Robins LN. A follow-up study of Vietnam veterans' drug use: the transition to civilian life. *J Drug Issues*. 1974(4):61–63.

94. Stanton MD. Drugs, Vietnam, and the Vietnam veteran: an overview. *Am J Drug Alcohol Abuse*. 1976;3(4):557–570.

95. Zinberg NE. Heroin use in Vietnam and the United States. A contrast and critique. *Arch Gen Psychiatry*. 1972;26(5):486–488.

96. Drug center opens at Long Binh. *Army Reporter*. 25 October 1971:4.

97. Stanton SL. *The Rise and Fall of an American Army: US Ground Forces in Vietnam, 1965–1973*. Novato, Calif: Presidio Press; 1985.

98. Jones FD. Disorders of frustration and loneliness. In: Jones FD, Sparacino LR, Wilcox VL, Rothberg JM, Stokes JW, eds. *War Psychiatry*. In: Zajtchuk R, Bellamy RF, eds. *Textbooks of Military Medicine*. Washington, DC: Department of the Army, Office of The Surgeon General, Borden Institute; 1995:63–83.

99. Kolb D, Nail RL, Gunderson EK. Differences in family characteristics of heroin injectors and inhalers. *J Nerv Ment Dis*. 1974;158(6):446–449.

100. DeHart RL, Sorrentino JP. Experience with drug abuse. *Mil Med*. 1973;138(5):294–297.

101. Kojak G Jr, Canby JP. Personality and behavior patterns of heroin-dependent American servicemen in Thailand. *Am J Psychiatry*. 1975;132(3):246–250.

102. Nelson KE. Quoted in: Bentel DJ, Crim D, Smith DE. Drug abuse in combat: the crisis of drugs and addiction among American troops in Vietnam. *J Psychedelic Drugs*. 1971;4:23–30.

103. Nelson KE, Panzarella J. *Preliminary Findings—Prevalence of Drug Use in Enlisted Vietnam Returnees Processing for ETS Separation, Oakland Overseas Processing Center*. Presidio, San Francisco, Calif: Letterman General Hospital; March 1971. Report for Department of the Army. [Final report available at: Alexandria, Va: Defense Technical Information Center. Document No. AD A743162.]

104. Robins LN, Helzer JE, Davis DH. Narcotic use in southeast Asia and afterward. An interview study of 898 Vietnam returnees. *Arch Gen Psychiatry*. 1975;32(8):955–961.

105. Helzer JE, Robins LN, Davis DH. Antecedents of narcotic use and addiction. A study of 898 Vietnam veterans. *Drug Alcohol Depend*. 1976;1(3):183–190.

106. Frenkel SI, Morgan DW, Greden JF. Heroin use among soldiers in the United States and Vietnam: a comparison in retrospect. *Int J Addict*. 1977;12(8):1143–1154.

107. Kuzmarov J. *The Myth of the Addicted Army: Vietnam and the Modern War on Drugs*.

Amherst and Boston, Mass: University of Massachusetts Press; 2009.

108. Holloway HC, Sodetz FJ, Elsmore TF and the members of Work Unit 102. Heroin dependence and withdrawal in the military heroin user in the US Army, Vietnam. In: *Annual Progress Report, 1973*. Washington, DC: Walter Reed Army Institute of Research; 1973: 1244–1246.

109. Howe RC, Hegge FW, Phillips JL. Acute heroin abstinence in man, I: Changes in behavior and sleep. *Drug Alcohol Depend*. 1980;5(5):341–356.

110. Howe RC, Hegge FW, Phillips JL. Acute heroin abstinence in man, II: Alterations in rapid eye movement (REM) sleep. *Drug Alcohol Depend*. 1980;6(3):149–161.

111. Robinson MG, Howe RC, Varni JG, Ream NW, Hegge FW. Assessment of pupil size during acute heroin withdrawal in Viet Nam. *Neurology*. 1974;24(8):729–732.

112. Bourne PG. *Men, Stress, and Vietnam*. Boston, Mass: Little, Brown; 1970.

113. Sanders CR. Doper's wonderland: functional drug use by military personnel in Vietnam. *J Drug Issues*. 1973;3:65–78.

114. Bentel DJ, Crim D, Smith DE. Drug abuse in combat: the crisis of drugs and addiction among American troops in Vietnam. *J Psychedelic Drugs*. 1971;4:23–30.

115. Hampton PT, Vogel DB. Personality characteristics of servicemen returned from Viet Nam identified as heroin abusers. *Am J Psychiatry*. 1973;130(9):1031–1032.

116. Nace EP, O'Brien CP, Mintz J, Ream NW, Myers AL. Drinking problems among Vietnam veterans. *Curr Alcohol*. 1977;2:35–324.

117. Solomon R. The rise and fall of the Laotian and Vietnamese opiate trades. *J Psychedelic Drugs*. 1979;11(3):159–171.

118. Tureen LL, Stein M. The base section psychiatric hospital. In: Hanson FR, ed. *Combat Psychiatry*. Washington, DC: US Government Printing Office; 1949: 105–134.

119. Harris FG. Some comments on the differential diagnosis and treatment of psychiatric breakdowns in Korea. *Proceedings of Course on Recent Advances in Medicine and Surgery*. Army Medical Service Graduate School. Washington, DC: Walter Reed Army Medical Center; 30 April 1954: 390–402.

120. Lee RA. The army "mutiny" of 1946. *J Am History*. 1966;53(3):555–571.

121. Ingraham LH. "The Nam" and "The World." Heroin use by US Army enlisted men serving in Vietnam. *Psychiatry*. 1974;37(2):114–128.

122. Imahara JK. Quoted in: Allerton WS, Forrest DV, Anderson JR, et al. Psychiatric casualties in Vietnam. In: Sherman LJ, Caffey EM Jr. *The Vietnam Veteran in Contemporary Society: Collected Materials Pertaining to the Young Veterans*. Washington, DC: Veterans Administration; 1972: sec. III: 54–59.

123. Linden E. The demoralization of an army: fragging and other withdrawal symptoms. *Saturday Rev*, 8 January 1972:12–17, 55.

124. Baker SL Jr. US Army heroin abuse identification program in Vietnam: implications for a methadone program. *Am J Public Health*. 1972;62(6):857–860.

CHAPTER 10

Preventive Social Psychiatry and Command Consultation: Who Is the Patient— The Soldier or His Military Unit?

. . . [U]nit commanders rely heavily on the psychiatrist to assist them in removing problem [soldiers]. The removal of the characerological is necessary to the functioning of the unit. From one standpoint the referral to the psychiatrist means a breakdown of group integrity. Sometimes it is not clear whether the patient does not feel a part of the group or whether he is not perceived as such. The passive aggressive, of course, was our stock in trade. With these referrals I had to consider whether the referral was honestly made. I think this is an important point because with time people's secret motives become apparent. . . . [For example, it] was quite commonplace for a unit to refer an alcoholic because he had said or done something while under the influence of alcohol. . . . [T]here were many referrals in which the [first] sergeant was angry, felt that he had to do something, and a compromise was to send them to the psychiatrist [as punishment].[1]

Captain Harold SR Byrdy, Division Psychiatrist
1st Cavalry Division (Airmobile)
Vietnam (August 1965–June 1966)

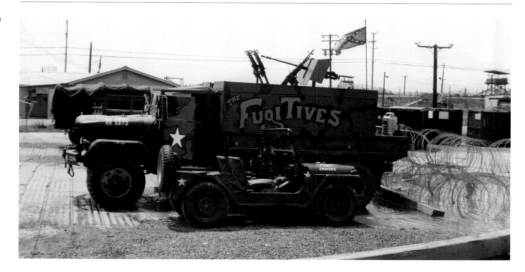

Armed two-and-a-half-ton truck with rebel flag. In this 1971 photograph, both the name on the side of the truck ("The Fugitives") and its Confederate battle flag, which was predictably a racist taunt to black troops, are consistent with the morale and discipline crisis that faced the Army in Vietnam during the last years of the war. Photograph courtesy of Norman M Camp, Colonel, US Army (Retired).

The subject of this chapter—social/community psychiatry, prevention, and command consultation—is a natural extension of the two preceding chapters: Chapter 8, which reviewed the psychiatric problems in Vietnam that were not specifically combat related, especially those associated with the radical decline in soldier morale and discipline, and Chapter 9, which examined the epidemic drug and alcohol problems that evolved. Taken together these two chapters not only described accelerating rates for psychiatric conditions and behavior problems among individual soldiers, but they also indicated that over time a social/institutional crisis developed within the US Army in Vietnam—a dangerous decline in soldier identification with their unit, its members, and its mission, along with a failure of military leaders to devise countermeasures. They also suggested that under those deteriorating circumstances (1) many of the referred soldiers who did not have evident preservice character defects could have been thought of as (combat theater) deployment stress reactions in addition to whatever conventional psychiatric diagnoses they warranted, in order to take into account the unique and generally overwhelming collection of stressful circumstances in the theater; and (2) many of the units from which they were referred could have been thought of as having inverted morale (ie, morale had dropped so low that military "commitment and cohesion" had fragmented and was replaced with cliques based on opposition to military authority as well as heavy drug use and other forms of misconduct and defiance).

After the war some senior psychiatric leaders concluded that the rock-bottom morale and the sheer volume of psychiatric and drug abuse casualties jeopardized combat readiness in Vietnam as much as the high incidence of combat stress casualties in earlier wars.[2] Military psychiatry planners certainly did not anticipate this outcome in the years preceding the war. In fact, they were quite confident about the future based on the cross-fertilization that had developed between the traditional principles of military psychiatry, which were reviewed in earlier chapters, and the growing community psychiatry movement (also referred to as social psychiatry) in civilian psychiatry[3–6]—a movement that was shifting psychiatry away from its traditional emphasis on individual psychopathology to one that identified the patient as someone who was unable to adapt because of a pathological transaction with his "community." This new model suggested that the most effective military psychiatrist was somewhat less involved in providing traditional direct services to the symptomatic soldier (ie, through diagnosis and treatment) and more involved in providing indirect services (ie, through supervision and consultation) to those individuals, especially military leaders, who could have a wider effect on soldier maladjustment and associated social/community failures. As it turned out, the Vietnam War presented a rich opportunity to test this model.

This chapter explores the available psychiatric literature pertaining to mental health consultation/liaison with healthcare providers, commanders, and other military leaders in Vietnam. Regarding command consultation specifically, it also draws from the Walter Reed Army Institute of Research (WRAIR) psychiatrist survey data in an attempt to fill in missing information.

BACKGROUND

In the decade between the Korean War and the Vietnam War, Army Regulation (AR) 40-216, *Medical Service: Neuropsychiatry* (dated 18 June 1959)—the Army regulation governing psychiatric care—was issued, which directed psychiatrists and allied mental health professionals to aid command in conserving the mental health of Army personnel.[7] This regulation further stipulated that the responsibilities of psychiatrists included the provision of prevention, diagnosis, and treatment of emotional and personality disorders, mental illness, and neurological diseases; specialized leadership for allied health professionals and paraprofessionals; and consultation to commanders regarding factors affecting the morale and mental health of their troops. Within the regulation's directives the primacy of prevention, the idea of the pathologic community and the premium placed on command consultation are distinguishable from direct treatments. These mutually reinforcing elements were drawn from three conceptual streams:

1. preventing the occurrence of conditions is more efficient than treating them after they have formed;
2. utilizing mental health personnel as consultants to military leaders and agencies has more impact in prevention than waiting for cases to arrive at a treatment facility; and
3. within the relatively healthy military population, applying a community psychiatry approach is more effective than one based on individual psychopathology.

Preventive Psychiatry and Military Populations

Even though the concept of prevention in psychiatry sounds intuitive, it can be confusing because the Army has historically considered that all activities of Army psychiatrists fall into one of three levels of prevention: primary, secondary, and tertiary, a concept that was borrowed from civilian psychiatry.[8]

Primary Psychiatric Prevention

Primary psychiatric prevention refers to efforts designed to reduce the generation of psychiatric conditions through advice to military leaders regarding overall morale and stress reduction. This is true prevention and takes the form of program-centered command consultation. According to Brigadier General William C Menninger, senior Army psychiatrist and Psychiatric Consultant to the Surgeon General of the Army during World War II,

> The most important functions of military psychiatry are primary preventive: to give counsel and advice regarding the attitude of military men toward their jobs; to minimize environmental stresses which tend to impair the efficiency of the personality; [and] to increase environmental supports to the personality.[9(p337)]

More about command consultation will follow.

Secondary Psychiatric Prevention

Secondary psychiatric prevention refers to early intervention and treatment designed to minimize symptoms for affected soldiers, with the goal being that of the prevention of greater disability. The model of secondary prevention would include the Army's traditional doctrine for management and treatment of combat stress casualties, which was reviewed in Chapter 7 (ie, proximity, immediacy, expectation, and simplicity, also known as "PIES"). To reiterate, this doctrine emphasizes the principles of prompt treatment of the symptomatic soldier as near his unit and the fighting as possible ("proximity" and "immediacy"), coupled with a treatment approach that encourages him to adapt to his combat environment and circumstance and reinforces his identify as a soldier and his loyalty to his military comrades ("simplicity" and "expectancy"). In instances when treatment personnel have established a liaison with an affected soldier's command cadre, this has been referred to as case-centered command consultation.

Tertiary Psychiatric Prevention

Tertiary psychiatric prevention refers to the treatment of psychiatrically disabled soldiers out of their duty setting, as in hospitals or other medical treatment facilities, with the goal being that of rapid recovery and return to duty function and the prevention of chronic disability.

Joining Community Psychiatry and Military Psychiatry

Since World War I and World War II, Army psychiatry has emphasized the importance of psychiatrists and allied mental health personnel developing an active liaison with unit commanders. Appreciation of the importance of the soldier's (small) group in stress reduction derived especially from experience in World War II. The following are conclusions drawn by Menninger:

> The psychiatrist who worked in the field had to know the Army and its mission; he had to be able to identify himself closely with the Army; he had to reorient from his interest in treating one person to the prevention of mental ill health in groups; he had to attempt to apply the best of his psychiatric knowledge to the social situation in which he worked.[9(p487)]

Also, according to Albert J Glass, senior Army psychiatrist and military psychiatry historian, the most important psychiatric problems in military populations—again, with the model being that of combat breakdown—were "situationally induced emotional disorders" (in contrast to endogenously derived civilian disorders). He wrote:

> The most significant contribution of WW II [World War II] psychiatry was recognition of mutually supportive influences by participants in combat or other stress situations. WW II clearly showed that interpersonal relationships and other external circumstances were at least as important as personality configuration or the assets and liabilities of the individual in the effectiveness of coping behavior. For example, the frequency of psychiatric casualties seemed to be more related to the characteristics of the group than the character traits of the individual . . . [ie,] the social determinants of adaptation.[10(p507)]

Incorporation of the community psychiatry perspective—one that located the symptomatic individual within his social and circumstantial context—was defined more broadly during the Korean War to include the causes of other types of soldier symptoms that might come from dysfunctional groups or units.[4] The community psychiatry model was found to be especially apropos both because military populations are composed of relatively psychologically healthy individuals, and because the military is a closed social system, that is, members are not free to quickly move in and out at will as are civilians. Thus behavioral determinants based on personality features, while significant, were believed to rarely be decisive in pathogenesis.[10]

Codification of the command consultation model especially took root when psychiatric expertise was extended to military trainers at stateside posts during World War II through a system of mental health consultation services (MHCS) for the purpose of "aiding newly inducted soldiers to adjust to separation from family, lack of privacy, fragmentation, unaccustomed physical activity and other deprivations and changes incident to the transition from civil to military life."[10(p505)] The MHCS model seemed validated by the fact that psychiatric disability was considerably reduced among the troops served by the new system.[10]

Principles of Command Consultation in the Vietnam Era

Command consultation especially included the process of apprising commanders of factors that reduced soldier morale and motivation—circumstances that often led to psychiatric conditions and discipline problems, in other words, primary prevention.[11] It also included (as secondary prevention) outreach activities that fostered early and more effective intervention for dysfunctional soldiers: the case-centered consultation. To mediate between the soldier and his primary group, that is, his enlisted cohorts as well as his more immediate military leaders, the proficient psychiatric consultant needed to understand the soldier's military environment. Effective consultation also required that the consultant appreciate the fact that the commander was ultimately responsible for the well-being of his troops and retained the prerogative of ignoring the consultant's advice.[12] According to AR 40-216, *Medical Service: Neuropsychiatry*:

> The majority of factors which affect the mental health and morale of troops fall within the responsibility of command, [for example], providing proper leadership, training, assignment, reassignment, incentive, motivation, rest, recreation, and elimination of the unsuitable, inept, and the unfit.[7(§1,3b(1),p1)]

Particularly useful in program consultation would be an epidemiological or public health perspective involving collecting and monitoring various data pertaining to problematic behaviors that may signal lowered morale. Examples would include rising rates for disciplinary incidents, trainee maladjustment, accidents, diseases, and other indicators of unit and individual dysfunction. Regarding accidents and diseases, certain actions, or inactions, by soldiers that increase their odds of having these can represent conscious or unwitting efforts to exempt themselves from participating in combat, that is, as "voluntary casualties"[13(p52)] (similar to Jones' "evacuation syndrome"—soldiers who are motivated to manipulate the system to get relief from foreign deployment and, perhaps, combat risks[14]). And the onus is on command to prevent of all of these. Thus through the epidemiologic approach, the consultant could provide a commander guidance regarding military policies and planning, screening, indoctrination and training, physical conditioning, morale and leadership, enhancement of social supports, and even decisions surrounding combat tactics.[15–17] Although it was difficult to prove that earlier prevention efforts produced favorable results, a wide-ranging review of existing programs among all service branches by the Group for the Advancement of Psychiatry in 1960 concluded that soldier ineffectiveness had been reduced, even if there was not evidence to indicate that emotional difficulties had been reduced.[18]

VIETNAM

As noted in Chapter 3, specific guidelines regarding the provision of psychiatric services for Army personnel operating in the combat theater of South Vietnam was contained in US Army Republic of Vietnam (USARV) Regulation 40-34, *Medical Services: Mental Health and Neuropsychiatry*[19] (Appendix 2 to this volume). This regulation served to reinforce and extend the principles found in the aforementioned Army regulation, AR 40-216, pertaining to psychiatric care, and both had been influenced by the preventive/community psychiatry movement in civilian and military psychiatry. USARV Regulation 40-34 indicated that the function of the mental hygiene unit was to prevent psychiatric problems from arising, as well as treat them if they did. Consultation with unit commanders was to be emphasized over direct psychiatric care. When direct treatment was necessary, outpatient management was preferred to inpatient management, if at all possible. These stipulations were consistent with the Army's belief that the soldier's unit had greater ability to help him recover than did a psychiatric treatment facility, and that it was the mental health consultant's role to help the commander "improve his influence on the members of the unit. . . ."[19(¶4a,p2)] In this regard commanders were urged to monitor various indicators of failing unit morale (ie, rising rates of "accidents, security breaches, disciplinary actions, racial incidents, drug and alcohol abuse, drunkenness, [and] apathy and other defective attitudes"[19(¶3e,p1)]).

USARV Regulation 40-34 reiterated the fact that the commander was primarily responsible for the management of the personnel within his unit to include "effective human relations among individuals and groups."[19(¶3a,p1)] To accomplish this he needed to have:

> . . . facility in the management of groups; which implies experience with the use and effects of rivalry among groups, the development of informal cliques and group pressures, the social uses and dangers of scape-goating and hero-making, and methods of integrating soldiers into the group as members who render useful duty, whether as close-knit buddies or isolates.[19(¶3c,p1)]

Psychiatrist Preparation

During the war newly commissioned psychiatrists attended the medical officer's basic training at the Medical Field Service School (MFSS) and received the handout "Introduction to Military Psychiatry." This document reminded participants of the often-dangerous circumstances faced by soldiers and informed them of the fact that the soldier's commanding officer was primarily responsible for his mental health. It also encouraged them to expand their etiologic considerations for soldiers to include pathogenic social dynamics:

> In the highly integrated social system of the Army, the early detection of emotional problems and mental illness has special significance. The close association and inter-dependence that is characteristic of the system make the epidemiology of psychiatric symptoms a more urgent consideration. The capability of soldiers to employ tremendously destructive forces also adds to the requirement for early recognition.

> Since mental health is a command responsibility, detection of severe emotional problems is also a necessary part of this obligation . . . and employing such resources for the early detection of mental illness is a function of the psychiatric service.

> *Psychiatric symptoms and emotional problems are not the exclusive property of the individual but are the result of a transaction or process with the environment* [emphasis added]. Consequently, the problem may often be dealt with as a problem of this transaction, or of the environment, rather than as a problem of individual pathology. In the latter instance, the emphases should be on evaluation of what is going on between the soldier and his environment, and [as treatment], environmental manipulation may have its greatest effectiveness—to reestablish a more healthy communication. Many times the group focuses its problems on a scapegoat. Other times poor management makes simple problems complex; malassignment and utilization are not especially rare and unit leaders have been known to be sadistic or inept. The question often arises as to who has the problem? Over and over again, the troubled soldier is a symptom of the pathology of the group, poor leadership, or detrimental policies or procedures. [Consequently] the psychiatrist must be thoroughly familiar with [the soldier's] "community."[20(pp2–3)]

Finally, to be an effective consult/liaison psychiatrist in the context of the Army, participants in the medical officer's basic training at MFSS were instructed to be fully aware of "any situation concerning policy, procedure, or practice within an organization or between organizational elements in which human behavior was a principle concern."[20(p11)]

Obstacles in Providing Command Consultation

On a practical basis, several potential problems existed for the psychiatrist who would undertake to provide program-centered and case-centered command consultation in Vietnam.

Inaccessibility of Senior Commanders to Psychiatric Opinion

As Army Regulation 40-216 indicated, division psychiatrists were not on the commander's staff but on that of the division surgeon:

[The Army psychiatrist was] to *assist the surgeon in advising the commander* [emphasis added] in matters pertaining to the morale of troops and the impact of current policies upon the psychological effectiveness of troops.[7(p1)]

This meant that organizationally he was not in a position to directly address command but was required to pass his advice through the division surgeon, who may or may not agree. It is uncertain from the available literature from Vietnam whether deployed division psychiatrists felt stymied by not having direct access to division commanders, but Colonel Clotilde D Bowen's End of Tour Report (Appendix 14 to this volume) from the period 1970 to 1971 did include the recommendation that the (staff) status of the division psychiatrist be elevated to that of the division surgeons. This suggested that there was a tendency for division surgeons to oppose or minimize the influence of their division psychiatrists.

In a similar vein, throughout the war mental health specialists had no direct organizational connection to the commanders of nondivisional combat and noncombat support units. Furthermore, no organizational modifications in this misalignment were made, even though they outnumbered the troops in the divisions by a factor of 2 to 3 and it was becoming increasingly apparent that support troops were sustaining higher psychiatric casualty rates.

Opposition of Commanders to Programmatic Psychiatric Attention

A subtle and usually not acknowledged factor is that many line commanders have a tendency to be wary of psychiatric input because they believe it has the potential to "weaken the fighting man."[21(p154)] By way of illustration, midway through the war, an article was published in *Military Medicine* and disseminated in Vietnam through the *USARV Medical Bulletin* by General William Westmoreland, the commander of the armed forces in Vietnam (US Military Assistance Command, Vietnam or USMACV) entitled "Mental Health—An Aspect of Command." Amidst General Westmoreland's otherwise encouragement of commanders to utilize behavioral science theory and military mental health support, he included this curious and clearly ambivalent passage:

Your psychiatrist should be encouraged to socialize every opportunity they get with the commander, the lower unit commanders and the other members of the staff. Let them see he is not the "weirdo" the comic books sometimes lead us to believe. Frankly, some commanders and many soldiers are leery of anyone or thing that smacks of "head shrinking." The psychiatrists I have met appear to be ordinary fellows (although I am not a psychiatrist) who do have specialized skills and knowledge and are trying to contribute to the conservation and utilization of manpower.[12(p213)]

Insufficient Preparation and Training in Command Consultation

A large proportion of the psychiatrists in Vietnam had no working familiarity with the Army before their assignment. As noted in Chapter 5, during the first half of the war, almost a quarter of psychiatrists arrived in Vietnam shortly after completing their civilian residency training. In the second half of the war, the percentage jumped to over half. Furthermore, the program at the MFSS, where they received their initial Army training prior to their first assignment, included neither instruction nor training as to how to obtain entrée to a unit as a consultant. As noted by McCarroll et al, development of command consultation skills requires an apprenticeship under an experienced psychiatrist.[21] In addition, the WRAIR survey data indicated that roughly half of the participants began their assignment in Vietnam with no overlap with the psychiatrist whom they had replaced. In an effort to remedy the situation, Lieutenant Colonel Robert L Pettera, a division psychiatrist in Vietnam, published an article in the *USARV Medical Journal* in early 1968 providing very basic advice as to how to develop a dialogue with unit leaders to facilitate primary and secondary command consultation[22]; however, its distribution in Vietnam at the time is uncertain, and it does not appear to have been circulated among the cohorts of replacement psychiatrists in the years that followed.

Case-Centered Command Consultation in Vietnam

Overview

From their vantage point of reviewing the theater-wide trends in Army psychiatry over the first two-thirds of the war, Colbach and Parrish touted the preventive mental health emphasis in Vietnam. However, according to their description, the record seemed mixed. ("Some mental health personnel have been quite effective in going into a unit, finding areas of interpersonal friction and correcting them before members of the unit become psychiatric casualties, [but] in the area of racial problems . . . this technique has been underused."[23(p340)]) In particular they chided the hospital-based psychiatrists for being more like traditional civilian psychiatrists ("hospital- and office-oriented rather than field-oriented"). According to Colbach and Parrish, "The large numbers of small support units have had much less group identity than the combat divisions, and mental health personnel have responded to this in part by staying in their offices. Although there have been exceptions, preventive psychiatry has been at a minimum at this level."[23(p336)]

In fairness to the nondivision psychiatrists, Colbach and Parrish also described how practicing preventive psychiatry in the combat divisions followed easily:

. . . For those [soldiers] returned to duty, follow-up has been easy because of the scattering of mental health personnel throughout the division.

Because of their many contacts throughout the division, mental health personnel at this level are quite adept at preventing problems before they arise. They generally have the power to manipulate the environment in many different ways and probably their main contribution has been in the area of preventive psychiatry.[23(p335)]

Reports From the Field

The psychiatrists' reports (again, almost exclusively from the first half of the war) generally indicated that in the divisions, mental health consultation with battalion surgeons and other medical personnel, as well as with unit leaders, was a regular activity that appeared to effectively reduce psychiatric attrition and morbidity. On the other hand, perhaps validating the observation by Colbach and Parrish, there is little information available to indicate that the psychiatrists with the hospitals and psychiatric specialty detachments functioned similarly. Intriguingly, 15 years after Colbach published with Parrish, he wrote another piece in which he agonized over his experiences in Vietnam:

In fact we did not do a whole lot of command consultation [at the 67th Evacuation Hospital and the 935th Psychiatric Detachment]. Being

hospital based, we were somewhat isolated. Also I don't think we really knew how to do command consultation, and we weren't exactly deluged with request for this from various commanders.[24(p259)]

As for the division psychiatrists, Byrdy, who served with the 1st Cavalry Division during the first year of the war (1965–1966), described feeling uncomfortable in "selling" mental health services to unit commanders ("as though we were drumming up business"[1(p47)]), even though he did take pains to become acquainted with them. In fact, he found some commanders were dismissive based on their prediction that there would be negligible psychiatric casualties in the division because it was Airmobile (and that he and his staff were "unnecessary baggage"). However, once cases began to appear, case-centered command consultation began to follow. ("[M]ore complicated cases were best handled when some closure was affected by personal contact with the unit. This might be a telephone call, a visit by me or the social worker to the CO [commanding officer] or the XO [executive officer], or a visit by a tech."[1(p50)]) But elsewhere he said:

We lacked any substantial follow-up on the execution of our recommendations. Doubtless the percentage of those acted upon is different from that in garrison, but not necessarily much smaller as one might expect. Unit commanders in the field, if they have time for the paper work, are eager to get rid of unpredictable personnel; whereas non-combat commanders, at times, unreasonably discourage the loss of manpower for any reasons, even for the most pressing.[25(p5)]

Over the course of the following year, functional relationships between division psychiatrists and commanders in Vietnam became more fluid, at least the case-centered command consultation approach. Perhaps this occurred because by then the divisions had established their operational bases and patterns of functioning in the novel environment and knew what types of casualties to expect and the value of the mental health advice and support. Captain John A Bostrom, who served with the 1st Cavalry Division a year or so after Byrdy (1967–1968), touted the unit consultation approach they utilized, but he did not mention primary prevention. He used two hypothetical case examples (one a soldier with psychosomatic back pain and the

---

EXHIBIT 10-1. Command (Program) Consultation to a Combat Unit by an Enlisted Social Work/Psychology Technician

This is Part 2 of a set of observations by Specialist 6th Class Dennis L Menard, an enlisted social work/psychology technician, from his consultation work with a 1st Infantry Division battalion in November 1967. This was undertaken because of an unusually high mental hygiene referral rate, and it entailed a week-long study of "the morale, interactions of the men, and the difficulties of the unit in the combat situation." (Part 1: Troop Living Conditions in the Field is in Chapter 1, Exhibit 1-2.)

[Besides the high mental health referral rate], the courts martial rate was very high . . . about 15 in the past month. Offenses included AWOL [absent without leave] and desertion, disobeying movement orders, refusal to go on ambush patrol or listening post, and careless handling of weapons resulting in personal injuries.

Consultation with a platoon leader was made about his relationships with the men . . . concerning how a good, confidence-inspiring leader can function on the level of his men [so as to] build trust, respect and friendship. This platoon leader does try to work and play with his men, and he avoids appearing that he is a rigid, aloof, and a demanding type of officer. He offered an explanation for some of the battalion's problems. It has had three commanding officers in the past 8 months. The first was described as very aggressive, aloof, and "hard core"; trying to make garrison troops of his men and following regulations to the letter. The men disliked him and his policies. The second commander was portrayed as just the opposite . . . a passive leader who was not a good decision maker. The men feared his shortcomings, which generated mistrust and low morale. The new commander is a young "Kennedy type." He is a dynamic, knowledgeable, and inspiring leader who makes sound tactical decisions. In addition, he lends an ear to his more experienced and proven officers and allows them to advise and suggest. He insists on discipline and has been "cracking down," giving Articles 15 and Courts Martial like they were "going out of style." But the men are somewhat apprehensive about him; fearing him as the unknown. Will he get them in more trouble . . . more inappropriate fire fights? Can he handle a crisis situation? From the standpoint of the average soldier . . . they consider him still unproven and are waiting and testing.

In general, soldiers bitch a lot when frequent moves require work . . . digging in, filling sandbags, etc. Nerves get tense and emotions reach explosive heights, and the men find it hard to take orders. Men complain in all wars about improper dissemination of information. Just not being informed about movements and operations may generate fear and dissension.

In the past there seemed to be a low morale in this battalion stemming from bad leadership, lack of faith in commanding officers, lack of identification with their unit, which resulted in an "I don't give a damn" attitude. This attitude can, of course, be a foundation for ineffectiveness and a low fighting spirit as exemplified in a high sick call rate prior to an operation and general shamming [pretending activity but without productivity] type complaints just before a patrol. If the morale is low and the men can find an escape, they tend to direct their efforts at avoiding duty. Of prime importance is the fact that any type of manipulating or "a way out" must be avoided and stopped as near the front as possible. Too many people being sent back for administrative or marginal sick call complaints tend to be detrimental to the "hardcore" soldier.

Conclusions: (1) Lack of confidence from past leaders. (2) Apprehension about the new battalion commander. (3) Irregularities in the battalion aid station felt to be the responsibility of the MSC [Medical Service Corps] officer. This promoted shamming and compromised medical care within the battalion. Results: The Division Psychiatrist made a field visit to check out the above formulation. As the Battalion Commander was so new, it was decided to pass over those aspects of the morale situation due to change in command. Regarding the problems at the aid station though, the Division Psychiatrist spent time with the Battalion Surgeon reviewing the administrative aspects of his job and discussing ways in which the MSC Officer had contributed to the aid station's problems [*Camp—ie, resulting in "evacuation syndromes"*]. The Battalion Surgeon "took charge" of the situation, which has since ceased to be a problem.

Source: Menard DL. The social work specialist in a combat division. *US Army Vietnam Med Bull.* 1968;(March/April):56–57.

---

other a "troublemaker") to demonstrate the effective use of case-centered unit consultation by his enlisted social work/psychology technicians.[26] That same year, Captain Gerald Motis with the 4th Infantry Division (ID), described an ambitious and effective program of forward-deployed enlisted social work/psychology

technicians whom he supervised regularly in the field, but apparently their consultation efforts were mostly with the battalion surgeons.[27]

The aforementioned article by Pettera was especially descriptive regarding the field consultation and treatment program implemented in the 9th ID the same year as

Bostrom and Motis.[22] He estimated that through their preventive approach they reduced psychiatric attrition in the division by a factor of three to five, but he provided no specifics on primary prevention interventions; his efforts apparently remained mostly centered on the management of emergent cases. Pettera described various types of defensive resistance exhibited by commanders, and he proposed strategies designed to achieve credibility and reduce obstacles to candid dialogue about cases and associated unit problems.[22] However, it must be assumed that Pettera's higher rank (lieutenant colonel) and military background enabled him to much more confidently liaise with the division's command cadres than Byrdy, Bostrom, and Motis (all with the rank of captain), who were civilian-trained psychiatrists.

Finally, Douglas R Bey, the division psychiatrist for the 1st ID (April 1969–April 1970) during the transition phase of the war, reported that he and his staff were very active in case-centered consultations with the command cadre who were responsible for the patients they treated (see a summary of Bey's activities in Chapter 3).

Several Army social work/psychology technicians provided reports indicating that they were very active in case-centered command consultation. Case 7-2 in Chapter 7, Staff Sergeant (SSGT) Victor, treated by SP6 Dennis L Menard (who worked with Edward L Gordon, the division psychiatrist with the 1st ID), illustrated the invaluable role played by that division's social work/psychology technicians in bridging between the symptomatic soldier and his unit's command cadre. In the same respect, Chapter 3 includes descriptions of the work of SP5 David B Stern with the 9th Infantry Division, who described the technician-level psychiatric support he provided to two of the division's combat battalions that were part of the Mobile Riverine Force; SP5 Paul A Bender with the 11th Infantry Brigade (Light), who provided a critical link between the primary care medical system and the division psychiatrist and between the medical and psychiatric system and the soldier's unit; and SP5 Smith, who, with Bey, extended both primary and secondary psychiatric prevention activities to various 1st ID units. (Case 6-11, SP4 Papa, in Chapter 6 demonstrated how Smith provided both therapeutic counseling to a traumatized patient and effective consultation to his unit's command cadre and battalion surgeon.[28(p365)])

Program-Centered Command Consultation in Vietnam

Of course, the individuals who served as Neuropsychiatry Consultant to the Commanding General, US Army, Republic of Vietnam (CG/USARV) Surgeon practiced pure program-centered, command consultation in the course of carrying out their duties. Otherwise, except for the few examples described below, the available professional literature from Vietnam, both from the psychiatrists assigned to the combat divisions and those serving at the hospitals and with the psychiatric specialty detachments, did not document program-centered, primary prevention activities. During the first year of the war, Byrdy, with the 1st Cavalry Division, complained that practical impediments, especially transportation and communication obstacles, doomed his primary prevention efforts. ("The net result was that we responded to crises rather than 'heading them off at the pass.'"[1(p50)]) However, during the ensuing years in Vietnam, additional factors likely served to limit primary prevention activities such as the increased pressure to provide direct treatment of soldiers or supervise allied mental health and medical personnel (for an example, see Alessi in Appendix 9, "Principles of Military Combat Psychiatry").

Program-Centered Command Consultation by Division Mental Health Personnel

Menard, a social work/psychology technician who served with the 1st ID during the peak phase of combat intensity, provided detailed documentation of his unit consultation that was a model of primary prevention activity by an enlisted specialist.[29] According to Menard's report, in November 1967, he spent a week becoming familiar with each company in an infantry battalion in order to search for systemic causes for higher than expected mental health, medical, and disciplinary problems (Exhibit 10-1).

The innovative command-consultation work by Bey and his staff in the 1st ID 2 years later exemplified primary prevention activities by division psychiatry personnel and set a standard in this regard. Their publications are rich in particulars, such as their routine of monitoring selected parameters of the division's battalions (eg, sick call and mental hygiene referrals as well as rates for nonjudicial punishments and courts-martial, Inspector General complaints, accidents, venereal disease, and malaria) in order to select at-risk units for a formal organizational case study and unit

---

EXHIBIT 10-2. Command (Program) Consultation by Division Psychiatry Personnel

This is a postwar account by Douglas R Bey, who served in Vietnam as Division Psychiatrist for the 1st Infantry Division (April 1969–April 1970).

We kept records of our cases and noted that periodically we would receive several referrals from the same unit at approximately the same time. We also monitored the number of chaplain visits, accident rates, sick call rates, mental health visits, Inspector General complaints, Article 15s, court-martials [sic], and malaria rates (this was a command indicator because it reflected unit discipline—if men didn't take their pills as ordered they got malaria). When the stress indicators for a unit increased, we contacted the battalion commander and battalion surgeon about the unit and [made] arrangements to meet and discuss our observations. If command concurred that there were problems in a specific company we would meet with the company commander and the executive officer. If it appeared that further evaluation was warranted, we would interview members of command and assign a [social work/psychology] technician to the unit to live and work with the enlisted men while gathering information about the unit's stresses. Afterwards we would report back to the unit starting at the top in written and oral form. Sometimes we could give specific recommendations to try to help reduce the unit's stress and in other situations, the process itself seemed to help the unit focus on the emotional aspects of the organization and solve the problem.

By graphing the stress indicators for each unit and by going to units to discuss organizational factors that were producing stress within the units we were able to identify a few organizational stress periods. For example, one unit that stood out was a dump truck company that had a high incidence of drug related problems such as referrals to sick call, referrals to psychiatry, arrests, and Article 15s. We consulted with the key members of the company and [social work/psychology technician] Specialist 5th Class Smith stayed with the unit to gather information. He found that the company commander put his own promotion above the welfare of his men and refused to give the men breaks or even Christmas Day off. There was also a chronic shortage of tires and spare parts which motivated drivers to steal the needed equipment from neighboring units. The unit did not have safety cages to protect men working on high pressure tires, and one driver was killed as a result. Armed guards were not provided to protect the truck convoys and drivers had to keep their M-16s in plastic bags to prevent them from getting jammed by dust. The AK-47s used by the VC [Viet Cong] did not jam with dust and the VC would use the dust as cover when mounting ambushes. The drivers were frightened and jumpy and had killed some Vietnamese children who were digging into an old well near the road. Although the children were looking for food and salvageable items in the [Army] trash, the drivers thought they were withdrawing hidden weapons from a cache. Another problem was that the first sergeant of the unit was a chronic alcoholic who was hard on drug users. When the findings, largely obtained from Specialist Smith's investigation, were conveyed to command some positive changes took place. New spare parts and a steel cage were ordered for the unit. The commanding officer was replaced and the first sergeant was medically evacuated for chemical dependency treatment.

Reproduced with permission from: Bey D. *Wizard Six: A Combat Psychiatrist in Vietnam.* College Station, Tex: Texas A & M University Military History Series, 104; 2006: 166–167.

---

consultation (Exhibit 10-2). Particularly notable are their efforts at educating unit commanders and others about special combat group stress points (ie, change of command and the introduction of a new unit member) as well as common stressors affecting individual soldiers (ie, "short-timer's syndrome" and soldiers having less education, being foreign born, or having a language handicap).

With respect to noncombat troops, Bey noticed that the morale of the support unit soldiers appeared to suffer compared to that of the combat troops. When he studied the psychiatric referrals from one support company, he discovered that most had character and behavior problems, and a high percentage were high school dropouts. This led to a morale-boosting collaborative effort with the Army Education Center that helped 26 soldiers pass their general educational development (GED) test.[30]

However, Bey also underscored the potential difficulties in providing primary prevention in a combat division:

From a practical point of view most field units want to get the job done and most [commanders] realize that the psychiatrist probably doesn't know his way around the military and will help him carry out his job. However, unless the psychiatrist has the support of key officers who understand the military

EXHIBIT 10-3. Command (Program) Consultation by Specialized Psychiatric Detachment Personnel

This is an account written by John A Bowman, a military-trained psychiatrist who served in Vietnam as the first commander of the 935th Psychiatric Detachment (KO) near Saigon (December 1965–October 1966).

The area that the 935th [Psychiatric Detachment] moved into [on the large US Army post at Long Binh, 30 miles outside of Saigon] was sparsely populated when we got there (January 1966). There was the 93rd Evac Hospital, the 616th Clearing Company, the 624th Quartermaster Company, 3rd Ordnance, and a few scattered engineer companies up and down the highway. By the time I left a year later, there were 131 different units there. And this necessitated our developing a mental hygiene consultation-type approach. I broke the [psychiatric detachment personnel] into two levels in the two sections in the outpatient clinic. Both were headed by social work officers. One social work officer and several enlisted men would make trips to the nearby military units in jeeps. The reason I say "nearby" is that there were many places which were unsafe to go to; but, to those areas that were unrestricted and to which we had free travel, we would make unit contacts in the field. The second social work officer and other social work specialists worked primarily in the clinic and they saw the many 'walk-ins' there. The reason we had 'walk-ins' was that helicopters were used to transport these patients from outlying units or inaccessible areas and the helicopter would bring 3 or 4 orthopedic or surgical cases to the hospital and also would put a psychiatric case on the helicopter and bring him as well. This worked out quite well for us. In the units that we were able to study in the surrounding area there were a few problems of morale and leadership that were reflected in the rate of psychiatric evaluations. We discovered this by having our men go out to the units. An example was a place at which there was an engineer unit. We were getting a very high rate of referrals from the unit. On a visit our social work officer found that as a matter of routine newly arriving men reporting into that engineer unit would report to the commanding officer. He had footprints drawn on the floor where these men would stand and then he would chew them out. This was on arriving in Vietnam! In working with the commanding officer and trying to help him become less rigid, we were able to lower the referral rate.

    In another unit, a signal unit, we'd got quite a few of their senior-ranking NCOs [noncommissioned officers]. I think that when you get senior-ranking NCOs coming in, it's good evidence that there's something wrong in the unit. Well, what was going on? This was a newly-arrived unit in Vietnam and the commanding officer had posted on the troop bulletin board that he wanted each man to work so hard that at the end of the day he'd be so exhausted that he would never ask for any post pass to go into the nearby town. Then a couple of his men who were on post pass got into difficulty. They were picked up at an Off-limits area, so he said, "From now on post passes are eliminated because I will not give post passes until the men in the unit learn how to deal with the Vietnamese culture and also the American military rules." The men in his unit reacted by saying, "How can we learn about military rules or about the Vietnamese culture unless we're given post passes and are allowed to go out?" Those caught in the middle, the NCOs, were the ones that developed the symptoms. They would come in with depressions, frustrations and anxiety. This was the unit that fell under Second Field Forces (Field Forces II) which had its own medical unit. I was able to work through the Second Field Forces surgeon, working in the field with this signal battalion, until eventually their referral rate fell off.

Source: Bowman JA. In: Johnson AW Jr, Bowman JA, Byrdy HS, Blank AS Jr. Panel Discussion: Army psychiatry in Vietnam. In: Jones FD, ed. *Proceedings: Social and Preventive Psychiatry Course, 1967*. Washington, DC: Government Printing Office; 1968: 63–64. [Available at: Defense Documentation Center, Alexandria, Virginia, Document AD A950058, 1980.]

he is very likely to find himself frustrated and unable to carry out his job. Thanks to the medical officers in our division . . . we did not have these difficulties and in fact can say that no program or effort on our part to provide new programs or additional services to the men in our division were ever thwarted because of red tape or lack of support from the medical battalion.[31(ChapV,pp6–7)]

Although Bey is the only division psychiatrist who described primary prevention as a discrete professional activity,[28,32] it could be said that, apart from some unique preparatory experiences he had before his assignment in Vietnam, he might have had more time for these activities because of the somewhat lower combat intensity by that point in the war.

Program-Centered Command Consultation by Psychiatric Personnel Assigned to the Hospitals and Specialty Detachments

    Exhibit 10-3 provides an example of program consultation during the first year of the war by John A Bowman, an Army-trained psychiatrist, and the personnel assigned to the 935th Psychiatric Detachment.[33]

Bowman's unpublished account of his experience with the 935th team, "Recent Experiences in Combat Psychiatry in Viet Nam," also underscored the clinical importance of a working liaison with the soldier/patient's unit leaders (Appendix 11 to this volume).

Two years after Bowman's year-long rotation was completed, John A Talbott's "community psychiatry" team, which was also based out of the 935th Psychiatric Detachment, offered outreach services and consultation (primary and secondary prevention care) for the USARV Stockade, 10 primary care medical dispensaries, the post chaplains, and commanders, primarily of support units and related agencies, most of which were located on and around the Long Binh post. The team was composed of six mental health professionals (psychiatry, psychology, and social work) and 10 enlisted social work/psychology technicians. They especially targeted units (and their supporting dispensaries) who showed unusually high rates for psychiatric referral, sick call visits, and stockade confinement.

Talbott's team's orientation was community-centered, that is, based on a belief that a soldier's problems often reflected difficulties within the military unit, and they offered recommendations regarding how a unit might better "structure the environmental situation"[34(p1235)] and reduce the incidence of psychiatric conditions and behavior problems. Although there were no outcome measures, the consensus seemed to be that this demonstration project had been effective in reducing case incidence and disability. Of note, however, Talbott added that the "successful practice of community psychiatry required considerable enthusiasm and interest, and persons not interested will not succeed."[34(p1235)]

It is interesting that contemporaneously with Talbott, Jack R Anderson, a Lieutenant Colonel with many years of Army experience and the commanding officer of Talbott's unit, argued that the social psychiatry/unit consultation model had proved only marginally successful in Vietnam compared to the patient-oriented, professional consultation model. However, his focus was on the division psychiatrists, and he opined that they would be more effectively utilized if they were reassigned to the hospitals and psychiatric detachments to provide tertiary echelon care.[35] H Spencer Bloch, who worked with Anderson, seemed to agree that primary prevention efforts proved to be inefficient at best (see Appendix 19, "Psychiatric Consultation in the War Zone: The Professional Consultation Model").

Finally, following his service in Vietnam and his publication (with Johnson) of the overview of the psychiatric problems in the Vietnam War, Jones concluded that primary preventive activities with the noncombat troops was even more important in Vietnam, especially during the drawdown. This was because the types of disorders that typically occur in that population—disaffection, indiscipline, and dysfunction—are more difficult to treat than combat stress disorders. According to Jones, commanders of support units should emphasize discipline and morale-enhancing activities for their troops as well as provide ample recognition of their critical role. In addition, a relationship should be established between support troops and the combat troops they support; and support troops should be allowed temporary assignments to combat units. More controversial, he also posited that disciplinary infractions could be dealt with through *forward* (in the direction of the fighting), rather than rearward, evacuation in order to minimize secondary gain from misconduct.[36] Somewhat in support of Jones, Spector, a military historian, reported that some commanders in Vietnam sought to get support troops more involved in activities related to combat to diffuse these tensions, that is, they were included in reaction squads or perimeter defense, and that this improved morale and lowered the rate of incidents.[37(p55)] However, overall there is no evidence that any of these ideas were institutionalized in Vietnam, and there is no documentation that the deployed psychiatrists were utilized as consultants regarding these matters.

WALTER REED ARMY INSTITUTE OF RESEARCH PSYCHIATRIST SURVEY FINDINGS: COMMAND CONSULTATION/SOCIAL PSYCHIATRY ACTIVITIES IN VIETNAM

The following extends the summary of findings from the 1982 WRAIR postwar survey of Army psychiatrists who served in Vietnam that was begun in Chapter 5. Specifically, it presents findings from responses to survey questions that explored participants' impressions of the extent to which they engaged in command consultation, apparent results, and potential impediments.

Frequency of Command/Program Consultation Efforts and Success

The preceding material highlighted the evident value of command consultation as a means by which

FIGURE 10-1. Estimated frequency of command consultation efforts: mean extent of survey psychiatrists' agreement on 1-to-5 point scale from 1 = very infrequent to 5 = very frequent for three questions [N = 61–83].

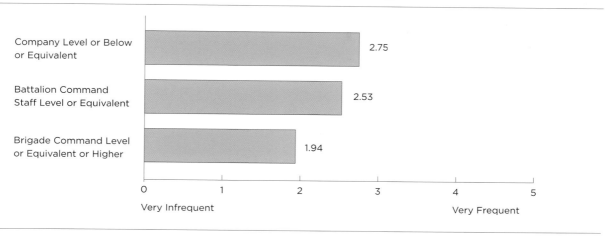

the military psychiatrist or other mental health specialist can apply principles of social/community psychiatry to military groups in order to reduce the occurrence and severity of soldier maladjustment or psychiatric conditions. The WRAIR survey psychiatrists were asked to estimate the frequency of their efforts in command consultation, as well as perceived success, with small (company level or below), medium (battalion command staff level), and large units (brigade command staff level or higher).

Figure 10-1 presents response means from questions regarding survey participants' estimations of the frequency they or their staff made efforts to provide command consultation to units according to three levels of unit size (company or lower, battalion or lower, or brigade or higher). The results suggest a trend in which the higher the level of the command, the less frequently psychiatrists provided command consultation. A similar set of questions asked about frequency of success in command consultation ("perceived some reduction in anticipated psychiatric casualties") for each of these command levels and the results were almost identical to the values for the items regarding frequency of command consultation efforts. Taken together these results suggest that command consultation was a relatively low priority (all means were less than 3), and furthermore, that the results from these activities were uncertain. Indications of low priority are consistent with results presented in Chapter 5, Figure 5-2 showing that survey psychiatrists estimated they devoted a limited percentage of their professional time to command consultation (12.1%

when they served in the combat divisions and 10.7% as hospital psychiatrists).

Survey psychiatrists' answers to four questions (ie, pertaining to their recalled efforts, and to their perceived success, in command consultation with small [company]- and with medium [battalion]-sized units) correlated substantially with each other. These items were subsequently combined into one four-item factor, and a regression analyses was conducted using three principle psychiatrist dichotomous variables: (1) phase of the war served (early vs late); (2) type of assignment in Vietnam (with any combat unit vs only with a hospital); and (3) the presence or absence of pre-Vietnam military experience. (This is a variation on the civilian vs military-trained distinction used in earlier analyses. Participants designated as "military experience" are those who had either Army psychiatric residency training or a military assignment before Vietnam, and those designated as "no military experience" had neither). The regression model included the main effects of these three predictors as well as all first-order interactions between them.

Two statistically significant main effects involving this factor were found and presented in Figures 10-2A and 10-2B (the factor is scaled such that a value of "0" corresponds to average or the "typical" psychiatrist's score). They accounted for 10% of the variation in the "efforts and successes" composite outcome.

Figure 10-2A depicts the relationship between reported frequency and success in command consultation and military experience before assignment in Vietnam. A high score implies greater frequency and greater success

FIGURE 10-2A. Factor analysis results of Survey Psychiatrists' estimates of frequency and success in command consultation, by pre-Vietnam military experience (p <.06). Low score indicates low frequency and success.

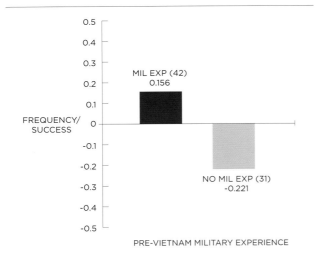

PRE-VIETNAM MILITARY EXPERIENCE

MIL EXP: presence of predeployment military experience (a psychiatrist with either Army psychiatric residency training or a military assignment before Vietnam) (number of respondents)

NO MIL EXP: refers to absence of predeployment military experience (a psychiatrist who had neither Army psychiatric residency training nor a military assignment before Vietnam) (number of respondents)

FIGURE 10-2B. Factor analysis results of Survey Psychiatrists' estimates of frequency and success in command consultation, by assignment type in Vietnam (p <.07). Low score indicates low frequency and success.

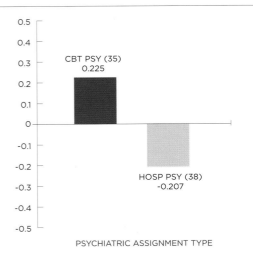

PSYCHIATRIC ASSIGNMENT TYPE

CBT PSY: at least one combat unit assignment in Vietnam (number of respondents)

HOSP PSY: no combat unit assignment in Vietnam (number of respondents)

in command consultation. These results suggest that psychiatrists with military experience before assignment in Vietnam report greater frequency and success in command consultation than do psychiatrists without military experience before assignment in Vietnam. (Psychiatrist rank differences were unlikely to explain these findings and those that follow because, apart from a few exceptions, the "military experience" group generally did not outrank their colleagues who had no pre-Vietnam military experience)

Figure 10-2B similarly depicts the relationship between frequency and success in command consultation and assignment type in Vietnam. These results imply that psychiatrists had greater frequency and success in command consultation if they served in a combat unit assignment as opposed to those who had only hospital assignments.

The higher estimates of perceived efforts and success in command consultation for both of these groups (ie, psychiatrists with either Army psychiatric

residency training or a military assignment before Vietnam and psychiatrists who had at least one combat-unit assignment in Vietnam) appear to coincide with impressions from earlier wars. They suggest that through either of these experiences, the psychiatrists who served in Vietnam were more likely to identify with the military and its goals and more regularly and successfully serve as consultants to commanders (see discussion in Chapter 5).

Factors Perceived as Interfering With Command Consultation Efforts or Success

Survey psychiatrists were also asked to speculate regarding instances when command consultation was not successful. They were asked to indicate the extent of their agreement for a series of forced-choice statements about factors perceived as interfering with command consultation. The results are presented in Table 10-1.

Visual inspection of the findings presented in Table 10-1 indicates that the majority of means for individual items lie just above the midpoint of the response scale

TABLE 10-1. Factors Perceived as Interfering With Command Consultation

Factors Interfering With Command Consultation	Mean
(8) Leaders were not receptive to inquiry and advice from outside of their chain of command	3.35
(2) Leaders feared the consultant would reveal and broadcast their deficiencies	3.27
(7) Leaders were not receptive to consultants who were unfamiliar with, or unidentified with, the military culture	3.18
(1) Leaders were not interested in a behavior science perspective from any source	3.17
(4) Consultants were not trained in community psychiatry or military psychiatry	3.08
(3) Psychiatric opinion had limited usefulness under the circumstances	3.08
(6) Leaders denied most of the problems within their unit	2.85
(5) Leaders were not committed to their troops or their problems	1.97

Mean extent of survey psychiatrists' agreement along a 5-point scale with 1 = very infrequent and 5 = very frequent (N = 61–83). (Numbers) refer to order of the item in the survey questionnaire.

(3) and are tightly clustered around this midpoint. Taken together, these means suggest an absence of strong feelings among the survey participants regarding factors interfering with command consultation. More complex statistical approaches were avoided because of small sample sizes. Nonetheless, from a purely descriptive point of view the trends warrant some comment. The two leading factors interfering with command consultation, items 8 and 2, suggest either command parochialism (ie, commanders would be unreceptive to advice from outside the unit's chain of command) or suspiciousness (ie, commanders would fear the consultant would broadcast their real or imagined deficiencies).

To some degree, the next lower item (7), lack of receptivity to the outsider consultant, may stem from the same source, but it could also suggest a communication problem shared by both consultant and consultee. Still, these three items (8, 2, and 7) appear to define the barrier consultants could have faced if they were not part of the organization ("organic") to which they would offer consultation. In this regard, although not tested, it is natural to assume that the psychiatrists who served in the combat divisions would have encountered these obstacles less often than the hospital and psychiatric specialty detachment psychiatrists, which would be consistent with findings presented in Figure 10-2B.

The second set of three items, 1, 4, and 3, appear to center on ignorance of the value of social psychiatry, which could reside in either the consultant or the consultee. Either would surely be regrettable, but they are potentially solvable through education and training. In consideration of the consultant psychiatrists, although the extent of their training in community psychiatry and organizational consultation during their pre-Vietnam psychiatric training was not explored in the study, it can be said that mastery of these skills was not generally a standard educational requirement in psychiatric training programs of the times. Also as noted, the Army provided no system-wide program for training them in command consultation either. Fortunately, the remaining two prospective obstacles (6 and 5), which could be seen as command denial and lack of commitment, clearly ominous, are ranked by the survey psychiatrists as the least likely to have been influential.

In conclusion, the low level of command consultation activity represented in Figure 10-1 and the extent of endorsement of various impediments presented in Table 10-1 are only suggestive. However, considering that preventive and social psychiatry had been emphasized by senior Army psychiatrists in the decades leading up to the war, these results imply that more could have been done to promote command consultation in Vietnam, that is, to train mental health personnel in situ, ensure receptivity by commanders, and monitor outcomes.

SUMMARY AND CONCLUSIONS

Army psychiatrists have historically been exhorted to support commanders by sharing their expertise through command consultation regarding risk factors for individual and group psychopathology. It was believed that a psychiatrist–commander dialogue could promote the conservation of manpower through prevention of soldier ineffectiveness and psychiatric disability. Such an approach was consistent with the commander's primary responsibility for minimizing the various environmental and situational stress factors that could lower the morale and mental health of his troops. It also rested on theories regarding the powerful stress-buffering potential of the soldier's community, that is, the small military unit with which he related and from which he drew his self-esteem.

At the time America entered the war in Vietnam, principles of program-centered (primary prevention) and case-centered (secondary prevention) command consultation were well established in the literature of military psychiatry and in the regulations governing Army psychiatrists and the provision of mental health-care. However, endorsing the community psychiatry/command consultation model does not ensure that the deployed psychiatric personnel are skilled or committed to command consultation, nor does it guarantee their entrée to a unit's command cadre. This chapter reviewed the available literature in order to explore the implementation of command consultation in Vietnam and evidence of its utility. The following summarizes the more salient findings:

- **At least through the buildup phase of the war (1965–1968), there is ample evidence from the available literature that the psychiatric personnel in the combat divisions, that is, professionals and paraprofessionals (social work/psychology technicians), actively and productively engaged in case-centered command consultation with unit leaders (officers and NCOs) and medical personnel in the interest of minimizing soldier disability from psychiatric and related problems.**

- **With regard to nondivisional combat and combat support/service support units, which constituted the majority of Army personnel in Vietnam, there is little evidence from the literature of case-centered command consultation by the psychiatric personnel responsible for the care of these troops.** This appears to be corroborated by the WRAIR psychiatrist survey finding in which the psychiatrists who were assigned only to hospitals reported lower frequency of effort and success in command consultation than did the psychiatrists who had combat unit

assignments. Apparently both the solo psychiatrists at the evacuation and field hospitals and the psychiatric personnel at the psychiatric detachments functioned more often in a reactive mode, responding to clinical demand from their hospital base. The first requirement of these professionals was to provide 3rd echelon, hospital-level treatment. When possible, they also provided 2nd echelon, outpatient evaluation and treatment services. Evidently, most often they communicated with unit leaders and dispensary medical personnel through patient health records and other formal means. Likely explanations for their limited case-centered, command consultation include:

- geographical remoteness was compounded by transportation and communication obstacles;
- solo psychiatrists at the evacuation and field hospitals did not have specialized staff to pursue active liaison with units;
- personnel at the psychiatric specialty detachments were often pressed to provide 3rd echelon care for troops who had been evacuated a long distance from their parent unit, and as a result they had little time and capability to provide unit consultation; and
- organizational divergence led to both formal and functional separateness.

- **Apart from some noteworthy exceptions, the available literature suggests that the more specialized program-centered command consultation was not routinely undertaken by psychiatrists and other mental health personnel in Vietnam.** Furthermore, the WRAIR survey responses suggest that overall the psychiatrists assigned in Vietnam were uncertain as to whether they had anything to offer the commander of a military unit on a programmatic level and likewise whether the commanders would welcome their advice. The question of whether commanders in Vietnam were trained to utilize the expertise of the available military psychiatrists and welcomed their input is unanswerable; however, explanations bearing on the psychiatrist side of the equation may include the following:

- most assigned psychiatrists had not received formal training in community psychiatry;

- the majority of psychiatrists had no military background and no training in consulting with a (nonmedical) line unit. The pertinence of this was suggested by the WRAIR survey finding that psychiatrists with no pre-Vietnam military experience reported lower frequency of effort and success in command consultation than did the psychiatrists who had some pre-Vietnam military experience; and

- roughly half of the psychiatrists had no overlap with their predecessor in Vietnam and had little opportunity for on-the-job training by the leaving psychiatrist.

- **Many of the activities of the nine USARV Psychiatry Consultants would certainly meet the definition of program-centered, primary prevention; however, there is almost no surviving documentation of their efforts or results.** By extension, considering the fact that the war became a drawn-out, unconventional/guerrilla war—and one to which the American public became increasingly opposed—the available evidence indicates there were no associated field studies or research regarding the impact of these stressors on the replacement troops and their units that would have guided the Psychiatry Consultants in providing consultation at the central, that is, USARV, level. At the very least, an epidemiologically based system for monitoring the various (changing) indices reflecting the widespread and growing demoralization and dysfunction in the theater should have been utilized. Such a dedicated preventive medicine approach could have informed command of stressors progressively undermining the force, which in turn could have led to timely command consultation by the psychiatric contingent to smaller units regarding possible psychosocial remedies. It also could have provided grounds for modification of the system of mental health resources and the selection and preparation of replacement psychiatrists for Vietnam. Compounding these matters, as noted in Chapter 4, during the final 2 years in Vietnam, when morale and drug problems reached extreme levels, the Army assigned psychiatrists as the USARV Psychiatry Consultants who had demonstrably less experience as military psychiatrists than had been the case earlier in the war.

- **The accumulated evidence strongly suggests that no matter how meritorious the combined principles of community psychiatry and military psychiatry are, their implementation in Vietnam was spotty at best and primarily dependent on individual initiative and advantageous background experience of the assigned psychiatrists as opposed to being institutionalized.**

REFERENCES

1. Byrdy HSR. In: Johnson AW Jr., Bowman JA, Byrdy HSR, Blank AS Jr. Panel discussion: Army psychiatry in Vietnam. In: Jones FD, ed. *Proceedings: Social and Preventive Psychiatry Course, 1967*. Washington, DC: Government Printing Office; 1968: 41–76. [Available at: Alexandria, Va: Defense Technical Information Center (Document AD A950058, 1980).]

2. Jones FD, Johnson AW. Medical and psychiatric treatment policy and practice in Vietnam. *J Soc Issues*; 1975(31):49–65.

3. *Symposium on Preventive and Social Psychiatry*. 15–17 April 1958, Walter Reed Army Institute of Research. Washington, DC: Government Printing Office; 1958.

4. Tiffany WJ, Allerton WS. Army psychiatry in the mid-60s. *Am J Psychiatry*. 1967;123:810–821.

5. Caldwell JM. Military psychiatry. In: Freedman AM, Kaplan HI, eds. *Comprehensive Textbook of Psychiatry*. Baltimore, Md: Williams and Wilkins Co; 1967: 1605–1612.

6. Hausman W, Rioch DMcK. Military psychiatry: a prototype of social and preventive psychiatry in the United States. *Arch Gen Psych*. 1967;16:727–739.

7. US Department of the Army. *Medical Service: Neuropsychiatry*. Washington, DC: DA; 18 June 1959. Army Regulation 40-216.

8. Caplan G. *Principles of Preventive Psychiatry*. New York, NY: Basic Books; 1964.

9. Menninger WC. *Psychiatry in a Troubled World*. New York, NY: Macmillin Co; 1948.

10. Glass AJ. Military psychiatry and changing systems of mental health care. *J Psychiat Res*. 1971;8:499–512.

11.	Glass AJ, Artiss KL, Gibbs JJ, Sweeney VC. The current status of Army psychiatry. *Am J Psychiatry*. 1961;117:673–683.

12.	Westmoreland WC. Mental health—An aspect of command. *Mil Med*. 1963;128(3)207–214.

13.	Rothberg JM. Psychiatric aspects of diseases in military personnel. In: Jones FD, Sparacino LR, Wilcox VL, Rothberg JM, eds. *Military Psychiatry: Preparing in Peace for War*. In: *Textbooks of Military Medicine*. Washington, DC: Office of The Surgeon General, US Department of the Army, Borden Institute; 1994: 51–60.

14.	Jones FD. Traditional warfare combat stress casualties. In: Jones FD, Sparacino LR, Wilcox VL, Rothberg JM, Stokes JW, eds. *War Psychiatry*. In: Zajtchuk R, Bellamy RF, eds. *Textbooks of Military Medicine*. Washington, DC: Department of the Army, Office of The Surgeon General, Borden Institute; 1995: 37–61.

15.	Ursano RJ, Holloway, HC. Military psychiatry. In: Kaplan I, Sadock BJ, eds. *Comprehensive Textbook of Psychiatry IV*. Baltimore, Md: Williams and Wilkins; 1985: 1900–1909.

16.	Marlowe D. The human dimension of battle and combat breakdown. In: Gabriel RA, ed. *Military Psychiatry: A Comparative Perspective*. Westport, Conn: Greenwood Press; 1986: 7–24.

17.	Belenky GL. Varieties of reaction and adaption to combat experience. *Bull Menninger Clin*. 1987;51:64–79.

18.	Group for the Advancement of Psychiatry. *Preventive Psychiatry in the Armed Forces: With Some Implications for Civilian Use*. New York: Group for the Advancement of Psychiatry; 1960. Report 47.

19.	US Department of the Army. *Mental Health and Neuropsychiatry*. March 1966. US Army Republic of Vietnam Regulation 40-34. [Full text available as Appendix 2 to this volume.]

20.	Medical Field Service School. *Introduction to Military Psychiatry*. Fort Sam Houston, Tex: Medical Field Service School Department of Neuropsychiatry; distributed July 1967. Training document GR 51-400-004-064.

21.	McCarroll JE, Jaccard JJ, Radke AQ. Psychiatric consultation to command. In: Jones FD, Sparacino LR, Wilcox VL, Rothberg JM, eds. *Military Psychiatry: Preparing in Peace for War*. In: Zajtchuk R, Bellamy F, eds. *Textbooks of Military Medicine*. Washington, DC: Office of The Surgeon General, US Department of the Army, Borden Institute; 1994: 151–170.

22.	Pettera RL. What is this thing called "field consultation" in psychiatry. *US Army Vietnam Med Bull*. 1968;January/February:31–36.

23.	Colbach EM, Parrish MD. Army mental health activities in Vietnam: 1965–1970. *Bull Menninger Clin*. 1970;31:333–342.

24.	Colbach EM. Ethical issues in combat psychiatry. *Mil Med*. 1985;150(5):256–265.

25.	Byrdy HSR. Division psychiatry in Vietnam (unpublished); 1967. [Full text available as Appendix 8 to this volume.]

26.	Bostrom JA. Psychiatric consultation in the First Cav. *US Army Vietnam Med Bull*. 1968;January/February:24–25.

27.	Motis G. Freud in the boonies: a preliminary report on the psychiatric field program in the 4th Infantry Division. *US Army Vietnam Med Bull*. 1967;September/October:5–8.

28.	Bey DR, Smith WE. Mental health technicians in Vietnam. *Bull Menninger Clin*. 1970;34:363–371.

29.	Menard DL. The social work specialist in a combat division. *US Army Vietnam Med Bull*. 1968;March/April:48–57.

30.	Bey D. *Wizard 6: A Combat Psychiatrist in Vietnam*. College Station, Tex: Texas A & M University Military History Series 104; 2006.

31.	Bey DR. Division Psychiatry in Vietnam (unpublished); no date.

32.	Bey DR, Smith WE. Organizational consultation in a combat unit. *Am J Psychiatry*. 1971;128:401–406.

33.	Bowman JA. In: Johnson AW Jr, Bowman JA, Byrdy HS, Blank AS Jr. Panel discussion: Army psychiatry in Vietnam. In: Jones FD, ed. *Proceedings: Social and Preventive Psychiatry Course, 1967*. Washington DC: Government Printing Office; 1968:41–76. [Available at: Alexandria, Va: Defense Technical Information Center (Document AD A950058, 1980).]

34.	Talbott JA. Community psychiatry in the Army: history, practice and applications to civilian psychiatry. *JAMA*. 1969;210:1233–1237.

35. Anderson JR. Psychiatric support of III and IV Corps tactical zones. *US Army Vietnam Med Bull.* 1968;January/February:37–39.

36. Jones FD. Psychiatric lessons of war. In: Jones FD, Sparacino LR, Wilcox VL, Rothberg JM, Stokes JW, eds. *War Psychiatry.* In: Zajtchuk R, Bellamy F, eds. *Textbooks of Military Medicine.* Washington, DC: Office of The Surgeon General, US Department of the Army, Borden Institute; 1995: 1–33.

37. Spector RH. *After Tet: The Bloodiest Year in Vietnam.* New York, NY: The Free Press; 1993.

CHAPTER 11

Operational Frustrations and Ethical Strain for Army Psychiatrists: "Crushing Burdens and Painful Memories"

. . . [As Vietnam veterans, it] was easy for us to get ourselves accepted as long as we maintained, for instance, that there was absolutely no excuse for American soldiers to be in any overseas theater, that military doctors were crude and inhuman, that poverty and misery in the U.S. was far more important and more horrible than such problems anywhere else in the world, that the Communists were not serious competitors of ours, and that the less we learned from Asia, Africa, and South America the better. For the home Americans seemed to "know" from the media that the Vietnam war was more immoral than the Civil War, the Spanish American War, or World War II. They explained how we soldiers should feel guilty for fighting such an immoral war.[1(p2)]

Colonel Matthew D Parrish, Medical Corps
3rd Neuropsychiatry Consultant to the Commanding General
US Army, Republic of Vietnam (1972)

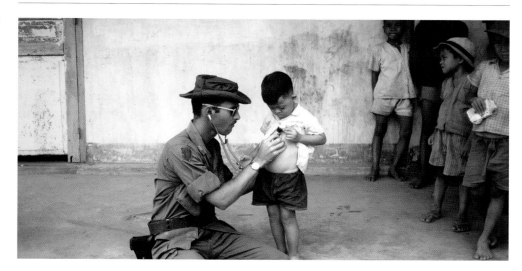

Photograph of Army trained psychiatrist Major Richard D Cameron, Medical Corps, division psychiatrist with 1st Cavalry Division (March–October, 1970), providing general medical care for local civilian children during his free time under the MILPHAP (Military Public Health Action Program). These programs were designed to "win the hearts and minds" of the Vietnamese; however, they brought only qualified success. Photograph courtesy of Richard D Cameron, Major General, US Army (Retired).

Psychiatrists are specialized physicians who enter military service already committed to their profession's humanitarian ethical values, which emphasize care of the individual. However, like all soldiers, while serving in the military they also function in the ethical shadow of the institution's enormous and strict hierarchy, the central organizing principle of which is the subordination of individual values to those of the organization[2]—presumably for the benefit of society. It follows that, in time of war, Army psychiatrists incur an obligation to support the US Army Medical Department's mission of contributing to the accomplishment of the combat mission, which means the clinical priority centers on the recovery of the individual soldier's combat function. In instances when humanitarian values (treatment of the sick and wounded) come into conflict with those of force conservation, elimination of otherwise tolerable symptoms among soldiers who are capable of returning to the battle becomes of secondary importance. As stated by Colbach and Parrish with respect to Vietnam, "[i]t is expected that soldiers in a combat zone will experience varying degrees of discomfort. This is a sacrifice that society expects them to make, and mental health personnel are guardians of this painful reality."[3(p341)]

Nonetheless, during and after the war in Vietnam, the ethical foundation for the Army's combat psychiatry forward treatment doctrine, a regimen in which basic physical and psychologically supportive treatments are utilized to encourage rapid resumption of combat duty function, was vigorously challenged by many in medicine and psychiatry, despite its historical validation as effective and ethical. These new critics opposed a treatment regimen designed to induce symptomatic soldiers to believe that facing further combat risks would be in their best interest or that of the nation. In particular they objected to the elements in the doctrine that would expect (the accusation was, coerce) psychologically traumatized soldiers to return to combat exposure if they were opposed or if they would be vulnerable in subsequent combat.[4] Furthermore, in that a much wider range of psychotropic medications was available to military psychiatrists and other physicians in Vietnam compared to earlier wars, these objections became even more pointed.

This chapter explores the ethical challenges surrounding military service as a psychiatrist during wartime and reviews the available literature to consider their effects (personally as well as professionally) on those who served in Vietnam. It also utilizes selected results from the Walter Reed Army Institute of Research (WRAIR) survey of Vietnam veteran psychiatrists to complete the picture.

BACKGROUND

The Historical Ethical Foundation for Military Psychiatrists

As indicated above, military psychiatrists who serve in a combat theater may have to contend with an exquisite and absolute contradiction of professional values.[4] Whereas their clinical decisions can have far-

reaching consequences, they may face organizational expectations that they function in ways that may be perceived, at least by others, if not by themselves, as violating the basic ethical tenets of psychiatry serving the welfare of the individual. This may become even more of a problem for civilian-trained psychiatrists. Brigadier General William C Menninger, the Army Surgeon General's Chief of the Neuropsychiatry Branch during most of World War II, had this to say about what was required of civilian psychiatrists in uniform:

> As civilian doctors they had to understand and correct abnormal reactions to normal situations. As medical officers they had to help normal personalities maintain their integration under horribly abnormal conditions. The Army psychiatrists saw war as a pathological activity which tended to force the development of psychopathology in its participants.[5(p49)]

However, before the Vietnam era, conflict between military and civilian psychiatric value systems was rarely mentioned in the professional literature,[6] even if it was implied.[7-9] The potential conflict pertained especially to the application of the forward treatment doctrine's principle of "expectancy," which referred to the overarching treatment attitude recognized since World War I to be essential in helping combat-stressed soldiers recover and return to duty (discussed in Chapter 7). For example, Peterson and Chambers acknowledged the discomfort their colleagues experienced in satisfying military priorities during the Korean War:

> It is easy to evacuate a soldier from combat and difficult to do the reverse. It is easier to say, "this man should never have been drafted," than to help him adjust to his duties. It is easier to send a frightened young soldier, who reminds one of one's self or one's own son, to the rear than to return him to combat duty. . . . One's own feelings of guilt over returning another to combat duty, make it difficult for the psychiatrist to function effectively and without anxiety.[7(p253)]

The daunting moral weight associated with having to send soldiers back into battle from one's position of relative safety is surely no more burdensome for the military psychiatrist than it is for the military leader, but in being a professional soldier, the military leader may be far more prepared. In this regard, as was pointed out in

Chapter 5, in previous wars the psychiatrists who were new to the military and who had not been sufficiently "indoctrinated" in the modified goals and methods of military psychiatry failed to understand both sides of the soldier's struggle to overcome his fear. As a result, they overly empathized with his heightened self-protective tendencies and overdiagnosed psychiatric disturbance. Furthermore, such outcomes had negative implications for both overall combat readiness and increased morbidity among individual soldiers. Although by this description the ethical strain for military psychiatrists—balancing the needs of the individual and those of the organization—is specific to combat circumstances, in fact, many of the professional responsibilities of military psychiatrists carry this ethical contradiction, even if latent and in derivative form.

As will be described, it was only after the war in Vietnam became so bitterly controversial that a frank and impassioned debate arose within psychiatry concerning the proper role for psychiatrists, especially military psychiatrists, in time of war. To understand how this value clash arose it is necessary to appreciate how the military distinguished between psychiatric reactions to combat and similar civilian casualties during the Vietnam era. As discussed in Chapter 6 and Chapter 7, the combat stress reaction was regarded by military psychiatry as a "normal" and typically reversible reaction to an abnormal circumstance, at least in its acute stages. Although not necessarily the primary etiology, the combat stress reaction could express the soldier's "refusal to fight"[10(p11)] in instances when he had reached the point where his fear, and perhaps his own ethical conflict,[11,12] overshadowed his combat motivation.

In a wartime context it followed that, even if such a soldier was reluctant, he had a duty on recovering to return to function and risk further sacrifices, perhaps to the point of giving his life. The military psychiatrist treating such a patient would be in a similar position. Also a soldier, he would be expected to aid his patient in fulfilling this duty—even if the psychiatrist was reluctant. More specifically, because the military psychiatrist's foremost responsibility in a combat theater is that of stemming the flow of individuals who manifest a temporary psychological incapacity or reluctance to soldier, he may be obligated to deny a psychologically traumatized soldier's anticipation of relief from further exposure to combat (or from a court-martial) to conform to the military's need for him to return to the battle if he could function, even if he has some persisting (if not

disabling) psychiatric symptoms or was opposed to returning.[13] The profound nature of this quandary was etched into America consciousness through Heller's 1961 best-selling farce about World War II, *Catch-22*.[14]

Dual Agency as a Problem for the Military Psychiatrist

A full appreciation of the military psychiatrist's potential for ethical strain requires acknowledgment of the dual or double agency nature of his position. This can be summed with the question: for whom does he work—the individual patient or the military organization? This dilemma may affect any physician when patient responsibilities contradict obligations to a third party and can affect treatment decisions (as well as those of allied mental health professionals).[15] As will be demonstrated, with regard to treatment of the combat soldier it can be seen as the choice between serving humanitarian values (treatment of the sick and wounded) versus a collective one centered on force conservation. There are at least two reasons why balancing loyalties can become more difficult for psychiatrists than for other types of military physicians. Not only are military psychiatrists more often required to make clinical decisions in which both advice (ie, patient-centered) and control (ie, organization-centered) functions are intertwined,[16] but there is a greater degree of professional disagreement about mental health norms.[17] Furthermore, the clinical decisions of military psychiatrists may also be affected by their personal ideology,[18,19] training, and experience,[20] as well as changing social contexts.[21]

The Importance of the Nation's Sanction and the Approval of One's Colleagues

The historical accounts of World War I, World War II, and the Korean War indicate that thousands of military psychiatrists—primarily mobilized civilians—performed their professional and military duties with a sustained allegiance to military objectives, and they accepted that their clinical goals and techniques would be altered by expediency associated with fighting those wars.[2,22] Although, as Albert J Glass noted, in contrast to World War I when America seemed eager to fight, in World War II there was greater reluctance within organized psychiatry to contribute to a war effort; nonetheless, once mobilization was a reality, commitment to supporting the military forces and their colleagues in uniform was evident within psychiatry.[9,23]

Psychiatrists perceived that these American wars were necessary and thus, like society, they expected soldiers to "do their part."[24(p242)] Any remaining doubt the psychiatrists in uniform may have had that the forward treatment doctrine was humanitarian was negated by convincing data indicating that in most cases of combat breakdown, the longer the soldier was hospitalized or the farther he was evacuated from his combat unit and comrades, the more intractable his symptoms became.[25(p731)] They apparently suffered little ethical conflict because they believed that they were simultaneously serving the best interests of their soldier-patients, the military, American society, and their profession.

The following is an especially elegant rationale for the forward treatment doctrine written during the Korean War by David McK Rioch, a distinguished neuropsychiatric researcher:

> [R]apid diagnosis, treatment, and return to duty of men with tolerable [stress] symptoms itself represents a significant communication to the group as a whole. In addition to demonstrating the serious consideration the Army has for the soldier's personal welfare, this policy establishes the importance of the individual to the group by the unequivocal implication that his presence and effort are more highly valued than comfort. That this policy represents a positive support and is not merely an inhibitory threat is indicated by the fact that reduction in the rate of evacuation for psychiatric causes has not been accompanied by a compensatory increase in other categories. The policy is "tough" in the sense that it assesses the personal worth and abilities of men at a higher level than many have been confident they could maintain. It is by no means "tough" in the sense of expressing personal disregard and contemptuous punishment for failure.[26]

VIETNAM

As indicated earlier in this volume, it was not new to observe in Vietnam that some soldiers with combat stress-generated psychiatric symptoms struggled with a conflict between self-protective motives and those representing feelings of obligation to their military comrades and mission (see Case 6-2, PFC Golf and Case

6-6, PFC Love in Chapter 6). In fact, this was anticipated in how medical and psychiatric care was structured in Vietnam, including the promulgation of the forward treatment doctrine. However, what was new during Vietnam were accusations that the doctrine, which was intended to limit the former (self-protective motives) and bolster the latter (feelings of obligation to military comrades and objectives), was harmful—challenges that became more pointed as the antiwar and antimilitary sentiment in America grew more strident.[15]

Operational Frustrations for Mental Health Personnel

As indicated in the individual reports by the psychiatrists and other mental health personnel reviewed in Chapter 3 and Chapter 4, the deployed mental health personnel in Vietnam often encountered substantial practical impediments and operational frustrations. Many of these overlap with ethical challenges if not conflicts per se; however, only a few examples will be mentioned in passing. For example, probably the most repetitive complaint was from the division psychiatrists who noted that not being issued a jeep severely hampered their clinical and command consultation capability. A more specific example was Franklin Del Jones' exasperation from when he accompanied the 25th Infantry Division (ID) to Vietnam and found he was not provided the essential equipment to do his job—"a jeep, a typewriter, a general-purpose medium tent and tent frame . . . to house [my] mental health clinic, a desk, and a locking file cabinet."[27(p1008)]

Much later in the war, Joel H Kaplan, with the 98th Psychiatric Detachment, objected to the fact that according to Army policy he was unable to ensure the confidentiality of soldier records for those in treatment for marijuana use—a deviation from civilian standards that he felt negatively affected their treatment.[28] And Nathan Cohen, with the 98th Psychiatric Detachment 2 years after Kaplan, expressed extreme frustration that the Army management and treatment program for heroin users in Vietnam, the amnesty program, was poorly conceived and implemented, and that this negatively impacted the treatment and recovery of many soldiers.

Ethical Strain Among Mental Health Personnel in the First Half of the War

In general, the information provided during or shortly after their tours in Vietnam by psychiatrists and other mental health personnel who served in the first half of the war suggested that they did not *experience* ethical strain while there.

Psychiatrists Assigned to the Divisions

Because most of the reporting division psychiatrists served in the first half of the war, the period of the greatest combat intensity, ethical dilemmas could have potentially been greater among that group. However, it seems noteworthy how unfazed they appeared to be. For example, John A Bostrom, with the 1st Cavalry Division (1967), advocated a treatment model that supported the combat soldier's return to duty function through minimizing his regressive urges (by downplaying the protective/"maternal" message) and strengthening his duty-centered, progressive ones (ie, by emphasizing the aggressive/"paternal" message). In his report there was no evidence that he was doubtful that this approach was in the soldier's best interest.[29] But lack of evidence for ethical strain does not prove that ethical conflicts aren't influential. As was discussed in Chapter 3, when the reported experience of Army-trained Jones was compared with his counterpart, civilian-trained Byrdy, during the first year of the war, Byrdy greatly exceeded Jones in the percentage of referrals that he hospitalized and the percentage that he evacuated out of the division (see Table 3-5 in Chapter 3). This is consistent with observations from earlier wars that civilian-trained psychiatrists are likely to be more protective of the combat stress casualty. The later experience of civilian-trained Bey (also in Table 3-5), whose rates for hospitalization and evacuation also exceed those of Jones, appear to provide further substantiation. However, his rates are substantially lower than Byrdy's, which could be partially explained by his having had an offsetting year of pre-Vietnam military experience, which "reoriented" him to the clinical priorities of the wartime military.

Psychiatrists Assigned to the Hospitals and Psychiatry Specialty Detachments

In contrast, some of the psychiatrists assigned to the KO detachments in the first half of the war did indicate that they were affected by ethical strain. Because they controlled the two choke points for medical evacuations out of Vietnam, they may have been more burdened than the other psychiatrists in Vietnam who could at least know that the final decision for medically exempting a soldier from further exposure to seemingly unbearable stress was not theirs to make. For example, during the first year of the ground war, John A Bowman, an experienced, Army-trained psychiatrist (October 1965–October 1966), indicated that he and his colleagues at the 935th Psychiatric Detachment returned approximately 90% of all hospitalized soldiers back to duty; however, as illustrated by his moving description in Chapter 7, this could be an exquisitely difficult process. Here are some further recollections of the personal repercussions he and his psychiatrist colleagues sustained in holding that line:

> The staff did not allow evacuations from the combat zone or transfers within the combat zone unless it was medically indicated or militarily feasible. Due to our *rigidity* [emphasis added] on evacuation policy our colleagues in the BOQ [bachelor officer quarters] frequently referred to us as "tough guys" and whimsical but pointed remarks about "Catch 22 were aimed in our direction.[30(p5)]

Elsewhere Bowman commented further:

> Some of my own personal experiences in dealing with the [Psychiatric Detachment] were to convince the team that, even though the patient was technically a psychiatric casualty, he wasn't necessarily to be considered sick. My [colleagues], I think, tended initially to view them in a most classical way, as being sick, but ended up at the year more "hard-nosed" than I was. They used to refer to me as a tough guy, but I'm sure that [they] became tougher than I was, or we found ourselves changing roles somewhere around the middle of the tour.[31(p65)]

Bowman's counterpart with the 98th Psychiatric Detachment, Louis R Conte, a civilian-trained psychiatrist, and his team presented an interesting contrast. They reported that they returned only 40% of hospitalized cases to duty—apparently as a consequence of their efforts to provide "humanness, giving, and feeding."[32(p165)] Yet they indicated they were pressured by military priorities and unsure if they were striking the right balance between protection and expectancy for their soldier-patients:

> How much "feeding" in a combat zone is appropriate was never clearly established in the minds of those concerned. We could never fully decide how comfortable we wanted to make it for

the patients . . . [for fear they would] cathect the patient role and then have separation problems when they were *asked* [emphasis added] to return to their duty unit.[32(p165)]

Bowman and Conte served early in the buildup years in Vietnam, and the higher attrition rate reported by civilian-trained Conte is consistent with the earlier observation regarding civilian-trained Byrdy, who served as a division psychiatrist. Otherwise there is no evidence that the clinical attitudes of Bowman or Conte were influenced by the beginning antiwar movement in the United States; however, this would soon change among the cohorts of replacement psychiatrists who followed (for example, see Chapter 5, Exhibit 5-2, "The Jones–Dr A Correspondence"). In the winter of 1967, the second USARV Psychiatry Consultant, Arnold W Johnson Jr, acknowledged the emerging criticism of the doctrine as applied in Vietnam and provided a vigorous defense using historical data from earlier wars. He also reiterated the preeminence of the military mission:

> It may be initially pointed out in answering these criticisms that, even if they were true, the action was justified since in combat whether an individual is ill, injured or psychiatrically disabled, the criterion for return to duty is not comfort or complete absence of symptoms but rather ability to perform.[33(p44)]

Defense of the doctrine was extended by Johnson in a follow-up article in 1969 when he suggested that the high morale and low psychiatric rate in Vietnam was partially based on patriotism ("doing one's part for one year as a good citizen in a common cause"[34(p336)]), and he reminded the reader that this was consistent with masculine virtues. ("There is the opportunity [for the soldier in Vietnam] to prove oneself a man and a chance to take part in helping those who need help."[34(p336)]) For those serving in medical roles, he acknowledged the added ethical weight brought about by the antiwar movement and offered a reassuring rationale: "[Medical personnel can] justify their presence in Vietnam on the basis of upholding the medical tradition of helping where needed, even if unsure about the war as a whole."[34(p337)]

Medical Field Service School Preparation

In July 1967, psychiatrists who received their basic Medical Corps orientation and training at the Army's Medical Field Service School (MFSS) were told, "The ultimate aim of any Army is to destroy the ability and will of the enemy to fight, [and] each soldier must have the capability of using the firepower of the modern army to destroy the enemy while preparing himself to defend himself from a similar attack."[35(p9)] They also were taught that military psychiatry's unique objective is to supplement the military mission through maintenance of the soldier's psychological effectiveness—to "conserve the fighting strength." However, the MFSS faculty felt it necessary to add the following:

> Junior psychiatrists . . . [i]n their first flush of humanitarian enthusiasm, crusading against incomprehension and intolerance [by the Army], may regard every patient with a grievance as a victim of an impersonal system. They identify themselves with the individual gallantly resisting dehumanizing and destructive pressures, and forget that they have an obligation equally as important— to serve the best interests of the organization.[36(pp3–4)]

And by way of a solution, they provided the following:

> . . . [Whereas the military psychiatrist] had to know the point of view of the men in the Army . . . he had to identify with the Army to the extent of believing in it, wanting to contribute constructively to it, and feeling a sense of pride in being part of it.[37(p4)]

Evidently, even at that early stage of the war, the Army had become concerned with growing opposition to the war and worried about its impact on military physicians, including psychiatrists. (Also see Chapter 5, Exhibit 5-1, "Potential Identity Problems Facing the Drafted, Civilian-Trained Psychiatrist.")

Widening Criticism of Military Psychiatry

As increasing numbers of Americans denounced the conflict in Southeast Asia, military psychiatry and its doctrine came under direct attack, indicating a shift in professional attitudes from the more sanguine early war period to the late war enmity.[38] Criticism came both from psychiatrists and other physicians who had served in Vietnam as well as from those who had not served there. With regard to those who had served in Vietnam, at least three former Army psychiatrists, including Dr A, provided their names and identified themselves as physicians in the war protest document, *Vietnam*

Veterans Against the War: Vietnam Veterans, Stand Up and Be Counted.[39] Robert J Lifton, a prominent psychiatrist with experience with military populations, veterans, and survivors of extreme military and civilian stress, is an example of a critical psychiatrist who had not served there. In his opinion, the military psychiatrists in Vietnam were "technicist" professionals who had colluded with an "absurd and evil organization."[40(p808)] In a subsequent publication he equated them with the German physicians who worked in Nazi death camps.[41]

> It turned out that many of these [Vietnam veterans I worked with] had experienced a mixture of revulsion and psychological conflict . . . and were taken to either a chaplain or a psychiatrist . . . [who] would attempt to help the [soldier] become strong enough to overcome his difficulties and remain in combat, which in Vietnam meant participating in or witnessing daily atrocities. . . . In that way, the chaplain or psychiatrist, quite inadvertently, undermined what the soldier would later come to view as his last remnant of decency in that situation.[41(p464)]

Lifton theorized that one reason psychiatrists became ethically corrupted was that they assumed that because they were practitioners of a healing profession, whatever they did served to heal. He also believed that "psychiatrists returning from Vietnam to their clinical and teaching situations had experienced psychological struggles no less severe than those of other Vietnam veterans."[41(p464)]

While not as starkly judgmental, Brass reviewed Peter G Bourne's *Men, Stress, and Vietnam* for the *Journal of the American Medial Association*, including Bourne's description of the practices of military psychiatrists in Vietnam, and inquired incredulously,

> If the soldier is seriously enough disturbed to require hospitalization or evacuation, is it good medicine to treat only his symptoms and then reexpose him to the cause of his breakdown? Just how well does a [soldier] on tranquilizers (a) fight, and (b) look after his own skin? One would like to know the comparative casualty figures of soldiers on tranquilizers against those not taking prescribed drugs.[42(p1473)]

Disputes Between Civilian and Military Psychiatrists Regarding the Ethical Treatment of Troops in Vietnam

Levin vs Arthur and Strange

Whereas the private disagreement between Jones and Talbott presented in Chapter 5 was centered on the morality of the war, there were public disputes that focused specifically on professional ethics. The debate between EC Levin, a civilian psychiatrist from Berkeley, California, and Robert E Strange and Ransom J Arthur, both Navy psychiatrists, illustrated the growing split between military psychiatrists and those in civilian positions. In 1967 Strange and Arthur published a report in America's leading psychiatric journal summarizing their experience with Marine and Navy personnel hospitalized aboard the USS *Repose* off the coast of South Vietnam between February and August 1966.[43] Levin reacted with a letter to the editor condemning the Navy's utilization of the forward treatment doctrine:

> Psychiatrists in general pride themselves on their ability to see their patients holistically and humanistically . . . [b]ut nowhere in their article do Cdrs. Strange and Arthur present any evidence for their having done anything more than see their patients as defective cogs in the military machine, to be repaired as quickly as possible so that they could be speedily returned "to combat and possible death or mutilation." I presume that the authors were too busy or too enamored with the task of secondary and tertiary prevention to ponder what primary prevention might have meant to the 13,000 Americans and the uncounted Vietnamese who have already died in the war.
>
> . . . Might not the greatest mark of personal and professional maturity lie in the willingness to work to lead men out of battle rather than into it?[44(pp1137–1138)]

The rebuttal by Arthur and Strange was equally sharp:

> Whether it is easier to evade war's realities in a hospital ship off Viet Nam or in a consultant's office in Berkeley, we leave to the readers of the *Journal* to judge. Based on our clinical experience and data from follow-up studies by the Navy [it

is evident that] . . . premature discharge from the Armed Forces for psychiatric reasons may in itself exert a life-long deleterious effect on the individual; and that provided the patient is not too ill, every effort should be made to enable him to complete his obligation to his nation and his comrades. In our paper we pointed out the necessity for early therapy oriented toward helping the patient marshal enough ego resources to finish his task. A psychiatrist does not need even a single day's experience in military medicine to understand the importance of this approach, with its attendant preservation of self-esteem.[45(p1138)]

Maier vs Bloch

More specific to the Army is the dispute between psychiatrists H Spencer Bloch and T Maier, which was also in the *American Journal of Psychiatry*. In 1969 Bloch wrote an article describing the psychiatric goals and methods used in Vietnam at the 935th Psychiatric Detachment (1967–1968).[46] A civilian-trained psychiatrist in uniform, Bloch confidently explained how his team adapted the Army's traditional doctrine for the treatment of combat casualties to fit the unique features of the low-intensity, counterinsurgency combat theater there. He also highlighted the value of previously unavailable psychotropic medications, like Thorazine, in their treatment.

Maier, a psychiatrist who treated psychiatric casualties from Vietnam while serving in the Army in Japan (1965 to 1967), reacted in a letter to the editor that was intensely critical of the ethics and practices of military psychiatrists in Vietnam. Maier concluded,

By acting to 'conserve the fighting strength' in this war of boundless immorality, [the military psychiatrist] partakes of the passive complicity that is the mark of guilt in our time. . . . Whatever else Army psychiatry may be, I see neither moral nor scientific justification for the dignity of its definition as clinical psychiatry.[47(p1039)]

Bloch rebutted that in his experience in Vietnam, soldiers who struggled with concerns regarding the morality of the conflict typically were driven by under-lying, pre-Vietnam psychological conflicts. He also defended the goals and methods of military psychiatry in Vietnam:

If reality is that America's youth are now fighting, then they deserve the best psychiatric care that can be afforded them. Such care neither oversimplifies issues nor encumbers and compromises the evaluation or treatment setting by intrusion of the psychiatrists' moral judgments and emotions.[48(p1040)]

War-Related Ethical Dilemmas Facing Other Psychiatrists

A number of Vietnam-era authors also explored the ethical dilemmas inherent for military psychiatrists that were indirectly linked to the combat theater.[18,19,49–53] For example, Daniels referred to the military psychiatrist as a "captive professional."[50(p255)] Friedman saw him (or her) as "the overseer of a system of social control which is distinctly nonmedical in its character."[51(p122)] Kirshner suggested that when evaluating and treating dissenting soldiers military psychiatrists were antitherapeutic because of obstacles based on the psychiatrists' unresolved identity issues.[54]

Locke, who provided a personal account of his stateside tour with the Army in 1969, contended that psychiatrists who served with the military systematically dehumanized the soldier, prosecuted the war, and betrayed their individualist values. As a consequence, the military psychiatrist was transformed into "a soft policeman, a pacifier, an institutional ombudsman, a mystifier, and the official stereotyper and narcotizer."[55(p20)] Locke's personal solution was his "third alternative," that is, active participation in the antimilitary soldiers' movement.[55]

Barr and Zunin proposed a different remedy. They suggested that military psychiatrists be redesignated "psychiatric military officers" (PMO) to warn drafted psychiatrists and soldiers of the subordination of their medical ethics to those of the institution. The authors argued that lack of confidentiality, emphasis on returning disordered patients to duty and conformity, and the unavoidable real role the psychiatrist has in the military organization of his patient serve to create medical, ethical, and moral dilemmas for the psychiatrist, distortions in the treatment relationship, and tendencies for patients to try to maximize their advantage through exaggeration of symptoms.[56] Similarly they were doubtful of the therapeutic effectiveness of military psychiatrists: "[Because] the PMO owes his primary allegiance to the military service . . . therapy is clearly secondary to returning a man successfully to duty."[57(p19)]

Concern for these potential ethical dilemmas was not confined to the role and activities of the psychiatrists serving in the military services. A number of civilian psychiatrists indicated that they were deeply troubled by conducting evaluations of young draft eligible men with symptoms that apparently arose in response to the threat of being drafted,[54,58–63] and several were overtly suspicious of allegiances of their colleagues in uniform. For example, Ollendorff and Adams defined the military-oriented "establishment" psychiatrist as one who is corrupt and who "declares as fit everybody who is not dead."[58(p89)]

Operational and Ethical Strain Among Mental Health Personnel in the Second Half of the War

Compared with the more confident accounts by psychiatrists who served in the first half of the war, several who went during the second half, such as Camp (as quoted in Ingraham and Manning,[64] also see Prologue), Char,[65] Joseph,[66] Ratner,[67] and Fisher (Navy/Marines),[68] expressed more frustration and cynicism (Figure 11-1). Collectively they gave the impression that conventional military psychiatric structures and doctrine were not adequate to address the avalanche of psychiatric and behavioral problems of the later years of the Vietnam conflict. Nonetheless, specific reference to ethical conflicts did not appear to be central in their reports—but perhaps it was implied. Two nonpsychiatrist individuals, one who served in the transition phase of the war and the other during the drawdown, warrant mention because they openly opposed the war and the Army's psychiatric treatment doctrine while they were in Vietnam.

Protest by Major Gordon S Livingston, Medical Corps

Livingston, a West Point graduate who volunteered to serve in Vietnam, was not a psychiatrist at the time he was assigned there as a medical officer in 1968; however, he did pursue psychiatric training after he left the Army. Livingston's postwar account[69,70] of the moral outrage he developed while serving as a regimental surgeon (a general physician who is also a staff officer) is noteworthy because of his specific reference to the combat psychiatry doctrine:

> I was confronted with several cases of "combat neurosis" who told me that they saw nothing in what they were doing that justified the risks they

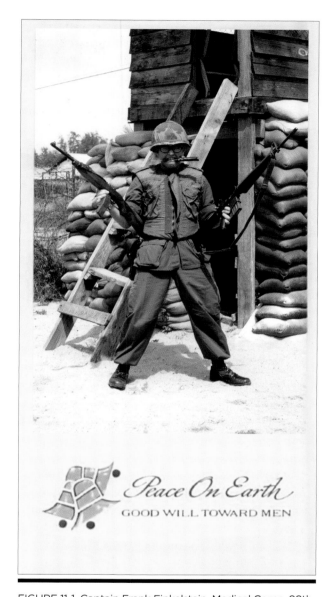

FIGURE 11-1. Captain Frank Finkelstein, Medical Corps, 98th Psychiatric Detachment (September 1969–September 1970). Finkelstein was a civilian-trained psychiatrist, and his holiday card's evident cynicism suggests that he endured role-related operational and ethical strain, especially that stemming from a clash between his physician's commitment to serve humanity and his wartime obligation to serve military expediency. Finkelstein was not unique in this regard, even if he was more demonstrative; this problem arose among many mental health providers assigned in Vietnam, particularly those who served in the latter half of the war and who had no prior military experience. Photograph courtesy of Frank Finkelstein.

were being asked to take. In effect, they had seen enough of death to know that they preferred life. What was I to do with deviant behavior like that? They were given a brief respite and returned to their units; the fighting strength was conserved. How many were later killed I do not know, nor do I wish to.[69(pp268–269)]

Livingston made numerous allusions to his belief that the psychiatric doctrine as practiced in Vietnam was hypocritical, and he concluded that because "without medical support the prosecution of this war would not have been possible. . . . [Physicians therefore are being used] to sanction and perpetuate one of the most anti-life enterprises of our time."[69(p272)] To solve his ethical conflict Livingston "disqualified" himself from future military service by disseminating the following satirical prowar prayer to the press at the change of command ceremony for Colonel George S Patton III.

God, our heavenly Father, hear our prayer. We acknowledge our shortcomings and ask thy help in being better soldiers for thee. Grant us, O Lord, those things we need to do thy work more effectively. Give us this day a gun that will fire 10,000 rounds a second, a napalm which will burn for a week. Help us to bring death and destruction wherever we go, for we do it in thy name and therefore it is meet and just. We thank thee for this war fully mindful that while it is not the best of all wars, it is better than no war at all. We remember that Christ said, "I came not to send peace, but a sword," and we pledge ourselves in all our works to be like Him. Forget not the least of thy children as they hide from us in the jungles; bring them under our merciful hand that we may end their suffering. In all things, O God, assist us, for we do our noble work in the knowledge that only with thy help can we avoid the catastrophe of peace which threatens us ever. All of which we ask in the name of thy son, George Patton. Amen.[70(p23)]

As a consequence he was relieved of his duties, evaluated psychiatrically, returned to the United States ("as an embarrassment to the command"[70(p23)]), and administratively discharged from the Army.

Protest by Captain Floyd (Shad) Meshad, Medical Service Corps

Meshad was assigned as an Army social work officer to the 98th Psychiatric Detachment during the drawdown phase. In his account he described the mounting soldier despair and dissent he encountered and its impact on him and his functioning as an Army mental health professional. According to Meshad, he sustained intolerable frustration while attempting to provide psychosocial assistance to soldiers and their leaders in a war he believed was wrong. As the narrative progressed, he increasingly identified with the confused, frightened, and often traumatized soldiers he met, which produced in him severe, role-linked guilt. ("It could have been me. I'd watch them and I'd have to ask myself, 'do I have the balls to do what they're doing?' Meanwhile, I'd be sitting there counseling them about their problems—the main problem being the same thoughts I was grappling with."[71(p98)])

In time he decided that the chief problem was that the soldiers, as well as himself, were victims of military authority. ("We were on a tight wire balanced between the chaos of war and the madness of military regulations . . . I began to think my biggest service to them was to help them manipulate the system."[71(p24)]) He became a maverick mental health officer who believed in passionate advocacy on behalf of soldiers and against military authority and the war. In the end he martyred himself by provoking the Army to court-martial him for the length of his mustache.[71]

The Reactions of Organized Psychiatry

Mental health organizations also reacted strongly to the war's increasing unpopularity. In March 1971, 67% of American Psychiatric Association (APA) members responding to a poll indicated that they wanted the US government to terminate all military activity in Vietnam.[72] This was followed by APA Board of Trustees' passing official resolutions that condemned the war and argued for an American withdrawal[73] and the APA eliminating the military psychiatry section of its annual convention as an expression of protest.[38]

In July 1972, the American Psychological Association joined seven other mental health associations in the following public statement, "We find it morally repugnant for any government to exact such heavy costs in human suffering for the sake of abstract conceptions of national pride or honor."[74(p1)] In raising questions about the morality of the US military intervention in Vietnam, these organizations increased the ethical tension for psychiatrists, psychologists, and social workers in uniform, yet they neglected to acknowledge that there was a dilemma of these proportions facing their members or to provide guidelines for addressing it. Psychiatry in particular left its military colleagues in uniform to struggle alone amidst the insinuated collective disapproval and open collegial criticism and scorn.

Defending Military Psychiatry

There were a few publications in the latter half of the war and afterward that sought to justify the role, doctrine, and methods used by military psychiatrists in Vietnam. Generally, these were authored by career military psychiatrists such as Arthur[22] and Brown,[38] both Navy psychiatrists; Hays,[75] an Air Force psychiatrist; and Parrish,[1] Johnson,[34] and Gibbs,[76] Army psychiatrists—all of whom were more restrained than their critics.

One notable exception on both counts was the review by Bey and Chapman.[77] Bey, who served in Vietnam with 1st ID (April 1969–April 1970), and Chapman rebutted those who would criticize the methods of military psychiatrists as dehumanizing and unethical by pointing out that, "While war is indeed immoral,"[77(p344)] all citizens become responsible by association for its destructive consequences.[77] They were unapologetic in declaring that in support of wartime mobilization the military psychiatrist's first priority must be the predominance of collective goals and values over those of the individual, and they enumerated 15 critical differences between military and civilian psychiatry. These centered around differences in the populations served (because individuals serving in the military have been selected and screened, they are generally healthier than those typically seen by the civilian psychiatrist); altered clinical goals (in a combat situation the military psychiatrist's task is to help normal individuals adjust to an abnormal situation); and revised allegiances and priorities (as an employee and agent of the organization the priority for the military psychiatrist is to be a management consultant to command and allied medical personnel regarding matters of morale, organizational stress, and psychiatric disorders and behavior problems; his secondary role is providing direct clinical care).

According to Bey and Chapman, in the combat theater the provision of psychotherapy—as well as diagnoses—is contraindicated because it encourages secondary gain and thereby interferes with effective adaptation of the soldier. The authors were not opposed to the absence of privileged communication between the military psychiatrist and his patient. They also were accepting of the fact that whereas the military psychiatrist often makes recommendations to a commander regarding the disposition of a soldier with character and behavior disorder, the commander has the option of disregarding it.

Finally, there also were some authors who felt it was crucial that the individual psychiatrists who served in Vietnam be distinguished from the implementation of the military psychiatry doctrine there and the criticism it provoked because of the war's unpopularity. They argued that a more realistic consideration would acknowledge the impossible clash of military and professional obligations faced by military psychiatrists under those circumstances. For example, Boman said, "The role of the military psychiatrist in a conflict like Vietnam encompasses so many ambiguities and moral dilemmas that one would not be surprised at his lapsing into almost a state of frozen ambivalence."[78(p124)] London, an ethicist, went further by challenging the new "moralistic 'right think'" of those who would fault military psychiatrists for not actively opposing the military in Vietnam: "it is unseemly, if not immoral, to retrospectively condemn the doctors of last decade's war for doing what then looked like their duty."[79(p250)]

POST-VIETNAM

Lingering Postwar Criticism of the Military Psychiatry Doctrine

Following the cessation of hostilities in Southeast Asia, the large numbers of veterans reporting post-Vietnam psychiatric symptoms and adjustment difficulties led some critics to fault the use of the forward treatment doctrine in Vietnam through speculating that it had served to mistreat psychiatric casualties in favor of questionable military and political goals.[40,80–83] These criticisms fell into three overlapping areas: (1) the incomplete treatment of combat troops and their premature return to duty, (2) the undisciplined use of psychotropic medications, and (3) the mislabeling of psychiatrically affected troops as character and behavior disorders.

Accusations of Incomplete Treatment and Premature Return to Duty

Australian military psychiatrists Spragg[84] and Boman[78] were very critical of the US combat psychiatry doctrine based on their experiences with Australian troops in Vietnam. Boman thought that reading US Army psychiatry literature from Vietnam was "hair raising."[78(p111)] Kolb, a posttraumatic stress disorder (PTSD) investigator, was especially disturbed because military psychiatrists had exhibited satisfaction in quickly returning combat stress-affected soldiers back to duty. He argued that such practices were etiologically influential in causing delayed PTSD in Vietnam veterans.[83] Similarly, Abse commented:

> Such [PTSD] patients in my experience have not received early effective treatment with emphasis on cathartic psychotherapy. On the contrary, they received, while in Vietnam, treatment which emphasized massive psychotropic medication, followed by crowding out with sundry recreational activities any focus on their essentially traumatic and pathogenic experiences. Such temporary suppressive treatment invited the reinforcement of dissociation though it may have worked for the while, while the soldier was in active service overseas.[81(p20)]

Accusations of the Undisciplined Use of Psychotropic Medications

A related concern was voiced after the war regarding the ethics associated with prescribing psychotropic medications for combat troops in Vietnam. Grossman,[85] Holloway,[86] and Abse[81] wondered if the suppressive use of pharmacotherapy contributed to delayed PTSD in veterans, and Gabriel[87] worried that the military was skating on ethical thin ice by prescribing such drugs as a prophylactic measure against disabling fear in soldiers.

Accusations of Mislabeling Affected Troops as Behavior Disorders

Like Renner, a Navy psychiatrist who expressed concern for the "hidden casualties" in Vietnam,[88] Australian military psychiatrist Boman similarly argued that Army psychiatrists systematically, if inadvertently, mistreated combat-generated psychiatric casualties in Vietnam by labeling them character disorders—a practice that served to disguise soldiers' true pathology in favor of a more expedient administrative (and prejudicial) disposition.[78] Similarly, Radine, a professor of sociology,

was critical of the principles and means utilized by Army psychiatrists in Vietnam based on the published record and opined that the Army induced mental health professionals to minimize treatment of true mental disorders in the service of "deviance control."[89] He noted that, "Even at the [psychiatric detachment] level, diagnosis and treatment seem to have been casual and brief."[89(p165)]

Questionable Evidence for Inadequate Treatment

In Chapter 2 it was noted that in the mid-1980s the government-sponsored National Vietnam Veterans Readjustment Study (NVVRS) found that large numbers of veterans (approximately 30% of male and 27% of female study participants) acknowledged PTSD symptoms at some point since serving in Vietnam, and that for many PTSD had become persistent and incapacitating (15% and 9% of study participants, respectively).[90] However, correlation between combat-associated psychiatric difficulties, psychotropic prescriptions, or character and behavior disorder diagnosis *while in Vietnam*, and postwar PTSD or other psychiatric or adjustment problems among veterans was apparently not systematically explored by these investigators.

On a more informal basis, (as noted in Chapter 2) Arthur S Blank Jr, former Army psychiatrist in Vietnam, and later the National Director for the Department of Veterans Affairs Readjustment Counseling Centers, noted that acute combat stress reactions did not typically meet the criteria for PTSD and did not generally evolve into diagnosable PTSD later.[91] And senior Army psychiatrist and Vietnam veteran Franklin Del Jones indicated that overly sympathetic attitudes toward Vietnam veterans have led some civilian psychiatrists to misunderstand the typically temporary and reversible nature of combat stress reactions and to fail to appreciate the increased risk for psychiatric morbidity (including PTSD) if treatments while in the field do not promote symptom suppression and rapid return to military function and comrades.[92]

On the other hand, Palinkas and Coben interpreted the results of their postwar study of all Marines who received psychiatric hospitalization in Vietnam, which was described in Chapter 7, as suggesting that strict implementation of the military treatment doctrine by Navy psychiatrists, including the use of modern psychotropic medications, may have resulted in inadequate treatment and impaired combat performance.[93] Obviously much more study of these questions was warranted.

Lingering Postwar Conflict Among Mental Health Professionals Who Served in Vietnam

This chapter opened with Parrish's poignant account of the ordeal that faced Vietnam returnees. His observations and reactions depicted substantial guilt-producing societal pressure on veterans, including medical and mental health professionals. With this in mind, it is not surprising to find that military psychiatrists and allied professionals may have struggled with unmitigated self-recrimination over the years following their service there (or defensive blame of society, the government, or the military). For some, the associated self-doubts would especially surround the ethics of doing one's job.

Major Edward M Colbach, Medical Corps

Colbach was civilian-trained in psychiatry and had no experience as a military physician before being assigned in Vietnam in October 1968, shortly following the enemy's pivotal Tet '68 offensives. During most of his year he was assigned as a solo psychiatrist to the 67th Evacuation Hospital in Qui Nhon (sometimes assisted by Raymond R Crowe, an Air Force psychiatrist). Based on his tour, Colbach published a pair of articles regarding clinical challenges in treating drug abuse (see Chapter 9). Upon his return to the United States in October 1969, he served as Assistant Psychiatry Consultant to the Office of The Surgeon General, US Army, and while there published an article on Army criteria for compassionate reassignment.[94] Also, along with Parrish, the Psychiatry Consultant, he published an overview of US Army mental health activities in Vietnam through mid-1970. Among other factors their review credited the clinical attitude of "expectancy" and the use of psychoactive medications in promoting a commendably high return-to-duty rate. They also included justification for the combat psychiatry doctrine used there:

> Mental health personnel have been criticized for their involvement in Vietnam. It has been implied that to maintain the fighting strength in such a controversial war, by sending reluctant, nervous soldiers back to duty and possible harm, is both inhumane and unethical. As has been stated, the military mental health worker is first and foremost

a guardian of reality. And the reality is that we are fighting in Vietnam, and someone has to carry a gun there, even though very few men actually choose to do so. If one soldier is relieved of this duty, another will have to replace him. And the soldier replaced by another will have to live a long time with the realization that he was so "sick," so weak, that someone else had to take over for him when the chips were really down.[3(p341)]

Fifteen years after his service in Vietnam, Colbach wrote a personally and professionally wrenching retrospection on his role and activities there—experiences that evidently haunted him long after his return. Throughout his narrative there were expressions of psychological conflict and regret. For example, he believed that his anger at being sent to Vietnam interfered with his empathy for his soldier-patients: "in many ways I was a failure in actually reaching out to those fellows and touching them and alleviating their suffering."[21(p265)] Similar to Bloch, Colbach was resigned to being the "guardian of reality"; however, this position seemed to give him little relief from his role-linked guilt. "I tried to help my patients learn that lesson [that all of life is a struggle], not to quit but to go on. Probably a few of them did learn that, *if they survived* [emphasis added]."[21(p265)] Ultimately, he found an ethical position he evidently hoped would bring him peace of mind:

> . . . Whether the Vietnam conflict fits these criteria [of a just war] or not is really beyond me to say. I did accept it as a just war when I agreed to serve in it.
> . . . I then had to accept that my obligation to my individual patient was far superseded by my obligation to the military and, eventually, to my country.[21(p265)]

Second Lieutenant Roger A Roffman, Medical Service Corps

A similar postwar lament came from Roffman. Early in 1967, he traveled by troop ship to Vietnam with the 9th ID as the division social work officer. He had received his commission in the Army several months after being awarded his master's degree in social work, and he completed 1 year of military service at Fort Riley, Kansas, before arriving in Vietnam. After serving with the 9th ID, Roffman was assigned to the 935th Psychiatric Detachment, where he conducted a pioneering survey of drug and alcohol use among enlisted confinees of the USARV Installation Stockade ("Long Binh Jail") as well as a similar one (with Ely Sapol, an Army psychologist,) with soldiers departing Vietnam, which was described in Chapter 9. In his unpublished manuscript, *Tilting at Myths: A Marijuana Memoir*, which was written four decades after his service in Vietnam, he included the following:

> . . . I told [the new 9th ID psychiatrist] how ambivalent I felt when, following military psychiatry protocol, we sent traumatized soldiers back to their units after a few days of rest and reassurance that they'd get through this very normal reaction to a very tragic experience.
>
> I also ranted about contrasts that seemed incomprehensible in a war zone, maybe even obscene. American kids in their teens and twenties were losing limbs when stepping on land mines, being impaled on stakes in punji pits, and being decimated in ambushes. Yet, many of us had had dinners in superb riverfront French restaurants in Bien Hoa, spent hours at an officers' swimming pool, and enjoyed "happy hour" in the roof-top bar of a Saigon hotel.[95(p27)]

Second Lieutenant Raymond M Scurfield, Medical Service Corps

Another example is that of Scurfield, also a social work officer, who was assigned in Vietnam to the 98th Psychiatric Detachment in March 1968, on the heels of the Tet offensives. He spent his year in the outpatient clinic serving as clinician and the detachment's administrative officer. He received his commission in the Army shortly after being awarded his master's degree in social work, and he completed 10 months of military service at Fort Bliss, Texas, before being assigned in Vietnam. Thirty-five years later he published *A Vietnam Trilogy: Veterans and Post Traumatic Stress: 1968, 1989, 2000*,[96] which included references to the guilt he carried from serving in Vietnam.[96(p127)] The following quotation serves to exemplify his ethical strain associated with implementing the combat psychiatry treatment doctrine:

> Some soldiers, convinced that they were going to die or be maimed or go crazy if they stayed any longer in the war zone, would do and say anything to try to build a case that they were "crazy" and had to be evacuated out of Vietnam. It was our responsibility

as psychiatric gate keepers to keep that gateway from blowing open.[96(p43)]

It should be noted that Scurfield's perspective was not only based on his experiences in Vietnam; it was also influenced by his many years of work with veterans while affiliated with the Veterans Administration and the Readjustment Counseling Service. Scurfield believed that the Army's system for dealing with emotionally troubled soldiers in Vietnam was neglectful and apparently resulted in large numbers of veterans developing chronic PTSD and other psychiatric conditions. In particular, he blamed commanding officers for being unsympathetic and punitive and not referring soldiers for psychiatric care. He also faulted them for discharging soldiers from the Army for nonmedical conditions, that is, character and behavior disorders, which denied them timely treatment. He held the psychiatrists responsible for enabling this process and for providing minimal psychiatric treatment and sending traumatized soldiers prematurely back to duty:

> The vast majority of soldiers who suffered extraordinary reactions to extraordinary events were not hospitalized psychiatrically, nor evacuated out of their duty stations. They received minimal or no psychiatric treatment, and were sent back to duty within several hours.[96(pp34–35)] . . . The overall mission in Vietnam was the same as the military medicine mission everywhere else—to conserve the fighting strength. This is extremely important in that our mission was not to do what was necessarily in the best interests of the longer-term mental health of the individual soldier.[96(p36)]

To prove his assertion that combat troops in Vietnam received inadequate psychiatric treatment, Scurfield alluded to seven cases (referring to examples provided by former Army psychiatrist, Arthur S Blank Jr); however, his assertion seems arguable because of the scant amount of information he included.[96(p35)] These consisted of either seemingly adequate treatment (one soldier was "subdued with injections of Thorazine,"[96(p35)] and another "slept for 22 hours and subsequently was completely clear and non-anxious"[96(p35)]), or were brief and dramatic descriptions of circumstances surrounding their admission without definitive information regarding treatment, clinical course, or disposition. Mostly, however, he blamed the situation in which he found himself:

> The internal conflicts this policy [ie, the forward treatment doctrine] raised in the medical, psychiatric and social work personnel fed an anger, indeed a rage, that we suppressed: rage at the government, at the country, at being in a Catch-22 situation. Freudian-based psychiatric theory was at best being unwittingly used by well-intentioned military mental health officers and at worst was being perversely misused to justify a military policy that was far more concerned about "the mission" than about the men and women who carried out the mission.[96(p42)]

Apparently Scurfield ultimately bolstered his psychological defenses through his career activities in veteran mental health:

> Any guilt that may be mine from having been so naïve I channel into purpose and conviction and drive to attempt to make the system and society more responsive to the real needs of vets and the real psychiatric legacies of war.[96(p127)]

Major Douglas R Bey, Medical Corps

Also pained were postwar comments by Bey, despite his defense of military psychiatry outlined earlier. Bey served later in Vietnam as the division psychiatrist for the 1st ID (April 1969–April 1970). He trained in psychiatry in a civilian program and during the period before his arrival in Vietnam he was assigned to the Army Hospital at Fort Knox, Kentucky. Bey served with distinction in Vietnam and authored or coauthored numerous articles regarding his experiences there as well as wrote a memoir. The following comments, also charged with guilt and blame, are from his personal account, some of which was published 35 years after he left:

> While in Vietnam I saw considerable waste of American lives, equipment, and money. I had little understanding of the mission of the 1st Infantry Division. The Civic Action Program didn't seem to make much sense medically. I saw that the Vietnamese people were suffering greatly. Our presence contributed to the disruption of the family structures, we corrupted their daughters who sold themselves for money, their sons who sold stolen goods and pimped for their sisters. We damaged their crop lands with our bombs and military equipment and we treated them like lesser beings (running over them on the roads, barging into their fine restaurants in boots and fatigues, had them burn our shit and do menial labor).[97]
>
> My impression was that soldiers in World War II had the feeling they were morally in the right and were supported by the folks back home. Men who avoided service were shunned.[98(p260)]
>
> . . . After my return from 'Nam, I tried to forget the whole experience. I didn't wear anything green for several years. I carried my own load of guilt going into Vietnam. In addition, I felt a vague sense of guilt in response to the criticism by the antiwar groups—particularly those from my colleagues in psychiatry.[98(p265)]

Bey indicated that over the years he had made peace with his role in the Vietnam War. For part of this, he credited a renewed religious spirituality. He also considered helpful his near-death experience from a heart attack, his industrious professional life, including scholarship regarding psychiatry in Vietnam, and his relationship with his wife and children. He concluded his account with the following:

> From all the stories of drinking, throwing optometrists through doors [sic], and such, the reader may conclude that I have been flawed by my experience in Vietnam and that perhaps I'm one of the many supposed victims of PTSD. . . .
>
> We weren't greeted warmly when we returned, but I have no regrets and am proud that I served. I support my son's wish to enlist. I feel it is important to support our military and our government in these troubled times. I make a special effort to welcome and praise our returning veterans.[98(pp256–257)]

A Challenge to Reconcile the Ethical Dilemmas Associated With the Military Forward Treatment Doctrine

In 2011 the Army Surgeon General's Office published a comprehensive update of military psychiatry, *Combat and Operational Behavioral Health*.[99] However, despite including chapters describing the contemporary organizational structure for responding to combat and operational stress problems,[100] psychiatric medications in military operations,[101] ethical conflicts in military mental health,[102] and the subject of stress on military health care providers,[103] there was no acknowledgment of the critical—and evidently latent—ethical dilemmas associated with the combat psychiatry forward treatment doctrine apart from a brief mention in this author's review chapter of the psychiatric experience in the Vietnam War.[104] Almost 20 years earlier this author had written the lead article in the *American Journal of Psychiatry* reviewing the doctrine's contradictory ethics and urging leaders in military and civilian psychiatry to reconcile the dilemmas that became so torturous for practitioners, both civilian and military, during the Vietnam War.[4] The following material is borrowed from that review to illustrate the value conflicts that surrounded the implementation of the doctrine in Vietnam.

A Case Example From Vietnam

Case 2-1, the case of SP4 Delta, presented in Chapter 2, will serve as an example of the management and treatment of a combat stress casualty in Vietnam. According to the hospital record, upon his admission to the 93rd Evacuation Hospital/935th Psychiatric Detachment in 1967, he was in a severely disorganized and dysfunctional combat stress-induced state. In the course of his treatment, he talked about the painful loss of his buddies and his revulsion toward the killing. He also declared he could not return to the field. Nonetheless, the treatment staff encouraged him to see his duty through, and he was quickly returned to his unit without recurrence of symptoms, at least as far as the 935th Psychiatric Detachment knew. Except for the substitution of the tranquilizer, Thorazine, for sedatives and hypnotics of an earlier era, he would have been managed similarly by military psychiatrists during the latter phases of World War I, in World War II, or in the Korean War, and probably with the same rapid return to duty.[46] As previously noted, in those wars there was consensus regarding the military doctrine's effectiveness in providing satisfactory treatment.[64] Thus, by Army standards, the treatment of SP4 Delta was a success because it was felt to serve both the needs of force conservation and those of this individual.[105,106]

However, just as legality is not a sure test of morality, neither is apparent treatment effectiveness a sure test of ethical treatment. Anti-Vietnam War sentiment and the new Vietnam-era humanitarian sensibilities would question whether this example of the implementation of the Army psychiatry doctrine there

demonstrated its harmfulness. Should the psychiatric team at the 935th be faulted for crossing an ethical line in exhorting SP4 Delta to return to more combat duty despite his opposition? Once returned to his unit, did reactivated psychiatric symptoms reduce his combat effectiveness and contribute to his becoming killed or wounded? Because his treatment was abbreviated to return him quickly to fight again, did he later develop post-Vietnam psychiatric symptoms or adjustment difficulties?[107] The accusations that the forward treatment doctrine was unethical centered on two confounding claims:

1. It primarily served, as some believed, the prosecution of an immoral or unjust war; and
2. It served military expediency or political objectives at the expense of the soldier's interests or welfare.

The Question of Participating in an Unjust War

Regarding the first question, whether SP4 Delta's treatment and disposition according to the forward treatment doctrine was unethical because it primarily served, as some believed, the prosecution of an immoral or unjust war, it is logically straightforward. Any professional activity by military psychiatrists that contributes to an immoral or unjust war would be categorically immoral and unethical. Although many came to believe that America's intervention in Vietnam was unjust and immoral,[12,108] such a conclusion remains controversial.[109] Some felt it was justified based on the principles of international law established after World War II by the military tribunal at Nuremberg.[110] Certainly specific combat activities, such as atrocities, may be readily distinguishable as immoral. But a link between particular immoral combat activities and the specific clinical activities of military psychiatrists may be very difficult to establish.

The Challenge of Distinguishing Harm and Benefit

The second question is a more general one and highlights the psychiatrist's obligation to the soldier. It is also complicated and has implications for the use of the military treatment doctrine in any war. In short, because of the double agent position, the military psychiatrist faces a complex array of competing values and influences and is held responsible for the effects of his treatments in terms of the balance of harm and benefit.[111] These can be examined along the following three lines: (1) the question of harm to the soldier, (2) the question of benefit to the soldier, and (3) the question of coercive treatment and the benefit to society.

The Question of Harm to the Soldier. Is it likely that SP4 Delta was harmed by the combat psychiatry treatment approach because it put him in unreasonable jeopardy in subsequent combat? If he was only partially treated, or if he was still under the sedating effect of Thorazine, or because of his already demonstrated susceptibility, his vulnerability in combat may have been greatly increased. As was mentioned previously, the question of the effects of the neuroleptic and anxiolytic drugs on the performance (or vulnerability) of combat soldiers who served in Vietnam was not studied. However, the aforementioned study by Palinkas and Coben[93] did suggest that, at least for some diagnostic groups, returning soldiers to combat exposure after psychiatric hospitalization, apparently including the administration of psychotropic medications, may have increased their risks.

The Question of Benefit to the Soldier. Is it likely that SP4 Delta benefited by being treated according to the combat psychiatry doctrine? As noted in Chapter 7 and this one, psychiatric morbidity in prior wars was greatly reduced among soldiers affected with combat stress reaction who were treated and managed according to the traditional doctrine[112] because it apparently (*a*) reinforced the soldiers psychological defenses against subsequent breakdown in combat and (*b*) opposed the fixation of his symptoms into a "self-protective disabling neurotic compromise."[8(p731)] It was the impression of the earlier military psychiatrists that through suppressive and repressive clinical means, they could strengthen the affected combat soldier's investment in his combat comrades, leaders, and objectives, as well as reinforce his confidence in his own capabilities, thereby reestablishing his primary psychological resistance against further combat-induced disorganization:

> [To adapt to combat the soldier must] fuse his personal identity with the new group identity, to form deep emotional relationships with his buddies and with his leader, in sharing boredom, hardship, sacrifice and danger with them, and whether by compromise or illusion, to become oriented with them toward the destructive goals which he understands to be necessary for the common good.[113(p365)]

Also, as noted in Chapter 7, deeper, longer, or more complicated treatments, and especially those occurring far from the soldier's original unit and in more comfortable surroundings, were found as far back as World War I to favor the development of chronic psychiatric disability.

The Question of Coercive Treatment and the Benefit to Society. Was SP4 Delta's treatment unethical because his combat reaction represented the combat refusal of a dissident or because it is normal not to want to return? By labeling him with the exclusively military diagnosis of combat exhaustion, disregarding his opposition to further combat, and imposing the military doctrine's treatment regimen, were his military psychiatrists "blaming the victim"?[50] Some writers have even referred to the soldier's new willingness to enter combat after such coercive treatment as an iatrogenic psychosis.[11,40]

The matter of informed consent or refusal is especially critical when psychiatrists are representing the interests of other parties in addition to those of their patients—the problem of dual agency.[114] In his presenting condition of near catatonia, he was not competent to understand an adequate consent process and there can be little doubt about the rightfulness of treating him as the military psychiatrists deemed necessary. However, on the following day, his regression and decompensation had largely resolved, and the situation became quite different. He was treated with more Thorazine and behavioral strategies, including exhortation of the duty side of his conflict, to sway him from his expressed (at least initially) opposition to killing, and he was rapidly returned to more combat duty.

No matter what efforts the treatment team might have expended to obtain SP4 Delta's consent, the existence of a powerful negative incentive, that is, the threat of a court-martial, eliminated the possibility of proper informed consent or refusal. Because these clinical techniques were imposed on an individual who was sufficiently competent and rational to cooperate with a consent process, SP4 Delta's treatment was technically coercive by definition and violated a "moral rule" (against causing pain and depriving freedom).[111]

There may, however, be overriding moral justification for coercive treatment when it is felt to serve the best interests of the patient (so-called paternalistic treatment[111]), but in civilian settings, the paternalism exception to the moral rule does not apply to rational, competent adults. However, because the rights of those

---

EXHIBIT 11-1. A Proposal to Reconcile the Ethical Dilemmas Surrounding the Army's Traditional Forward Treatment Doctrine

---

The following was included in an address ("The Vietnam War and the Ethics of Combat Psychiatry") by the author [NMC] made to the Department of Psychiatry, Walter Reed Army Medical Center, Washington, DC, 8 August 1993.

In lieu of further research addressing the short- and long-term consequences from implementation of the forward treatment doctrine and based on military psychiatrists' observations across three major wars and my own experience serving in Vietnam, I propose that the following principles should predominate in the treatment of combat stress casualties:

Once in military uniform, and especially once assigned in a combat theater, the military psychiatrist must entrust the military to define duty, his and the patient's—except in the most dire circumstances.

This is necessary because of the exceedingly strong tendency for various compromises to arise in the soldier's "will to fight," as well as in the clinician's "will to treat," under the extreme circumstances of war.

With regard to an ethical stance associated with the forward treatment doctrine:
- It is acknowledged that a behavior treatment milieu, such as the forward treatment doctrine, does violate the ethical principle of informed consent/refusal.
- Nonetheless, whereas compassion can be extended to affected soldier-patients, their expressed opposition to military performance requirements should be overridden if their basic mental functions are not impaired.
- Such rapid return to military function is justified by the preeminence of group/unit/national needs. It is incumbent on the military psychiatrist to function as if serving in a locum parentis-like capacity (ie, such as making parental decisions for an adolescent). Consequently the military psychiatrist would ordinarily direct soldier-patients toward completing their duty—even if additional combat hazards are predictable.

Among clinical populations:
- If the combat stress-generated condition is expressed in intractable and disabling psychiatric symptoms, it is necessary to provide protection and additional treatment.
- If it is expressed in treatable symptoms and accompanied by avoidance of resumption of duty, this may be briefly accommodated but with rapid return to duty as the explicit goal.
- If it is expressed in a situationally derived (eg, new) opposition to more combat exposure, no matter how logically constructed, this represents a self-serving rationalization. If it is taken at face value by treators, soldier regression and persisting "sick role" is encouraged, other soldiers often follow suit, and the "fighting force" may be degraded.

In other words, the military psychiatrist:
must take responsibility for expecting that the (competent) soldier resume his duty function—but *cannot* take responsibility for the outcome (risk).

---

in active military service have historically been abridged by law, these boundaries are less certain.[12] In fact, there are numerous military regulations and policies that shape the practice of psychiatry to represent the preeminence of institutional goals and values over those of the individual.[77,115] Besides the absence of a right to informed consent or refusal with regard to hospitalization or psychiatric treatment, there are also limitations in the service member's rights to privileged communication[116] and to psychiatric due process.[117]

There also may be overriding moral justification for coercive treatment when the treatment is deemed necessary for the welfare of others (so-called utilitarian value). Was there sufficient benefit to society to justify treating SP4 Delta according to the combat psychiatry doctrine? That is, in overriding his autonomous choice and quickly returning him to fight again in spite of some additional risk to him, was his treatment team serving a superseding value representing the welfare of the American people? As a soldier, was he obligated to unconditionally sacrifice his self-interest for the common good? On the other hand, some would argue that a treatment approach that purports to sacrifice the interests of the individual soldier for the good of society might simply coincide with the military's value of teamwork and combat efficiency in some situations. The military's values can diverge from those of society, as many believe was the case in Vietnam.

Practical Realities in Treating Combat Stress Casualties

It seems reasonable to say that in practice it is unrealistic to believe that the individual combat psychiatrist can distinguish at any given time whether the military treatment doctrine serves essential public welfare or only conforms to military objectives, political goals, or a war's popularity. Furthermore, this uncertainty may compound the already difficult task of determining clinically whether a soldier who is opposed to returning to combat is suffering from a mental disorder or expressing a rational refusal.[17] Brill's comment from World War II illustrated the influence of the seeming utilitarian values on clinical judgment: "It was difficult to define exactly how much of such patients' ineffectiveness was due to illness and how much to lack of desire to do their part."[24(p242)] During the Vietnam era, Baker took a more disparaging attitude when he speculated that the soldier with a prolonged postcombat recovery had "consolidated his adaptation on a *parasitic* basis (emphasis added)."[112(p1835)] Since American troops were withdrawn from Vietnam, the ethical dilemmas surrounding the combat psychiatry forward treatment doctrine have remained unreconciled between civilian and military psychiatry. In an effort to help military mental health professionals avoid getting lost in these value crosscurrents, this author [NM Camp] proposed a set of ethical principles in an address in 1993 to the Department of Psychiatry of Walter Reed Army Medical Center (Exhibit 11-1); however, this had no measurable effect. Until official ethical guidelines can be established for the psychiatric management and treatment of combat casualties, it will regrettably remain incumbent on each individual psychiatrist who serves in the combat theater to bear a greater burden of conscience in performing his/her duties, just as was the case for those who served in Vietnam.

WALTER REED ARMY INSTITUTE OF RESEARCH PSYCHIATRIST SURVEY FINDINGS: OPERATIONAL FRUSTRATIONS AND ETHICAL DILEMMAS FOR MENTAL HEALTH PERSONNEL IN VIETNAM

The following extends the presentation of findings from the Walter Reed Army Institute of Research postwar survey (1982) of Army psychiatrists who served in Vietnam that was begun in Chapter 5. Under the heading of subjective reactions to service in Vietnam, the survey psychiatrists were asked to indicate on a scalar range of 1-to-5 the strength of their "disagreement" (1) or "agreement" (5) with 31 statements referring to their attitudes, dilemmas, and frustrations as a result of assignment and functioning in Vietnam. The section also included open-ended questions and a general invitation to make marginal notations that would further explain their personal reactions. Notably, the number of psychiatrist participants who responded to these questions ranged from 78 to 85, the highest response rate among all sections of the questionnaire.

Qualitative Responses

Participant responses to open-ended questions are arranged below according to dominant patterns. Overall a large proportion of the study psychiatrists emphasized that they felt quite strongly—typically negatively—about the war and their participation in it. This was especially true for those who had civilian training in psychiatry and those who served after the midpoint in the war in general. Whereas it has been noted throughout this work that the psychiatrists who served in the second half of the war published relatively little describing their experiences in Vietnam, when prompted by the survey they were vigorously outspoken, often bitter, and also defensive. As will become evident, the psychiatrists of this latter period were also more likely to complain of inequities and to be critical of their preparation and utilization by the Army.

Reactions to the Walter Reed Army Institute of Research Survey

Participants' reactions to the questionnaire and to the research more generally were quite variable and often passionate. The majority of comments about the research questionnaire were positive; however, there were also a number of comments that in one way or another could be considered negative. Quite a few participants expressed gratitude that the research had provided them with an opportunity for remembering and catharsis. One respondent also sent his inpatient log and copies of clinical summaries he had collected from his tour in the event that such data might support other research. (Only three participants gave an affirmative response to the question of whether they brought back clinical records.)

Many participants remarked on the extent of time that had passed between when they completed their year in Vietnam and when they were contacted for the study (ranging from 10 to 17 years). A small number expressed regret that some questions asked for more detail than their memory could provide, and others volunteered that they had been aware of trying to forget their Vietnam experiences. Several were more specific in stating that they had not spoken of their Vietnam tour since they returned—in spite of an appreciation that it was one of the most important experiences of their life. One participant provided the following explanation for his "clinical amnesia." He wrote, "A curious thing about my Vietnam experience is that I recall my personal—as opposed to clinical—experience more vividly. . . . I suspect the personal trauma of isolation from home and family made the actual work secondary in importance."

A number of other participants emphasized a bitterness that it had taken so long for someone to ask for their impressions, which led to a cynicism that any positive changes would come from the study. For example, one participant wrote, "this study is about 15 years too late. . . . My social work officer and I did attempt to collect [clinical] data at the time we served, but I got only static from the Army when I attempted to find out what happened to the [patients] I had seen."

Another psychiatrist declined to participate in the study, referring to the project as "pseudo-recollective science at its worst." He felt so strongly that he wrote the editors of several psychiatric journals to warn them about the study. Another example was that of a psychiatrist who faulted the study design as a poor epidemiological approach because of the lengthy interval for recollection. He suggested that a better approach would be to get the case records from those who were there. He acknowledged that he retained such records and expressed a willingness to analyze them if the Army would pay him. Ultimately he completed the questionnaire, indicating that he had carefully consulted his records. He remarked, "[seeking] the truth about our experiences in Vietnam is now the most valuable professional goal in the service of our country."

One psychiatrist returned an unmarked questionnaire with the following unsigned statement, "Many of us who served as medical officers in Vietnam were as deeply affected and carry as lasting reactions as any of the other men who served there. I have yet to find the peace of mind that would allow [me] to watch any of the Vietnam War movies, or talk about the war without threat of loss of control."

A final example is the participant who offered a general, but obviously also personal, justification for the psychiatrist's participation in the war in Vietnam. After acknowledging his efforts at forgetting the associated painful memories, he revealed his residual bitterness and cynicism. He wrote,

> [My memories] are now quite dim and probably repressed. . . . I believe our government made a political error in going to Vietnam, but once the Army is sent somewhere, it does what it is supposed to do . . . and support people—like psychiatrists— do what they do . . . [therefore this study] strikes me as rather unimportant, something like focusing attention on a skin blemish and ignoring a cancer.

Reactions to Being Assigned to Vietnam

Participant reactions to questions regarding attitudes about being assigned to Vietnam, preparation for serving, and perceptions of one's counterparts patterned especially around the distinction between pre-Vietnam military and civilian psychiatric training.

Attitude About Being Sent to Vietnam

Civilian-Trained Psychiatrists. The civilian-trained participants included little about how they happened to go to Vietnam despite their often profuse and usually emotional expressions of regret and resentment for having served there. Only one civilian-trained psychiatrist spontaneously indicated that he was truly a volunteer. Perhaps this contributed to his apparent conflicts about the war and his role in it. He wrote, "I was there early in the war when there was no stigma. I volunteered to be assigned . . . and wanted to go because I was curious. I came away more cynical about life and institutions [like the Army], but that's a good effect." Perhaps another participant spoke more clearly for the civilian-trained group when he simply said, "Most of us were drafted."

Somewhat related were the several comments by civilian-trained psychiatrists reflecting feelings of dismay about a perceived inequity in the relative proportion of military-trained psychiatrists required to serve in Vietnam. As one wrote, "I noted that few career Army psychiatrists went to Vietnam. They got out of it in various ways—threatening to leave the Army, etc." A similar complaint by another civilian-trained participant emphasized his feelings of relative inexperience. He stated, "Note that so many career military psychiatrists avoided Vietnam [thereby] leaving it to neophytes like me." Another spoke about how he was reassigned to Vietnam from his stateside post, only to be replaced there by an Army-trained psychiatrist "who was single."

Evidently, he, too, believed that the Army-trained psychiatrist had a greater obligation, but this feeling was compounded with a similar one about those with fewer family obligations.

Military-Trained Psychiatrists. Generally there was somewhat less regret and resentment expressed by the group of military-trained psychiatrists. Perhaps it can be presumed that having been trained by the military generated some sense of commitment to support the military mission. Still, negative reactions to having been sent to Vietnam predominated. A small minority of military-trained psychiatrists spontaneously commented on how they became assigned to Vietnam. A few of these indicated that they had some eagerness to professionally support the war effort. For example, one psychiatrist wrote, "Having chosen to 'identify with the enemy' by joining the Army in my senior year of medical school, I took my internship and residency with the full expectation that I would be assigned in some capacity in Vietnam if the war was still going on—as it was."

More common, however, were military-trained participants who recalled a frank regret at having been made to go. This feeling was commonly linked to a resentment of Army colleagues who succeeded in avoiding a Vietnam assignment. Others seemed to have experienced a combination of eagerness and reticence. An example of such apparent mixed motivations can be seen in this comment by one military-trained participant, "I volunteered because we were told that 80% of [graduating Army residents] were going anyway, and that volunteers would get [special] consideration for a next assignment. I was also a patriot, and a Europe assignment seemed as boring as Ft. [Knox]. Basically, I was curious." This individual went on to highlight his feeling of being cheated because he was the only one of his graduating class to be sent.

Another military-trained psychiatrist voiced a similar concern for fairness, only in this instance he included an explanation for the perceived inequity. He stated, "It did not help my morale nor that of most other MDs [medical doctors] to know that [late in the war] only the 'losers' were sent to Vietnam. I felt that I was sent there as punishment for having antagonized my superiors during the [Army] residency."

Apparently it was not only late in the war that such feelings of being punitively assigned to Vietnam affected the military-trained psychiatrist. One who served early commented, "I was assigned to Vietnam [because] I turned down several attractive offers for continuance with the Army [and] indicated I was going to resign my commission. Needless to say, this did cause some bitterness on my part."

Another military-trained psychiatrist spoke with some resentment about the fact that of his graduating class of eight, two of the three psychiatrists without children were assigned to Vietnam, with the third being assigned to Korea. In his estimation, the intent to evade Vietnam by his colleagues was transparent in that in several cases their wives became pregnant for the first time as the class began its last year of training.

Lastly were the remarks of a very experienced Army psychiatrist who also expressed dismay about inequity. Yet in his instance, the comparison was with the Army psychiatrists who also had extensive military backgrounds. He wrote, "My disappointment was solely due to what I thought was discrimination. I had already served two hardship tours, one in heavy combat and one in a combat zone, while over half of my peers had [not]."

Professional Preparation for Vietnam

Civilian-Trained Psychiatrists. Study participants were asked several questions about the specifics of their professional preparations for service in Vietnam, such as unique training environments or personal study. Most of the civilian-trained subjects either left this question blank or indicated they had none. However, a number did comment on training experiences that they felt overlapped with the clinical challenges in Vietnam, as in crisis intervention, community psychiatry, industrial psychiatry, and psychoanalytic anthropology.

Several of the civilian-trained psychiatrists felt they were well prepared because a particularly influential faculty member in their residency program had served in a prior war and had shaped the program in the direction of a social psychiatry model. An example was the following comment: "I probably adapted easier than most to the needs of the service and the philosophy (early return to duty) because that is how I was trained in my residency by a very senior and experienced retired Army psychiatrist." One individual highlighted that his civilian training was in a Veterans Administration center where he learned about combat stress. Lastly, quite a few commented, much more so than those trained in the military, that they had prepared for their tour by reading books and articles about the Vietnamese people and culture or other works exploring the history and geopolitics surrounding the war.

Military-Trained Psychiatrists. Among those trained in military settings, many acknowledged that their training was to some extent a specialized preparation, and they generally highlighted their exposure to the classical writings in combat psychiatry. A few, however, expressed dismay that their training was in fact not distinguishable from civilian training. One participant acknowledged that while there were aspects of his military residency that emphasized combat theater psychiatry, his training was nonetheless "anecdotal, minimal, adjunctive, and self-taught." Another similarly affected psychiatrist commented, "Being lucky, I was assigned [in Vietnam] to a hospital and not [to do] field psychiatry so I did not feel the effects of my lack of training . . . a marked deficit."

Only one among the military-trained group commented that he felt more prepared because he had been exposed specifically to soldiers who had been evacuated from Vietnam. Especially notable was a comment by a psychiatrist who had trained both in civilian and military programs (only two participants had this hybrid training). To the question asking if his training was in part directed to special considerations of the combat theater, he emphasized, "No, not even in [my Army training] program."

Retrospective Conclusions About Preparation

At the end of the questionnaire participants were asked, "Knowing now what you know, what would you have done better to prepare for Vietnam service?" Of all the questions, this one evoked the greatest collection of remarks expressing strong personal sentiments about having served in Vietnam. They ranged from highly emotional to quite rational and included suggestions for professional preparation as well as comments relating to Army policies and methods. These did not split so strongly between civilian and military training

background, suggesting that those who trained in a military setting did not automatically incur a functional familiarity with the Army culture and its ways and means.

In analyzing the responses it was sometimes difficult to distinguish the often bitter and resentful feelings from practical suggestions about preparation. Many participants, especially the civilian-trained ones who served later in the war, dismissed the question with pithy sarcastic answers such as, "Not go!"; "Go to jail, or Canada"; "Joined the Navy!"; "Switched to surgery!"; and "Get a good lawyer!" The comment of another— "I'm not sure anything would have helped!"—was echoed by several colleagues. One psychiatrist combined both personal and practical reflections in his response, "[I would] vote against LBJ (President Johnson)—I was adequately prepared for a bad situation." Similarly, another said, "I don't think there was much I could have done to prepare for Vietnam. It was a stressful and harrowing experience." Yet a third chose to speak more explicitly about his personal side when he suggested his "preparation" would be "to not get married or certainly not have children."

With respect to professional preparation specifically, the predominant refrain was that of having needed beforehand the distilled experience and wisdom of those psychiatrists who preceded them. The implications in this, and in a few cases explicitly stated, were (*a*) that the orientation and training at the MFSS for the psychiatrists deploying to Vietnam was not adequate, and (*b*) that the psychiatrists in central roles in the Army failed to serve a critical function by not systematically "debriefing" each returning psychiatrist so as to extract practical information for use in preparing subsequent cohorts of replacements. As one participant stated, "MFSS did a decent job of preparing one for medical unit duty, but not for combat unit duties." Another said, "MFSS is not the answer. Some sort of training with previous field (not [psychiatric detachment]) psychiatrists would have been helpful." The perceived need to have been briefed before arrival in Vietnam was often intertwined with frustrations at never having been debriefed following their own tour.

Other comments made under the heading of preparations included the wish to have had specific training and practical experience with the types of clinical problems that were the most challenging for the psychiatrist during his tour. Not surprisingly, several spoke of having needed more information on the treatment of combat stress reactions. Others spoke of needing more expertise with such problems as toxic psychoses, sociopathy, drug abuse, and addiction, as well as with treatment modalities such as narcotherapy and hypnotherapy. One participant spoke of needing "clearer training in psychiatric treatment options [in the combat setting] and when to use them."

Even some of the civilian-trained psychiatrists who had pre-Vietnam military assignments noted how they might have enhanced their preparation by tailoring their activities toward the Vietnam assignment. One such participant wrote, "[I would have] practiced more unit consultation at Ft. [Knox]." Another wrote, "I should have spent the year at Ft. [Riley] entirely with the division so that I could have known the middle level command people better."

Several participants highlighted their initial unfamiliarity with Army policies and methods. Although one psychiatrist spoke of his great appreciation for how quickly his enlisted staff helped to orient him, another spoke instead of a negative experience. He commented, "I needed more experience being in the military before going directly to a war zone. Being so dependent on a [sergeant] for basic military knowledge made me feel inadequate. The way it really operates is not in the books." Some also alluded to the need for a more functional familiarity with the "line" Army [nonmedical units] so as to have facilitated primary prevention interventions, that is, command consultation. Lastly, and in some contrast to the specific recommendations above, were a number of comments emphasizing how necessary it was to actually become a part of the combat theater environment before mastering it. One subject put it this way, "No [further preparation would have helped]! The actuality of the Vietnam experience was in no way comparable to the stateside view of it. Furthermore, the unpredictable nature of [Vietnam] negates the possibility of greater preparation." Another commented, "I really don't know [how to have better prepared]. What I did not know, I learned very quickly."

Stateside Military Experience as Preparation for Vietnam

Civilian-Trained Psychiatrists. Several civilian-trained psychiatrists indicated that their pre-Vietnam Army assignment had served several important preparatory functions. It provided a general process of enculturation, taught them critical differences in the perspectives and goals of civilian versus military psychiatry, and provided a context for the goals of military psychiatry within the institution of the Army. Several civilian-trained psychiatrists also mentioned the benefit of their having grown up with a father who had been in the military. They remarked on their comfort and familiarity in the military culture as well as an appreciation for the objectives of the military.

Military-Trained Psychiatrists. The military-trained participants who served in military assignments before service in Vietnam said very little about how those experiences affected their preparation for the tour in Vietnam. However, one commented, "I felt my skill was adequate. Part of my comfort lay in knowing personally some of the important medical commanders [before arriving in Vietnam], and in having served in the Far East before having to participate in actual combat."

Finally, a psychiatrist who served as the USARV Psychiatry Consultant late in the war provided the following observation pertaining to psychiatrist preparation, "The Surgeon General's Office seemed to be more busy filling slots rather than seeing to it that the assignees were provided with the literature, training, overlap, and especially time to get ready for the job." One could assume that this allegation would have its greatest impact on the civilian-trained psychiatrist with no prior military assignment.

Perceptions of One's Counterparts

Civilian-Trained Psychiatrists. More than one civilian-trained psychiatrist commented on his perception that the career Army psychiatrists were questionably competent. One participant emphatically declared: "None were adequately militarily trained!" Another commented, "Too many of the Army doctors above the rank of Major with whom I had contact both in Vietnam and [in the United States] were incompetent both as doctors and as administrators, and they seemed to have chosen to stay in the military because they could not make it in the real world."

Contrasting that perspective were the remarks of a civilian-trained psychiatrist who referred to himself as "a right-wing nut." He wrote, "Not only was I completely persuaded to patriotic virtue and the extraordinary ability of career military [psychiatric] people. I was also highly impressed with [their] professional competence."

Military-Trained Psychiatrists. One experienced military psychiatrist wrote,

We did not adequately prepare [the civilian-trained] psychiatrists for Vietnam, nor were they given adequate senior role models . . . [consequently] they never did fully identify themselves as part of the Army. A lot of their emotional energy was expended in expressing their frustration with the "system" and this attitude was frequently communicated to patients and was not constructive.

Overall Reactions to Having Served in Vietnam

Participant responses to questions regarding reactions to having served in Vietnam, including recollections of ethical conflicts, strongly patterned around which half of the war the psychiatrist served. These comments are presented below without commentary to allow the reader to fully appreciate their individual poignancy.

Early-War Psychiatrists

- "[I regret not receiving] any recognition for patriotically having done [my] duty at great personal expense."

Late-War Psychiatrists

- "[I wish] I would have been 10 years older and post psychoanalysis."
- "[I wish] I would have been psychoanalyzed."
- "Overall I have felt then and now that it has been one of the most interesting and best experiences of my professional life . . . a very gratifying experience."
- "I would never choose to go to . . . Vietnam. However, the experience was valuable from a psychiatric viewpoint because of the intensity and myriad of feelings generated by all in such an environment but best understood and recognized by a psychiatrist. One recognizes more so one's own mortality and accepts the proximity to death, rationalizes away fear in order to survive and not be paralyzed by it."
- "I was afraid of dying."
- "Would I go again? I don't know. Hopefully I will never have to make that decision. The whole Vietnam debacle had its ravages on us all."

Ethical Conflicts
Early-War Psychiatrists

- "I did have personal emotional trauma to the extent that I identified with individual needs when they conflicted with the needs of the service."

Late-War Psychiatrists

- "Psychiatrists need to accept the age old notion that 'war is hell' . . . all the preparation and best on the spot treatment we can give will increase the efficiency of the military's function, at best, [but] will not in my opinion significantly reduce the psychiatric casualties—sorry."
- "I'm proud to have served. I wish I had done more for the troops. I'm left with the feeling of having contributed very little. The war was close and yet I seemed safe enough. I almost wish I'd been exposed to more danger. I carry a legacy of painful memories and a crushing burden of the image of carnage, yet I perceive that others experienced far worse than I."
- "Didn't the practice of returning individuals with combat related disorders to duty as expeditiously as possible prove deleterious in the long run?"

Adaptations
Early-War Psychiatrists

- "What I did was get clear in my mind that my job was to meet the needs of the system as the first priority."
- "I had to decide that this was my job, but I didn't like it."
- "As my year in Vietnam passed my ethical dilemma increased some, but I was hired by the Army, not the specific patient. The second fact was that I knew if I wanted to try to do something for a specific person, someone else would have to come to Vietnam to take his place."

Late-War Psychiatrists

- "I was only partly trained—but that was the Army's choice, not mine."
- "I accepted my assignment as an obligation despite my conviction as early as 1964 that our involvement was stupid, would fail, would be a disastrous waste of wealth, power, and lives, and was unjustified politically, historically, and morally. I did not feel strong ethical conflict over my role in the Army in RVN [Republic of Vietnam] . . . the therapeutic technique of psychiatry is inimical to the military cast of mind and would probably undermine morale and exacerbate disciplinary problems with many soldiers."
- "I did not feel it was my business to greatly dwell on moral or ethical issues of our involvement in Vietnam. Rather I felt like an orthopedic surgeon at the bottom of a ski slope—there was a great deal

of clinical necessity for my presence and to this I put my attention. Wars occur, people are injured, doctors take care of the sick [therefore] I should be there."

- "I soon adapted by realizing I could only be of use by cooperating with the military in most ways. To have tried to be another Ghandi [sic] would have been pointless and would have deprived those few I could help with my expertise."

- "My attitude was apolitical and patriotic."

- "I had no [ethical] dilemma but I sure as hell wasn't neutral and didn't perceive what I did as neutral. I believe what I did was a positive contribution to the war. I'm proud I did it and I'd do it again tomorrow."

- "I wasn't neutral, I treated patients and rooted for us to win."

- "My values are clear to me—I wasn't a 'double agent' [in Vietnam], I didn't return [my patient-soldiers] to combat. I medevac'd them to Japan."

Recriminations
Early-War Psychiatrists

- "I think it is significant that the whole experience did personally affect me for many years. I was active in the [antiwar movement], practically from the moment I received my discharge. Even though my combat experience in Vietnam was minimal, I am, like many Vietnam veterans, still horrified by the stupidity of that particular war; and I have generalized that experience to war in general. I am sure that my years in the antiwar movement could be termed a posttraumatic stress syndrome."

- "The injuries and deaths which I felt resulted from the [individualized 1-year assignments] far outweighed the low psychiatric casualty rate. My efforts to convey this impression to people in Saigon and later in the US [United States] met with the result I expected—nothing. This was because, my guess, this was a politically expedient decision."

- "[To have prepared for the assignment I would] have learned some Vietnamese history, and then probably not have gone. You hint at but don't get at the constant double talk that went on from the Ia Drang battle on . . . phony body counts, phony optimism . . . double accounting . . . war crimes . . . military cover-ups. . . . It was a deception [beginning with] the Gulf of Tonkin."

Late-War Psychiatrists

- "A war has to be fought with full support, including folks back home. We all felt so alone and isolated."

- "There was absolutely no leadership, either from the medical commanders or the Consultant, or myself."

- "If ever I am called again, I will not accept an assignment that entails great discrepancy between responsibility (great) and authority (little)."

- "Where in the hell were all the other Army shrinks when I was over there?"

- "Hell, none of us should have been there."

- "I'd have been more motivated to go, to function as a shrink, if the US [United States] had been more positive about winning!"

- "My [Army] residency did little or no formal teaching about combat psychiatry. I received good psychiatric training, but miserable military training. My preparation for Vietnam consisted of being handed a little booklet called 'This is Vietnam' when I boarded the plane at Travis AFB [Air Force Base]. [I had asked not to be assigned away from my family because of serious marital problems, yet] I was told I was the only member of my class that they could trust to send out from residency directly to a responsible assignment in the field. Two of my classmates had avoided [Vietnam] by applying for child fellowships. [Once in Vietnam] I learned how little I really knew about the Army and how poorly my training had prepared me for a role as a military psychiatrist."

- "Vietnam was an experience for which I was poorly prepared personally or professionally. I have never been more depressed, [and] I did not understand why for months after my service obligation was over. To some extent I am still bitter. I felt poorly prepared by the Army for what I was to do. I did not understand the dilemma of being treated like the 'enemy' by my side. I felt I was given propaganda and not information. I felt poorly valued by the military and that the majority of psychiatric problems could have been handled by a social-worker."

Quantitative Responses

Operational Frustrations and Ethical Dilemmas

The WRAIR survey participants were provided 31 forced-choice statements intended to address a range of potential operational frustrations and ethical dilemmas associated with assignment and professional functioning in Vietnam and asked to indicate the extent of their agreement while they were there. Table 11-1 presents the summaries of the statements, which are arranged according to the means of participant responses for each item (right-hand column).

Responses to these items were further submitted to factor analysis, which yielded the following observations:

- The factor analysis of the responses to the set of 31 items generated four factors (W, X, Y, and Z) composed of 23 items. The four factors were interpreted and named as Factor W: "Patient Allegiance and Ethical Conflict" (30% of the variance); Factor X: "Civilian Professional Allegiance and Psychiatrist Burnout" (27% of the variance); Factor Y: "Opposition to the War and Compassion Fatigue" (23% of the variance); and Factor Z: "Opposition to Military Medical Structure and Policies" (20% of the variance). These are indicated in the column on the left side of Table 11-1.
- The clustering of participant responses into these four factors indicated that many psychiatrists experienced the set of items comprising each of the factors similarly and distinct from the items comprising the other factors; and
- Only one of the factors, Factor W, explicitly centered on ethical conflict.

Two of the eight items not included in the four factors warrant additional emphasis: survey participants agreed that more career military psychiatrists should have served in Vietnam (3.24), and they disagreed that Vietnam was a constructive experience for them (1.93). The others are self-explanatory. Further analysis of the responses to the item regarding the value of the guidance from the senior Army psychiatrist in Vietnam, that is, the US Army Republic of Vietnam (USARV) Psychiatry Consultant, will follow.

Multiple regression analysis was also performed using each of the four factors as the dependent variable while the three psychiatrist dichotomous variables, that is, key distinctions between psychiatrists, served as the independent variables: (1) phase of the war served (early vs late), (2) type of assignment in Vietnam (with *any* combat unit vs *only* with hospitals), and (3) site of psychiatry residency training (military vs civilian). The regression model included the "main effects" of these three predictors as well as all interactions of the three

variables. The relationship between each factor and each of these predictors is visually depicted in Figures 11-2, 3, 4, and 5. Considering the small sample size and the exploratory nature of the analysis, the main and interaction effects presented below include those that reached the level of significance of $p < .10$ and below [note that in these figures, the dependent variable has been scaled such that "0" corresponds to the "average" or "typical" psychiatrist's score].

Factor W: Patient Allegiance and Ethical Conflict. A high score means the psychiatrist *did not* primarily serve in Vietnam out of patriotism and felt conflict over implementing the military forward treatment doctrine there. Among the reasons for this conflict were because a patient's need for refuge from combat or deployment stress could clash with the collective need to "conserve the fighting strength," restoring patients to military function could force dissenting soldiers to conform and vulnerable ones to return to more trauma, and commanders could exercise military authority to manipulate clinical decisions. With regard to the multiple regression analysis, Figure 11-2 depicts a statistically significant interaction only when all three of the psychiatrist dichotomous variables, that is, key distinctions between psychiatrists, and their two and three-way interactions, were included.

During the second half of the war, when moral and ethical ambiguities were increasing, all psychiatrists reported some heightened patient allegiance and ethical conflict, especially the military-trained psychiatrists who worked in the hospitals. This latter finding could represent the combination of (*a*) the higher prevalence for demoralization among noncombat troops (the majority of the troops treated by the hospital psychiatrists) during the second half of the war because of drawdown stress, and (*b*) a greater susceptibility for ethical conflict among the military-trained psychiatrists because they possessed a greater loyalty to military goals, structure, and discipline.

More difficult to explain are the findings for the first half of the war, that is, those military-trained psychiatrists assigned to the combat units and the civilian-trained psychiatrists who worked in the hospitals reported greater ethical conflict. In that the stress during the first half of the war was borne more by combat troops because of the overall higher levels of combat activity at that phase of the war, the military-trained psychiatrists who were assigned to the combat units

TABLE 11-1. Recollections of Operational Frustrations and Ethical Dilemmas in Vietnam

Factor Loadings	Subjective Reactions of Army Psychiatrists in Vietnam	Mean Value
	5 = STRONGLY AGREE	
-0.58 (W)	I accepted assignment in Vietnam out of a sense of duty and obligation	4.08
	4 = AGREE	
0.63 (W)	Psychiatric care for troops is not always neutral and humanitarian	3.64
0.55 (Z)	I reacted negatively to notification of my assignment to Vietnam	3.53
0.64 (X)	Officers or senior NCOs needing care rarely sought it nor were referred	3.45
	More military-trained psychiatrists should have served in Vietnam	3.24
	3 = INTERMEDIATE	
0.51 (Y)	Soldiers and unit leaders expected magic from mental health team	2.98
0.68 (W)	It was difficult to reconcile Army requirements (group needs) vs soldier expectations (who wished to avoid their military situation)	2.94
0.80 (Y)	Before serving in Vietnam I felt American involvement there was counterproductive and destructive	2.89
-0.77 (Y)	Before serving in Vietnam I felt American involvement there was justified	2.84
0.49 (X)	The military in Vietnam paid insufficient attention to human factors	2.81
0.73 (W)	A psychiatric diagnosis may help in Vietnam but cause harm as a veteran	2.76
	Guidance from the senior Army psychiatrist (USARV Consultant) was timely and beneficial	2.71*
0.57 (X)	I may have misled soldiers as a "double agent," ie, by also representing military priorities	2.68
0.55 (Z)	Military psychiatrists cannot guarantee confidentiality for soldiers	2.68
0.51 (W)	Restoring a patient to duty status may mean returning him to more trauma	2.62
	I reacted to notification of my assignment in Vietnam with ambivalence	2.61
0.73 (Z)	A character disorder diagnosis left the commander responsible for the disposition	2.56
0.66 (W)	Following the military psychiatry doctrine (PIES) meant some soldiers were inadequately treated and vulnerable when returned to combat	2.48
0.66 (X)	Psychiatric clinical need exceeded clinical capability in Vietnam	2.48
0.67 (W)	Commanders pressured me to act contrary to my clinical judgment	2.42
0.53 (Z)	I had a real position, ie, as an officer, in the social system of patients and thus may not have been trusted	2.42
0.61 (W)	I felt obligated to clinically coerce some patients into military conformity	2.29
0.65 (Z)	My decisions may be reversed by physicians up the evacuation chain	2.23
0.83 (X)	I felt troubled in Vietnam by social condemnation of those serving there	2.18
0.78 (Y)	Before serving in Vietnam I perceived US involvement there to be immoral	2.17
	I reacted to notification of my assignment in Vietnam with eagerness	2.03
	2 = DISAGREE	
	Vietnam was a constructive experience for me	1.93
	General medical officers had too much authority in psychiatric decisions	1.90
	Enlisted social work/psychology techs had too much clinical authority	1.85
0.76 (X)	I felt troubled by professional condemnation of military psychiatrists	1.85
	Ethical doubts stemmed from treating patients who insinuated atrocities	1.79
	1 = STRONGLY DISAGREE	

These 31 items were ranked by means of survey participants' agreement using a 1-to-5 scale where 1 = "strongly disagree" and 5 = "strongly agree." (N = 78 to 85). In the left column are the four factors (W, X, Y, and Z) from the factor analysis of responses (23 items) along with the factor loading for the items included in each factor.

Factor W: Patient Allegiance and Ethical Conflict

Factor X: Civilian Professional Allegiance and Psychiatrist Burnout

Factor Y: Opposition to the War and Compassion Fatigue

Factor Z: Opposition to Military Medical Structure and Policies

PIES: proximity, immediacy, expectancy, simplicity

USARV: US Army Republic of Vietnam

*Further analysis is provided in text.

FIGURE 11-2. Multiple regression results for Factor W: Patient Allegiance and Ethical Conflict, by three-way interaction of war phase, type of psychiatry training, and type of assignment in Vietnam (p <.01).

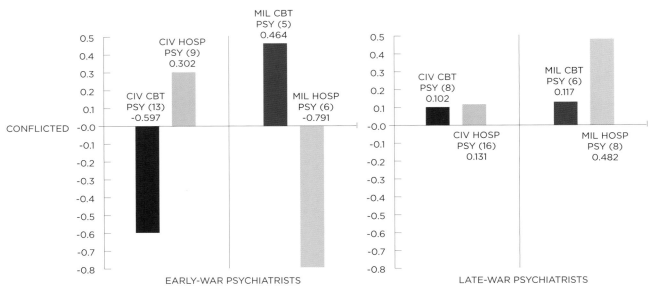

EARLY-WAR PSY: psychiatrist arrived in Vietnam before mid-1968

LATE-WAR PSY: psychiatrist arrived in Vietnam after mid-1968

CIV CBT PSY: psychiatry training was in a civilian program and psychiatrist served with at least one combat unit in Vietnam

CIV HOSP PSY: psychiatry training was in a civilian program and psychiatrist served only with a hospital or psychiatric detachment in Vietnam

MIL CBT PSY: psychiatry training was in a military program and psychiatrist served with at least one combat unit in Vietnam

MIL HOSP PSY: psychiatry training was in a military program and psychiatrist served only with a hospital or psychiatric detachment in Vietnam

may have been more sensitive to the ethical dilemmas than their civilian-trained counterparts. However, that the civilian-trained psychiatrists who served in hospitals would report more ethical conflict than their civilian-trained counterparts assigned to the combat units seems counterintuitive. It may indicate that the civilian-trained psychiatrists assigned to the combat units were buffered by combat unit membership. Recall from Chapter 5 that 21% of psychiatrists (18) in the WRAIR survey indicated that they served only with their original combat division and declined a mid-tour rotation to a safer and more comfortable hospital facility. These psychiatrists were almost exclusively civilian-trained and served during the first half of the war. Many indicated they eschewed reassignment because of their strong allegiance to their combat unit and comrades. It also may be the result of an unstable estimation due to the small sample size.

Factor X: Civilian Professional Allegiance and Psychiatrist Burnout. For this factor, a high score means the psychiatrist felt distress from social and professional opprobrium for serving in the war, being a "double agent" with patients due to his (the psychiatrist's) military rank and authority, the military's paying insufficient attention to human (risk) factors in Vietnam and providing inadequate psychiatric care, and the unwillingness of military leaders to access psychiatric care for themselves. This factor's inclusion of the item "Psychiatric clinical need exceeded clinical capability in Vietnam" suggests that psychiatrist "burnout," that is, exhaustion from an overwhelming workload,[103] was important in this factor. With regard to the multiple regression analysis, Figure 11-3 depicts the statistically significant main effect of phase of the war in which the psychiatrist served, with distress secondary to this factor increasing among Army psychiatrists serving in Vietnam after the war passed the midpoint and American resolve to achieve victory was replaced with an urgency to pull out. Neither the setting of one's psychiatry training nor assignment with a combat unit in Vietnam apparently buffered these late-war feelings.

Factor Y: Opposition to the War and Compassion Fatigue. For this factor, a high score means the psychiatrist felt the war was not justified, was immoral and destructive, and that the expectations of the mental health personnel in Vietnam by both soldiers and their leaders were grossly exaggerated. This factor's inclusion of the item "Soldiers and unit leaders expected magic from mental health team" suggests that "compassion fatigue" (emotional distress among those caring for traumatized individuals consequent to secondary traumatization[103]) was important in this factor. With regard to the multiple regression analysis, Figure 11-4 depicts a statistical trend regarding the interaction between the phase of the war in which the psychiatrist served and the type of assignment he had in Vietnam. This suggests that among those who served during the first half, neither the combat nor the hospital psychiatrists expressed a high score for this factor (ie, exceeding 0.0), but on a relative basis the combat psychiatrists indicated more opposition to the war and compassion fatigue than the hospital psychiatrists. However, this relationship strongly reversed among the psychiatrists who served during the second half, that is, the hospital psychiatrists expressed strong opposition to the war and compassion fatigue compared to the combat psychiatrists who did not. Whereas it is expectable to find a higher overall opposition to the war among psychiatrists who served in the second half of the war, the low score for the psychiatrists assigned to the combat units is noteworthy. Perhaps this finding is explained by the lowered combat activity in the second half of the war and a morale-buffering effect from psychiatrist membership in a line, that is a nonmedical, unit. Inversely, the high scores for the hospital psychiatrists are consistent with the late-war shift in psychiatric challenge to the support units and the hospitals who served them.

Factor Z: Opposition to Military Medical Structure and Policies. For this factor, a high score means the psychiatrist was averse to assignment in Vietnam and felt frustrated in the practice of psychiatry because enlisted patients mistrusted those with rank, evacuation decisions could be reversed by unsympathetic military physicians

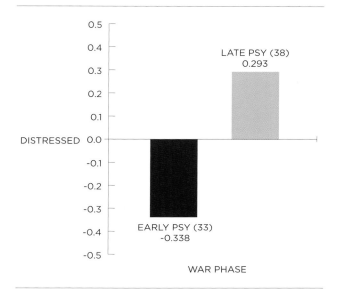

FIGURE 11-3. Multiple regression results for Factor X: Civilian Profession Allegiance and Psychiatrist Burnout, by war phase (p <.007).

EARLY PSY: psychiatrist arrived in Vietnam before mid-1968
LATE PSY: psychiatrist arrived in Vietnam after mid-1968

(insinuating military-loyal psychiatrists) further up the evacuation chain, and line commanders decided the final disposition of soldiers diagnosed with character disorder. With regard to the multiple regression analysis, Figure 11-5 depicts the statistically significant main effect of type of the psychiatrist's pre-Vietnam psychiatric training. Compared to their Army-trained counterparts, civilian-trained psychiatrists were frustrated throughout the war by the unique policies pertaining to patient care that represented the preeminence of military expediency.

In conclusion, analysis of the Army psychiatrists' responses to statements pertaining to subjective reactions to service in Vietnam produced a number of interesting and provocative findings. The following impressions seem notable; however, because of small sample size and the delay between service in Vietnam and participation in the survey, the results are only suggestive.

• The results coincide with the strong negative reactions to service in Vietnam that were expressed by many of the survey participants in their answers to the open-ended questions and their voluntary comments, especially the psychiatrists who served in the second half of the war.

FIGURE 11-4. Multiple regression results for Factor Y: Opposition to the War and Compassion Fatigue, by two-way interaction of war phase and type of assignment in Vietnam (p <.08).

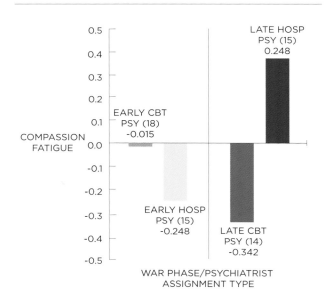

EARLY CBT PSY: psychiatrist arrived before mid-1968 and served with at least one combat unit in Vietnam

EARLY HOSP PSY: psychiatrist arrived before mid-1968 and served only with a hospital or psychiatric detachment in Vietnam

LATE CBT PSY: psychiatrist arrived after mid-1968 and served with at least one combat unit in Vietnam

LATE HOSP PSY: psychiatrist arrived after mid-1968 and served only with a hospital or psychiatric detachment in Vietnam

- Only one of the four factors produced by the factor analysis clearly defined ethical dilemmas (Factor W: Patient Allegiance and Ethical Conflict). The other three factors acknowledged stress in the performance of psychiatric duties in Vietnam but were apparently experienced by the survey psychiatrists as discrete from ethical conflict. This suggests that, whereas there may be conceptual agreement that an ethical dilemma is present in a given clinical event based on its particular circumstances, the experience of the individual clinician involved may be affected by additional variables, some of which can be measured separately, that may exacerbate, mitigate, or have no effect, on their experience of it as an ethical

dilemma. Some of this variability was found to be associated with principal distinctions between the deployed Army psychiatrists (ie, Army vs civilian psychiatry training, era of the war served, and assignment with a combat unit in Vietnam). In other words, an Army psychiatrist who served in Vietnam could be opposed to the war, feel at odds with civilian colleagues about clinical priorities, feel overwhelmed by the psychiatric challenges or by compassion fatigue, or object to Army medical policies that served military expediency, and yet not feel ethically conflicted while implementing the military forward treatment doctrine. Of course, as one respondent indicated, it is also possible that some may have experienced little ethical strain because they opposed and subverted the doctrine.

- Having received one's psychiatric training in an Army program did not necessarily protect psychiatrists from experiencing ethical strain; in fact, it may have exacerbated it. Figure 11-2 suggests that the military-trained group was more strained when serving in combat divisions during the first half of the war and when serving in the hospitals in the second half. This seems notable because the clinical challenges were heightened in both of those settings depending on the phase of the war.

Finally, although it has been demonstrated that clinician values can affect clinical decision making,[18,19] there were no studies of the effects of such values on clinical outcomes either in Vietnam or among Vietnam veterans. Still, the divergence of perspectives between subgroups of psychiatrists represented here is striking. Were clinical decisions of some late-war psychiatrists affected by doubt and demoralization? As the nation turned progressively against the war, did they, perhaps especially those with civilian training, lean more in the direction of a protective, sympathetic overdiagnosis (at least from the military's point of view) and overevacuation of soldiers as suggested by Jones,[118] even though in past wars such a clinical attitude threatened force conservation and contributed to sustained disability among soldier-patients? Future research should systematically explore clinical outcome as it relates to the organizational, personal, and interpersonal dimensions that affect orientation to service in military psychiatrists (and allied mental health personnel).

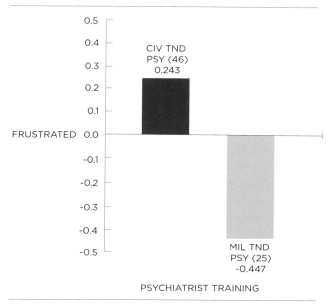

FIGURE 11-5. Multiple regression results for Factor Z: Opposition to Military Medical Structure and Policies, by type of psychiatry training (p <.005).

CIV TND PSY: psychiatry training was in a civilian program
MIL TND PSY: psychiatry training was in a military program

Perceived Caliber of Leadership From the US Army Republic of Vietnam Psychiatry Consultant

The questionnaire asked respondents to rate (on a 5-point scale) the extent of their agreement or disagreement with the statement "I found the guidance from and input to the Vietnam theater Psychiatric Consultant timely and beneficial" (ie, the senior Army psychiatrist in Vietnam). The mean for 79 participants (excluding the Consultants) was 2.75 (SD = 1.41), suggesting an absence of strong feelings about this question.

However, to look closer at this question from the perspective of military chronology, the study participants were divided by three phases of the war: the buildup phase (n = 31), the transition phase (n = 25), or the drawdown phase (n = 23). Means for the psychiatrists of the early (3.13), middle (2.88), and late (2.09) stages of the war suggest decreasing confidence in the leadership of the theater Psychiatry Consultant. This was substantiated in an analysis of variance (ANOVA) conducted on the three means (F = 4.07, df = 2,76, p < .052). Further confirming this impression, the most

conservative post-hoc multiple range test of differences among these groups (Scheffe's) revealed significant differences (p < .05) between the late and early groups and between the late and middle groups.

This finding—that as the war proceeded, the deployed psychiatrists felt less allied with, and supported by, their theater Psychiatry Consultant—appears to be important. As Menninger pointed out regarding World War II, one of the most valuable functions of the command consultant was to improve the morale of his colleagues in the field:

> The consultant brought status and prestige to the clinician who often felt neglected and forgotten. . . . A renewed sense of a professional identity was gained in addition to the military model to which most [of the psychiatrists] were overwhelmingly and scrupulously loyal, even though discouraged about their own activities.[119(p82)]

Of course, the progressive decline in confidence in their consultants among the Vietnam psychiatry respondents must be considered as affected by all the other declining features in the second half of the war: the rise in clinical demand, the eroding public and professional support for the war, the declining morale among Army personnel in Vietnam, and the role uncertainties in psychiatrists. That is, one can speculate that their waning confidence in the Psychiatry Consultant was in part a reflection of waning confidence in themselves. But these differences could also be explained by the declining levels of pre-Vietnam military psychiatry experience among successive Psychiatry Consultants (see Chapter 4). One senior Army psychiatrist wrote, "There was a tendency [in the last years] to assign less than the best we had as [USARV Psychiatric] Consultant—it was more a game of 'who can we get/force to take the position,' [rather] than 'who is our most qualified.'" It does seem logical in retrospect that, under such deteriorating circumstances, consultants with more practical experience should have been provided, perhaps even in greater strength, or with an augmented staff. The evidence indicating a seriously declining confidence in the clinical and administrative leadership of the theater Psychiatry Consultant is even more noteworthy when recalling that the psychiatrists who served in the latter half of the war were themselves less experienced.

Post-Vietnam Psychiatrist Retention

Sixty-five percent (52 of 80) of the WRAIR survey participants indicated that they left the Army within the year following their service in Vietnam, and an additional eight left after their third year (reaching a total of 75% out of uniform within 3 years of completing their tour in Vietnam). The interpretation of this finding is uncertain as these individuals represented various career paths (starting with military vs civilian psychiatric training) and obligations with the Army (such as the Berry Plan deferment) that influenced post-Vietnam retention. However, the subjective data reviewed earlier indicating considerable bitterness toward the Army among the psychiatrists who served in Vietnam would explain an overall disinclination for further service beyond one's irreducible obligation. Such a drain on Army psychiatry's most experienced individuals would have been detrimental for subsequent needs of the Army, especially for training and preparation of future mental health providers and leaders.

SUMMARY AND CONCLUSIONS

This chapter began with a review of the rationale for military psychiatry's traditional forward treatment doctrine and its associated ethical quandaries. It also explored the subjective experience of the Army psychiatrists who served in Vietnam with an emphasis on the military policies and circumstances that affected their professional activities and shaped the ethical frame within which they functioned. The following summary of this chapter's observations and findings includes a reiteration of selected historical features. All references to hospital psychiatrists are intended to also include those who were assigned to the psychiatric specialty detachments.

Historical Context

- **The rationale for the traditional military forward treatment doctrine brought to Vietnam was pragmatically derived from the preceding main force wars.** Although the doctrine is illustrated in this chapter using the example of the management and treatment of the soldier with a combat stress reaction, many other clinical activities of military psychiatrists in the combat theater are variations of the model.

  - The typical combat exhaustion casualty manifests a stress-induced condition that appears to be reversible, at least in its acute stages. Because it arises under the unique circumstances of warfare, it is considered to be distinct from similar stress reactions seen among civilians (acute stress reaction). In its inception, it is not a PTSD.

  - Although there are other pathogenic contributions, overall it is presumed to represent a final common pathway in which the overwhelmed soldier's self-protective motivation has eclipsed his commitment to his combat buddies and his unit.

  - Nonetheless, it is the soldier's duty to recover as quickly as possible and return to duty status—even if he is hesitant, expresses a moral opposition to killing, or faces additional physical and psychological risks.

  - The military forward treatment doctrine serves that objective by providing the affected soldier simple but abbreviated physical and psychosocial support near his unit and the fighting—including exhortation that he resume his duty function.

  - The military forward treatment doctrine is justified as a wartime necessity, that is, supporting force conservation and national defense.

  - In a paternalistic sense, it also is justified based on past observations that such a treatment approach reduces chronicity (morbidity) among combat-affected soldiers.

- **There are potential ethical conflicts that surround the military psychiatrist in the implementation of the doctrine.**

  - The psychiatrist is also a soldier and subject to the authority and hierarchical values of the military.

  - He is obligated to aid his patient in fulfilling his duty *if he can function*—even if the psychiatrist is reluctant.

  - Symptom elimination is *not* the clinical priority as would be the case in civilian medical practice.

  - "Tender" individualist values, that is, ideals of humanitarian care of the sick and wounded, can be at crossed purposes with "tough" collectivist values, that is, those favored by the military in the service of combat objectives.

• **This ethical conflict is theoretical until war begins. Under wartime circumstances military psychiatrists can feel placed in an ethically difficult position because of a clash of values.**
   ■ Accomplishment of military objectives is crucial to victory.
   ■ Severe losses are predicted and critical manpower shortages are anticipated.
   ■ Overall combat effectiveness may be eroded by excessive numbers of unrecoverable psychiatric casualties.
   ■ Some traumatized soldier-patients may incur further harm if they are incompletely treated and face more combat exposure, that is, if not protected.
   ■ Some soldier-patients may incur increased psychiatric morbidity if treatment is prolonged, that is, if they are overprotected.
   ■ The Army expects military psychiatrists to distinguish between these two possibilities and to implement the forward treatment doctrine when appropriate.
   ■ The profession of psychiatry may or may not endorse use of the doctrine.

• **In the more popular wars before Vietnam, the Army's forward treatment doctrine rested on a foundation of mutually reinforcing ethical positions that seemed sufficiently humanitarian.**
   ■ Military psychiatrists felt they were conforming to the expectations and values of the military.
   ■ There was congruence between what was perceived to be best for the soldier and best for America. The doctrine appeared to not only contribute to national defense but also represent the most effective, scientifically based regimen for protecting soldiers from further combat traumatization and from chronic psychiatric disability.
   ■ Military psychiatrists were apparently also conforming to the expectations and ethical values of the profession of psychiatry.
   ■ The psychiatrist who failed to understand both sides of the soldier's struggle to overcome his fear or moral doubt could overly

empathize with his self-protective tendencies, "overdiagnose" and "overevacuate," thereby increasing his psychiatric morbidity and jeopardizing the military mission.

Vietnam Observations and Impressions

• **Army psychiatrists assigned to Vietnam late in the war experienced demoralization in sympathy with the troops.** Many psychiatrists (and allied mental health personnel) who served in the second half of the war appear to have been greatly affected by the psychosocial deterioration there. As indicated in earlier chapters, these later cohorts of replacement psychiatrists faced an accelerating array of more complex, and in many ways unique and unanticipated, problems in Vietnam. Furthermore, many apparently shared the demoralization and antiwar passions of the dissenting soldiers that they served, personally if not publicly objecting to US objectives in Vietnam, and became uncertain of their own goals and procedures, including the forward treatment doctrine. More specifically they questioned the treatment regimen that would induce soldiers to believe that further exposure to combat, or even the hardships associated with service in the theater, was in their best interests; and they evidently worried they might "expect" soldiers to risk their lives or their mental stability without moral justification.

• **Military psychiatry and military psychiatrists were openly challenged by civilian psychiatrists regarding the ethical justification for the forward treatment doctrine.** The alignment of justifying moral principles for combat psychiatry's doctrine that had held throughout the earlier wars was precariously balanced. During Vietnam, opponents of military psychiatry argued that the doctrine's treatment goals and methods violated psychiatry's humanitarian principles by neglecting the needs of the soldier in order to wage an unjust war. They alleged that psychiatrists in uniform corrupted the principles of humanitarian care (violated the principle of primum non nocere), opposed the vital interests of American society, and principally served political interests and military expediency while coercing symptomatic soldier-patients to face further risks.

- The proportion of civilian-trained psychiatrists assigned in Vietnam increased in the latter half of the war, and overall they were less convinced of the preeminence of military values and policies. They had come directly from a fractious American society and were surrounded by a professional climate hostile to military psychiatry.

- Although the psychiatrists assigned in Vietnam were influenced by powerful, potentially competing value systems, they could not realistically assess some of the most important factors affecting the balance of harms and benefits associated with their treatment decisions. Army psychiatrists serving in Vietnam functioned in the dark. Although they knew of the successful implementation of the military treatment doctrine in past wars, they had no reliable information about whether their patients might face unacceptable risks because of its use in Vietnam. Nor could they comprehend whether the doctrine truly served public welfare. Even if the conflict met objective standards for a just war,[12] its morality for the psychiatrist in Vietnam, just as for the soldier or citizen, may have been far more subjectively determined.

- The ethical burden for Vietnam's military psychiatrists was magnified because they struggled with these issues alone. Civilian psychiatry failed to recognize their dilemma; monitor the institutional regulations, policies, and treatment doctrine that affected the practice of military psychiatry; or provide them with ethical guidelines. Furthermore, the tendency for critics to equate the questions about the institutional abuse of psychiatry with those regarding the conduct of the individual psychiatrist greatly added to the burden associated with the military psychiatrist's role.

Walter Reed Army Institute of Research Survey Results

The robust responses to the survey, both qualitative and quantitative, indicated that despite the 10 to 17 years since their service there, most of the psychiatrist participants had strong feelings—typically negative—regarding their tour of duty in Vietnam. The general impression was that many still sustained substantial personal and professional anguish as a result.

Qualitative Responses
- Many of the study psychiatrists indicated they still felt bitter about the war and their role in it.

- Psychiatrists with civilian training in psychiatry generally, and psychiatrists who served in the second half of the war regardless of training background, appeared to have the most role-linked psychological conflict. Data reviewed in earlier chapters suggest more specifically that as the war prolonged, they increasingly felt overwhelmed by the challenges associated with the raging drug epidemic, racial tensions and incidents, and outbreaks of violence; betrayed by the Army because of their poor preparation and support in the theater; and blamed by their stateside colleagues and countrymen for doing the job it was their duty to do.

- The responses also suggest wide variability in adapting to these pressures. Some acknowledged the ethical and personal strain, some said they felt none, while others indicated that their solution was to intentionally shield patients.

Quantitative Responses
The factor analysis of participants' responses to a set of statements pertaining to professional frustrations and ethical dilemmas in Vietnam yielded four statistically distinct clusters (factors). This suggested that the deployed psychiatrists could have been stressed in their professional roles from compound sources, and interpretation of the stress could have differed considerably among them. However, multiple regression analysis yielded significant differences among psychiatrists for each of the four factors based on the three key dichotomous distinctions between psychiatrists: (1) in which half of the war they served, (2) whether their residency training in psychiatry was in a civilian or military setting, and (3) whether they served in a combat unit at some point or exclusively in a hospital. Findings included:

- Psychiatrists were stressed by ethical conflict (Factor W):
  - Second half of the war: Regardless of site of residency training or assignment type in Vietnam, psychiatrists overall indicated some measure of frank ethical conflict in their role

of "conserving the fighting strength." This was especially true for the psychiatrists with military training who were assigned to the hospitals. The increasing ethical conflict is predictable as opposition to the war increased. The rising clinical challenge among the support troops and the psychiatrists working in the hospitals who served them in the second half of the war may be predictable also. The military-trained psychiatrists who worked in the hospitals may have experienced more ethical strain because of greater loyalty to military values, structure, and discipline adopted during their Army residency training.

- First half of the war: Greater ethical conflict was also reported by those who served in the first half of the war who had military training and were assigned to the combat units, and by those who had civilian training and were assigned to the hospitals. Greater combat-generated clinical challenge could be found in the combat units in the first half of the war because of higher combat intensity and stress, which could explain greater ethical conflict for psychiatrists assigned to combat units. But the greater ethical strain among the psychiatrists with military training may again be due to greater loyalty to military values, structure, and discipline. Hospitals were not exempt from having increased combat-generated clinical challenges as they were required to treat the more intractable cases from the combat units. However, it seems plausible to explain the increased ethical strain among the civilian-trained psychiatrists assigned with the hospitals based on their not being afforded the morale-buffering effect that the combat psychiatrists seemed to derive from their membership in a line, that is, a nonmedical unit.

- Psychiatrists were stressed by the criticism of civilian colleagues and professional exhaustion (Factor X): In general, psychiatrists who served in the second half of the war indicated they felt greater criticism from civilian peers for doing their job and depleted by the challenges they faced compared to those who served in the first half of the war. This is true regardless of whether their residency training in psychiatry was in a civilian or military institution

and whether they served in a combat unit or in a hospital.

- Psychiatrists were stressed from feeling opposition to the war and from feeling overwhelmed by the suffering they encountered (Factor Y):
  - Second half of the war: Psychiatrists assigned to hospitals expressed more opposition to the war and compassion fatigue than their counterparts with combat units as well as all early-war psychiatrists. This is consistent with the increasing antiwar spirit among Americans and troops in Vietnam as the war lengthened. It also is consistent with the dramatic rise in psychiatric and behavior problems among noncombat troops, the majority of whom would be treated by hospital-based psychiatrists.
  - First half of the war: Psychiatrists with combat units expressed relatively more opposition to the war and compassion fatigue than early war hospital psychiatrists. This is consistent with apparently greater levels of psychiatric and behavior problems within combat units because of the higher combat intensity in the first half of the war.

- Psychiatrists were stressed by having to conform to military medical and psychiatric policies (Factor Z): Throughout the war, compared to military-trained psychiatrists, civilian-trained psychiatrists were bothered more by the organizational modifications of the structure of medical and psychiatric care that favored military expediency.

- Survey respondents indicated that over the course of the war there was a significant decline in confidence in leadership provided by the successive USARV Psychiatry Consultants, the senior Army psychiatrists in Vietnam.

REFERENCES

1. Parrish MD. *A Veteran of Three Wars Looks at Psychiatry in the Military*. [Draft of paper provided to the author (NMC).]
2. Brown SL. Some observations on the role of an Army psychiatrist. *Am J Psychiatry*. 1953;110(2):110–114.

3. Colbach EM, Parrish MD. Army mental health activities in Vietnam: 1965–1970. *Bull Menninger Clin.* 1970;34(6):333–342.

4. Camp NM. The Vietnam War and the ethics of combat psychiatry. *Am J Psychiatry.* 1993;150(7):1000–1010.

5. Menninger WC. *Psychiatry in a Troubled World: Yesterday's War and Today's Challenge.* New York, NY: Macmillan; 1948.

6. Maskin M. Something about a soldier. *Psychiatry.* 1946;9:189–191.

7. Peterson DB, Chambers RB. Restatement of combat psychiatry. *Am J Psychiatry.* 1952;109:249–254.

8. Glass AJ. Psychotherapy in the combat zone. *Am J Psychiatry.* 1954;110:725–731.

9. Glass AJ. Lessons learned. In: Mullens WS, Glass AJ, eds, *Neuropsychiatry in World War II.* Vol 2. *Overseas Theaters.* Washington, DC: Medical Department, US Army; 1973: 989–1027.

10. Kormos HR. The nature of combat stress. In: Figley CR, ed. *Stress Disorders Among Vietnam Veterans: Theory, Research and Treatment.* New York, NY: Bruner/Mazel; 1978: 3–22.

11. Veatch RM. The psychiatrist's role in war. In: Veatch RM, ed. *Case Studies in Medical Ethics.* Cambridge, Mass: Harvard University Press; 1977: 245–251.

12. Walzer M. *Just and Unjust Wars: A Moral Argument With Historical Illustrations.* New York, NY: Basic Books; 1977.

13. Johnson AW Jr. Combat psychiatry, I: A historical review. *Med Bull US Army Europe.* 1969;26(10):305–308.

14. Heller J. *Catch-22.* New York, NY: Simon and Schuster; 1961.

15. Hastings Center Report. *In the Service of the State: The Psychiatrist as Double Agent: Special Supplement.* Washington, DC: The Hastings Center Institute of Society, Ethics and the Life Sciences; 1978.

16. Lomas HD, Berman JD. Diagnosing for administrative purposes: some ethical problems. *Soc Sci Med.* 1983;17(4):241–244.

17. Sider RC. Mental health norms and ethical practice. *Psychiatric Ann.* 1983;13(4):302–309.

18. Sullivan PR. Influence of personal values on psychiatric judgment: a military example. *J Nerv Ment Dis.* 1971;152(3):193–198.

19. Weitzel WD. A psychiatrist in a bureaucracy: the unsettling compromises. *Hosp Community Psychiatry.* 1976;27(9):644–647.

20. Camp NM, Carney CM. US Army psychiatry in Vietnam: preliminary findings of a survey, I: Background and method. *Bull Menninger Clin.* 1987;51(1):6–18.

21. Colbach EM. Ethical issues in combat psychiatry. *Mil Med.* 1985;150(5):256–265.

22. Arthur RJ. Reflections on military psychiatry. *Am J Psychiatry.* 1978;135 Suppl:2–7.

23. Glass AJ. Army psychiatry before World War II. In: Glass AJ, Bernucci R, eds. *Neuropsychiatry in World War II.* Vol 1. *Zone of the Interior.* Washington, DC: Medical Department, US Army; 1966: 3–23.

24. Brill NQ. Hospitalization and disposition. In: Glass AJ, Bernucci R, eds. *Neuropsychiatry in World War II.* Vol 1. *Zone of the Interior.* Washington, DC: Medical Department, US Army; 1966: 195–253.

25. Hausman W, Rioch D McK. Military psychiatry. A prototype of social and preventive psychiatry in the United States. *Arch Gen Psych.* 1967;16(6):727–739.

26. Rioch D McK. Problems of Preventive Psychiatry in War. Talk given to the Army Medical Service Graduate School, Walter Reed General Hospital, Washington, DC, October 1954.

27. Jones FD. Experiences of a division psychiatrist in Vietnam. *Mil Med.* 1967:132(12):1003–1008.

28. Kaplan JH. Marijuana and drug abuse in Vietnam. *Ann N Y Acad Sci.* 1971;191:261–269.

29. Bostrom JA. Management of combat reactions. *US Army Vietnam Med Bull.* 1967;July/August:6–8.

30. Bowman JA. Recent experiences in combat psychiatry in Viet Nam (unpublished); 1967. [Full text available as Appendix 11 to this volume.]

31. Bowman JA. In: Johnson AW Jr, Bowman JA, Byrdy HS, Blank AS Jr. Panel discussion:

Army psychiatry in Vietnam. In: Jones FD, ed. *Proceedings: Social and Preventive Psychiatry Course, 1967*. Washington, DC: GPO; 1968: 41–76. [Available at: Alexandria, Va: Defense Technical Information Center. Document No. AD A950058.]

32. Conte LR. A neuropsychiatric team in Vietnam 1966–1967: an overview. In: Parker RS, ed. *The Emotional Stress of War, Violence, and Peace*. Pittsburgh, Penn: Stanwix House; 1972: 163–168.

33. Johnson AW Jr. Psychiatric treatment in the combat situation. *US Army Vietnam Med Bull*. 1967;January/February:38–45.

34. Johnson AW Jr. Combat psychiatry, II: The US Army in Vietnam. *Med Bull US Army Europe*. 1969;26(11):335–339.

35. Medical Field Service School. *Introduction to Military Psychiatry*. Fort Sam Houston, Tex: Department of Neuropsychiatry, Medical Field Service School; distributed July 1967. Training Document GR 51-400-004, 064.

36. Pozner H. Common sense and military psychiatry. *J Royal Medical Corps*. 1961;107(3):157. In: Medical Field Service School. *Philosophy of Military Psychiatry*. Fort Sam Houston, Tex: Department of Neuropsychiatry, Medical Field Service School; distributed July 1967. Training Document GR 51-400-006, 045.

37. Menninger WC. *Psychiatry in a Troubled World*. New York, NY: Macmillin Co; 1948: 487. In: Medical Field Service School. *Philosophy of Military Psychiatry*. Fort Sam Houston, Tex: Department of Neuropsychiatry, Medical Field Service School; distributed July 1967. Training Document GR 51-400-006, 045.

38. Brown DE. The military: a valuable arena for research and innovation. *Am J Psychiatry*. 1970;127(4):511–512.

39. *Vietnam Veterans Against the War: Vietnam Veterans, Stand Up and Be Counted* [position statement, undated]. Available at: http://www.vvaw.org/veteran/article/?id=1717, accessed 9 April 2013.

40. Lifton RJ. Advocacy and corruption in the healing professions. *Conn Med*. 1975;39(3):803–813.

41. Lifton RJ. *The Nazi Doctors: Medical Killing and the Psychology of Genocide*. New York, NY: Basic Books; 1986.

42. Brass A. Medicine over there. *JAMA*. 1970;213(9):1473–1475.

43. Strange RE, Arthur RJ. Hospital ship psychiatry in a war zone. *Am J Psychiatry*. 1967;124(3):281–286.

44. Levin EC. Evading the realities of war? [letter] *Am J Psychiatry*. 1968;124:1137–1138.

45. Arthur RJ, Strange RE. Cdrs. Strange and Arthur reply [letter]. *Am J Psychiatry*. 1968;124:1138.

46. Bloch HS. Army clinical psychiatry in the combat zone: 1967–1968. *Am J Psychiatry*. 1969;126(3):289–298.

47. Maier T. The Army psychiatrist: an adjunct to the system of social control [letter]. *Am J Psychiatry*. 1970;126:1039.

48. Bloch HS. Dr. Bloch replies [letter]. *Am J Psychiatry*. 1970;126:1039–1040.

49. Clausen RE Jr, Daniels AK. Role conflicts and their ideological resolution in military psychiatric practice. *Am J Psychiatry*. 1966;123:280–287.

50. Daniels AK. The captive professional. Bureaucratic limitations in the practice of military psychiatry. *J Health Soc Behav*. 1969;10(4):255–265.

51. Friedman HJ. Military psychiatry. Limitations of the current preventive approach. *Arch Gen Psychiatry*. 1972;26(2):118–123.

52. Dubey J. The military psychiatrist as social engineer. *Am J Psychiatry*. 1967;124(1):52–58.

53. Perlman MS. Basic problems of military psychiatry: delayed reaction in Vietnam veterans. *Int J Offender Ther Comp Criminol*. 1975;19:129–138.

54. Kirshner LA. Countertransference issues in the treatment of the military dissenter. *Am J Orthopsychiatry*. 1973;43(4):654–659.

55. Locke K. Notes on the adjustment of a psychiatrist to the military. *Psych Op*. 1972;9(6):17–21.

56. Barr NI, Zunin LM. Clarification of the psychiatrist's dilemma while in military service. *Am J Orthopsychiatry*. 1971;41(4):672–674.

57. Barr NI, Zunin LM. The role of the psychiatrist in the military service. *Psych Op.* 1973;10(1):17–19.

58. Ollendorff RH, Adams PL. Psychiatry and the draft. *Am J Orthopsychiatry.* 1971;41(1):85–90.

59. Frank IM, Hoedemaker FS. The civilian psychiatrist and the draft. *Am J Psychiatry.* 1970;127(4):497–502.

60. Liberman RP, Sonnenberg SM, Stern MS. Psychiatric evaluations for young men facing the draft: a report of 147 cases. *Am J Psychiatry* 1971;128:147–152.

61. Moskowitz JA. On drafting the psychiatric "draft" letter. *Am J Psychiatry.* 1971;128(1):69–72.

62. Roemer PA. The psychiatrist and the draft evader [letter]. *Am J Psychiatry.* 1971;127(9):1236–1237.

63. Robitscher J. *The Powers of Psychiatry.* Boston, Mass: Houghton Mifflin; 1980.

64. Ingraham L, Manning F. American military psychiatry. In: Gabriel RA, ed. *Military Psychiatry: A Comparative Perspective.* Westport, Conn: Greenwood Press; 1986: 25–65.

65. Char J. Drug abuse in Vietnam. *Am J Psychiatry.* 1972;129(4):463–465.

66. Joseph BS. Lessons on heroin abuse from treating users in Vietnam. *Hosp Community Psychiatry.* 1974;25(11):742–744.

67. Ratner RA. Drugs and despair in Vietnam. *U Chicago Magazine.* 1972;64:15–23.

68. Fisher HW. Vietnam psychiatry. Portrait of anarchy. *Minn Med.* 1972;55(12):1165–1167.

69. Livingston GS. Medicine in the military. In: Visscher MB, ed. *Humanistic Perspectives in Medical Ethics.* Buffalo, NY: Prometheus Books; 1972: 266–274.

70. Livingston GS. Letter from a Vietnam veteran. *Saturday Rev.* 1969;(September 20):22–23.

71. Meshad S. *Captain for Dark Mornings: A True Story.* Playa Del Rey, Calif: Creative Image Associate; 1982.

72. APA members hit meeting disruptions in opinion poll results. *Psychiatric News.* 3 March 1971;6:1.

73. Tarjan G. Highlights of the 124th annual meeting. *Am J Psychiatry.* 1971;128(1):137–140.

74. Psychologists, MH groups attack Vietnam war. *Psychiatric News.* 5 July 1972;7:1.

75. Hays FW. Lest we forget. *Mil Med.* 1977;142:263–267.

76. Gibbs JJ. Military psychiatry: reflections and projections. *Psychiatr Opinion.* 1973;10(1):20–23.

77. Bey DR, Chapman RE. Psychiatry—the right way, the wrong way, and the military way. *Bull Menninger Clin.* 1974;38:343–354.

78. Boman B. The Vietnam veteran ten years on. *Aust N Z J Psychiatry.* 1982;16(3):107–127.

79. London P. Quoted by: Veatch RM. The psychiatrist's role in war. In: Veatch RM, ed. *Case Studies in Medical Ethics.* Cambridge, Mass: Harvard University Press; 1977: 250.

80. Shatan CF. How do we turn off the guilt? *Human Behav.* 1973;2:56–61.

81. Abse DW. Brief historical overview of the concept of war neurosis and of associated treatment methods. In: Schwartz HJ, ed. *Psychotherapy of the Combat Veteran.* New York, NY: Spectrum Publications; 1984: 1–22.

82. DeFazio VJ. Psychoanalytic psychotherapy and the Vietnam veteran. In: Schwartz HJ, ed. *Psychotherapy of the Combat Veteran.* New York, NY: Spectrum Publications Medical & Scientific Books; 1984: 23–46.

83. Kolb LC. Post-traumatic stress disorder in Vietnam veterans [editorial]. *N Engl J Med.* 1986;314(10):641–642.

84. Spragg GS. Psychiatry in the Australian military forces. *Med J Aust.* 1972;1(15):745–751.

85. Grossman DA. *On Killing: The Psychological Cost of Learning to Kill in War and Society.* New York, NY: Little, Brown; 1995.

86. Holloway HC. Vietnam military psychiatry revisited. Presentation to: American Psychiatric Association Annual Meeting; 19 May 1982; Toronto, Ontario, Canada.

87. Gabriel RA. *No More Heroes: Madness & Psychiatry in War.* New York, NY: Hill and Wang; 1987.

88. Renner JA Jr. The changing patterns of psychiatric problems in Vietnam. *Compr Psychiatry.* 1973;14(2):169–181.

89. Radine LB. *The Taming of the Troops: Social Control in the United States Army.* Westport, Conn: Greenwood Press; 1977.

90. Kulka RA, Schlenger WE, Fairbank JA, et al. *Trauma and the Vietnam War Generation: Report of Findings From the National Vietnam Veterans Readjustment Study*. New York, NY: Brunner/Mazel; 1990.

91. Blank AS Jr. The longitudinal course of posttraumatic stress disorder. In: Davidson JRT, Foa EB, eds. *Posttraumatic Stress Disorder: DSM–IV and Beyond*. Washington, DC: APA; 1993: 3–22.

92. Jones FD. Chronic post-traumatic stress disorders. In: Jones FD, Sparacino LR, Wilcox VL, Rothberg JM, Stokes JW, eds. *War Psychiatry*. In: Zajtchuk R, Bellamy RF, eds. *Textbooks of Military Medicine*. Washington, DC: Department of the Army, Office of The Surgeon General, Borden Institute; 1995: 409–430.

93. Palinkas LA, Coben P. Psychiatric disorders among United States Marines wounded in action in Vietnam. *J Nerv Ment Dis*. 1987; 175(5):291–300.

94. Colbach EM. Psychiatric criteria for compassionate reassignment in the Army. *Am J Psychiatry*. 1970;127(4):508–510.

95. Roffman RA. *Tilting at Myths: A Marijuana Memoir* (unpublished manuscript).

96. Scurfield RM. *A Vietnam Trilogy: Veterans and Post Traumatic Stress: 1968, 1989, 2000*. New York, NY: Algora Publishing; 2004.

97. Bey D. *Wizard 6* (unpublished memoir); no date.

98. Bey D. *Wizard 6: A Combat Psychiatrist in Vietnam*. College Station, Tex: Texas A & M University Military History Series, 104; 2006.

99. Ritchie EC, ed. *Combat and Operational Behavioral Health*. In: Lenhart MK, ed. *Textbooks of Military Medicine*. Washington, DC: Department of the Army, Office of The Surgeon General, Borden Institute; 2011.

100. Brusher EA. Combat and operational stress control. In: Ritchie EC, ed. *Combat and Operational Behavioral Health*. In: Lenhart MK, ed. *Textbooks of Military Medicine*. Washington, DC: Department of the Army, Office of The Surgeon General, Borden Institute; 2011: 59–71.

101. Schneider BJ, Bradley JC, Christopher HW, Benedek MD. Psychiatric medications in military operations. In: Ritchie EC, ed. *Combat and Operational Behavioral Health*. In: Lenhart MK, ed. *Textbooks of Military Medicine*. Washington, DC: Department of the Army, Office of The Surgeon General, Borden Institute; 2011: 151–162.

102. Howe EG, McKenzie DO, Bradford C. Ethics and military medicine: core contemporary questions. In: Ritchie EC, ed. *Combat and Operational Behavioral Health*. In: Lenhart MK, ed. *Textbooks of Military Medicine*. Washington, DC: Department of the Army, Office of The Surgeon General, Borden Institute; 2011: 727–746.

103. Pechacek MA, Bicknell GC, Landry L. Provider fatigue and provider resiliency training. In: Ritchie EC, ed. *Combat and Operational Behavioral Health*. In: Lenhart MK, ed. *Textbooks of Military Medicine*. Washington, DC: Department of the Army, Office of The Surgeon General, Borden Institute; 2011: 375–389.

104. Camp NM. US Army psychiatry legacies of the Vietnam War. In: Ritchie EC, ed. *Combat and Operational Behavioral Health*. In: Lenhart MK, ed. *Textbooks of Military Medicine*. Washington, DC: Department of the Army, Office of The Surgeon General, Borden Institute; 2011: 9–42.

105. US Department of the Army. *Military Psychiatry*. Washington, DC: HQDA; August 1957. Technical Manual 8-244.

106. Neel SH. *Medical Support of the US Army in Vietnam, 1965–1970*. Washington, DC: GPO; 1973.

107. Scurfield RM. Post-traumatic stress disorder in Vietnam veterans. In: Wilson JP, Raphael B, eds. *International Handbook of Traumatic Stress Syndromes*. New York, NY: Plenum Press; 1993: 285–296.

108. Falk RA, Kolko G, Lifton RJ, eds. *Crimes of War*. New York, NY: Random House; 1971.

109. Butterfield F. The new Vietnam scholarship. *NY Times Mag*. 1983;(February):26–35, 45–47, 52–58.

110. Ferencz BB. War crimes law and the Vietnam war. *Am U Law Rev*. 1968;17:403–423.

111. Committee on Medical Education, Group for the Advancement of Psychiatry. *A Casebook in Psychiatric Ethics*. New York, NY: Brunner-Mazel; 1990.

112. Baker SL Jr. Traumatic war disorders. In: Kaplan HI, Freedman AM, Sadock BJ, eds. *Comprehensive Textbook of Psychiatry*. 3rd ed. Baltimore, Md: Williams & Wilkins; 1980: 1829–1842.

113. Bartemeier LH, Kubie LS, Menninger KA, Romano J, Whitehorn JC. Combat exhaustion. *J Nerv Ment Dis*. 1946;104:358–389.

114. American Psychiatric Association. *The Principles of Medical Ethics: With Annotations Especially Applicable to Psychiatry*. Washington, DC: American Psychiatric Association; 1985.

115. Bitzer R. Caught in the middle: mentally disabled Vietnam veterans and the Veterans Administration. In: Figley CR, Leventman S, eds. *Strangers at Home: Vietnam Veterans Since the War*. New York, NY: Praeger; 1980: 305–323.

116. Ursano RJ, Holloway HC. Military psychiatry. In: Kaplan I, Sadock BJ, eds. *Comprehensive Textbook of Psychiatry IV*. Baltimore, Md: Williams and Wilkins; 1985: 1900–1909.

117. Grant WH, Resnick PJ. Right of active duty military personnel to refuse psychiatric treatment. *Behav Sci Law*. 1989;7(3):339–354.

118. Jones FD. Traditional warfare combat stress casualties. In: Jones FD, Sparacino LR, Wilcox VL, Rothberg JM, Stokes JW, eds. *War Psychiatry*. In: Zajtchuk R, Bellamy RF, eds. *Textbooks of Military Medicine*. Washington, DC: Department of the Army, Office of The Surgeon General, Borden Institute; 1995: 37–61.

119. Menninger WC, Farrell MJ, Brosin HW. The consultant system. In: Glass AJ, Bernucci R, eds. *Neuropsychiatry in World War II*. Vol 1. *Zone of the Interior*. Washington, DC: Medical Department, US Army; 1966: 67–96.

CHAPTER 12

Lessons Learned: Linking the Long, Controversial War to Unsustainable Psychiatric and Behavioral Losses

. . . [I]t is important that the psychiatric experience of Vietnam and its aftermath be subjected to continuous re-evaluation utilizing new source material, operational concepts and conceptual procedures so that the important lessons in military psychiatry hidden within the heart of human tragedies like Vietnam be perceived and applied to the mitigation of human suffering in the practice of psychiatry and in future conflicts.[1(p19)]

Harry C Holloway, MD
Senior Research Psychiatrist
Colonel, US Army (Retired)

This is a photograph of Sergeant First Class Keith Abrahams, a senior enlisted social work/psychology specialist, in an encounter with a Vietnamese man at a Cham temple near Nha Trang in 1969. Their apparent interpersonal remoteness is emblematic of a widespread problem. Because friend and enemy alike were both indigenous (within Vietnam) and exotic (to Americans), US government and military leaders, as well as the troops, did not comprehend their historical and cultural set, the complexity of their motives, and their capabilities. Photograph courtesy of Richard D Cameron, Major General, US Army (Retired).

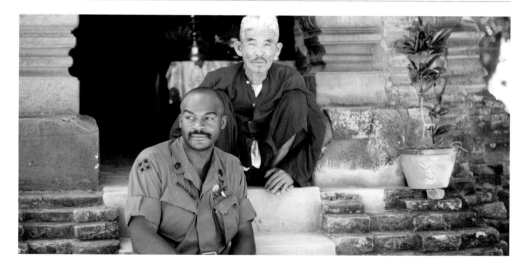

aterial presented in the preceding chapters provides the basis to characterize the Army's psychiatric experience in Vietnam, propose lessons learned, indicate lingering questions (of which there are many), and offer recommendations in retrospect. Despite four decades having passed since the end of hostilities in Vietnam, this information may prove especially worthwhile considering:

- **America fought a new type of war in Vietnam—a counterinsurgency/guerrilla war.** Vietnam was a protracted, divisive, bloody, irregular, counterinsurgency/guerrilla war in which US forces utilized superior weaponry, communication, medical care, and transportation, especially heliborne. This was in striking contrast to the preceding high-intensity wars, which were of shorter duration and accompanied by full mobilization and censored public knowledge. Thus in certain important respects Vietnam appears to have presaged the type of American wars that have arisen so far in the 21st century and that may become more common in the future.

- **The US military went to war in Vietnam armed with new psychopharmacologic capabilities.** Vietnam provided military medicine with its first set of physicians—especially psychiatrists—routinely trained in the use of neuroleptic and anxiolytic tranquilizing medications and the tricyclic antidepressants. These compounds had revolutionized the practice of psychiatry generally, including military psychiatry. More specific to the combat environment, in contrast to the sedatives used sparingly in earlier wars, these new medications were widely utilized in Vietnam as therapeutic agents because they were far less likely to produce sustained central nervous depression and interfere with military performance.

- **Vietnam ultimately became a lost cause.** Despite great effort and sacrifice, the United States failed to achieve its political and military objectives in Vietnam. Withdrawal was ultimately forced by opposition at home, not military defeat, and became a lengthy and tentative process that produced thousands of additional casualties, widespread soldier demoralization and dissent, and unprecedented numbers of psychiatric and behavioral problems.

This work is a composite of published and unpublished reports by psychiatrists and other medical and mental health personnel describing their activities, observations, or studies while there, as well as documents pertaining to soldier morale and mental health in the theater. This approach was taken because the Army Medical Department failed to develop in a timely fashion a historical summary of psychiatry in Vietnam or systematically study the related problems that arose there for "lessons learned." Furthermore, in contrast to World War I, World War II, and the Korean War, the lack of archival material from Vietnam prohibited database analyses. Potential primary source material was evidently lost, abandoned, or destroyed at the conclusion of hostilities (see Appendix 13, Parrish's postwar commentary on why this happened). Some of the deficits in this alternative approach were offset by findings from the 1982 Walter Reed Army Institute of Research (WRAIR) survey of veteran Army psychiatrists (N = 115 of the estimated 135 Army psychiatrists

who were assigned in Vietnam). Although there are limitations to this study that have been previously noted in each chapter, patterns have emerged that appear to be especially instructive.

THE UNEVEN PSYCHIATRIC LEGACY FROM VIETNAM

The existing psychiatric literature that came out of Vietnam is fragmented and misleading. This is primarily because it mostly rests on individual psychiatrists' motivations to publish their accounts, and these are heavily skewed toward the first and more optimistic half of the war. Overall the only consensus is that there was a relatively low incidence of acute combat exhaustion (also known as combat stress reaction [CSR]) casualties in Vietnam (estimated to be 6–7 cases/1,000 troops/year). Otherwise rival claims as to the predominant clinical conditions and their causes and treatment have come from psychiatrists whose vantage points may have been affected by time and role differences and, in some instances, political perspective. The following are illustrative examples:

- *Disorders of frustration and loneliness.* Jones, in his overview (with Johnson) of the Army psychiatric experience in Vietnam, emphasized that "disorders of loneliness"—alcohol, venereal disease, and drug problems—predominated in Vietnam over combat stress-related disorders.[2] In his opinion, neither combat stress nor soldier dissent was of overriding importance. Instead, low combat intensity led to lowered unit cohesion, which produced "nostalgia" casualties (disabling homesickness), especially among noncombat troops, which led to various forms of military ineffectiveness and misconduct. ("[T]he disenchantment toward the end . . . may not have been as important a factor in generating nostalgic casualties as the loss of unit cohesion."[3(p67)]) But Jones was likely affected by having served as a division psychiatrist in the first year of the war where he reported he treated no combat fatigue cases nor encountered soldier dissent.[4]

- *Character and behavior disorders.* During roughly the same time frame as Jones, Bourne, a WRAIR research psychiatrist operating in the theater, noted that the predominant cause for psychiatric attrition in Vietnam was the character and behavior disorder; however, he determined that many of these soldiers, at least those who were hospitalized, were exaggerating their symptoms to secure a socially acceptable path to avoid hardships and combat risks.[5]

- *Psychological reactions from antiwar attitudes.* Two years later, Talbott served in Vietnam as a hospital psychiatrist and subsequently declared that all of his (nonpsychotic) cases were primarily affected by opposition to serving in Vietnam ("a widespread negative sociologic phenomenon"[6]). Notably, Talbott had been strongly against the war before he was assigned in Vietnam and became a prominent antiwar activist following his return.

- *Psychological reactions from fighting guerrilla warfare.* Serving 2 years after Talbott (1969), Renner, a Navy psychiatrist, saw many of the same symptomatic behaviors among Marine psychiatric casualties as the others, but he was convinced that they were primarily affected by the pernicious nature of the counterinsurgency/guerrilla warfare.[7] He also proposed that their pathodynamics were further influenced by the growing antiwar movement in the United States. ("Our troops in Vietnam have not been able to rely on socially reinforced rationalizations [that existed in earlier wars] to help them justify their . . . doubts about the morality of their actions."[7(p172)])

- *Drug problems and dissent.* This author's observation (presented in the Prologue)—that the Army in Vietnam was disabled by a social disorder and the collapse of military discipline—was certainly affected by serving the following year (1970–1971), when the new heroin epidemic took center stage along with myriad antimilitary behaviors, including soldiers threatening to assassinate their leaders.

- *Minimal use of psychotropic medication.* As reviewed in Chapter 7, the available literature amply documented that Vietnam represented the first effective use of modern psychotropic medications under combat circumstances (ie, the anxiolytics, neuroleptics, and tricyclics—drugs without a high sedating potential); yet a recent review of the military use of psychotropics written under Army auspices failed to acknowledge that the use of these medications in Vietnam was historically unique.[8] By way of contrast, Stewart L Baker Jr,

senior Army psychiatrist and Neuropsychiatry Consultant to the Army Surgeon General during the latter years of the war, summarized the vital role served by those medications in the theater as follows: "[In Vietnam] *most combat syndromes* [emphasis added]—including acute agitation, hysterical episodes, and even psychosomatic problems—responded encouragingly within 48 hours to heavy doses of Thorazine coupled with nighttime sodium amobarbital sedation. Thereafter, medication could be rapidly reduced, and psychotherapy could profitably be undertaken."[9(p1836)]

- *Posttraumatic stress disorder.* In one sense this is really a postwar feature in that posttraumatic stress disorder (PTSD) did not exist as a defined diagnostic entity during the war but was later devised to account for the high prevalence of psychiatric and behavior symptoms among Vietnam veterans. Many psychiatric observers came to believe that PTSD was a unique readjustment problem borne by Vietnam veterans—despite the evidence for large numbers of similarly affected veterans from earlier wars.[10] However, this led to conflation of the clinical concept of PTSD with that of combat exhaustion (or combat stress reaction), which many took to mean that PTSD was the preeminent condition arising *in the theater.*

In fact, psychiatric problems in Vietnam cannot be easily characterized by a single salient feature. As the following synopsis illustrates, the war consisted of two halves, each the inverse of the other: a "good" war—in which the US military was effectively fighting the enemy, followed by a "bad" war—in which the US military was fighting itself. Each occurred under distinctly different military and sociopolitical circumstances and with a totally different set of personnel. Also in each, psychiatric resources were dominated by different professional challenges.

SYNOPSIS OF CRITICAL PSYCHIATRIC AND BEHAVIORAL FINDINGS FROM VIETNAM: FROM CONFIDENCE TO CRISIS

During the first half of the Vietnam ground war (mid-1965 through mid-1968) the deployed Army psychiatrists and allied medical and mental health personnel effectively treated an array of problems, and according to their individual reports the overall morale in the theater stayed positive, the numbers of referrals were manageable, and prevention and treatment of combat stress-related disorders (granted in modest numbers) remained the priority. Then, as described in Chapter 1 and Chapter 2, the military and political events that occurred in 1968 not only ended America's resolve to win in Vietnam, but also led to radical changes in strategy, tactics, and troop attitudes—as well as overall social dynamics. During the second half (mid-1968 to mid-1972) the military drawdown saw a dramatic drop in Army morale along with unprecedented levels of dissent, misconduct, drug use, and psychiatric referrals. Despite reduced combat activity, a huge proportion of previously functional soldiers (replacements) became psychiatric and behavioral casualties. In time military order and discipline became marginal while military leaders, law enforcement, and mental health services were all severely challenged. The following is a more detailed list of prominent findings:

- *Psychosocial disorders progressively outweighed combat-generated ones.* In contrast to prior American wars in the 20th century, acute psychiatric casualties generated by the stress of combat (ie, shock trauma) were not the predominant clinical conditions requiring professional attention. They also did not become a force conservation problem during the war. On the other hand, noncombat-related psychiatric and behavior problems accelerated despite declining combat intensity.

- *Insidious stressors were associated with fighting counterinsurgency/guerrilla warfare.* Evidence suggests that the enemy's guerrilla strategy and tactics and the bloody, ambiguous, protracted, and often discouraging nature of fighting provoked large numbers of troops to develop diffuse behavioral, psychological, and psychosomatic reactions that remained mostly unrecognized for what they were—partial trauma and strain trauma (ie, emotionally taxing events—singular or recurring— that were not of sufficient intensity at the time to make them disabling, but that were nonetheless psychologically damaging). It is further speculated that these more subtle factors affected the health and adjustment of many veterans as well.

- *Psychotropic medications were commonly prescribed and highly valued.* Among troops who suffered with various psychiatric symptoms in Vietnam, including combat-related ones, new psychotropic medications assumed a primary role in facilitating their treatment, restoring them rapidly to function, and minimizing disability. However, prescribing physicians had no systematic way to measure short-term and long-term risks associated with their use.

- *Morale, conduct, and mental health problems started to climb between mid-1968 and mid-1970.* The two years following the enemy's Tet offensives, which occurred in the winter and spring of 1968, saw a rise in numbers of troops, including those with no combat exposure, referred for disciplinary problems, racial disturbances, challenges to military authority, drug abuse, and character and behavior disorder diagnoses.

- *Low morale and associated conduct problems became disabling from mid-1970 through mid-1972.* During the last 2 years of the drawdown, various forms of misconduct increased dramatically, especially heroin use (although most users were not addicted) and assassination attempts (or threats) on superiors. These appeared to express both the individual, "(combat theater) deployment stress reaction," and the group, "inverted morale" (eg, when the requisite military culture of commitment and cohesion retrogresses into a pathological, antimilitary one with features suggesting a class war between lower ranks and their superiors). This was somewhat more common among support and service support units. The resultant fulminating antimilitary spirit among the younger troops and the heroin epidemic failed to yield either to efforts to strengthen military leadership, commitment, and cohesion or conventional psychiatric approaches. In time administrative and law enforcement measures had to be intensified until the remaining troops were withdrawn.

- *Coordination between Army leaders and psychiatrists in Vietnam was uncommon.* As the war progressed, matters bearing on military morale and soldier mental health became quite entangled, and yet those primarily responsible for the former, that is, military commanders, and those responsible for the latter, that is, mental health personnel, did not typically maintain a running dialogue, especially in instances of divergent command structures. This was verified from the WRAIR survey findings indicating that with few exceptions, the psychiatrists operating in the field had only limited success with efforts at primary prevention, that is, program consultation with line commanders, in an effort to prevent psychiatric casualties and behavior problems. Furthermore, it is especially regrettable that no documentation survives as to the efforts of those individuals assigned as Psychiatry Consultant to the Commanding General/US Army Republic of Vietnam (USARV) to influence senior Army leaders.

Thus, despite a promising beginning, the Army ultimately underwent an alarming psychosocial and institutional decline in Vietnam that was only indirectly related to fighting the enemy (but most certainly had to do with Vietnam being a theater of combat operations) and mostly did not produce the expectable types of psychiatric disorders. Regrettably following the war there was little apparent interest in studying what went wrong there, certainly by Army psychiatry. However, even at this late date it would seem foolish to assume that the political/social/environmental circumstances that led to the morale, discipline, and mental health failure in Vietnam were so historically unique, that the US military's experience there can be discounted as unlikely to repeat.

EPIDEMIOLOGIC CONSIDERATIONS: TROUBLING QUESTIONS WITH FEW ANSWERS

In the spirit of prevention, could more have been done by medical/psychiatric leaders to maintain esprit, bolster military order and discipline, preserve the mental health, and, by extension, help maintain combat readiness in Vietnam? During the drawdown did the medical leadership in Vietnam overlook early signs of mounting problems and fail to adjust psychiatric perspectives or modify the selection, preparation and training, and distribution/organization of mental health personnel to meet these challenges?[11,12]

Linked to these questions about the specific activities of military medicine and psychiatry in the theater (micro) are equally important questions about where they fit in the bigger picture (macro). The unprecedented high levels for psychiatric disorders and behavior problems during the last 2 years in Vietnam should prompt epidemiologic considerations that acknowledge a pathogenic pathway reaching back to decisions by the US government and military leaders regarding whether, and how, to fight in Vietnam, as well as to the administration's management of public relations during the war—decisions that indirectly but powerfully affected the mental health risks for the troops who fought there.

Indirect Influences on Troops Fighting in Vietnam (Macro)

Questions Regarding the Effects of Decisions Originating in Washington

- Was the initial decision to commit American ground forces in Vietnam, which was justified as necessary to oppose the worldwide spread of communism, a mistake?[13(p177)] (Or, put another way, should the commitment to go to war have had a higher threshold, that is, be limited to circumstances when the threat to the nation is more imminent?[14])
- Was it a mistake to rely on a strategy of winning via enemy attrition, that is, measured by body counts and kill ratios? (Should the United States and its allies instead have opted to fight for territorial pacification and control?[15,16])
- Were the force management policies implemented, which included the extensive reliance on conscription, 1-year tour limitations, and individual rotation schedules (vs full mobilization of US forces, including Reserves and National Guard, unit-based deployments, and individual tours, if not "for the duration" as in earlier wars,[11(p177)] at least by a rotation system based on hardship and risk)?

According to Bourne, apart from the means by which the administration sold the war to the American people, specific policy decisions were made, including those regarding the selection and deployment of forces, for the sole purpose of minimizing public opposition and dissent. These would include gradualism in the force deployment, minimization of perception of national sacrifice, avoidance of media censorship, exempting Reserves and National Guard units, 1-year tours, etc. The government's objective was to have the public feel that in most important regards in the United States, it was business as usual. These proved to be colossal miscalculations—mistakes that had equally enormous consequences for the attitudes of the American public toward the war and, ultimately, for each soldier whose fate it was to serve there.[17]

Questions Regarding the Effects of Failed Public Relations

An equally important question was whether America's adversaries in Vietnam were more adept at psychological warfare than the US government and military. (Psychological warfare includes ways in which the soldier's perception of the reality of his situation is altered to varying degrees by the enemy's disinformation, and, in the case of the US military in Vietnam, by that coming from home and the antiwar movement—which also may have been manipulated by the enemy.) Particularly crucial in this respect, what should be assumed as to the public relations effect on the American people, as well as the troops, following the 1968 surprise Tet offensives in which the enemy, despite the Johnson administration's assurances of imminent defeat, launched coordinated attacks on cities and towns throughout South Vietnam? Although militarily unsuccessful, these attacks, along with the simultaneous siege of the Marine base at Khe Sanh and the extended battle for Hue, encouraged the American media to effectively make the case that the war could not be won at any reasonable cost.[18] The resultant reversal of public and political support for the war demoralized both those at home and those sent there to fight, which in turn powerfully affected the war's outcome.

In addition to these critical decisions that indirectly influenced soldier morale and mental health, the following are some of the more predominant stress-inducing and stress-reducing features in the theater that directly affected the morale, performance, and mental health of Army troops.

Direct Influences on Troops Fighting in Vietnam (Micro)

Stress-Inducing Features in the Buildup Years

- Vietnam was a very long way from home.
- Troops had to master formidable environmental and cross-cultural challenges.
- They had to tolerate the hardships associated with serving in a theater of combat operations.
- Because of the enemy's perseverance and elusiveness, no location was completely safe.

- Combat troops had to contend with a complex combat ecology that was dictated by the enemy's guerrilla strategy and tactics. Apparently for some troops this provoked excessive combat aggression.

Stress-Reducing Features in the Buildup Years

- Most troops (65%–75%) had noncombat assignments.
- The fighting was typically intermittent.
- US troops utilized helicopter mobility and other technological advantages including superior communications, individual weapons, and ordnance systems.
- Combat forays were of limited scope and staged from secure enclaves that were relatively comfortable and easily resupplied.
- Psychiatric observers praised the professionalism of the troops and the high caliber of leadership.
- There was an abundance of supplies, equipment, and support, especially medical support.
- Alcohol (legal) and marijuana (not legal) were available and used frequently. Although they obviously differ in important respects, evidently for most users these served as a safe means of stress-reduction and bonding (but for some they were disabling).
- The Army replacement policy of fixed, 1-year tours apparently had mostly a stress-reducing effect in the early years by allowing soldiers to anticipate the end of their tour.

Additional Stress-Inducing Factors in the Drawdown Years

- Prolongation of the war, the perception of military setbacks, and the growing numbers of casualties were ultimately extremely morale depleting.
- Also demoralizing were divisive US politics and corresponding shifting, sometimes contradictory, government and military policies for prosecuting the war and pursuing the peace.
- The young men who fought in Vietnam were affected by increasingly confrontational antiwar and antimilitary passions in America, which resulted in a reversal of national will regarding the war and a redefinition of patriotism—with honor becoming associated with opposing induction into, or cooperation with, the US military.
- They also were strongly influenced by incendiary social tensions in the United States, especially

the radicalized, liberal, "counterculture" youth movement (the "generation gap"); racial polarization; and widespread antagonism toward American institutions, especially the US military.

- Before deployment, replacement troops were surrounded by the rapidly expanding youth drug culture, which included more dangerous drugs.
- In 1970 indigenous South Vietnamese established an efficient heroin trafficking system throughout the country that greatly expanded heroin accessibility to soldiers in the field.
- The thousands of miles separating Vietnam from the United States were easily bridged by jet-speed transmission of discordant stateside attitudes as media representatives shuttled back and forth and the full complement of troops was replaced annually.
- The Army replacement policy of fixed, 1-year tours had more of a stress-inducing effect as the war wore on because it compromised unit cohesion and commitment as well as depleted the leadership pool of experienced officers and noncommissioned officers.
- Public scorn for those serving in the military, including returning veterans, became open and commonplace.

No data are available that would help answer questions as to whether military psychiatrists, or social scientists for that matter, had any influence on either the decisions made by the US military in Washington or regarding the administration's management of public relations. Also no evidence exists that the assigned military psychiatrists were able to influence any of these stress-inducing features in Vietnam. Still, in the spirit of "lessons learned," if it is not possible to agree that these two levels of phenomena are epidemiologically linked—macro-decisions regarding the "whether" and "how" a war is fought, and micro-influences pertaining to the experience of the individual soldier—then future military psychiatrists (and later those associated with the Veterans Administration [VA]) will, as was the case with Vietnam, mostly serve at the sump end of a long, complex, and sorry ordeal, relegated to providing sympathy and psychological/medicinal balms. (As one of the WRAIR survey psychiatrists commented, "waiting at the bottom of a ski slope").

NOVEL MENTAL HEALTH RISK FACTORS IN VIETNAM

Among these lists of principal psychiatric and behavioral findings and epidemiologic influences, six areas of mental health risk deserve elaboration as novel for US troops serving in Vietnam: (1) conventional troops fighting counterinsurgency/guerrilla warfare; (2) troops fighting for a divided America; (3) fixed, individual, 1-year assignments; (4) deterioration of military morale and discipline near the tipping point, with troops opposing military authority and the military mission (inverted morale); (5) soldier-patients treated by military psychiatrists with limited military experience and allegiance; and (6) Vietnam veterans returning to a rejecting society.

Conventional Troops Fighting Counterinsurgency/Guerrilla Warfare

As discussed in Chapter 6, the mental health effects for conventional ground troops fighting a mostly irregular type of warfare were not systematically addressed by military psychiatry in Vietnam. Overall combat intensity remained relatively low (measured by the wounded-in-action rate), and this correlated with the low rate for acute, disorganizing combat exhaustion cases (roughly estimated at less than 25% of rates seen in earlier, high-intensity wars). Furthermore, the record indicated that by military standards, combat exhaustion cases were effectively treated using a modified version of the traditional forward treatment doctrine, which included liberal use of pharmacotherapy. However, additional evidence suggested that the psychological toll for combat troops was greater than that measured by the combat exhaustion casualty rate. Renner, the Navy psychiatrist mentioned earlier, was the first to suggest that among the growing numbers of psychosomatic disorders, cases of misconduct, drug and alcohol problems, soldiers diagnosed as character and behavior disorders, and veterans with postdeployment PTSD, many were in fact "hidden casualties" of fighting counterinsurgency/guerrilla warfare (ie, they sustained partial trauma or strain trauma).

Anecdotally, some of the Army psychiatrists, as well as some individual case records, appear to corroborate this proposition. US combat units employed aggressive search-and-destroy tactics and other means to isolate the enemy in Vietnam; however, the enemy proved to be patient and elusive and utilized a variety of ruses to dictate the tempo of the fighting. Over time, the gradual attrition of American troops resulting from the enemy's hit-and-run tactics (ambushes, sniping, mortar and rocket fire, and nighttime infiltration by sappers) and indirect means of attack (mines, punji sticks, and booby traps), as well as their terrorism toward civilians, apparently psychologically traumatized and demoralized uncounted numbers of US troops—like the "death by 1,000 cuts." Also, the principle US strategy of enemy attrition, that is, body counts and kill ratios, employed through the first half of the war appeared to be uniquely stressful for troops as well.

Troops Fighting for a Divided America

Chapter 1 described how the growing American opposition to the war rapidly accelerated following the events in early 1968 to become highly charged and confrontational. To fully appreciate the effects of this shift on the soldier fighting in Vietnam, one has to also take into account that this was the first televised war, and the Johnson administration chose not to suppress news coverage. After the war, Baker addressed the epidemiologic effects on the soldiers in Vietnam generated from the home front from his vantage point as the Neuropsychiatry Consultant to the Army Surgeon General during the latter years of the war. According to Baker,

> Simply, war cannot be waged successfully by the military alone. War can be waged successfully only by a united nation. During the Vietnam War, the painful absence of such unity was emphasized by the news media and was reflected to the units in the combat zone as diminished support and discredited performances.[9(p1837)]

Baker spoke of "the shock theater of combat,"[9(p1837)] referring to the public's experience with immediacy of "battlefield color television,"[9(p1837)] which provoked them to have a sense of their own, that is, vicarious, participation in the war, particularly identification with the destructive behavior by the US forces in the field. He felt that this generated guilt in the public psyche, which in turn evoked an urgency to withdraw from Vietnam. ("The public mind becomes . . . defensive [, tending] to abrogate any corresponding personal discipline or geopolitical responsibility."[9(p1837)]) Also, because they corresponded with military personnel in Vietnam

("strongly negative feedback"[9(p1837)]), such reactions, particularly those coming from friends and loved ones, contributed to some troops developing "incapacitating emotional disorders."[9(p1837)] According to Baker, the overall effect on the troops serving in Vietnam was, "chronic anxiety . . . often associated with a progressive feeling of alienation, isolation, decreased self-esteem, and inexpressible anger at the institutional aspects of combat—the structure of the military service, its standard policies, the political meaning proposed for the war effort, and so on."[9(p1837)]

Fixed, Individual, 1-Year Assignments

The military planners for Vietnam evidently assumed that fixed, individual, 1-year assignments would be the most efficient and effective method of force management and would also bolster morale and reduce attrition from psychiatric disorders and behavior problems, that is, it would be stress-mitigating in spreading the risk and hardship. Early in the war the merits of this policy were even defended by Matthew D Parrish (July 1967–July 1968), the third USARV Psychiatry Consultant.[19] According to Parrish, maximum effectiveness for a specific combat ecology was achieved when a soldier became symbiotic with his work group or infantry unit and its technology ("man-team-environment"[19(p9)]), which created, "the ultimate weapon for work or war."[19(p9)] He argued that the individualized replacement system in Vietnam was the least disruptive to the team's task adaptation (ie, it assimilated new members with the least disequilibrium to the group's effectiveness).

However, the record from Vietnam indicated that the rotation policy was increasingly problematic as the war prolonged, both from the standpoint of impairing the stress-reducing potential derived from soldiers bonding with fellow soldiers and unit leaders (cohesion) and the broader dimension of commitment to the unit's history and its mission. Baker concluded after the war that morale in Vietnam had been seriously degraded by the combination of the individualized, 1-year tour and the relative ease of communicating with home. This was problematic in that "[the soldier's] adjustment was often marked by an intense *personalized* (emphasis added) struggle to survive . . . [such that] he developed no great concern about the outcome of the war and, in the main, felt only personal relief when he left Vietnam."[9(p1836)]

Deterioration of Military Morale
Near the Tipping Point

The reduction in combat activities and the perception of demobilization surely explains some of the rise in psychiatric conditions and behavioral problems after 1968. In this regard, the skyrocketing medical evacuation rate in Vietnam for soldiers whose urine tested positive for heroin breakdown products in 1971–72 may reasonably be considered a collective form of the "evacuation syndrome" (ie, they were motivated to manipulate the system to get relief from foreign deployment and, perhaps, combat risks).[20] However, beyond these sorts of reactions to demobilization familiar from earlier wars, the troops in the latter part of the Vietnam War were unique in that they bonded around their intense opposition to military authority and the mission—an attitude that coincided with the virulent antiwar, antimilitary feelings of those at home. The unprecedented rates for psychiatric conditions and behavioral problems evidently expressed soldier resentment of being asked to make sacrifices to salvage America's lost cause there while surrounded by the moral outrage and blame of the US public. It has been suggested that these soldier behaviors collectively represented a "macromutiny."[21] Considering that many of the antimilitary authority behaviors were passive or covert, for example, "search and avoid" combat missions[16(p97)] and "shamming" (the pretense of activity but without productivity), and considering that young soldiers commonly referred to the Army as "the green machine,"[16,22] perhaps sabotage is a preferable term to mutiny.

Regardless of the terminology, the disturbing truth is that by the end of the war many soldiers had more or less disabled (or demobilized) themselves through mental disorders, drug use, and other symptoms and forms of misconduct. Although clearly some soldiers brought preservice personality susceptibility to the theater that facilitated their acting out their frustrations in these ways, the exceptionally high incidence of these problems among previously functional soldiers ("epidemic") and the very reduced levels of combat activity at the time suggest more. In this author's opinion, a full pathodynamic explanation must include a recognition that a social disorder—a crisis of the collective—was a principle contributor to the disturbed functioning of these soldiers (eg, that a social–psychiatric "disorder" emerged, such as in Goffman's pathogenic "total institution,"[23] Fleming's "sociosis,"[24]

or Rose's "macromutiny"[21]), as opposed to one primarily centered on individual psychology. In other words, these were symptoms of a failure of adaptation at the level of the group. They arose from a complex interaction of personal circumstance and powerful biological (often including drug-induced), psychological, and social stressors (in Vietnam as well as from home) —stressors that became progressively onerous for sequential cohorts of replacement soldiers as the war wound to its bitter conclusion.

Fortunately, American military readiness in the last few years of the Vietnam War was not seriously tested by the enemy, leaving moot the question of the degree and consequences of force erosion stemming from public doubt, low troop morale, opposition to the military mission, and widespread "evacuation syndromes." In retrospect it seems plausible that the enemy didn't challenge the remaining US forces for one compelling reason: the US military was at war with itself. However, the potential for disaster seems indisputable.[25]

Soldier-Patients Treated by Military Psychiatrists With Limited Military Experience and Allegiance

Among the psychiatrists who served during the second half of the war, the few who wrote about it reflected increasing frustration in applying traditional military psychiatry models and structures in response to the changing nature and scope of the behavioral and psychiatric challenges. Even if in many respects these problems were insoluble, at least on any terms pertaining to clinical psychiatry, possibly contributory were:

- Theater psychiatric statistics collected by USARV utilized a taxonomy that was too limited.
- In the latter half of the war when other data emerged that reflected deteriorating troop morale, discipline, and performance, timely modifications in the selection, preparation, deployment, and organization of psychiatric assets were not devised to address these challenges.
- The morale of many of the psychiatrists who served in the latter half of the war suffered a serious decrement that paralleled that of the typical soldier. It also appeared that they lost confidence in their objectives, structure, methods, and results.
- As theater problems deteriorated and opposition to the war increased, the Army deployed fewer

psychiatrists with postresidency military experience and familiarity with military priorities and structures. Also, replacement psychiatric leaders (USARV Psychiatry Consultants) had less military psychiatry experience than those who had preceded them. Furthermore, many of the civilian-trained psychiatrists were inclined to be more alienated from the mission.

- After the war many of the veteran psychiatrists were troubled by their role in Vietnam and expressed feeling inadequate and betrayed because they were ill prepared and unsupported by the Army in Vietnam. This occurred despite the fact that, overall, the Army psychiatrists assigned in Vietnam had an unprecedented degree of formal psychiatric training.

- Whereas the remarkable prevalence of problems that arose suggests the effects of a social disorder, especially the intense, adversarial relationship between soldiers and leaders, the psychiatric training of the times—somewhat so in Army residency programs but more so in civilian ones—did not emphasize social pathology and interventions nor provide sufficient practical training.

Apart from these features, it also seems safe to say that as the war lengthened, the deployed Army psychiatrists were affected by the public disapproval of the war and the increasing criticism of military psychiatry's priorities by psychiatrists in the civilian professional community. What is less certain is how much these influences may have affected the clinical decisions of the deployed psychiatrists. Ethical and moral reactions to a war and its politics have been shown to shape military psychiatrists' diagnosis and disposition of cases (eg, encourage what the military would describe as sympathetic "overdiagnosis" and "overevacuation"—clinical decisions believed in past wars to contribute to chronicity in combat-affected soldiers as well as jeopardize force conservation).

Did psychiatrists who believed the war was unjust perceive that participation was a primary etiologic factor in the pathogenesis of their soldier-patients? Were clinical perception and judgment affected by alignment between the soldier-patient's desire to be removed from combat duty, or the theater, and the psychiatrist's doubt about military necessity? Were psychiatrists with limited pre-Vietnam military psychiatry experience more prone

to identify with their symptomatic soldier-patient's antimilitary sentiments in Vietnam? By extension, could the rising hospitalization rate in the second half of the war have also expressed identification of some psychiatrists with symptomatic soldiers? At least some of the WRAIR survey participants acknowledged that they sought to protect soldiers by exaggerating the diagnosis in order to get them evacuated from the theater. In the same vein, following the war some civilian psychiatrists raised concerns that the military may have harmed soldiers because of incomplete treatment and premature return to duty in Vietnam.

Vietnam Veterans Returning to a Rejecting Society

As noted earlier, a comprehensive review of postdeployment difficulties among Vietnam veterans is beyond the scope of this work. However, it is worth considering that a deployed soldier invariably worries about how he will be treated when he reenters stateside life, and this strongly influences his adjustment within the theater. Once back stateside it then becomes necessary for him to master and assimilate "his" war (his ordeal, reactions, and losses, and their meaning to him). If he succeeds, he is likely strengthened.[26] If not, he may make costly psychological compromises and remain more or less permanently affected or even disabled (Figure 12-1). For all who served in the theater, but surely more so for the veterans of the combat itself, his cherished premilitary self-image may have become damaged if circumstances contributed to his concluding that he had faced his personal ordeal as a coward, or as a savage.

Recovering his mental equilibrium as a veteran in large part depends on positive relationships, that is, social supports. His effort to reconcile his own moral dilemma about killing (or being an accessory to the killing[27]) and the war's destructiveness is a process that is especially affected by the manner in which he is treated by his family and the nation. Is there affirmation, redemption, as if he is a hero? Or is there disregard (or worse), as if he's a pariah? Reconciling his experience becomes more difficult for the citizen-soldier who, following his enlistment, leaves the military and its generally supportive culture.[28] It seems safe to say that when it is all over no one is the same as before it began. With regard to Vietnam, the clash of values over the war not only encouraged widespread problems among veterans, but it can additionally be said that sooner

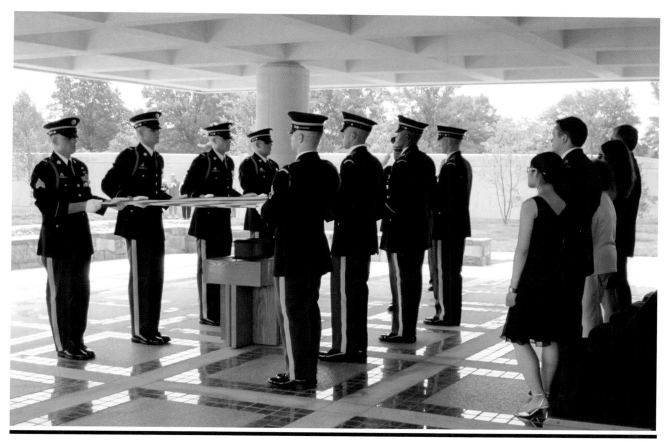

FIGURE 12-1. Military funeral at Arlington National Cemetery for Vietnam veteran Chris McGinley Schneider (2010). Although a female veteran, she is emblematic of thousands of soldiers, combat and noncombat, who became hidden casualties of the war—individuals who left Vietnam apparently unscathed but whose wounds, physical and psychological, emerged months to years later. Schneider volunteered to go to Vietnam as a nurse and served selflessly and with distinction at the 95th Evacuation Hospital in 1970–71. Soon after returning to civilian life she developed chronic posttraumatic stress disorder that was so severe she abandoned nursing as a career. In 2009 she was diagnosed with leukemia, which was suspected to be the consequence of her exposure in Vietnam to the herbicide Agent Orange and other environmental biohazards.

or later every soldier who served there had to contend with the added psychological burden of knowing he participated in, and sacrificed for, a lost and socially repudiated cause.

Some perspective regarding the unique psychosocial burdens affecting Vietnam veterans came from Richard P Fox, a Navy psychiatrist, who reported on his study of Vietnam returnee clinical referrals who had severe reentry symptoms and behavioral problems. Fox argued that, as a group, the troops returning from Vietnam were demonized by American society. In earlier wars, wounds to the soldier's self-esteem, which were the predictable consequence of participating in combat, were buffered by the "adulation" of those at home. Under those circumstances only soldiers

with predisposing personality deficits would suffer sustained postwar disability. In contrast, for the soldiers who fought in Vietnam, the public opposition to the war meant that the adulation was instead directed to those who resisted the draft or in other ways avoided Vietnam. Families were pleased to see their sons and husbands return, but there were few heroes' welcomes. "The reluctance of family and friends to listen to the war stories the returnee had to tell not only added to his sense of isolation but also deprived him of [the adulation required for him to repair his self-esteem, which was traditionally] accorded the returning warrior."[29(pp810–811)]

In this respect, Dave Grossman, a retired Army Ranger and former West Point professor of psychology, offered a compelling model for understanding the studies pointing to higher than expected PTSD levels among some Vietnam veterans whose exposure to combat may have been limited. According to Grossman's perspective, the process and experience of veterans reintegrating to stateside life is etiologically equivalent to, and interacts with, the ordeal he sustained in the combat zone because it either mitigates it or aggravates the psychological sequelae of his war experience. Grossman proposed the following complemental series for returnees from any war: that there is a sliding functional relationship between experiences in the combat zone ("combat trauma") and those upon returning to the United States ("social support") that shapes their postwar adjustment. For instance, soldiers with a high degree of combat exposure in World War II received a strong societal embrace and affirmation for what they saw and did because of the popularity of that cause, and may, consequently, have lower PTSD levels. In contrast, those who had a much lower degree of combat exposure in Vietnam nonetheless felt scorned and blamed for serving in the war upon their return because of that war's great unpopularity and, as a consequence, sustained higher PTSD levels.

Grossman's explanation for this included the proposition that if society turns on the war effort and reacts to it as morally unjustified, then in simply having been "in the midst" of the killing in the combat theater, the soldier is made into an accessory to murder. Quoting one veteran, "society didn't make any distinction who they spat on."[27] This is a model espoused by Bourne as well.[30] (This author [NM Camp] would further add that there is no such thing as "lack of support" for the veteran, or "nonsupport," suggesting a neutral or indifferent response. To the veteran, any ambiguity or nonsupport is experienced contextually as blame and condemnation, provoking a deeply troubling sense of being a social outcast.)

The perspective offered by Theodore Nadelson, Chief of Psychiatry at the Boston VA Medical Center, seems especially poignant:

> In Vietnam, where the usual guides to behavior disappeared and women and children killed also, some young combatants lost their moral center. They were forced to discover their competence in situations of mortal risk where loyalty to friends was most valued. It was, for most of them, in very young adulthood, a time of greatest sensitivity

to such a strong force. In killing some of them celebrated their combined youthful strength, their survival and dominance and that of their nation. On return home they discovered only anomie, devaluation of their wartime experience, and rejection of their skill and loyalties.[31(p135)]

> . . . (Furthermore) these returned veterans have an awareness that something happened to them as a result of exposure to intense and addicting experiences dissonant with expectations "back home," in the "real world," in "so-called civilization." They experience further difficulty because of a sense of betrayal regarding their sacrifice and risk, the deaths of their buddies, and a failure on the part of the nation to reciprocally reinforce the ancient mutual loyalty to its warriors by appropriate "expiatory rituals" for killing.[31(p139)] (See also Exhibit 12-1: Post-Vietnam Challenges to the Military Psychiatry Forward Treatment Doctrine.)

RETROSPECTIVE CRITIQUE

The preceding review of stress-inducing and stress-mitigating phenomena affecting American troops in Vietnam compels a belated effort to consider remedies. The following list of recommendations pertains to the mental health activities of the Army Medical Department in Vietnam, especially its mental health specialists. The items are roughly arrayed in three categories: (1) prevention; (2) adaptation; and (3) documentation. However, as remedies they are limited as they would require corresponding efforts by USARV and the Department of the Army. Clearly, for lessons learned in military psychiatry to have any broad impact, they must be linked to lessons learned on the leadership side; but to this author's knowledge, there has been no official review from that vantage point.

Prevention

- **A preventive medicine-like system to monitor the various (changing) indices indicating the rising incidence of psychiatric and related medical disability, unit demoralization, and flagging soldier performance in Vietnam should have been employed by the Army.** The taxonomy used by USARV to collect psychiatric information from the medical treatment facilities was too limited to account for the growing complexity in the theater. Also, evidently there was insufficient integration of the gleaned psychiatric information with data from major commands and other medical, administrative, and law enforcement sources pertaining to related problems. What was needed was a dedicated epidemiologic field team to collect, analyze, and disseminate information regarding a wide array of often initially innocuous indices of psychiatric and behavior dysfunction as well as flagging morale and group performance. This information would have permitted the early detection of deteriorating psychosocial and psychiatric circumstances and provided clinicians and commanders a timely map of the psychosocial "terrain" regarding stressors and their effects. In turn this could have triggered development of preventative and intervention measures. It also would have satisfied historical, planning, training, research, and treatment goals. (An example is the model program provided by Douglas R Bey and Walter E Smith with the 1st Infantry Division [1969–1970]. The list of unit parameters they monitored to identify troubled units was especially useful.[32]) At the very least the USARV Psychiatry Consultants should have teamed up with preventive medicine personnel to target specific dysfunctional units or problem areas for special attention by major unit commanders and their mental health assets.

- **During the buildup phase, Army medicine/ psychiatry should have detected the rising incidence of covert psychiatric symptoms and behavior disturbances among combat troops and sought to modify systems of prevention at the unit level as well as treatment approaches by medical and mental health personnel.** From the standpoint of soldier stress, the Army was unprepared for the type of combat encountered in Vietnam, where many soldiers apparently sustained widespread but more subtle psychological and psychosocial effects, (ie, partial trauma and strain trauma) than that found in earlier wars. This was a consequence of fighting an irregular, drawn-out, bloody guerrilla/ counterinsurgency war—a war fought on the far side of the world against a determined and resourceful enemy while using mostly citizen-soldiers and having to contend with intense controversy about the war at home. Recognition of these differences should have prompted a search for

new strategies for prevention, early detection, and treatment of these types of casualties.

- **During the drawdown phase, Army medicine/ psychiatry, as well as Army leadership, should have applied a social psychiatry model to aid in the early detection, prevention, and treatment of the growing numbers of psychiatric and behavioral casualties.** The Army, like the psychiatric component, failed to anticipate the unprecedented psychosocial strain associated with disengagement after years of stalemated and controversial war in Vietnam. What was needed was an overarching multivariate model of combat "theater" breakdown (as opposed to one limited to combat stress reaction [CSR]). Such a model would have encompassed both symptomatic soldiers (ie, those with "deployment stress reaction") as well as dysfunctional groups of soldiers (eg, units with inverted morale), and prompted a search for new strategies for prevention, early detection, treatment, or countermeasures.

Adaptation

- **Adjustments should have been made in the distribution of mental health assets as the situation deteriorated in Vietnam.** The mounting and changing psychiatric demands in Vietnam went unchallenged by adaptive strategies for the organization of psychiatric care. The Army initially deployed a pair of fully staffed psychiatric treatment centers (ie, the KO team/psychiatric specialty detachments). The establishment of these freestanding, but in many instances geographically isolated, centers, which provided mostly conventional, hospital-based, in- and outpatient services, was predicated on the Army's pre-Vietnam war experience; however, questions can be raised as to the wisdom of retaining this structure over the course of the war. The flood of combat-generated stress responses that was anticipated never materialized. Over time, the breakdown of morale and discipline became the greater hazard to combat readiness—especially through noncombat-related psychiatric disorders and behavior problems, and especially among noncombat units. As a result the initial distribution of mental health assets that favored the combat divisions became problematic because the center of effort shifted to nondivision support and service-support units, which went underserved.

EXHIBIT 12-1. Post-Vietnam Challenges to the Military Psychiatry Forward Treatment Doctrine

The historical narrative of military psychiatry leading up to Vietnam repeatedly observed that the lessons learned in previous wars had been forgotten between wars, and that in the next war there was a costly delay before mental health specialists were placed in forward positions and the combat psychiatry forward treatment doctrine was reinstituted in order to limit evacuations among otherwise recoverable combat stress casualties.[1-3] Unfortunately, this may be happening again.[4] In particular, at this point in time (late 2013), and even in the wake of two recent military engagements with similarities to Vietnam but on a smaller scale—Iraq and Afghanistan—civilian/humanitarian sensibilities, that is, consistent with Department of Veterans Affairs–oriented protective ones, have served to challenge the traditional forward treatment doctrine because the latter is based on the primacy of force conservation for the sake of mission accomplishment. This shift has arisen because of the convergence of four trends:

1. There was never a serious shortage of fighting personnel in Vietnam because of the draft. Even though the adaptation of the doctrine in Vietnam appears validated by this work, this carries only so much weight because force conservation was never a critical dimension during the war.
2. America's social and cultural wounds consequent to losing the war in Vietnam were expressed through sympathies for its physical and mental casualties, especially through the establishment of the new psychiatric diagnosis, posttraumatic stress disorder (PTSD). Although the PTSD concept drew much needed medical attention to the treatment needs of Vietnam veterans, it simultaneously served to discredit veteran complaints of contributory mistreatment by society, the government, and the military. Furthermore, as discussed in Chapter 2, a number of investigators and clinicians with experience with military veterans came to question the validity of the PTSD diagnosis. Also, clinical confusion often arose when distinguishing combat-generated acute stress reactions from PTSD. Nonetheless public opinion has been strongly shaped by suggestions that the America's military activities in Vietnam and since have produced unacceptable levels of PTSD.
3. The revolutionary change in the American taxonomy of psychiatric disorders in 1980, the 3rd edition of the *Diagnostic and Statistical Manual of Mental Disorders* (DSM-III), served by extension to cast doubt on earlier, empirically derived theories of causation for combat stress casualties—theories that encompassed predisposition, psychosocial disturbances, and psychic conflict. The resultant vacuum led some to favor neurophysiologic theories as alternatives. For example, William P Nash, a Navy psychiatrist, recently challenged the traditional military forward treatment doctrine—what he referred to as the "demedicalized" or "normalization" model—because it expected combat-exposed service members to withstand their strains and traumas predicated on an assumption that combat aversion and stress reactions were natural accompaniments to combat deployment.[5,6] According to Nash, the doctrine meant that there were frequent instances of combat stress-generated neurologic "injury" at the molecular and cellular level, especially from glutamate neurotoxicity, that were overlooked (he is not referring to soldiers with blast-generated traumatic brain injuries). He further argued that the traditional forward treatment doctrine caused combat-exposed troops with mental difficulties to be unnecessarily subjected to a military culture of stigma and shame and to consequently fail to seek timely care. Nash admitted that if combat stress casualties were instead treated according to his injury model, "Military leaders and public policy makers may fear [an increase in] the risk for epidemics of stress-injured [soldiers] seeking evacuation from war zones or disability compensation from the Dept. of Veterans Affairs"[6(p794)]; however, he provided no solution for this disturbing possibility. Thus in effect, Nash appears to have reverted to the abandoned World War I model of shell shock with its disastrous potential for unsustainable psychiatric attrition, unnecessary and high soldier morbidity, and the risk of military defeat.
4. Military psychiatry has increasingly turned toward an occupational medicine model as opposed to one centered on the (psychiatric) risk/benefit ratio required in accomplishing the combat mission. During the four decades since Vietnam, the US military has been fortunate in being able to sustain itself using an all-volunteer force. Through augmentation of active units with Reserve units and National Guard units, and by redeploying military personnel, fighting military America's major engagements, for example, the Persian Gulf War, and Iraq and Afghanistan, has not required full mobilization and conscription. The result, however, is that deployment stress, as well as combat stress, have come to be viewed simply and dispassionately as "hazardous exposures in the workplace," with the associated mental health objective being to "define levels of acceptable exposure to those hazards."[7] This paradigm shift has been led by Charles Hoge (an Army-trained psychiatrist and epidemiologist) and his colleagues at the WRAIR Department of Psychiatry and Behavioral Sciences. In the publication "Priorities for Psychiatric Research in the US Military: An Epidemiologic Approach," they repeatedly used the adjective "occupational" to allude to the soldier's adaptational

EXHIBIT 12-1. Post-Vietnam Challenges to the Military Psychiatry Forward Treatment Doctrine (continued)

challenge (as in "occupational . . . functioning," ". . . dysfunction," ". . . attrition"; "the highly structured occupational environment in the military"; and "the occupational burden of mental disorders"). On the other hand, the unique psychological requirements associated with combat, such as duty, valor, commitment to a unit's mission and fellow soldiers, or sacrifice, are omitted.[8] Equally illustrative of this new mindset are publications by Hoge et al of results of their surveys of military personnel before and after deployment in Iraq and Afghanistan exploring soldier mental health and behavioral complaints and self-reported extent of contact with the enemy.[9] Although their approach is laudatory as a preliminary study of the psychological and psychosomatic consequences of combat theater deployment, it is also misleading both because it is more consistent with the treatment objectives of the Department of Veterans Affairs than that of an army at war, and because it fails to account for the true nature of war with its complex physical and psychosocial challenges. In effect, by relying on participant self-reports without corroboration from the field (objective measures and clinical findings), the authors studied these troops as if they were simply individuals who had been exposed to high occupational risk that was now in the past (as one might do with disaster workers), and as if those who reported psychological wounds were primarily victims, that is, tantamount to civilians who sustained unforeseen trauma. They seem not to comprehend that every soldier struggles to manage the conflict between his self-protective instincts and his desire to honorably and selflessly perform his military duty (eg, through loyalty to comrades, unit, and country); that increased psychological symptoms under those circumstances are the predictable consequence of that strain; that for many it is how their psychological perturbations are managed at the time and later (referring especially to the quantity and quality of available social supports, both in-country and at home) that makes the difference in psychological sequelae; and that, for the sake of the mission, commanders invariably worry that too much attention can be paid to mild to moderate symptoms among troops that stem from the heightened dangers, hardships, uncertainty, and homesickness that arise in a combat environment.

In conclusion, this volume's study of Army psychiatry in Vietnam strongly suggests that the country owes it to the troops to keep in mind the history of military psychiatry and *(a)* employ a complex model of combat stress, breakdown, and recovery—one that is fully bio\psycho\social in nature, and *(b)* retain the military psychiatry doctrine that was validated through America's earlier wars in the modern era. Although the traditional doctrine carries with it a sometimes regrettable requirement that in extreme circumstances the protection of individual soldiers must be subordinate to military necessity, the failure to envision a future, large-scale war requiring full mobilization and reinstitution of the draft—a war that may again become unpopular and bring with it widespread combat aversion and evasion and require psychosocial treatments supporting force conservation—may put American military forces, and thus the nation, at more risk than the nation is willing to accept.

REFERENCES
1. Hausman W, Rioch DM. A prototype of social and preventive psychiatry in the United States. *Arch Gen Psychiatry*. 1967;16:727–739.
2. Glass AJ. Military psychiatry and changing systems of mental health care. *J Psychiat Res*. 1971;8:499–512.
3. Johnson AW Jr. Psychiatric treatment in the combat situation. *US Army Vietnam Med Bull*. 1967;January/February:38–45.
4. Levin A. Will PTSD by any other name bring more troops to treatment? *Psychiatric News*. July 2012;47(13):1,6.
5. Nash WP. US Marine Corps and Navy combat and operational stress continuum model: a tool for leaders. In: Ritchie EC, ed. *Combat and Operational Behavioral Health*. In: Lenhart MK, ed. *Textbooks of Military Medicine*. Washington, DC: Department of the Army, Office of The Surgeon General, Borden Institute; 2011: 107–119.
6. Nash WP, Silva C, Litz B. The historic origins of military and veteran mental health stigma and the stress injury model as a means to reduce it. *Psych Annals*. 2009;39:789–794.
7. McFarlane AC. The duration of deployment and sensitization to stress. *Psych Annals*. 2009;39:81–88.
8. Hoge CW, Messer SC, Engel CC, et al. Priorities for psychiatric research in the US military: an epidemiologic approach. *Mil Med*. 2003;168(3):182–185.
9. Hoge CW, Castro CA, Messer SC, McGurk D, Cotting DI, Koffman RL. Combat duty in Iraq and Afghanistan, mental health problems, and barriers to care. *N Engl J Med*. 2004;351:13–22.

- **Greater attention should have been given to training and mentoring psychiatrists in command consultation.** Participants' responses to the WRAIR survey (corroborated with anecdotal data) indicated that program-centered command consultation, that is, true primary prevention, was not routinely provided. When psychiatrists did engage in program-centered command consultation, they reported greater success if they had some military experience before being sent to Vietnam (either a military residency or a pre-Vietnam assignment) or had been assigned at some point in Vietnam to a combat unit. This is an important finding regarding the saliency of a military background and familiarity in teaching the psychiatrist the value of a socioenvironmental preventive approach for reducing both incidence and morbidity of psychiatric problems among soldiers. Psychiatrists without this background should have been systematically taught these critical skills in Vietnam by those who had the requisite experience.

- **As implementation of the military psychiatry forward treatment doctrine in Vietnam became more ethically burdensome the assigned psychiatrists should have received specific support in managing the strain.** The major goal of this work was to illuminate a history of the Army's effort to fight and win in Vietnam through the lens of military psychiatry's twin and sometimes clashing values: "conserve the fighting strength" and "care of the sick and wounded" (humanitarian values). In this regard it is necessary to remind the reader that although it is desirable that humanitarian values be served, military medicine was born of the necessity for the prevention and restoration of battle casualties. The priority for military psychiatrists has historically been to promote maximal psychological endurance among soldiers committed to combat through preventive advice to their commanders and the effective treatment and rehabilitation of those whose personal resources have been exceeded by the circumstances.[33] Yet the psychiatric literature and the WRAIR survey participants indicated that when it came to fighting in Vietnam, maintaining this values hierarchy was more difficult than in earlier wars.

  Whereas Army psychiatrists serving during the first half of the war did not appear to struggle with operational or ethical strain, those who served in the second half, and despite falling combat

activity, indicated the opposite. More specifically, to varying degrees they were affected by stresses of: *(a)* being overworked (burnout), *(b)* provider fatigue (or compassion fatigue), *(c)* opposition to Army medical policies that favored military expediency over patient rights, and *(d)* true ethical strain (having protective impulses toward soldier-patients, ie, civilian values, in opposition to military ones that would urge soldiers to quickly return to duty).

- **Policies and procedures for selection, preparation, and deployment of psychiatrists and other mental health professionals and paraprofessionals for Vietnam should have been revised and strengthened by Army psychiatry leaders.** The unmitigated increase in psychosocial casualties among the US Army troops in Vietnam raises questions about decisions and policies made at the level of the Psychiatry Consultant, Army Surgeon General, pertaining to: *(a)* the selection and preparation of psychiatrists, especially in the second half of the war, and *(b)* the assimilation of, and accommodation to, information from the theater. The Army's two residency training programs were able to provide for a substantial proportion of the deployed psychiatrists (roughly one-third); however, the median amount of postresidency experience among the respondents was only 4 to 6 months, and there were repeated expressions by the WRAIR survey respondents of feeling ill-prepared, especially among those with civilian training and those who served in the later half.

  The responses from the psychiatrist participants in the WRAIR survey do not suggest there was an official Army policy as to what constituted sufficient specific preparation or training for service as a psychiatrist in Vietnam. Nor for that matter was it apparent what were the requisite background factors for the selection of the USARV Psychiatry Consultants. It is clearly notable that greater numbers of psychiatrists with less military experience, especially those just graduated from civilian residencies, would be sent as replacements amidst the perceptibly deteriorating morale, psychological fitness, and military readiness in the second half of the war. It also seems puzzling that the USARV Psychiatry Consultants assigned in the drawdown phase would also have had appreciably less experience serving as military psychiatrists than their predecessors.

Compounding the matter, a critical deficiency was that there was no systematic debriefing of returning psychiatrists. Considering that the Army psychiatrists in Vietnam and the USARV Psychiatry Consultants were replaced annually, an aggressive program of debriefing the returning psychiatrists should have been implemented so as to impart to the replacement psychiatrists the gleaned wisdom and to guide modifications of the structures and policies in the theater. In fact WRAIR survey respondents repeatedly complained about wanting to have been informed about the actual conditions they would face in Vietnam before they deployed. In particular such a process could have prompted replacement psychiatrists to redirect some of their attention from a combat stress model toward a social stress model of psychiatric dysfunction.

Other structural adaptations as the war in Vietnam lengthened might have included: (*a*) development and distribution of operationalized diagnostic criteria and treatment guidelines for common psychiatric disorders, especially uniquely military conditions such as combat exhaustion; (*b*) extending the tours of each of the USARV Psychiatry Consultants beyond the standard year (as well as tours of other psychiatrists in leadership positions) to provide needed continuity; (*c*) increasing the level of seniority of the replacement military psychiatrists as the pool of experienced civilian psychiatrists unavoidably decreased; (*d*) linking numbers of deployed psychiatrists to epidemiologically documented need, rather than to overall troop strength or an outdated structure; (*e*) modifying the curricula of the Army psychiatric residency programs to reflect the changing nature of the challenge in Vietnam; (*f*) requiring that each recently graduated psychiatrist, regardless of the type of his/her original training, serve some time with a stateside military unit before departing for Vietnam (presuming such an arrangement otherwise did not interfere with overall mobilization requirements); and (*g*) providing for a 1- to 2-week overlap between the arriving and departing psychiatrists in Vietnam.

Documentation

- **Psychiatric research projects should have been devised and conducted in Vietnam throughout the war.** Considering the aforementioned list of unique risk elements comprising the combat or theater ecology, it seems logical that the Army Medical Research and Development Command should have conducted formal studies in Vietnam throughout the war on matters pertaining to stress, morale, and mental health. Among other possibilities, these could have addressed the impact on regular troops consequent to fighting an unconventional/guerrilla war and the short- and long-term effects of psychotropic medications.

- **The Army should have committed to maintaining a historical record of psychiatric matters in Vietnam.** A prominent and surprising finding of this review is that evidently throughout the war there was no centralized psychiatric information collected except for the theater-wide statistics mentioned earlier. This situation stands in stark contrast to published historical accounts of World War II. Bernucci and Glass described how they, in anticipation of writing a history and while hostilities were still under way, collected the relevant materials and documents. ("Key personnel and many of the consultants were periodically brought into the [Surgeon General's Office] to record their experiences before they were deployed elsewhere or released from the Army."[34(pxv)]) Equally important was the Army's ultimate decision to establish a formal dedicated position as editor for its historical account. As they described, initially the project failed under the assumption that it could be written with part-time leadership. Regarding any war, certainly Vietnam, it seems logical that there must be a before-the-fact commitment to a historical record—in the form of policies and structures for data gathering and storage, and an after-the-fact commitment of resources to analyze and present the salient facts.

As the record from Vietnam shows, assuming that the participating psychiatrists will, in time, publish their observations risks leaving a very incomplete or skewed record of what may turn out to be critical information. Responsibility for this failure with respect to Vietnam certainly lies with Army psychiatry and more generally with USARV. Disturbingly, some have speculated that it could have reflected the intentions of some politicians who sought to prevent such research.[35]

FINAL THOUGHTS

It has been arguably estimated that the Vietnam War was the most psychologically damaging of all of America's wars in the 20th century. This may, in fact, be the case if it includes not only psychiatric conditions and behavior disorders, especially among veterans, but also America's decades-long postwar malaise. Furthermore, wars with features similar to those that arose in Vietnam may become increasingly common in the future—protracted, low-intensity wars with limited goals that are surrounded by intense media scrutiny and political controversy. It was with this in mind that this review sought to reconstruct the experience of US Army psychiatrists who served in Vietnam and the record of care they provided there. Regrettably, it is a disheartening account. Following a commendable first few years, the enemy proved to be more formidable than expected and the war dragged on the American public withdrew its approval, and troop morale and mental health declined and ultimately dissidence and misconduct rose to near mutinous proportions. And throughout all this, the Army psychiatrists and their mental health colleagues in Vietnam were increasingly challenged, were too often stymied, and in many instances left Vietnam indelibly embittered.

However, Army psychiatry's story in Vietnam is only reflective of the larger story of the war. Although President Reagan later referred to it as a "noble cause,"[36] realistically there is no way to avoid acknowledging that the American war in Vietnam was a tragic failure. Whether history decides that this was because it was ill-conceived, was mismanaged, or became despised and repudiated—or all the above—a central truth is that this outcome also came about because of human sensibilities and limitations, not a lack of military might. Despite Secretary of Defense Robert McNamara's highly touted managerial strategy,[37] and despite the sustained and courageous effort by US military forces, America was ultimately forced to withdraw from Vietnam because of critical miscalculations regarding the American public's willingness to tolerate continued fighting, losses, and international criticism, and the military's incapacity to maintain discipline and a sense of purpose under those circumstances. In fact, perhaps the greatest lesson from Vietnam was the discovery that there were irreducible limitations in the forbearance of the American people, as well as those fighting in Vietnam, for the specific conditions of war faced there—a variable that needs to be seriously considered in planning for future wars.

What happened in Vietnam was only indirectly related to the role and task for the Army psychiatrists assigned in Vietnam, but it is tempting to wonder if some of this could have been averted if senior military psychiatrists and other behavioral and social scientists had been included in the original planning for the war. And what about the direct role of Army psychiatry in Vietnam—particularly with regard to the swelling number of referrals during the second half of the war? It is evident from this review that as the country lost its will to make sacrifices for the sake of fighting the war, soldiers became progressively demoralized and dysfunctional, and the psychiatrists sent to support them struggled as well. But could the psychiatrists and allied mental health personnel have played more of a role in reducing the psychological toll? Military psychiatry is unique among the other military medical specialties because of its interest in the mind of the soldier-patient and the influence of his social environment (past and present). These influences became critical in Vietnam because soldiers were not only operating under combat conditions in a remote and extreme setting, but they also had to contend with the harsh criticism from home.

The sobering truth is that over time the mental health system became swamped with troops referred for various expressions of disobedience, defiance, and dissent; performance failure; violent, antimilitary behaviors; racial incidents; drug abuse and addiction; etc., most of which were unrelated to combat stress. Furthermore, the demoralization and antagonism toward the military mission and authority that was at the heart of this misconduct epidemic was fundamentally untreatable (apart from detoxification). The few soldiers who might have been treatable through conventional approaches—those with symptoms stemming from endogenous forms of psychiatric disorders such as psychosis, depression, anxiety, or psychosomatic conditions—were perhaps still not rehabilitable in the theater. And because the US Army in Vietnam was a completely closed system (eg, soldiers could not simply walk away or easily quit) and yet those at home were urging them to oppose participation, the principal and thankless task borne by the later psychiatrists was that of sorting and labeling antagonistic, command-referred soldiers, and they had little else to offer (again, "waiting at the bottom of a ski slope"). Adding to the strain, commanders were equally overwhelmed and ardently hoped psychiatry would take the most unmanageable troops off their hands. In particular they wanted the mental health component to become the custodians for these troops and to label them character and behavior disorders so they could be expeditiously removed from Vietnam and eliminated from the Army—though this diagnosis was not usually warranted. In every respect the system was broken.

What about efforts at prevention by Army psychiatrists, that is, command (program) consultation? Evidently there was little commitment by the psychiatrists or military leaders to command consultation in Vietnam. This is despite the fact that during the Vietnam era senior Army psychiatrists had become quite taken with the idea that every military psychiatrist should utilize the new theories of social psychiatry in advising unit commanders to reduce the incidence of psychiatric conditions and performance failures. This does not mean that these principles had little potential utility in Vietnam, just that the psychiatrists assigned in the later years of the war had minimal training in this approach, limited practical familiarity with the Army, and little receptivity by line commanders.

It seems fair to say that the promise of military psychiatry was oversold with respect to the problems that arose in Vietnam. However, more truthfully, Vietnam proved that military psychiatry has limitations as a remedy for failed military and political leadership. Fitzgerald, a Vietnam War historian, put it poignantly:

> [T]he civilians may neglect or try to ignore it, but those who have seen combat must find a reason for that killing; they must put it in some relation to their normal experience and to their role as citizens. The usual agent for this reintegration is not the psychiatrist, but the politician. In this case [of Vietnam], however, the politicians could give no satisfactory answer. . . . [38(pp423–424)]

Although Fitzgerald limited his observation to postwar anomie, veterans, combat troops, and politicians, his point also applied to all troops in the theater, including noncombat troops, and to the overall military leadership.

In closing, it is important to acknowledge that by its nature, the medical specialty of psychiatry—and thus military psychiatry—generally concentrates on deficits while not fully addressing strengths and capabilities.

With respect to military personnel the latter would include such positive attributes as patriotism, bravery, loyalty, sacrifice, and devotion to the mission, among many. This work has in no way intended to overlook these qualities as they were demonstrated by the troops who served in Vietnam; in fact the majority of those assigned in Vietnam fulfilled their duty faithfully with courage and commitment. Despite the outcome of the war, America surely owed every one of them a heartfelt demonstration of gratitude for their effort and sacrifices. This certainly also applies to the Army psychiatrists and their professional and paraprofessional colleagues. Although this work has highlighted the many problems that arose in the theater, not enough can be said about their sustained devotion to providing the best care for the troops that they could, their willingness to overcome hardships in the service of that end, and their record of capable and commendable service.

REFERENCES

1. Holloway HC. Vietnam military psychiatry revisited. Presentation to: American Psychiatric Association Annual Meeting; 19 May 1982; Toronto, Ontario, Canada.

2. Jones FD, Johnson AW Jr. Medical and psychiatric treatment policy and practice in Vietnam. *J Soc Issues*. 1975;31(4):49–65.

3. Jones FD. Disorders of frustration and loneliness. In: Jones FD, Sparacino LR, Wilcox VL, Rothberg JM, Stokes JW, eds. *War Psychiatry*. In: Zajtchuk R, Bellamy RF, eds. *Textbooks of Military Medicine*. Washington, DC: Department of the Army, Office of The Surgeon General, Borden Institute; 1995: 63–83.

4. Jones FD. Experiences of a division psychiatrist in Vietnam. *Mil Med*. 1967:132(12): 1003–1008.

5. Bourne PG, Coli WM, Nguyen DS. A comparative study of neuropsychiatric casualties in the United States Army and the Army of the Republic of Vietnam. In: Bourne PG, ed. *The Psychology and Physiology of Stress: With Reference to Special Studies of the Viet Nam War*. New York, NY: Academic Press; 1969: 51–58.

6. Talbott JA. In: Allerton WS, Forrest DV, Anderson JR, et al. Psychiatric casualties in Vietnam. In: Sherman LJ, Caffey EM Jr. *The Vietnam Veteran in Contemporary Society: Collected Materials Pertaining to the Young Veterans*. Washington DC: Veterans Administration; 1972: III: 54–59.

7. Renner JA Jr. The changing patterns of psychiatric problems in Vietnam. *Compr Psychiatry*. 1973;14(2):169–181.

8. Schneider BJ, Bradley JC, Warner CH, Benedek DM. Psychiatric medications in military operations. In: Ritchie EC, ed. *Combat and Operational Behavioral Health*. In: Lenhart MK, ed. *Textbooks of Military Medicine*. Washington, DC: Department of the Army, Office of The Surgeon General, Borden Institute; 2011: 151–162.

9. Baker SL Jr. Traumatic war disorders. In: Kaplan HI, Freedman AM, Sadock BJ, eds. *Comprehensive Textbook of Psychiatry*. 3rd ed. Baltimore, Md: Williams & Wilkins; 1980: 1829–1842.

10. Glass AJ. Psychotherapy in the combat zone. *Am J Psychiatry*. 1954;110:725–731.

11. Neel SH. *Medical Support of the US Army in Vietnam, 1965–1970*. Washington, DC: GPO; 1973.

12. Colbach EM, Parrish MD. Army mental health activities in Vietnam: 1965–1970. *Bull Menninger Clin*. 1970;34(6):333–342.

13. Balkind JJ. *Morale Deterioration in the United States Military During the Vietnam Period* [dissertation]. Ann Arbor, Mich: University Microfilms International; 1978: 235. [Available at: *Dissertations Abstracts International*, 39 (1-A), 438. Order No. 78-11, 333.]

14. Haass RN. *War of Necessity, War of Choice: A Memoir of Two Iraq Wars*. New York, NY: Simon & Schuster; 2009.

15. Doyle E, Lipsman S, and the editors of Boston Publishing Co. *The Vietnam Experience: America Takes Over*. Boston, Mass: Boston Publishing Co; 1982.

16. Lipsman S, Doyle E, and the editors of Boston Publishing Co. *The Vietnam Experience: Fighting For Time*. Boston, Mass: Boston Publishing Co; 1983.

17. Bourne PG. The war. *Men, Stress, and Vietnam*. Boston, Mass: Little, Brown; 1970: 27–46.

18. Braestrup P. *Big Story: How the American Press and Television Reported and Interpreted the Crisis of Tet 1968 in Vietnam and Washington*. 2 vols. Boulder, Colo: Westview Press; 1977.

19. Parrish MD. Man-team-environment systems in Vietnam. In: Jones FD, ed. *M. D. Parrish: Collected Works 1955–1970*. Alexandria, Va: Defense Technical Information Center; 1981. Document No. AD A108069.

20. Jones FD. Psychiatric lessons of war. In: Jones FD, Sparacino LR, Wilcox VL, Rothberg JM, Stokes JW, eds. *War Psychiatry*. In: Zajtchuk R, Bellamy RF, eds. *Textbooks of Military Medicine*. Washington, DC: Department of the Army, Office of The Surgeon General, Borden Institute; 1995: 1–33.

21. Rose E. The anatomy of a mutiny. *Armed Forces Soc*. 1982;8:561–574.

22. Cincinnatus. *Self-Destruction: The Disintegration and Decay of the United States Army During the Vietnam Era*. New York, NY: Norton; 1981.

23. Goffman E. Characteristics of total institutions. In: *Symposium on Preventive and Social Psychiatry*, Walter Reed Army Institute of Research, Washington, DC; 15–17 April 1957: 43–84. Expanded as: Goffman E. *Asylums: Essays on the Social Situation of Mental Patients and Other Inmates*. New York, NY: Doubleday; 1990.

24. Fleming RH. Post Vietnam syndrome: neurosis or sociosis? *Psychiatry*. 1985;48:122–139.

25. Sorley L. *A Better War: The Unexamined Victories and Final Tragedy of America's Last Years in Vietnam*. New York, NY: Harcourt Books; 1999.

26. Bloch HS. The psychological adjustment of normal people during a year's tour in Vietnam. *Psychiatric Q*. 1970;44(4):613–626.

27. Grossman DA. *On Killing: The Psychological Cost of Learning to Kill in War and Society*. New York, NY: Little, Brown; 1995.

28. Stretch RH. Incidence and etiology of post-traumatic stress disorder among active duty Army personnel. *J Appl Soc Psychol*. 1986;16:464–481.

29. Fox RP. Narcissistic rage and the problem of combat aggression. *Arch Gen Psychiatry.* 1974;31(6):807–811.

30. Bourne PG. The Vietnam veteran: psychosocial casualties. *Psychiatry Med.* 1972;3(1):23–27.

31. Nadelson T. *Trained to Kill: Soldiers at War.* Baltimore, Md: The Johns Hopkins University Press; 2005.

32. Bey DR Jr, Smith WE. Organizational consultation in a combat unit. *Am J Psychiatry.* 1971;128(4):401–406.

33. Glass AJ. Military psychiatry and changing systems of mental health care. *J Psychiat Res.* 1971;8(3):499–512.

34. Bernucci RJ, Glass AJ. Preface. In: Glass AJ, Bernucci R, eds. *Neuropsychiatry in World War II.* Vol 1. *Zone of the Interior.* Washington, DC: Medical Department, US Army; 1966: xv–vxiii.

35. David McK Rioch, former Director, Walter Reed Army Institute of Research, personal communication, 5 September 1985.

36. Reagan R. Peace: restoring the margin of safety. Speech presented at: Veterans of Foreign Wars Convention; 18 August 1980: Chicago, Ill. Available at: http://www.reagan.utexas.edu/archives/reference/8.18.80.html. Accessed 8 August 2013.

37. Shapley D. *Promise and Power: The Life and Times of Robert McNamara.* New York, NY: Little, Brown; 1993.

38. Fitzgerald F. *Fire in the Lake: The Vietnamese and the Americans in Vietnam.* Boston, Mass: Little, Brown; 1972.

Acronyms and Abbreviations

17-OHCS	17-hydroxycorticosteroid
91-F	enlisted neuropsychiatric specialist
91-G	enlisted social work specialist
91-H	enlisted clinical psychology technician
ADAPCP	Alcohol and Drug Abuse Prevention and Control Program
AFB	Air Force Base
AFQT	Armed Forces Qualifying Test
AIT	advanced individual training
APA	American Psychiatric Association
AR	Army Regulation
ARVN	Army of the Republic of Vietnam
ASD	acute stress disorder
AWOL	absent without leave
BAS	battalion aid station
BCT	basic combat training
BG	Brigadier General
BOQ	bachelor officer quarters
CACCF	Combat Area Casualties Current File
Cav	Cavalry
CBT	combat
CG/USARV	Commanding General, US Army Republic of Vietnam
CID	Criminal Investigation Division
Cir	Circular
CIV CBT PSY	civilian-trained combat psychiatrist
CIV HOSP PSY	civilian-trained hospital psychiatrist
CIV TND PSY	civilian-trained psychiatrist
CO	commanding officer
COL	Colonel
CONUS	continental United States
COSR	combat/ongoing military operation stress reaction
CSR	combat stress reaction
D-MAACL	Daily Form, Multiple Affect Adjective Check List
DA	Department of the Army
DART	Drug Abuse Rehabilitation Therapy
DEROS	date of expected return from overseas
DMZ	demilitarized zone
DoD	Department of Defense
DSM	*Diagnostic and Statistical Manual*
DT	delirium tremors

DVA	Department of Veterans Affairs
EARLY CBT PSY	early war combat psychiatrist
EARLY HOSP PSY	early war hospital psychiatrist
EM	enlisted man, enlisted men
EXP	experience
FTA	f--k the Army
GED	general educational development
GI	"government issue"
GMO	general medical officer
HOSP	hospital
ICD-9-CM	*International Classification of Diseases, 9th Revision, Clinical Modification*
ID	Infantry Division
IG	Inspector General
IM	intramuscular
IQ	intelligence quotient
IV	intravenous
KIA	killed in action
KO	psychiatric specialty detachment
KP	"kitchen patrol"
LATE CBT PSY	late war combat psychiatrist
LATE HOSP PSY	late war hospital psychiatrist
LPC	Limited Privilege Communication
LRRP	long-range reconnaissance patrol
LSD	lysergic acid diethylamide
MAAG	Military Assistance and Advisory Group
MACV	Military Assistance Command, Vietnam
MD	medical doctor
MFSS	Medical Field Service School
MG	major general
MHCS	mental hygiene consultation services
MIA	missing in action
MIL	military
MIL CBT PSY	military-trained combat psychiatrist
MIL HOSP PSY	military-trained hospital psychiatrist
MIL TND PSY	military-trained psychiatrist
MOS	military occupational specialty
MP	military police
MSC	Medical Service Corps
NCO	noncommissioned officer
NCOIC	noncommissioned officer in charge
NLF	National Liberation Front
NP	neuropsychiatric
NVA	North Vietnam Army
NVVRS	National Vietnam Veterans Readjustment Study
OJ	opium joint
OTSG	Office of The Surgeon General
PIES	proximity, immediacy, expectancy, and simplicity

PMO	psychiatric military officers
PSY	psychiatrist
PTSD	posttraumatic stress disorder
PX	post exchange
R & R	rest and recuperation
REMF	"rear echelon mother f--ker"
RVN	Republic of Vietnam
SR	Special Regulations
TB	tuberculosis
TGIF	Thank God It's Friday
TM	Technical Manual
TO&E	Table of Organization and Equipment
UCMJ	Uniform Code of Military Justice
US	United States
USARV	US Army Republic of Vietnam
USDB	United States Disciplinary Barracks
USMACV	US Military Assistance Command, Vietnam
USO	United Service Organizations
VA	Veterans Administration
VC	Viet Cong
VE	Victory Europe
WIA	wounded in action
WRAIR	Walter Reed Army Institute of Research
WRGH	Walter Reed General Hospital
WW II	World War II
XO	executive officer

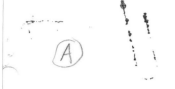

DEPARTMENT OF THE ARMY
98th Medical Detachment (KO)
APO SF 96349

AVBJ GC EE KO

THRU: Commanding Officer   TO: Colonel C. Bowen   FROM: Commanding Officer
95th Evac Hosp (Smbl)   Psychiatric Consultant   98th Med Det (KO)
APO SF 96349   USARV: AVHSU   APO SF 96349
                               APO SF 96375

SUBJECT: Report of Activities of the 98th Med Det (KO) for the six months
         ending 31 Dec 1970.

Dear Colonel Bowen,

    Hope this report answers any and all questions you might have regarding
the activities of the 98th Med Det (KO). This report was not sent with December's statistics because your letter of 26 Dec arrived after our statistics
had been mailed to you. Perhaps there was some delay in our receiving your
letter because it was mistakenly addressed to Major Mitchel Camp, APO 96337.
I hope this information is helpful in your grasping the overall picture.

                        Yours Very Truly,

                        NORMAN M. CAMP
                        MAJ, MC
                        Commanding

Enclosures
1-MHCS Policy Statement
2-Medical Technical Guidence, Drug Abuse
3-Requirements for Psychiatric Evaluation
   as part of AR 635-212 Provisions
4-Yearly Activities Report

AVBJ GC EE KO
SUBJECT: (Activities Report)

1. New Programs initiated in the 98th Med Det (KO) in the past 6 months.

   A. Staff Changes:
      1. Major Smith, C.O., was replaced by myself in Oct 70, with Major
         Cohen serving as temporary C.O. for 3 weeks prior to my arrival.
      2. Dr. Finklestein DEROS in Sept 70.
      3. Drs. Nathan and Barbara Cohen and Dr. Robinson, all fully trained
         psychiatrists, joined the 98th (KO) team in Aug 1970.
      4. In Oct 70, Cpt Meshad MSW and Cpt Van Remortel MSW, were rotated
         to other units in country and Cpt Nygaard, MSW, joined the (KO)
         team in Nov 70.
      5. In Oct 70, Cpt Olsen, psychologist, was rotated to the 935th (KO)
         team.
      6. In Dec 1970, SFC Abrahams, NCOIC of the Mental Hygiene Clinic
         DEROS and was replaced by SFC Ortopan. In Sept SSG Grant, NCOIC
         of the Psych Ward was Med-evacuated to Japan and was replaced in
         Dec 70 by SFC Merkley. In Dec 70, SFC McKinney DEROS and in con-
         junction with this , MSG Kersey, attached to the 98th from the
         95th Evac Hosp has become the 1st Sgt of the 98th Med Det (KO).
         MSG Kersey also serves the team doing Psychologicals on a limited
         scale and does much liason work between the 95th Evac Hosp and the
         98th (KO) team.
      7. Officer responsibilities are as follows: Maj N. Cohen is deputy
         C.O. and director of education and training. Cpt Nygaard is Det-
         achment Executive officer and MHC administrator. Maj B. Cohen is
         MHC Director. Maj E. Robinson is Psychiatric Ward Officer.
      8. In Nov 1970, all four psychiatrists attended a 2 day conference in
         Cam Rhan Bay of the psychiatrists in RVN. Also in Nov, Cpt Nygaard,
         SFC Abrahams and three social work specialists attended a 3 day
         social work conference in Cam Rahn Bay.
      9. Because of a shortage of technicians with 91G and 91F MOS, techni-
         cians with other 91 MOS and college degrees in social sciences have
         been attached to the 98th Med Det and given OJT in these areas.
         Also begun is a program of cross training in which 91G personnel
         are being rotated to the psychiatric ward for one month of intensive
         OJT and vice versa for 91F personnel. This has proven to be valuable
         in increasing the ability of these specialists in their respective
         primary areas of functioning, as well as adding a new dimension of
         flexibility to the K.O. team.
     10. In Oct a program of inservice education in basic psychology plus
         interview and counselling techniques was begun by Maj. N. Cohen on
         a once weekly basis.

AV~ GC EE KO
SU~ ~CT: (Continued)

B. Mental Hygiene Clinic Changes:
1. A program of specialization has been developed in order to stream-
   line clinic function and increase expertise. I am handling all legal
   and VIP cases, as well as community psychiatric and liason work. Drs.
   Cohen do all 212 evaluations. Dr. N. Cohen and myself do all inpatient
   consultations. Cpt Nygaard acts as clinic administrator, clinic triage
   and supervises closely the work of the technicians. All physicians
   share in general evaluation and therapy work.
2. Emphasis has been placed on education and information to referrer and
   referrees with the publication of documents by this MHC pertaining to
   MHC policy, drug information, drug amnesty program and requirements for
   212 evaluation.
3. Emphasis has been placed on more extensive supervision of work of social
   work specialists, but without destroying their position as the primary
   mental health worker for the patient and his unit.
4. Emphasis has been placed on acceleration of time between when the patient
   is referred and when first disposition is made or certification is rendered.
5. Emphasis has been placed on more accurate clinic statistics with major
   revisions in data collection methods, especially related to drug abuse
   cases.
6. Much time and energy has been expended in creating a viable physical
   structure within the two shell buildings assigned to us by the 95th Evac
   Hosp, most of the time and energy has been during time off from primary jobs by the enlisted men.
C. Psychiatric Ward Changes:
1. Since Major Robinson has become the Ward Officer, a multi-focused effort
   has been generated to create a dynamic milieu therapy ward from what was
   previously more or less a holding ward for patients waiting to be air-
   evacuated to other treatment facilities. Steps in this transformation
   include: The designation of one physician as ward director, the commencement of ward staff meetings to discuss patients including patient treatment plans, commencement of group therapy on a daily basis, emphasis of
   ward staff expectation that patients will be returning to duty, commencement of a viable supervised work therapy program, the commencement of a
   recreation therapy program, and a concerted effort to screen out character
   and behavior disorders before admission. These efforts have served to
   reduce ward census, increase hospitalization time while greatly increase-
   ing percentage being returned to duty and decreasing psychiatric morbidity.
2. Emphasis has also been placed on more complete and informative narrative
   summaries, more accurate statistics, especially those drug related cases
   and more active liaison with the patient's unit.
3. Also created is a program of out patient Nalline Provocative test for
   heroin addiction. This is performed on the ward under close scrutiny of
   physician and nurse. It has proven useful in screening out those patients
   not truly requiring hospitalization and therapy and there by reducing ward
   census and psychiatric morbidity. In ten cases over the past 6 weeks, we
   have seen only one positive result.

Nalorphine = used for challenge test to determine opioid dependence

AVBJ GC EE KO
SUBJECT: (Continued)

2. Community Psychiatry.

In general, a premium is placed on direct unit and program consultation as the method of choice for practicing preventitive psychiatry and reducing psychiatric morbidity. In the Danang area, this is difficult because of the very complicated command structure of the numerous non-divisional units, often from distances involving much travel on the part of patients, commanders or mental hygiene staff. It has been made even more complicated because of the very erratic and often non-existant telephone service and continual difficulties in maintaining the detachment's vehicles.

The major focus of our community psychiatry efforts has been through the local dispensaries which are attached to the 95th Evac Hosp and who serve the various compounds and commands in the Danang area. The personnel of these units represent second echelon mental hygiene and commanders are encouraged to consult with their unit physician before a man is seen by mental hygiene. With this in mind, a close relationship is maintained with these dispensary staffs for educational purposes and for case detection purposes. From these sources command consultations are stimulated; and mental hygiene representatives, along with dispensary staff are frequently part of planning councils for drug, racial and morale problems.

Also newly created is a USARV stockade consultation program on once weekly basis which includes group sessions with stockade counsellors, plus consultation with the dispensary physicians and evaluation of confinees, this program involves one psychiatrist and two technicians and has proved valuable in reducing the number of required evaluations, accelerating the processing time of 212 and Chapter 10 action and reducing the turmoil and potential for danger caused by having prisoners and guards with weapons congregating in the MHCS clinic.

3. Views on Amnesty Program, are covered in Maj Cohen's paper read at the I Corps Medical Society meeting, 2 Jan 71 (sent to you seperately). In general, the only drug users which are admitted are those which we are fairly certain have a significant physiological addiction. Following hospitalization, or outpatient evaluation, they are referred back to command for consideration for the Amnesty program, or for Administrative/Judicial action with a report of the extent of the problem and treatment rendered.

4. Suggestions for the Future of Military Psychiatry in RVN.

A. Closer communication with MedCom and your office, particularly concerning USARV policies and documents which are pertinent or helpful to our mission.

B. A very thorough in-country briefing of new psychiatrists and social workers pertaining to the various facets of the mission and with specific suggestions and guidelines as to how these may most expediciously and correctly be handled. Not only is "the Army way" often quite unique, butthe added factors specific to RVN must be assimilated into the professionals theoretical framework.

AVBJ GC EE KO
SUBJECT: (Continued)

The orientation at Ft Sam is very helpful in getting off on the right foot, but the rapidly changing exigences of Vietnam should be superimposed on that framework by those already in country and familiar with the problems and solutions or attempts at same. Along this line every effort at substantial overlap should be programmed into the replacement schedule.

C. More Army trained psychiatrists, or psychiatrists with a year or more of Army service should be sent to RVN in preference to drafted psychiatrists recently completing the MFSS basic course.

D. Also suggested is an additional slot under the Psychiatric Consultant for an experienced Army psychiatrist solely devoted to helping the various psychiatrists in country develop community psychiatric programs. This special community psychiatric consultant would have no other duties and would be free to stay in a given area or Division for as many weeks as necessary to help set up viable and practical programs, and would make periodic visits to assess the worthwhileness of these programs. In most cases, psychiatrists fresh from residencies have little or no community psychiatry experience and beyond that are bewildered by the Army organizational structure and procedures.

E. I feel stabilized tours for the entire year are a vital necessity. Military and combat psychiatry bear little resemblance to other branches of medicine when it comes to community relationships, therefore the temptation to rotate psychiatrists should be resisted. The one year tour in itself does enough to sow the seeds of apathy in Army personnel without exacerbating it with an even shorter tour. It has been well documented that in any system, it takes a minimum of three months and often longer to become familiar enough with that system in order to develop those areas which need change. Therefore to rotate psychiatrists every six months means a minimum of six months of the 12 month tour is familiarization time.

Appendix 2 USARV REGULATION NO. 40-34

USARV Reg No 40-34

HEADQUARTERS UNITED STATES ARMY VIETNAM
APO San Francisco 96375

REGULATION   15 October 1970
NUMBER 40-34

Medical Services
MENTAL HEALTH AND NEUROPSYCHIATRY

1. **PURPOSE**: To provide instructions and prescribe procedures for the maintenance of high standards of mental health and for the management of psychiatric
and neurologic problems in this command.

2. **DEFINITIONS**: a. Mental health is the adjustment of individuals to their
environment and to each other with as high a degree of mission effectiveness
and satisfaction as conditions permit.

   b. Psychiatry patients are individuals having a suspected or actual
emotional illness, who require or are undergoing appropriate observation,
evaluation or treatment.

   c. Neurology patients are individuals with suspected or actual disease
of the nervous system, who require or are undergoing observation, evaluation
or treatment.

3. **COMMAND RESPONSIBILITIES**: Commanders at all levels are responsible for
the following items of psychiatric import:

   a. The mental health and behavior of their troops to include effective
human relations among individuals and groups. For all these factors the
psychiatrist, social work officer, social work technician or other mental
health consultant is considered a staff resource who can offer guidance and
participate in command planning upon these responsibilities. Thus, the command is expected to utilize the best of modern human relations planning to
keep its human resources most effective.

   b. A personal knowledge of men which, in company size units, implies
knowing each man by name and having an estimate of his capabilities.

   c. Facility in the management of groups; which implies experience with
the use and effects of rivalry among groups, the development of informal
cliques and group pressures, the social uses and dangers of scape-goating
and hero-making, and methods of integrating soldiers into the group as members
who render useful duty, whether as close-knit buddies or isolates.

   d. Maximum use of manpower by providing proper incentive and such
reclassification, reassignment, recreation and relaxation as the military
situation permits.

   e. Constant appraisal of such indicators of unit morale as rates of
accidents, security breaches, disciplinary actions, racial incidents, drug
and alcohol abuse, drunkenness, apathy and other defective attitudes, as well
as such assets as improvisations, inventiveness, useful suggestions, conservation, self-improvement and reenlistment rates.

Reg No 40-34, HQ USARV, APO 96375, 15 Oct 70 (Cont)

c. Familiarity with procedures governing administrative separation contained in AR's 635-105, 635-206 and 635-212. Requests for psychiatric evaluation of individuals in the above administrative procedures will be forwarded to the psychiatrist by unit commanders or responsible agencies using the format in Appendix I as a guide.

4. <u>PSYCHIATRIC AND NEUROLOGICAL EVALUATION AND TREATMENT IN USARV</u>:

a. General: The mental hygiene unit's role involves prevention as well as treatment and includes close liaison with AMEDS members of the organization, as well as with unit commanders in order to prevent psychiatric problems from arising. Consultation with those responsible for the functioning of individuals and groups is emphasized over direct psychiatric care. Where some direct treatment is necessary, outpatient management is emphasized over inpatient. No psychiatric facility has as much ability to improve the functioning of a soldier for his natural duty as does his normal duty unit. Mental health consultants can help the unit commander work out ways to improve his influence on the members of the unit or utilize effectively some seemingly incorrigible individuals. Hospitalization is to be avoided except where patients are potentially dangerous to themselves or others, and then only because of mental illness. It is not to be used when personnel, who for administrative reasons or convenience, need only to remain overnight or await some administrative action. With rare exceptions, sociopathic soldiers (character and behavior disorders) are not to be admitted to hospitals. Medical facilities will not serve as substitutes for administrative action once the psychiatrist has recommended such action.

b. Organic psychiatric support:

(1) Psychiatric teams assigned to divisions and separate brigades provide consultation service, outpatient evaluations and treatment, and limited inpatient care. Soldiers whose condition requires consideration of out-of-country evacuation will be transferred to the appropriate in-country treatment center listed in para 4c(2), below.

(2) Organic psychiatrists and psychiatrists who serve as consultants to specific units hold a uniquely advantageous position in evaluating soldiers from their respective units. Frequently, they are intimately familiar with cases from their inceptions and are consistently best qualified to weigh the role stresses and other characteristics within both the unit and the patient. Accordingly, the command consultant's evaluation normally will be considered sufficient for courts-martial or board actions except in very special instances to be determined by the appropriate authority. When a sanity board is required (see para 5c) or a second opinion is requested, the nearest psychiatrist with qualifications equal to the first examiner will be employed wherever possible. A board of one physician only, a psychiatrist, is entirely proper.

c. Treatment facilities:

(1) Certain hospitals have a staff psychiatrist who has consultation contact with certain units, maintains an outpatient service, and to a limited

2

Reg No 40-34, HQ USARV, APO 9637/5, 15 Oct 70 (Cont)

extent depending on local facilities and policies, provides inpatient care. Non-emergency inpatients may then be treated commensurate with the evacuation policy of the command.

(2) There are two psychiatry and neurology treatment centers in this command. One is operated by the 98th Medical Detachment (KO), 95th Evacuation Hospital at Da Nang, APO 96337, which serves all Army units in I and II N Military Regions. The 935th Medical Detachment (KO), located at the 93rd Evacuation Hospital at Long Binh, serves III and IV Military Regions. Additionally, the 483rd Air Force Hospital serves units in II S Military Region. These centers are staffed and equipped to provide evaluation, care and treatment for all types of psychiatric patients as well as neurological patients. All psychiatry and neurology patients whose condition suggests the need for out-of-country evacuation will be transferred to one of these centers for evaluation.

5. ADMINISTRATIVE PROCEDURES, RECORDS AND REPORTS: a. General: Psychiatrists should be familiar with the AR's listed in para 3, as well as with TM 8-240, TM 8-244, and SR 40-1025-2. When psychiatric diagnosis is appropriate, psychiatrists will use only the standard nomenclature of the disease, as stated in AR 40-401, and give complete diagnosis with code, including description of severity, manifestations, predisposition, stress, LD and degree of incapacity, where applicable. Psychiatrists will forward reports of neuro-psychiatric examinations for administrative separations or sanity findings to the requesting agencies within five days following examination. Format shown at Appendixes II and III should be used as a guide.

b. Sanity Boards: Formal sanity boards, when required, will be initiated and conducted in accordance with para 121 of the Manual for Courts-Martial, United States, 1969 (Revised Edition); para 44, AR 40-3; para 19, TM 8-240; and para 11, TM 8-244.

c. Reports: Psychiatrists and neurologists are responsible for keeping accurate records of all outpatients and inpatients, and for coordinating with registrars so that accurate morbidity figures are obtained and forwarded. In addition to the aforementioned morbidity reports, USARV Form 55 (USARV Psychiatry and Neurology Morbidity Report) will be forwarded by courier in three copies through the commanding officer of the appropriate medical unit to this headquarters, ATTN: AVHSU-M, APO 96384, within five days following the end of each month. Reports Control Symbol AVHSU-31 has been assigned to this report (see Appendix IV).

d. Supplies: Psychiatrists and neurologists, through their unit medical supply officers, are responsible for maintaining adequate levels of medicine used in their practice, anticipating future needs and reordering when stocks are low.

6. REFERENCES: a. AR 40-3.

b. AR 40-401.

c. AR 635-105.

3

Reg No 40-34, HQ USARV, APO 96375, 15 Oct 70 (Cont)

    d. AR 635-206. *misconduct*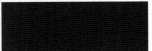

    e. AR 635-212.

    f. SR 40-1025-2.

    g. TM 8-240.

    h. TM 8-244.

    i. Manual for Courts-Martial, United States, 1969 (Revised Edition)

(AVHSU-M)

FOR THE COMMANDER:

OFFICIAL: CHARLES M. GETTYS
                                          Major General, USA
                                          Chief of Staff

Colonel, AGC
Adjutant General

4 Appendixes
    I   Format for Request for Psychiatric Evaluation
   II   Format for Psychiatric Reports for Administrative Type Separation
 III Format for Psychiatric Report for Sanity Findings
  IV Form for USARV Psychiatry and Neurology Morbidity Report

DISTRIBUTION:
B Plus
130 CG, USAMEDCOMV(P)
10 Surgeon, MACV
10 Surgeon, I FFORCEV
10 Surgeon, II FFORCEV
10 Surgeon, XXIV Corps
20 AVHAG-A
800 AVHAG-AP
1 Ref Library
6 CINCUSARPAC
1 USARPAC Hist Unit
1 MACV AG M&D Branch, APO 96222
1 AVHGF-M-(RCO)

4

USARV Reg No 40-34

APPENDIX I

FORMAT FOR REQUEST FOR PSYCHIATRIC EVALUATION

Request for Psychiatric Evaluation of

1. _____
   NAME   RANK   SSAN

   _____
   ORGANIZATION   ADDRESS   DATE

2. Purpose of referral: ( ) Psychiatric Treatment, ( ) Psychiatric
Evaluation for possible administrative separation under provisions of
AR_____ ( ), Psychiatric Evaluation prior to _____,
Court-Martial for charges of _____,

3. Personal Data: Years of Service_____, highest rank held_____,
No. of Art 15's_____, of Courts-Martial_____, of reductions_____,
of AWOLS_____, Latest ratings for conduct_____, efficiency_____,
physical profile other than 1_____.

4. Commander's statement regarding individual's performance and behavior
and rehabilitation potential._____

_____

_____

5. Commander's recommendations: ( ) Retention, ( ) Separation,
( ) Transfer, ( ) Other_____.

                                    _____
                                    Signature

                                    _____
                                    Title

USARV Reg No 40-34

APPENDIX II

FORMAT FOR PSYCHIATRIC REPORTS FOR ADMINISTRATIVE-TYPE SEPARATION

Heading - (Organization of Psychiatrist)

REPORT OF NEUROPSYCHIATRIC EXAMINATION

This is a report of neuropsychiatric examination in the case of (Name, Rank, SSAN, Organization) who was seen for (length of time) at (place and date). He was advised of his rights under Article 31, UCMJ prior to the interview.

Pertinent history: (State reason for referral, investigative or other reports available, and individual's account of the situation. Include pertinent past history).

Mental status: (Give symptoms and signs to substantiate diagnosis).

Physical examination: (Give only significant abnormalities).

Diagnosis: (Use Army Nomenclature, AR 40-401 and TB Med 15. When psychiatric diagnosis is indicated, give complete diagnosis).

Brief clinical abstract of findings: Examples:

  1. This soldier gives a history of marked social unadaptability prior to and during service. He uses poor judgement, is not committed to any productive goals, and is completely unmotivated for further service. It is believed that he will not adjust to further military service and further rehabilitative efforts probably will be nonproductive.

  2. There are no disqualifying mental or physical defects sufficient to warrant disposition through medical channnels.

  3. Private Doe was and is mentally responsible, able to distinguish right from wrong and to adhere to the right, and has the mental capacity to understand and participate in board proceedings.

Comments: (optional)

Recommendations:

  1. That individual be separated under provision of AR_____.

  2. Other, if applicable.

USARV Reg No 40-34

APPENDIX III

FORMAT FOR PSYCHIATRIC REPORT OF SANITY FINDINGS

Heading - (Organization of Psychiatrist)

REPORT OF NEUROPSYCHIATRIC EXAMINATION

This is a report of neuropsychiatric examination in the case of (Name, Rank, SSAN, Organization) who was seen for (length of time) at (place and date). He was advised of his rights under Article 31, UCMJ prior to the interview.

Pertinent history: (State reason for referral, investigative or other reports available and individual's account of the situation. Include pertinent past history. State whether formal investigation data was reviewed).

Mental status: (Give symptoms and signs to substantiate diagnosis).

Physical examination: (Give only signs to substantiate diagnosis).

Physical examination: (Give only significant abnormalities).

Diagnosis: (Use Army nomenclature, AR 40-401 and TB Med 15. When psychiatric diagnosis is indicated, give complete diagnosis).

Sanity findings:

1. At the time of the alleged offense, the accused (was) (was not) so far free from mental disease, defect or derangement as to be able to distinguish right from wrong concerning the particular acts as charged.

2. At the time of the alleged offense, the accused (was) (was not) so far free from mental disease, defect or derangement as to be able to adhere to the right concerning the particular acts as charged.

3. The accused (possesses) (does not possess) sufficient mental capacity to understand the nature of the proceedings against him and to conduct or cooperate intelligently in his own defense.

4. The accused (was) (was not) capable of forming the specific intent to commit the alleged offense.

Comment: (optional)

Recommendations: (optional)

(It is usual to make a comment as to whether from a psychiatric point of view the member would eventually be expected to perform adequate duty or whether administrative or medical separation would be indicated).

APPENDIX IV

USARV Reg No 40-34

USARV PSYCHIATRY AND NEUROLOGY MORBIDITY REPORT
(USARV Reg 40-34)

PERIOD ENDING: _____

REPORTS CONTROL SYMBOL
AVHSU-31

THRU: _____

TO: CG, USARV, ATTN: AVHSU
Psychiatric Consultant
APO 96384

FROM: _____

SECTION A - IN - PATIENT

CLASSIFICATION (final diagnostic category) (a)	ADMISSIONS		CONSULTATIONS (not NP Pts) (d)	IN-COUNTRY EVACUATIONS (e)	OUT-COUNTRY EVACUATIONS (f)	REMAINING	RTN TO DY (g)	MAN-DAYS IN HOSP (h)
	DIRECT (b)	BY TRANSFER (c)						
L I N E 1 PSYCHOTIC DISORDERS								
2 PSYCHONEUROTIC DISORDERS								
3 CHARACTER AND BEHAVIOR DISORDERS								
4 DRUG ABUSE								
5 STRESS REACTION								
6 COMBAT EXHAUSTION								
7 OBSERVATION NP (7930)								
NO PSYCHIATRIC DIAG								
8 TOTAL PSYCHIATRIC								
9 DISEASE OF NERVOUS SYS								

See over for definitions

SECTION B - OUT - PATIENT

CLASSIFICATION (a)	TOTAL NO OF PATIENTS (b)	EVALUATION (CERTIFICATES) (c)	TREATMENT VISITS (d)	RTN TO DY (e)	HOSPITALIZED (f)
L I N E 1 PSYCHOTIC DISORDERS					
2 PSYCHONEUROTIC DISORDERS					
3 CHARACTER AND BEHAVIOR DISORDERS					
4 DRUG ABUSE					
5 STRESS REACTION					
6 COMBAT EXHAUSTION					
7 OBSERVATION NP (7930)					
NO PSYCHIATRIC DIAG					
8 COMMAND CONSULTATION					
9 TOTAL PSYCHIATRIC					
10 DISEASE OF NERVOUS SYS.					

USARV Form 55 Revised 22 Aug 70 PREVIOUS EDITIONS OF THIS FORM ARE OBSOLETE.

USARV Reg No 40-34

INSTRUCTIONS FOR USARV PSYCHIATRY AND MORBIDITY REPORT (USARV FORM 55)

Item #2   Psychoneurotic Reaction. Include psychophysiologic and psychoso-
           matic reactions.

Item #3   Character and Behavior Disorder. Cases where drugs are responsible
           for inpatient/outpatient care should be listed in Item #4.

Item #4   Drug abuse, suspected or proven. Exclude cases where drugs are only
           incidental to care (outpatient/inpatient).

Item #5   Stress Reactions. Should include acute reactions not related to
           combat and those combat reactions not severe enough to be called
           combat exhaustion (as defined by Noyes and Kolb, American Handbook
           of Psychiatry, etc.).

Item #6 - Combat Exhaustion

Item #7   Observation Neuropsychiatric. Only those cases <u>discharged</u> with this
           diagnosis should be listed here. If admitted as observation N-P
           and a subsequent psychiatric diagnosis is made the case should show
           admission and disposition under that new classification only.

Item #8   (Inpatient) Total of all psychiatric evaluations.

           (Outpatient) Command Consultation to include evaluation for AR
           635-200, 635-212, 40-501, etc.

Item #9   (Outpatient) Total of all psychiatric evaluations.

Inpatient Remaining. Those cases remaining inpatient at the end of the reporting period. Previously the total of admissions did not equal the total
of dispositions.

Inpatient. Direct admissions should include (i) also those patients shown in
"Hospitalized" under outpatient section B in addition to direct admissions and
(2) only those patients admitted to the facility providing the report; a Medical
Battalion if the reporting unit is a Division or a Brigade; a hospital if the
reporting MHCS (e.g. if a division psychiatrist admits to a field or an evacuation hospital, then the inpatient report from the division will <u>not</u> include
these patients). They should be reported by the hospital.

A4-2

Appendix 3

NALLINE

AVHSU-PS   21 October 1970
SUBJECT: Procedure for Determining Narcotic Addiction - Tech Guidance

SEE DISTRIBUTION:

1. PURPOSE: To provide guidance for battalion surgeons, division surgeons/
psychiatrists, and MEDCOM physicians/psychiatrists in the evaluation, treatment, and processing of patients suspected of narcotic addiction.

2. The patient who is not overtly psychotic:

     a. If it is established that the last narcotics were taken more than 96 hours *4 Days*
prior to evaluation and the patient is asymptomatic, dependence is considered
unlikely.

     b. If the patient exhibits the following symptom complex the diagnosis of
physical dependence is established.

         (1) Sweating, yawning, lacrimation, rhinorrhea, mydriasis, tachypnea.

     c. For patients who do not exhibit the above findings but claim physical de-
pendence on narcotics, the following may be utilized to aid in the diagnosis of
dependence.

         (1) N-allylnormorphine (Nalline) 3 mgm will be given subcutaneously.

         (2) If the symptom complex described in para b(1) above is not displayed
within 20 minutes a second dose of 5 mgm will be given. If the withdrawal
symptom complex is not elicited within 20 minutes after the second injection
a third and final dose of 7 mgm will be given. If this last dose also fails to
elicit the symptoms and findings described in para b(1) above the test is considered negative and the patient will not be considered to be physically dependent on narcotics. The results of the test cannot be considered positive unless the overall symptom complex is characteristic; mere dilation of the pupil,
for example, without the other signs is not sufficient for a diagnosis of physical dependence.

NARCAN ®
"Endo" lab
.4 mg/cc

AVHSU-PS   21 October 1970
SUBJECT: Procedure for Determining Narcotic Addiction (cont.)

3. If physical dependence is established as outlined in para b(1) above, the patient should be hospitalized for treatment of withdrawal symptoms.

4. If physical dependence is not present the patient can be treated with tranquilizers and counselling on an outpatient basis, in consultation with mental health personnel as necessary.

FOR THE SURGEON:

███████████████████████

COL, MC
Deputy Surgeon

DISTRIBUTION: A

2

Appendix 4 INTERIM CHANGE TO AR 635-206

HEADQUARTERS UNITED STATES ARMY VIETNAM
APO San Francisco 96375

CIRCULAR
NUMBER 635-206-1

4 June 1971

(Expires 31 December 1971)
Personnel Separations
INTERIM CHANGE TO AR 635-206

Unclassified DA Message from AGPO, 122117Z, is quoted for your information and compliance.

"SUBJECT: Interim Changes to AR 635-212 and AR 635-206 (To Be Published as Changes)

1. AR 635-206, 15 Jul 66, is changed as follows:

Page 4, Paragraph is superseded as follows:

7. Medical Evaluation. A. When a unit commander determines that an individual under military control is to be processed for separation under this regulation, he will initially refer the individual to the servicing Army medical treatment facility and request a medical and mental status evaluation. The reason for considering this individual for separation will be furnished the medical treatment facility. The medical treatment facility providing dispensary care will accomplish the final-type physical examination and mental status evaluation. The individual will not be referred to a psychiatrist for a psychiatric evaluation except under the following circumstances:

(1) When psychiatric evaluation is specifically requested by the individual subject to separation action.

(2) When psychiatric evaluation is specifically requested by the commanding officer recommending separation action.

(3) When psychiatric evaluation is deemed necessary and appropriate by the medical examiner performing the requested medical and mental status evaluation.

(4) When a psychiatric evaluation is requested by the board considering separation action.

B. In all cases the physician performing the physical examination will accomplish the mental status evaluation. In the exceptional cases detailed in paragraph A above, reasons for specifically requesting a psychiatric evaluation will be provided to the psychiatrist. Under no circumstances will medical personnel be used as an investigative agency to determine facts relative to the individual's behavior.

C. In addition to the SF 88 (Report of Medical Examination) and the SF 89 (Report of Medical History) the medical treatment facility will

Cir No 635-206-1, HQ, USARV, APO 96375, 4 Jun 71 (Cont)

prepare a report of mental status evaluation as indicated in Figure 3.

        D. The medical treatment facility commander will forward the original of the evaluation report to the unit commander. A copy will be filed in the individual's health record."

2. Add Figure 3 to AR 635-206.

(AVHAG-PA(PS))

FOR THE COMMANDER:

OFFICIAL:

                                   CHARLES M. GETTYS
                                   Major General, USA
                                   Chief of Staff

Colonel, AGC
Adjutant General

1 Inclosure
Figure 3

DISTRIBUTION:
A Plus
 20 AVHAG-PA(PS)
500 AVHAG-AP
  6 CINCUSARPAC
  2 AVHAG-A
  1 USARPAC Hist Unit
  1 Ref Library
  1 AVHDR-MR(RCO)
  L HAV AG I&D Br

2

DEPARTMENT OF THE ARMY
98th Medical Detachment (KO)
AFO San Francisco 96349

AVBJ GC EE KO

SUBJECT: Requirements for Psychiatric Evaluation
as part of elimination of enlisted personnel
under the provisions of AR 635-212

I.   In accordance with Sec III, Para 8, AR 635-212. Psychiatric evaluation
of an individual at 98th Med Det (KO) will not be accomplished without a com-
-manding officer's report in letter form, furnishing the following:

a) Name, grade, service no., age, date of enlistment or induction, length of
term for which enlisted and prior service.
b) Reason for action recommended, general, nondescript terms will not be used.
c) Armed Forces Qualification Test (AFQT) score, aptitude test scores and duty
occupational military specialty (MOS).
d) Results of MOS evaluation testing, to include MOS in which evaluated and
evaluation score.
e) Record of counseling
f) Description of rehabilitation attempts.(List assignments and duties under
different officers and non-commissioned officers, in each organization or unit.
Include duration of each assignment.
g) Conduct and efficiency ratings.
h) Record of trial by court martial.
i) Record of disciplinary action(include company punishments)
j) A statement by the individual indicating that he has been advised of his
rights (para 10)
k) Any other information pertinent to the case.

II.   This information is vital to the formulation of a psychiatric opinion
regarding the individuals mental condition in relation to the conduct under
consideration, and the probable effectiveness of further rehabilitative efforts
as required by AR 635-212.

III.   In accordance with USARV Supplient 1 to AR 635-212. In the instance
that psychiatric services are not readily available, particularly in non-di-
-visional units and where the service of a psychiatrist would require great
distances of travel and loss of time in processing the AR 635-212 action, a
medical corps officer who does not have specialized psychiatric training, but
who is available locally to the unit, may complete the medical evaluation
portion normally completed by a psychiatrist.

NORMAN M. CAMP
MAJ, MC
Commanding

DEPARTMENT OF THE ARMY
HEADQUARTERS, XXIV CORPS
APO SAN FRANCISCO 96349

AVII-CS

SUBJECT: Administrative Elimination Under the Provisions of AR 635-212

SEE DISTRIBUTION

1. The Commanding General desires that all commanders under his General Court Martial jurisdiction personally review the following references which outline problems which continue to plague the effectiveness of our program for administrative elimination of undesirable or unfit soldiers:

   a. Letter, AVHAG-PA, Headquarters, United States Army, Vietnam, subject: AR 635-212 Eliminations for FY 1970, 5 December 1970, with 1st Indorsement, AVII-CG, this headquarters, 30 December 1970.

   b. Letter, AVII-JA, this headquarters, subject: Administrative Eliminations, AR 635-212, 28 December 1970.

   c. USARV Supplement 1 to AR 635-212, 23 April 1971.

2. The trend toward inappropriate elimination of drug abusers as "unsuitable" personnel, thus allowing the Board only the choice of an Honorable or General discharge certificate, appears now to be under control. Reports submitted to this headquarters by Special Court Martial convening authorities show that thus far this calendar year, no separations have been ordered for unsuitability by reason of drug abuse. Commanders must continue to give this point their personal attention to insure that past errors in this regard are corrected.

3. This headquarters provided the "Guide to Unit Commanders" for simplified interpretation of the subject regulations and stressed the urgent need for expeditious completion of these actions. To date, the average processing time in CY 71 for cases in which the respondent does not request a hearing before a board of officers is 26 days, compared with 40.5 days in the latter half of CY 70. This is an improvement — but is not good enough. Elimination actions must be completed in the maximum of 20 days where no board hearing is requested, and in 35 days when a board of officers is convened. This time frame is computed from the date of the unit commander's letter recommending elimination to the date of final action ordering separation. All discharge actions will be reported to this headquarters with a specific explanation provided in cases which required more than the alloted 20 or 35 day cumulative time standards.

AVII-CS
SUBJECT: Administrative Elimination Under the Provisions of AR 635-212

4. USARV policy requires that the immediate commander review the service record of each soldier who has been administered three judicial and/or nonjudicial punishments, and consider at that time, whether to retain him, recommend rehabilitative reassignment, or recommend administrative elimination. Senior commanders must take positive action to insure that these requirements are met. While it is not suggested that a record of three disciplinary actions automatically dictates elimination, it is of paramount importance that this course of action be taken when warranted. In this regard, it has been noted with concern that in several cases referred to this headquarters for elimination for unfitness, a well documented record is provided of shirking and/or frequent incidents of flagrant disregard of orders and regulations, to include contemptuous behavior toward superiors. In these same cases, however, the unit commander reported without comment that no disciplinary action had been taken or was pending against the offender. To permit such misbehavior to go unpunished lessens the chances of rehabilitating a recalcitrant soldier and merely hastens the day when he must be eliminated from the service. Administrative elimination is not a substitute for professional leadership.

5. Rehabilitative reassignments are appropriate when it appears some improvement may be expected. When the soldier's attitude clearly demonstrates that this is not the case, the commander should request that this requirement be waived.

6. Retention of those men who have demonstrated their unsuitability or unfitness for continued service in the United States Army is a grave injustice to the majority of our dutiful young soldiers. Moreover, retention of such men often seriously impairs our combat posture and is detrimental to the maintenance of good order and discipline. It is imperative that the provisions of AR 635-212 be invoked where warranted and that commanders personally insure strict adherence to the requirements of the regulations and policies, to include expeditious processing and staying within the time standards imposed.

7. The "Guide for Unit Commanders," published by reference 1b, will be revised in the near future in consonance with the additional USARV guidance contained in reference 1c.

Robert C. Hixon

ROBERT C. HIXON
Brigadier General, USA
Chief of Staff

DISTRIBUTION:
Special

2

Appendix 7 DIVISION PSYCHIATRY IN VIETNAM

Byrdy was assigned in Vietnam as the division psychiatrist with the 1st Cavalry Division (Airmobile), the first full division ordered into combat since the Korean War. He wrote this paper in 1967 shortly after his return to stateside civilian life. It is a candid and comprehensive overview of the challenges associated with the provision of psychiatric services within a newly deployed combat division during the buildup phase.

UNPUBLISHED PAPER: CAPTAIN HAROLD SR BYRDY, MEDICAL CORPS
DIVISION OF PSYCHIATRY, VIETNAM

History

The division arrived in Vietnam in two separate groups, the air-transported advanced party of 1,040 which arrived within a week and the main body of the division which traveled by ocean and arrived in mid-September.[1] The base camp to be established was to be near an old French military installation at An Khe in the central highlands of Vietnam.

The division psychiatrist traveled with the advanced party. Some sixteen days after signing in at Fort Benning, Georgia, he was treating psychiatric patients [in Vietnam] under a tree near a temporary aide station. The first month was a period of rapid transformation of the area, of literally carving out a working area in the jungle. During this time the division circular defining policies and procedures of the Psychiatric Service was distributed and the psychiatric holding facility was established. The circular simply re-interpreted the basic Army Regulation 40-216. The several principles of military psychiatry were adhered to as closely as possible. Planned lines of evacuation were followed, by and large, except when tactical operations brought engaged units closer to extra-divisional medical facilities. The division strength of 15,000 men was supplemented by 5000 in attached units. The composition of the division which incorporated the 11th Air Assault Division and the 2nd Division had a large percentage of regular army men in the enlisted ranks. Further, since the previous base of operations was Fort Benning, Georgia, there was a large southern element. A non-official report by a personnel officer was that the division was an even 20% Negro in strength.

Psychiatric Role and Capability

As defined in regulation the division psychiatrist has a broad range of responsibilities, which for some cast him as the prototype of the community psychiatrist. In brief, he is responsible for whatever types of psychiatric patients are generated, combat or otherwise; he is responsible for advising command in matters of morale, of establishing a preventive psychiatry program and he is available for board and disciplinary action.

The actual facilities that were evolved were an office in Headquarters, Headquarters Company and a ward in Headquarters of the Medical Battalion. In the latter, the psychiatrist was assisted by a social worker and three technical specialists. Though the division's table of operations and equipment allows for other ancillary staff, these five effectively served to staff the mental health consultation service and in-patient unit. After the psychiatric ward no longer handled the overflow of medical patients, we at no time had more than six in-patients.

Patient Source

Patients were referred either from any of the divisions' 44 physicians as "medical referrals" or were referred in through administrative channels. They were discouraged from presenting in any other way, that is, as self-referrals without going through their unit aide stations or by other agencies, such as special services or the chaplain.

The patients discussed here were seen between 30 August 1965, the date the first Vietnam patient presented, [and] 10 June 1966, a total of 252 days. During that period of time 503 patients were seen in 1,065 outpatient visits; 116 of these 503 were hospitalized.

Period of Adjustment

Flexibility, that oft magically invoked quality that is certain to carry many an American-trained psychiatrist through many ambiguous situations, was the hallmark in the execution of our services. Insofar as it was not clear how air mobility would effect the generation of psychiatric patients, no other orientation could be seriously maintained. Indeed, one unit commander expressed the opinion that a psychiatrist in an airmobile division was unnecessary because he felt that static tactical situations were remotely possible. That orientation overlooked the role of the Army psychiatrist as personnel officer. Eventually we evolved a service that combined the essence of a garrison mental health consultation service and a hospital, and which was to accommodate to any exigency that might present. With time, Camp Radcliff, as it was named, periodically manifested the temper of garrison life. During periods of heavy operations, the attitudes of the forward elements permeated the base camp. However, there were times when the units in the base camp would revert to the style of the garrison with its pre-occupation with polished boots and buckles. From the military standpoint, this reversion is entirely understandable; but from the standpoint of the trooper who had recently experienced contact with life threats and death, this seemed to some as bizarre. The lesson, presumably, is that obsessive rituals are not of equal value for all.

Military operations were in effect from the very beginning of troop arrival. However, the larger

operations during the period in which these cases were collected were in the Ia Drang Valley and in the Bong Son region. The former was in October and November 1965 and the latter in February and March 1966. It was during these two periods that the majority of the cases of combat exhaustion were generated. Personnel had so planned the rotation of men from the theater so that changes would begin within several months after the division had arrived. It was intended that a massive rotation of troops at one time be obviated. The loss of men through battle casualties and rapid replacement of them facilitated this intention.

Operating in a new division in the field were integrative as well as fragmenting forces. Promoting group identity which in the writer's mind is the true glue of any military unit of whatever size and whatever mission was the fact that the helicopter units had long trained together. There was a pervasive feeling of enthusiasm and expectation about what the new airmobile division could accomplish in combat. A centripetal force to the division's integrity was the fact that the official announcement of the division's formation occurred only six weeks before it moved out of the States, meaning that some units were rather abruptly incorporated into the division.

It was a clinical impression, on the basis of the arrival of the advanced party and then of the main body of the division, that the second week in the theater seemed to be the low point of adjustment to the situation. It seemed that then the novelty of the area wore off, the reality of a year's tour, and the incessant dangers became pre-occupations. However, with subsequently newly arriving troops this impression did not seem to be further substantiated.

Collection of Statistics

Unfortunately some of the conditions of being a new organization in the field preclude rigorously accurate and elaborate collection of psychiatric data. Indeed only through considerable effort was it possible to get rudimentary facts in a systematic way. Analysis of hospitalized populations must be more fruitful and in the history of the Second [World] War were the source of workable statistics. Certainly level of education, marital status, service category (Regular Army or draftee), and duration of duty (in the service and in the theater) would be illuminating social parameters to assess. The social parameters for the whole division

TABLE I. Analysis of Patient Population According to Rank

Pay Grade	Title	Number of Patients	Average age	% Negro	Number Hospitalized
E-1	Private	3	20.3	0	0
E-2	Private	51	22.2	41.2	4
E-3	Private First Class (-1)	199	21.3	21.6	46
E-4	Corporal (-1, 2)	108	23.2	20.4	32
E-5	Sergeant	80	29.5	26.2	20
E-6	Staff Sergeant	30	35.0	6.7	8
E-7	Platoon Sergeant or Sergeant First Class	8	34.1	0	3
E-8	First Sergeant or Master Sergeant	3	42.7	0	1
E-9	Sergeant Major	1	46.0	0	0
W 1-4	Warrant Officer	10	32.5	0	2
O-1	2nd Lieutenant	1	24.0	0	0
O-2	1st Lieutenant	5	24.2	0	0
O-3	Captain	3	29.3	0	0
O-4	Major	1	39.0	0	0
	TOTAL	503	24.7	21.7	116

1-lacks one designation of age
2-lacks one designation of race

would have been interesting, especially in light of congressional declination in modifying the draft laws. In psychiatric practice, at least, it became commonplace not only to encounter the high school drop out, but even the grammar school dropout.

Further we lack any substantial follow-up on the execution of our recommendations. Doubtless the percentage of those acted upon is different from that in garrison, but not necessarily much smaller as one might expect. Unit Commanders in the field, if they have time for the paper work, are eager to get rid of unpredictable personnel; whereas non-combat commanders, at times, unreasonably discourage the loss of manpower for any reasons, even for the most pressing.

Rank

93% of the patients came from the ranks E-2 through E-6 (see Table I), the greater burden, 61%, from PFC (E-3 and E-4). During the course of the year, some men were rapidly promoted because military policy in a combat area was conducive to rapid promotion. Further combat and medical losses within the individual units invariably opened "slots" for those

remaining. Despite combat familiarity, some of these men had difficulty in leading rank juniors who were often age peers or seniors.

Ranks E-2 through E-6 included all of the Negro patients. It is not readily apparent why 41.2% of the E-2[s] are Negro when the general incidence of Negro patients was 21.7%. New troops, before they are rapidly promoted, have that designation as do many who are demoted for infractions.

Diagnosis

Table II lists the incidence for the general diagnostic categories. Incidence is based on troops strength of approximately 20,000, that is, the 15,000 organic to the division and 5,000 attached troops. In fact, during this period, approximately 8,000 additional troops rotated in the division because of combat and medical casualties and termination of service. The numerical incidence is in all likelihood exaggerated therefore. The figure of 2.2 evacuees per thousand per year jibes with Tiffany's and Allerton's statistic of less than 3 per thousand per year which was based on the theater statistics for January 1966.[2] The percentage of patients seen in the various

TABLE II. Analysis of Patient population according to diagnosis

Diagnosis	Number of cases	Average Age	% Negro	Number Hospitalized	Incidence per 1,000 per year
1. Acute brain syndrome -1	22	22.3	18.2	21	1.6
2. Psychosis	12	22.2	41.5	11	.8
3. Psychophysiologic reaction	24	24.1	25.0	7	1.7
4. Psychoneurosis -1, 2	70	26.9	14.1	13	5.1
5. Personality disorder	203	24.2	24.6	35	14.7
6. Combat exhaustion	22	23.5	27.7	13	1.6
7. Adult situational reaction	18	25.5	5.5	9	1.3
8. Miscellaneous	132	24.2	21.2	7	9.6
TOTAL	503	24.7	21.7	116	36.0
Evacuees [out of division]	30	—	—	—	2.2

1-lacks one designation of age
2-lacks one designation of race

diagnostic categories would not be similar to an analysis of an evacuation hospital and are not.[3]

Familiarization with the situation in the field brings the realization that the kinds of referrals depend on the tactical situation. Homosexuals and discipline problems are rarely referred in from units under engagement. Hausman and Rioch note that during the Korean War that the term "combat exhaustion" was used to designate all psychiatric casualties to minimize the damage to evacuees who might read their diagnoses.[4] We very early and very quickly abandoned this all-inclusive designation for the far less ambiguous and more specific standard nomenclature. The former system worked, presumably, because everyone knew the signals. In the Vietnamese situation, clearly they did not.

Of the 12 psychoses, one man was manic, 7 were acute undifferentiated schizophrenics, and 4 were paranoid. One man who shot himself in the leg was grossly psychotic.

Anxiety (35 cases) and depression (27 cases) were the two most common neuroses. Depression in the older soldier became more common in the sixth month of the tour. This co-incided roughly with the second major operation of the division. Of the phobias to flying, 2 could be said to be combat connected, while three others showed up in non-combatant men just prior to their rotation back to the states.

As might be expected, passive-aggressive personality was the most common characterologica1 diagnosis. A number of these patients were seen for psychiatric clearance in criminal action. These were just a fraction of those referred in for administrative boarding. To this writer's mind, there is little way of assessing the assumption that the passive-aggressive personality, a devil in the camp, is an excellent soldier in the field. There was no rule of thumb in recommending for this sort of referral. The sociopath, however, was generally recommended for boarding. It was held that group integrity and safety in the unit was jeopardized by a man with a strong anti-social history.

No systematic effort was made in chronicling suicidal gestures. Some self-inflicted wounds were sent for evaluation after they had healed and were ready to be returned to duty. Suicides fell into the province of the military police. Only once was an effort made to involve the psychiatrist in a post-suicide investigation. There were very few suicidal gestures that were directly referred into the psychiatrist.

A large group of cases (26.2%) were classified as miscellaneous. Included here are No Psychiatric Disease and No Diagnosis Established. Medical problems, administrative cases needing psychiatric clearance, and referrals for counseling are the kinds of cases grouped here.

Disposition

Of the patients that were seen, an even 30 or 6% were evacuated "psychiatrically" from the division. This number included the 12 psychotics. Such patients as unresponsive combat exhaustion or those who merited further medical work-up, e.g., hypertensives, originally referred for headache, or seizure cases, would be evacuated. All others were returned to duty. Character disorders, the diagnoses most often invoked for administrative problems which were referred to the psychiatrist for disposition, did not routinely carry a recommendation for further administrative action, other than clearance. We quickly learned that there was no point executing our three day holding policy on psychotics. Two of these fellows were returned to the division, one the following day, the second after several months in a hospital setting. The latter again became fuminantly [*sic*] psychotic.

No patient was maintained as an out-patient on any psychotropic medication more potent than Librium. A consideration here was patient responsiveness in mortar attacks. Further, it was felt that if a patient merited Thorazine, he might best be accommodated in the psychiatric ward or out of the division.

The enuretics that were tried on Tofranil (Imipramine Hydrochloride) all failed to improve. Here again, discharge was not routinely recommended for enuresis. (It was for chronic encopresis). One man was referred in through his medic. He was three months shy of his three year tour and wet the bed frequently. He wanted some free medical help before he got out of the service. No one had known of his difficulty.

Of the 116 patients hospitalized, 27 were either acutely or chronically alcoholic. Unless these men were repeatedly hospitalized or were being considered for disciplinary or administrative action by their unit, they were merely 'dried out'.

Combat Exhaustion

The cases of combat exhaustion were engendered largely during the two major operations of the division.

The average age of these men was 23.5 years. By initial diagnosis there were 32 cases. However, ten of these diagnoses were changed on sign out. Two were psychoneurotic. There were one psycho-physiological reaction, one schizophrenic, two alcoholic agitations, and four who manifested characterological difficulties in the subsequent contacts.

These men were treated with bed rest and tranquilization where necessary. In general they responded well to treatment. Three, however, were evacuated eventually. Of those evacuated, two were psychotic and the other irrevocably psychoneurotic. Two men eventually were transferred out of combat units.

Morale

Morale is an elusive issue. It is perhaps more easily influenced than accurately assessed. Insofar as much of the division saw itself as new and experimental in warfare, there was considerable enthusiasm. In the very early days of the division, the mail and the daily allotment of two cans of beer, usually warm, was a crucial issue which was quickly perceived by command. Though priority [mail] became fairly regular. The Stars and Stripes became available. Special services movies were instituted before the arrival of the main body of the division (The troops especially liked war films). Eventually there were Red Cross Services Network, Saigon with "doughnut dollies" and a local radio station relaying the Armed Forces Network from Saigon and also broadcasting its own programs. Camp followers, in a very well organized fashion, quickly moved into the area. Depending on the rather complicated desires of command, the troops variably had access to them. There was an in-country and out-of-country "rest and relaxation" system the functioning of which varied vastly from unit to unit and from rank to rank, but which could have only a salutary effect on the troops who were far removed from the coastal cities.

That the tour was for a 12 month period rather than "for the duration" facilitated morale and enhanced endurance.

Realistic personal danger varied tremendously among the units, the line companies, of course, being pre-eminent. Breakdown of psychiatric cases by units within the division show the line companies pathetically far in the numerical lead.

Preventive Psychiatry

The re-institution of the psychiatrist into the division during the Second [World] War was effected because many of the psychiatric problems could be anticipated and handled at the local level. The task of the division psychiatrist in its multiple ramifications is vast and almost by definition an impossibility. In garrison, with the assigned technicians in full strength, the psychiatrist may have a more direct source of information about troop attitudes, and further he may have competent men to handle problems locally. However, there is a strong hypothetical aspect to the smooth functioning of such an operation.

In the Cavalry, the psychiatrist was able to meet the 44 doctors at some time. Certainly he was never able to meet a large percentage of the unit commanders. This was not feasible though possibly desirable. Contacts with the general medical officers were intended largely to clarify referral policy and [were] didactic only on invitation. In general, there was little need to re-iterate the policy of referral, already issued in the division directive. However, physicians, overburdened with the humdrum of sick call, might abruptly refer ambiguous cases in. Often the patient who did not improve according to expectation (from perhaps gastritis or punji stake wound) would be referred in. The locus of the hang-up between patient and physician would be shifted and usually could be broken since the psychiatrist might be able to afford the luxury of taking a history or putting a partially ambulatory man with a poorly healing wound at bed rest. One man was referred in for exaggerated complaining and had been seen by two physicians whose physical examination did not include palpation. The man had an obviously fulminant punji stake abscess in his gastrocnemius.

Contacts with units were made whenever possible and nearly always with difficult cases through either the psychiatrist, the social worker, or a technical specialist, usually a social work specialist. However, these contacts were both relatively infrequent and almost always after the fact. A number of referrals from one unit at one time would invariably mean that the unit was "housecleaning" after returning from a mission, or that there was trouble in leadership. Three men, Negroes, were referred in from one unit. By the time the third man, whose eye was swollen, was seen, the brigade commander had seen fit to relieve the Commanding Officer and First Sergeant of the company and rectified the situation.

Personal contact with units was not facilely accomplished in any systematic way insofar as telephone communication took up to 45 minutes sometimes, if at all. Vehicular transportation depended on loan; and helicopter transportation which was difficult to schedule was generously or grudgingly offered, depending on the tactical situation. The difficulties of transportation were primarily time-consuming rather than impossible.

Essentially we practiced preventive psychiatry on the secondary level, that is, early diagnosis and rapid treatment, and we relied on the usual evacuation and referral channels for our patient population. In general, it was not policy to sell psychiatry to anyone. Availability when the need arose was ample justification for the service.

The few central principles of military psychiatry were practiced systematically. Hausman and Rioch state these succinctly "Immediacy, proximity, expectancy, . . . concurrence, and commitment."[4] In the Vietnamese war, heavy reliance on the first three seemed the most fruitful. Here the psychiatrist's efficacy is at its greatest when his identification with the group is most conducive to the immediate goals of the group, specifically, its integrity and self-preservation.

[*Post script: Byrdy, in correspondence with this author on 11 August 1982, said: "In contrast to news accounts of what subsequently transpired in military units in Vietnam, during my year the morale in the 1st Cav was remarkably high; however, in the course of that year there was erosion. Tiger beer was the main substance abused. There was marijuana available, but, as far as I know, very little in the way of hard drugs."*]

References

1. Hymoff E. *The First [Air] Cavalry Division*. New York, NY: M.W. [Lads] Publishing Co.; 1967.
2. Tiffany WJ, Allerton WS. Army psychiatry in the Mid-'60s. *Am J Psychiatry*. 1967;123:810–819.
3. Strange RE, Arthur RJ. Hospital ship psychiatry in a war zone. *Am J Psychiatry*. 1967;124:281–286.
4. Hausman W, Rioch DM. Military psychiatry. *Arch Gen Psychiatry*. 1967;16:727–739.

Appendix 8 LIEUTENANT COLONEL ARNOLD W JOHNSON JR

Lieutenant Colonel Arnold W Johnson served in Vietnam (July 1966–1967) during the buildup of forces as the senior Army psychiatrist in the theater—the Neuropsychiatry Consultant to the CG/USARV Surgeon. He provides a granular account of the growing complexity of the Army's combat role in Vietnam from the vantage point of the psychiatric challenges encountered in the early years of the war.

PANEL REMARKS: LIEUTENANT COLONEL ARNOLD W JOHNSON JR
NEUROPSYCHIATRY CONSULTANT TO THE COMMANDING GENERAL/
US ARMY REPUBLIC OF VIETNAM SURGEON

. . . I do a certain amount of clinical work but I don't take too much time for that. Mostly the job consists of administrative and preventive work, staff work, working in terms of community psychiatry for all of the military communities in Vietnam and a great deal of traveling. I should be traveling about half the time in order to cover all of the obligations that are there. But there's a lot of office work, too, so sometimes it's hard to get away. The job is satisfying also from the point of view that the United States Army in Vietnam has an excellent level of morale and motivation. As far as my work is concerned, I get excellent cooperation not only from the medical people and the medical units, but also from the line people and the line units. In general, I think that the psychiatric system has been working well, and this also is satisfying.

. . . [I]n July of 1965 there were 31,000 troops in Vietnam, by January there were 128,000, by last July and August when I arrived there were about 170,000, and when I left the other day there were about 250,000 with more expected. It is growing very rapidly and will continue to grow for some time. You can begin to get some idea of the magnitude of the operation. . . . There are practical problems in Vietnam, things like communication, the telephone system. . . . The dial system that's been promised so long is gradually coming into being, but it's going to be a long time before telephone communication is very good. . . . Another practical problem is transportation. Land transportation is a little difficult. . . . I could travel out to see John Bowman at the 93rd Evac Hospital by car without too much difficulty, but he was about the only psychiatrist I could visit by automobile. In other cases I would ordinarily be flying. . . . Although the roads are passable and convoys go on satisfactorily, if you take a vehicle by yourself Charlie (Viet Cong guerrillas) is likely to stop you. Air transportation is good when you can get it, which depends on whether you have enough priority. I have enough priority so that I can usually get around without too much trouble, but once in a while I get bumped, too. The division psychiatrists, who are usually captains, sometimes have a great deal of difficulty getting the kind of transportation . . . they need to get them around to see the people whom they really ought to be seeing. As we get down into the Delta we'll probably be hearing more about water transportation. I think transportation in the Delta is going to be a problem; there won't be much land transportation down there.

For the last couple of months the climate has been pretty good. Sort of like fall, not terribly hot, but most of the year the weather is really quite hot, quite humid, quite wet and quite uncomfortable. There's a jungle with which to contend, and all the various kinds of fauna as well as flora.

One thing that must be getting clear to you by now from our conversations and from the pictures is that, differently from previous wars, all the hospitals are in permanent or semi-permanent buildings. The 93rd Evac is in Quonsets, the 3rd Field is in concrete permanent buildings and the 8th Field is in tropical, semi-permanent buildings, the 85th is in Quonsets, the 67th in some nice new concrete buildings, etc. The only exception is the 45th Hospital at Tay Ninh, which is the MUST unit made of inflatable buildings. Technically speaking, I suppose that makes them the only really mobile hospital. All of the others are being built in relatively permanent buildings. The rate at which they build hospitals is much better than it was in the days that John is describing, and they're learning something about holding off professional complement until things are sort of ready to go.

My job as consultant is partly an office job and partly a traveling job. The USARV Surgeon does not really command anything except a medical journal for Vietnam which General Wier, the USARV Surgeon, requested be established as a means of medical professional communication within Vietnam. Part of my job, along with that of the other Consultants who help me with this, is to get all the physicians around Vietnam to contribute the things that they ought to contribute in terms of communicating professionally within Vietnam. This puts me in touch with a lot of people besides psychiatrists, from my point of view as psychiatric consultant a very useful thing because it's an extra entree into a lot of areas that I wouldn't get into otherwise, or not as easily anyway.

I'm going to talk a bit more about the psychiatric aspects of this entire picture that I talked about before. We touched already somewhat on the evacuation system and I'm sure that you're aware that most of the medical evacuation is done by air, either by helicopter or by airplane. There is some land evacuation, but relatively little. There might be land evacuation under some circumstances from An Khe to Qui Nhon or from the Binh Son area to Qui Nhon, or from Saigon to Long Binh, or vice versa, from Di An to Long Binh. But by and large the roads that are really open and safe for an ambulance traveling alone are relatively few so that most of the medical evacuation is by air. Rather typically from a combat area a helicopter will pick up a patient and take him to a clearing station organic to the unit. If the patient needs to be evacuated further, a helicopter will then take him from the clearing station to the nearest hospital, perhaps a surgical hospital, perhaps an evac hospital. Then, if the hospital is in the forward area and the patient needs to be evacuated further, he'll probably be picked up by airplane, say from Pleiku or An Khe, and taken down to Qui Nhon to one of the evac hospitals there. Similar things go on in the Saigon area. Then, from Qui Nhon or Cam Ranh or Saigon, patients will be taken by airplane, sometimes directly to Okinawa or Japan, sometimes over to Clark Air Force Base in the Philippines and then trans-shipped to Japan or Okinawa from there, or perhaps sent directly back to the States. It used to be that all the psychiatric patients went either directly back to the States or to Clark and generally directly back to the States. Recently, however, this has been changed so that most of them are taken to Japan, given a certain amount of treatment there, and then sent back to the States later. There are about 3 hospitals in Japan that have psychiatric wards and a number of psychiatrists. . . .

The helicopter units that pick up patients are directly under the medical groups, the 55th Medical Group, the 43rd and the 68th. They are not assigned to the combat units. They don't have enough of them either, by the way, and as a result what usually happens is that the helicopters are assigned to cover a certain area, certain groups that are in that area. Hospitals also tend to cover an area. There are fixed hospitals; thus they can't follow any units around and they tend to cover the area that is close to them. Take as an example the helicopters stationed at Pleiku and the hospital at Pleiku. The helicopters will fan out and cover the combat units in that area. Transportation by air is simple if you can get it, but you can't always get it. Also, it's dangerous at times and this has contributed to the business of area coverage rather than medical care following the individual unit. As a result our psychiatric care has tended to become area coverage also. For instance, I have asked the division psychiatrist of the 4th infantry Division at Pleiku, Captain Randall, to cover the Pleiku area generally in addition to the 4th Infantry Division Headquarters and the 2nd Brigade of the 4th Infantry. Thus, he makes regular visits to the 18th Surgical Hospital at Pleiku, to the base camp of the 3rd Brigade of the 25th Infantry, and also support units of one kind or another that are based in the Pleiku area. In effect, he provides psychiatric coverage for all the Pleiku area. The psychiatrist at An Khe doesn't have quite as

as well as the 3rd Brigade of the 4th Division which is at nearby Dau Tien. These units are controlled by the 25th Division which renders medical support, including a psychiatrist. I just want to mention one thing. In general, the 25th Division has had very few psychiatric casualties; that is, the rate has been quite low, slightly lower than that which Dr. Byrdy described for the Air Cav. But this doesn't mean that they don't have any; they do have some. Operation Attleboro, as you remember, was one of the big operations last fall. Up at Tay Ninh at the medical clearing company of the 196th Brigade there's a social work specialist by the name of Mann, the only mental hygiene-kind of personnel in Tay Ninh. He has operated in such a manner that the medical people at Tay Ninh have gained all kinds of confidence in his ability to screen and work with psychiatric patients. Whenever a psychiatric casualty comes to attention in Tay Ninh, the medical people there have Mann see him. Mann has gained quite a reputation. He submits a report to me every month on the patients he sees and the work that he does. I talked with him about what happened during Operation Attleboro. We've mentioned the fact that there isn't any combat fatigue, etc. It isn't that there isn't any combat fatigue, there just hasn't been as much of it, and much of what has occurred has not been as severe as some that we've seen in the past. Either that or it's been handled much better. At the height of Operation Attleboro there were two companies of the 25th Division up in that area who got hit rather hard. Inside of a couple of days or so, Mann processed about 12 or 14 fellows from these two companies who essentially were a form of combat fatigue or combat exhaustion. These companies were hit very hard with a lot of casualties and a lot of people's buddies got killed. They worked hard during that period also. The way Mann described it, these were rather typically "shook up," and anxious, frightened and exhausted kids. He treated them in conjunction with the doctors there in the classical textbook fashion for combat exhaustion with a little rest, a little ventilation, a little reassurance, a little food, and sleep overnight. After 24 hours they all went back to duty and, as far as he could tell, they all did fine. So it isn't that these cases don't happen; it's that to some extent they are being handled perhaps better than they have at times in the past. This is a credit to the other physicians in the area, too, that they understand this process and are able to cooperate with it. At other times I've talked with individual physicians who understand this process very well all by themselves without any help

from any psychiatrists or social workers. At Di An is the 1st Infantry Division psychiatrist and perhaps this division has had more of what you might call combat fatigue right along than any other. They've had some operations which were lengthy in which the fellows stayed out in the jungle for long periods of time, and right along they've had, not a large number, but maybe up to 6 or 8 a month, a steady trickle of cases that they call combat fatigue, which has gotten back to the psychiatrist. There have been more that have been taken care of in the medical companies, sometimes by the social work technicians in conjunction with the doctors. But the psychiatrist will often receive them and take care of them for 2 to 5 days in the medical battalion, back at his headquarters, and then return them to duty. Very rarely do they actually get back as far as the hospital at Long Binh, although there have been a few. The team at Long Binh has trained some social work technicians. They've trained at least one for the 173rd Airborne Brigade at Ben Hoa and another one for the Cavalry. . . .

[Next,] I . . . want to show you some figures. [The] . . . trouble with these figures is that, as Captain Byrdy mentioned, the rates and figures are very difficult to arrive at in a situation like this. These figures, for instance, refer only to reports that I've received from psychiatrists. When you say this is the rate seen by the psychiatrist or these are the admissions done by the psychiatrists at the psychiatric facilities, they aren't really complete. The evacuation figure is perhaps more accurate than any, because this represents the rate for patients who have been evacuated by our psychiatrists. There have been a few that haven't, but we've evacuated a few of those of other services, too, so it probably comes out about even. The morbidity rate is a little more problematical because this is the figure that is reported by all of the registrars from all of the medical facilities around the country that have registrars. I found errors in that at times. On the other hand, I found errors in all these figures at times. You can't take this as gospel, but it gives you an idea as to how the rates go. You'll notice that the out-patient rate stays relatively the same. There was a little drop, probably representing a period when there were 2 or 3 of the psychiatrists out at the same time during which time a couple of the clinics weren't operating. While this rate has stayed in the same ball park, the population in the country has been rising steadily causing the number of outpatients to rise steadily. The psychiatric admission rate as reported by the psychiatric facilities at least stays roughly in the same general area but the number has been rising as the population in the country rises. You roughly double the population in the country and the numbers that are admitted to our psychiatric wards roughly doubles. The evacuation rate out of country was a little lower last summer than it has been for the last four months, but you'll notice how closely the evacuation rate has been the same for the last four months, quite low, around 2 per thousand per year. This figure is the percentage of the total evacuees out of country for the month. I didn't get the figure for the total December evacuations so I couldn't figure the percentages, but I have reason to think that the percentage of evacs for December is about the same as for November. Perhaps about 3 percent of all evacs were psychiatric. The morbidity is essentially lost time due to psychiatric diagnoses as reported by all the registrars. You'll notice that this rate is generally a little larger than the admission rate reported by psychiatrists. This you can expect because other people besides psychiatrists will make admissions for psychiatric reasons, and they won't all get to a psychiatrist necessarily. I think that these figures are slightly small but they're probably comparable to the figures that are reported in the command health report from the Department of the Army in which the CONUS rate for the first six months of 1966 varied from about 9 to 11, and the Army as a whole varied from about 9 to 11. Bill Allerton was telling me that the CONUS rate is up now. If you look at this you can see that, although we aren't having any unusual problem with combat fatigue, we aren't having any unusual problem with more psychiatric cases for any reasons in Vietnam than you might expect, yet we are having an amount of business that is comparable to the business that you get on a troop post in the United States. Perhaps this is not quite as high as a rate that you get out of a basic training camp; but it isn't that there aren't any psychiatric problems in Vietnam, it's just that the rate is not particularly unusual.

[A question-and-answer period followed Johnson's comments]

[Johnson, responding to a question.] I think there are many different factors involved in the psychiatric rate in Vietnam. The leadership by command in Vietnam is excellent and I'm sure that's a part of the picture. I'm sure that many of the facilities that have been established

for troops in this situation which weren't established in previous situations as well are a part of the picture, too. For instance, the mail situation is much better than that I experienced in Korea. Also, there are things such as the Armed Forces Radio, for any soldier in Vietnam who carries a little pocket radio can listen to the news and find out what's going on. The food is excellent in general. Often I'll travel up to the 4th Infantry Division in Pleiku and go out to a mess tent and eat a meal that is just as good as anything that I can get in Saigon . The leadership has established for the troops other things that make for good morale generally. I think another factor is the one-year rotation. I think that the trooper generally has the feeling that one year is a short while; and, if he can make it for a year he'll have it made and will sort of prove himself. I think this is a definite factor—the combat isn't endless. If one can make it for a year, he can get out of it. It isn't the hopeless feeling that one has when the combat is essentially endless and he expects that the unit is going to disappear entirely including himself. I think I have not answered your question well at all. I think there are many different factors, including the morbidity of the troops. I think on the positive side is the fact that one doesn't just sit in a defensive position and stand off attacks. Our units generally are on the attack all the time. They go out and attack and then come back and rest and then go out and attack. The rest between the periods of attack is important.

. . .[Johnson, responding to a question about slightly increased incidence of psychiatric evacuations in September of 1966.] Well, I think it refers to a lot of things. I think that at this point there were a lot more replacements arriving. The 4th Division was arriving at that time, but in addition there were a lot of others. You see, the big build-up started the previous summer and by September of 1966 a lot of the troops that had volunteered to come over here or were organic to a unit were being replaced by individual replacements some of whom were volunteers but some of whom were not necessarily volunteers. This increased replacement situation started in about September. I think this had something to do with the little jump in rate at that time.

[Johnson, responding to a question as to the low casualty rate in units arriving with good unit integrity; ie, soldiers who had served in the same unit for some time.] Definitely a factor. This, I feel, has been part of the thing about the low rates in the 25th Division and the 1st

Cav in the past which, I think, changes as the individual replacements begin to come in.

[Johnson, responding to the question, "If that's true, then why are some of the units split up so much? This seems like asking for trouble. I know this is a command problem; they've got some of the soldiers in three different spots."] The only thing I can say about the fact that the divisions are split up the way they are is that this was done because of military necessity. The divisions are built out of brigades specifically so that they can be flexible in response to military requirements. [Comment by another participant]: The three brigades conduct themselves quite independently from one another. Indeed, our major field problems envisage that they would be separated. One brigade would have no difficulty to go out into the field for a long period of time quite independent of the other two brigades and having its own internal cohesiveness and morale, which is, I think, pretty much separate from one another. They could go out into the field for a long period without the feeling that the division was fragmented. . . .

[Johnson, responding to the question, "[M]orale seems to be so high over there and [yet there is] the paradox [of] the activities [antiwar riots] at Berkeley. It would appear as though they're [the soldiers] getting either screened information or else they're getting all of it and handling it very well."] No, there's no screening of the information. The fellows over there just laugh about it, as far as I can tell.… On the plane on the way back I was listening to some of them talking and they were making jokes about the guys at Berkeley.

[Panel member comment]: . . . [I]n my experience with the divisions naturally we had no information for several months. We got a radio tape, I think, in the four months there. Mail service as yet hadn't had all the wrinkles ironed out, people really had to rely on letters from home and clippings from home for the first half of our tour. And then, our two sources of information, the troop sources of information, were the radio in Saigon and the *Stars and Stripes*. These radios told everything that was worthwhile, including rock and roll records. The *Stars and Stripes*, comparing it with clippings from the *Times*, tended to tone down somewhat the disclaimers of the war.

[Johnson, responding to a question as to U.S. soldiers being adversely affected in morale by Vietnamese intransigence.]: I don't really believe so. It seems to me that in most cases the relationship between the American troops and the Vietnamese people is quite good. I've made a number of friends among the Vietnamese myself and I observe many other people that do. I observed that the Privates and PFC's do also, and I observed very little in the way of real friction.

[Panel member comment]: In our division we were really isolated pretty much from the civilian population. Our base camp was set up in such a way as to be quite separate and maintain a large degree of integrity until those times when we thought that the integrity should be broken down somewhat. However, I think that many people have an attitude of unusual suspiciousness toward the local civilian population. In our division this was based on a number of incidents in which the local brush cutters laid out little signs about installations and that sort of thing. I think that we kept things going in an insulated manner mostly, but the attitude of suspiciousness prevailed and I assume that at least in our area it must still prevail.

[Johnson]: Let me say one more thing about the information business. By this time there are PX's in every unit around the country, and one can go into the PX to buy a *Time Magazine* or *Newsweek* or *Observer*, or whatever he wants. He can read anything that he wants to read. Sometimes it's a week or two late, but it isn't as it was back in September when it was two months late. In addition to which, particularly in Saigon, there are daily papers. I buy a paper every morning and read the news. The Vietnamese government censors some of the military news, but they don't do anything to censor the news that comes out of the United States. All of the draft card burners and Berkeley protesters are featured in the news over there daily, and I think it makes no particular problem.

[Johnson, responding to a question comparing troops in Korea with those in Vietnam]: . . . [O]ne of the factors in Korea is that it is essentially a defensive position. It was essentially a situation of sitting still and waiting for something to maybe happen. Also, it is essentially a garrison-type of situation with a certain amount of rigidity, "spit and polish," and so forth. We find that in Vietnam in the base camps when the soldiers are there for a while and things get a bit more rigid, there's more acting out. The troops enjoy being out in the field more. One would think that the rates would go up when they go out in the field to try to find Charlie, but that's when the rate goes down and everybody seems to feel quite good with relatively few problems. The problems return when they return to the post.

Source: Jones FD, ed. *Proceedings: Social and Preventive Psychiatry Course, 1967.* Washington, DC: GPO; 1968: 41–46, 73-76. [Available at: Alexandria, Va: Defense Technical Information Center. Document No. AD A950058.]

In: *Overview of Army Psychiatry in Vietnam, Soc and Preventive Psy Course*, Washington, DC, 1967

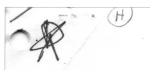

23d INFANTRY DIVISION
MENTAL HYGIENE CONSULTATION SERVICE
APO San Francisco 96374

AVDF-SU   20 November 1970

SUBJECT: Principles of Military Combat Psychiatry

SEE DISTRIBUTION

1. The large number of inappropriate referrals to the MHCS requires a
review of the principles of military combat psychiatry. It is recommended
that these principles be utilized at the unit level in the management
of emotional disorders, psychiatric, and drug disorders. These principles
were developed from the extensive experience of WW I, WW II, and the
Korean War. Several recent studies confirm the applicability of these
principles to the requirements of Viet Nam. These principles involve
immediacy, proximity and expectancy. They imply that the soldier should
be treated as soon as possible after developing symptoms. He should be
treated as close to his own unit and his comrades as possible. His treatment should be undertaken and maintained with the expectation that he
will improve and return to duty. The successful application of these
principles requires that every soldier with an emotional or drug problem
be effectively screened by his unit surgeon who must function as the
unit psychiatrist in the field. Only those emotional or drug problems
which the unit surgeon does not feel professionally qualified to manage
should be referred to MHCS. The division psychiatrist should be utilized
in the capacity of psychiatric consultant when possible.

AVDF-SU   20 November 1970
SUBJECT: Principles of Military Combat Psychiatry

2. <u>SPECIFIC PRINCIPLES OF MANAGEMENT OF PSYCHIATRIC OR EMOTIONALLY</u>

<u>DISTURBED PATIENTS</u>:

    a. <u>PSYCHOPHYSIOLOGICAL REACTIONS</u>: hyperventilation, syncope,

vomiting, incontinence, eneuresis, headaches and <u>HYSTERICAL REACTIONS</u>:

pains without organic disease, panicky feelings, freezing up, sleep-

walking, nerves. The management of the bulk of patients with these

disorders can be accomplished effectively at the unit level. Treat-

ment consists of emotional support, reassurance, the opportunity to

ventilate, and a tranquilizer (e.g. Mellaril 25 mg bid). The patient

should not be allowed to obtain secondary gain, such as coming out of

the field or relief from duty, which only serves to fix his symptoms

rather than relieve them. The further this type of patient is evac-

uated towards the rear, the more difficult will be his rehabilitation

and return to duty. A frequent problem with this category of disorder

concerns a judgement on the potential hazard of the soldier to his unit.

Such patients when evaluated by the MHCS, ordinarily will be returned to

their units for duty. Exceptions to this policy may be the individual

whose symptom manifestations have been documented as hazardous to his

unit. Thus hyperventilation after a firefight will not warrant a profile

limitation. The same reaction during a firefight, which jeopardized the

safety of the unit, would justify a profile limiting field duty. However,

such reaction should be substantiated in the individual's health record

prior to referral to the mental hygiene consult. Service decisions by

AVDF-SU   20 November 1970
SUBJECT: Principles of Military Combat Psychiatry

the MHCS on profile limitations are based on what the patient has done
and not on what he says he might do.

    b. <u>CHARACTER AND BEHAVIOR DISORDERS INCLUDING DRUG DEPENDENCE</u>:
The major portion of these disorders can be managed effectively in the
unit by appropriate rehabilitative and disciplinary action. Those individuals on the Drug Amnesty program can be provided support as described
in the SOP on the Amnesty program. Supplementary use of tranquilizers
may be indicated such as Mellaril, 25 mg bid-tid. Those who are considered physically dependent on barbiturates or narcotics should be referred
to MHCS for withdrawal over a 5-8 day period.

    c. <u>PSYCHOSES</u>: Delusions and/or hallucinations not related to drug
intoxication and <u>SEVERE NEUROSES</u>: hysterical paralysis, mutism, amnesia,
and compulsions which impair the ability of the individual to function.
Patients with these disorders should be referred to MHCS where a specific
treatment plan and/or limitation of duty will be recommended.

3. NON-PSYCHIATRIC EMOTIONAL PROBLEMS:

    a. <u>FEAR OF THE FIELD</u>: Fear of the field is a normal reaction. It
can be managed effectively by unit measures such as the "buddy system",
which keeps the individual close to an experienced soldier or NCO during
the initial period in combat action. It is important that the soldier
who manifests such fear joins his unit in the field as soon as possible.
The unit surgeon must reassure the soldier that his fear is normal and
can be overcome. Tranquilizers should not be prescribed if symptoms
of anxiety (outlined in b below) are not present.

AVDF-SU   20 November 1970
SUBJECT: Principles of Military Combat Psychiatry

normal CSR

   b. ANXIETY: No one should expect to feel comfortable and relaxed
in the combat field. Headaches, abdominal cramps, poor sleep, poor appetite, are normal symptoms in combat, and do not justify evacuation.
Again, the unit surgeon must reassure the soldier that most combat soldiers
at some time experience some or all of these symptoms and that they are
not indicative of emotional illness. In these cases, however, tranquilizers (e.g. Mellaril 25 mg b.i.d.) may be prescribed to help control
the overt anxiety.

   c. REFUSAL TO GO TO THE FIELD: When a soldier who has been in a
combat area refuses to return because of psychiatric reasons, he should
be evaluated by the unit surgeon to determine fitness. If he has been
able to perform his field duties in the past without presenting a hazard
to his unit, he is considered fit for field duty. He should be managed
administratively. When a man who has never been in the combat field
before refuses to go, he cannot claim psychiatric unfitness. Psychiatric evaluation of fitness is based upon actual performance in the field.
A trial of field combat duty is necessary before any determination of
fitness can be made.

4. MHCS REFERRALS: Most referrals to the MHCS will be accomplished by
the unit surgeon. Administrative referrals may be made directly to
MHCS by the unit commander for the following: 212, CO status, or court
martial proceedings. In such cases Americal Form 49 should accompany

AVDF-SU   20 November 1970
SUBJECT: Principles of Military Combat Psychiatry

the individual to MHCS.

Larry E. Alessi

DISTRIBUTION: LARRY E. ALESSI
1-Bde Surg, 11th Inf Bde   CPT, MC
1-Bde Surg, 196th Inf Bde   Division Psychiatrist
1-Bde Surg, 198th Inf Bde
1-Gp Surg, 16th CAG
1-Surg, Div Arty
4-Div Surg Off
4-Surgeons, Co A, 23d Med Bn
2-Surgeons, Co B, 23d Med Bn
2-Surgeons, Co C, 23d Med Bn
3-Surgeons, Co D, 23d Med Bn
1-Surg, 1-20 Inf Bn
1-Surg, 3-1 Inf Bn
1-Surg, 4-3 Inf Bn
1-Surg, 4-21 Inf Bn
1-Surg, 1-46 Inf Bn
1-Surg, 2-1 Inf Bn
1-Surg, 3-21 Inf Bn
1-Surg, 4-31 Inf Bn
1-Surg, 1-6 Inf Bn
1-Surg, 1-52 Inf Bn
1-Surg, 5-46 Inf Bn
1-Surg, 1-14 Arty Bn
1-Surg, 1-82 Arty Bn
1-Surg, 3-16 Arty Bn
1-Surg, 3-18 Arty Bn
1-Surg, 3-82 Arty Bn
1-Surg, 6-11 Arty Bn
1-Surg, 14 CAB
1-Surg, 123d Avn Bn
1-Surg, 1-1 Cavalry
1-Surg, 26th Engr Bn
100- Division Psychiatrist

Appendix 10 PSYCHIATRIC EXPERIENCE AT THE 3RD FIELD HOSPITAL

Captain Arthur S Blank Jr, Medical Corps, was a civilian-trained psychiatrist who served in Vietnam (October 1965–1966) during the first year that ground troops were deployed. He was initially assigned with the 1st Infantry Division, then with the 935th Neuropsychiatric Detachment (KO), and finally with the 3rd Field Hospital in Saigon. The comments below center on his experiences as a solo psychiatrist assigned to the 3rd Field Hospital (April–September 1966).

PANEL REMARKS: CPT. ARTHUR S BLANK JR.
3RD FIELD HOSPITAL, SAIGON

During my first few months in Vietnam I was the de facto First Division Psychiatrist in as much as Captain Perito did not arrive until the beginning of January 1966. After that the KO Team arrived and we worked together until I moved to the 3rd Field Hospital in Saigon in April 1966. I'd like to devote most of my comments to that latter six months which I spent at the 3rd Field Hospital. In doing so, I think I'm talking about an experience which is fairly typical for the psychiatrist who is stationed at an Evac or Field hospital where there is not a KO Team, not a psychiatric ward as such, and essentially no other psychiatric personnel. The 3rd Field and the 17th Field Hospitals in Saigon provide directed medical support for the 25,000, maybe now 30,000, troops in the Saigon area, our support troops, and also provide, along with the 93rd Evac Hospital, direct support for support and combat troops in the Delta, such as there are.

The work load was manageable, although I want to hasten to make the same points that Dr. Byrdy did, that matters of administration and communication take much longer in Vietnam than they do, I think, anyplace else in the world. We're going to have to take this into consideration. I would also say about these general statistics that these would represent roughly one-half of the business in Saigon during this period. Captain William Kenny is at the 17th Field Hospital. He was seeing approximately the same number of patients as was I, although not quite as many inpatients.

What I have in mind here is to demonstrate the kind of patients that are admitted to what might be considered a "middle-level" psychiatric facility, between field stations and the clearing company on the one hand, and the evac hospital or field hospital with the KO Team on the other hand. All the schizophrenic patients admitted during this period were eventually sent to the 93rd Evac Hospital and eventually evacuated from there. With exceptions of the few severely neurotic, severely depressed or severely anxious neurotic patients, the patients listed here as neurosis, situational reaction and combat exhaustion were admitted to the hospital by me. This was occasionally my procedure calculated to facilitate the evaluation. Many of these were patients from the Delta or from units out of town who could not be seen as outpatients. Also, some of them were admitted to be started on drugs. Now the patients with character disorders, chronic alcoholism and acute alcoholism were admitted by other people besides me to my service, and discharged by me as quickly as possible. I do not have a figure for the average length of stay down here but it was in the order of under 5 days. It was not substantially different for any particular diagnostic group.

On page three I have some numbers about where these patients came from. I think this will help to give you an idea of the complexity of evacuation channels in Vietnam and give you an idea of the fact that things really don't follow the traditional model so much in that, with certain exceptions, any medical facility tends to get patients from anywhere. As you see, I've got patients from battalion surgeons in the field, dispensaries in Saigon shipped to doctors off the coast, flight surgeons from aviation battalions in the Delta, and so on. Only two patients in the entire six months came in from clearing companies. These same proportions apply to my outpatient statistics for that period. Under the lower half of page three I have some miscellaneous comments about the patients admitted. Well, let's make the following additions. First of all, there was one successful suicide in a chronically depressed alcoholic, which, interestingly enough, generated two other outpatients who both were seen for some time. In one, the suicide of this sergeant precipitated a classical obsessional neurosis, while the other patient had a fairly severe transient anxiety reaction.

I'd like to add a couple of other things. From these 61 patients admitted, 8 had been previously psychiatrically hospitalized anywhere from 1 to 4 admissions and all of these hospitalizations had been before they came to Vietnam. In addition, another 17 of the 61 had had some kind of contact with a psychiatrist, ranging anywhere from one evaluation to extended outpatient therapy as a civilian before coming into the military. In all of these cases the previous psychiatric contact was before they came to Vietnam. I wasn't particularly conscious of this as I was seeing the patients over there, and I want to go into this in looking over my outpatients. It raises an interesting question about screening. I do not know what the baseline figures would be in this area. Even though these numbers are small and they're all from one facility, I wonder if the question is not raised here. Since these were patients who ended up in the hospital in Vietnam, perhaps attention should be paid particularly to previous psychiatric hospitalization and also outpatient contact as part of the screening process for deployment. I simply don't know what's being done along that line, and I would be interested to hear about it. Another fact I'd like to add concerning these inpatients is that there was in relation to their time in Vietnam, a small peak around 4 weeks in-country. But the largest group of

them had been in Vietnam about 5 months. I'm really not sure what this means; the time curve for outpatients at 3rd Field was studied by my predecessor there, Ed Huffman, and also by me; and most of the outpatients come in around 4 to 6 weeks in-country.

Finally, on the back page, there are some numbers about inpatient consults. These are patients referred to me during the six-month period by the medical and surgical services. What I mean by this is that initially the patient had been admitted for some sort of physical symptoms or some apparently organic problem. After the medical or surgical work up was completed and I saw the patient it was clear that it was a psychosomatic problem or a straight psychiatric problem that had been the reason for his admission into the hospital. This was the case in 12 out of 33 of the patients and in 18 out of the 33 it turned out that the psychiatric problem was either not existent or was incidental to what they had been admitted to the hospital for. Three of the patients were diagnostic problems who were subsequently evacuated from the country by the medical or surgical services for further work up. In going over these statistics, I found that I had recorded none of these 12 patients as psychiatric admissions. I remembered sometime early after arriving in Vietnam to monitor the discharges from other services in the hospital particularly for psychosomatic problems. I bring this up now because I suspect that this may be happening at other facilities and may be the experience of other psychiatrists besides myself. There may be in this area a certain percentage of covert psychiatric casualties. In the case of this six-month period at 3rd Field these 12 patients represent about 18 percent of the psychiatric admissions. The numbers refer only to the 12 consults whose admission was determined by psychiatric problems, and I don't think they need any particular explanation at this point.

I'd like to make a few general comments about the outpatients seen. Clinically the group of 300 or so outpatients fit closely with the kinds of problems described by Dr. Byrdy with the exception, of course, that in my situation the percentage of combat troops was only about 20 percent. Transient situational reactions were predominant. In addition, I saw a goodly number, probably around 70 or 80, out of this group of support troops who clearly had a passive dependent character and who had an anxiety syndrome in 4 to 6 weeks after they arrived in Vietnam. It appeared in most cases that these individuals were reacting to a combination of the stress of being there and particularly of the heavy work load which many of them had--12, 14, or 16 hours a day, 7 days a week. A combination of this kind of stress and the separation from their mothers, or their wives toward whom they related as a child to a mother. In general I found them to be eminently treatable. These were passive dependent characters who came to see the psychiatrist largely because of their discomfort, not because of somebody's dissatisfaction with their behavior. Some of them were treated with a combination of one or two interviews and thoroughly large doses of Librium which I used quite regularly and found extremely effective with this kind of person.

Well, I'd like to move on to some other topics about which I want to comment just briefly and perhaps about which we can talk more in the discussion. During the six-month period I saw 50 of the AR 635-212 cases, almost all of whom were from the Saigon area. It's interesting to compare this with my only other experience in the military, which has been at Fort Dix since I returned. It's interesting to compare the kinds of behavior patterns of administrative cases we see there with these 50 in Saigon. The majority of these 50 in Saigon had engaged in overtly hostile behavior. Instead of passive aggression a lot of it was aggressive aggression, and consisted of either directing repeated incidents of either verbal abuse toward superiors or all-out physical assault on superiors, usually while armed and often appearing with some degree of intoxication, but not always. I'm interested in the group and I'm trying to study my records on them. I don't have much of an idea of what they were like psychologically. In general, they had been in the service for a while, were RA and had a reasonable record as far as I could determine with reference to disciplinary problems and general performance before they came to Vietnam. Furthermore in the large majority of them there was a clear-cut absence of, or an infrequent presence of, the father's role in their development. I guess this is a common feature in certain groups of behavioral cases anyway. I had the impression there was something about being in Vietnam, something about the situation, something about the war, something about the invitation to violence, which was implied by the contract that had really changed the course of their relationship with the military.

I'd like to mention now something about terrorism. During the period 1 April to 30 September three major terrorist incidents occurred in Saigon—two mortar attacks in the Tan Son Nhut area, one in April and one in August, and the plastic explosion at the Victor BOQ in downtown Saigon in April. Additionally, the period April through June was relatively significant by reason of agitation by Buddhist groups and agitation by Catholic groups. In general the city was more tense during this three month period than it was any other time I was there. This resulted in an increase in the usual level of minor terrorist incidents—grenades thrown in jeeps, occasional sniping, burning of vehicles and so on. However, throughout this entire period only one patient was admitted to either hospital in Saigon in which the psychiatric syndrome was attributable to experience with a terrorist incident. This was a captain who had a transient psychotic reaction following the Victory blast and who was admitted to 17th Field Hospital for a few days. He cleared up quite rapidly. I saw two other patients myself during this time whose problems were in part attributable to terrorist activity—one fellow who had been chronically anxious for six months during his residence somewhere down in the Delta and who had an exacerbation of this just as he was about to return home. Shortly after arriving in Vietnam the other had been sniped at outside the Tan Son Nhut gate; it isn't clear by whom. He was upset about this. It seems clear that at least during the period I'm talking about there was really no direct connection between psychiatric admissions or psychiatric outpatient visits and terrorism. Bill Kenny did a questionnaire study of the officers at the Victory BOQ in April and found that a large majority of those near the blast reported subjectively experiencing anxiety and some preoccupation with the blast, all the usual symptoms of a mild traumatic state, for about two weeks afterwards. Interestingly, I made the same kind of observations in a more informal way. I observed the 3rd Field Hospital staff following the two mortarings at Tan Son Nhut. It was a jumpy one or two weeks afterwards with an increase in alcohol intake and so on. I'm not sure what the experience of others in the country has been, perhaps we can get into this later, but I think it's an important point that the terrorist activity of the VC has not generated any significant clinical problems as far as we're concerned.

I would like to close with a few brief and probably not very profound comments about the whole question of the war and its relationship to our work over there. I found that I've been asked many times what kind of patients does one see, what kind of problems does one see in relation to the political ambiguities of the war, the dissension of this country about it, and so on. Is there any connection? Does this seem to be a problem? Do the ambiguities of the war seem to be a problem for the soldiers? The answer to this is very simply, "No." I did not see single patient in whom I felt that any kind of conflict about the war on any level was primary in precipitating his visits to me or his admission to the hospital. A few patients happened also to be preoccupied with the question of the war and the politics involved, etc. In one way or another many patients and personnel, probably representing about the same proportion as that which one would find in the general public in this country, were less than enthusiastic about our national effort there. But again, this seemed to have no connection, really, with what was troubling them psychiatrically.

[*Reference is made in the proceedings to an incident in which one of Captain Blank's patients brought a grenade into his office and exploded it after warning Captain Blank to leave. The patient sustained some frontal lobe damage but lived, and Captain Blank was uninjured.*]

In: Johnson AW Jr, Bowman JA, Byrdy HS, Blank AS Jr. Panel discussion: Army psychiatry in Vietnam. In: Jones FD, ed. *Proceedings: Social and Preventive Psychiatry Course, 1967*. Washington DC: Government Printing Office; 1968:41-76. [See also Alexandria, VA: Defense Documentation Center (Document AD No. 950-058, 1980).]

Appendix 11 RECENT EXPERIENCES IN COMBAT PSYCHIATRY IN VIETNAM

UNPUBLISHED PAPER: JOHN A BOWMAN, MAJOR, MEDICAL CORPS
935TH NEUROPSYCHIATRIC MEDICAL SPECIALTY DETACHMENT

This paper (unpublished) provides an overview of the experiences of the 935th Neuropsychiatric Medical Specialty Detachment (KO), which was attached to the 93rd Evacuation Hospital on the Long Binh post 20 miles northeast of Saigon. It was written by its first commander, Major John A Bowman, Medical Corps, who was Army-trained in psychiatry, and spans between January 1966, when the 935th first deployed in Vietnam, and the following June. Bowman wrote this soon after he returned to the United States after completing his assignment in Vietnam. This material is published with the expressed permission of the author. Minor edits have been applied to the original.

The author, a Regular Army psychiatrist, served in Viet Nam from December 1965 to November 1966 as the Commanding Officer of the Psychiatry and Neurology Treatment and Evacuation Center [The 935th Medical Detachment (KO)]. This center was composed of a professional complement of three psychiatrists, one neurologist, two social workers, one clinical psychologist, and one male psychiatric nurse. Twelve to 15 enlisted men of various training, that is, social work specialists, clinical psychology technicians, and neuropsychiatric specialists, were members of the KO Team, thereby totaling 20 to 23 men.

The mission of the KO Team was to establish a center where soldiers in Viet Nam could receive psychiatric and neurological consultation and treatment for up to 30 days as inpatients, if necessary, prior to evacuation to the continental United States [CONUS] or return to duty. The KO Team served as the evacuation center for all Army psychiatry and neurology casualties in Viet Nam. To accomplish this mission the team was assigned to the 93rd Evacuation Hospital and functioned in Quonset buildings in an area 20 miles northeast of Saigon in close proximity to the "D" War Zone. A second function or mission soon became to establish an MHCS [mental hygiene consultation service] type facility for the many thousands of soldiers in the surrounding area who had no psychiatric services organic to their respective units. The combat units the KO team provided care for were the 25th Infantry Division, the 1st Infantry Division, the 1st Cavalry Division (Airmobile), and the 173d Airborne Brigade of the 101st Airborne Division. These were primarily Regular Army professional soldiers who were well motivated and skillfully led.

The purpose of this paper is to present a few of the experiences of the Combat Psychiatry Team (KO) operating in Viet Nam. The 935th Medical Detachment (KO) was activated at Valley Forge General Hospital in October 1965 and trained as a unit for combat before overseas deployment on 29 November 1965. Arriving in December 1965, the team became operational in January 1966. The statistics presented herein represent the six-month period from January through June 1966. This period was characterized by mass movements of personnel into Viet Nam and also by many search-and-destroy type combat missions, both of which may account for monthly variations in the psychiatry and neurology [P&N] morbidity reports. The data and statistics, therefore, are presented to reflect the type and amount of work accomplished, and we do not attempt to interpret the monthly fluctuations of various diagnostic categories or the total number of referrals evaluated. Overall it can be said that we encountered a very low rate of combat exhaustion and an increase in character and behavioral disorders as time progressed.

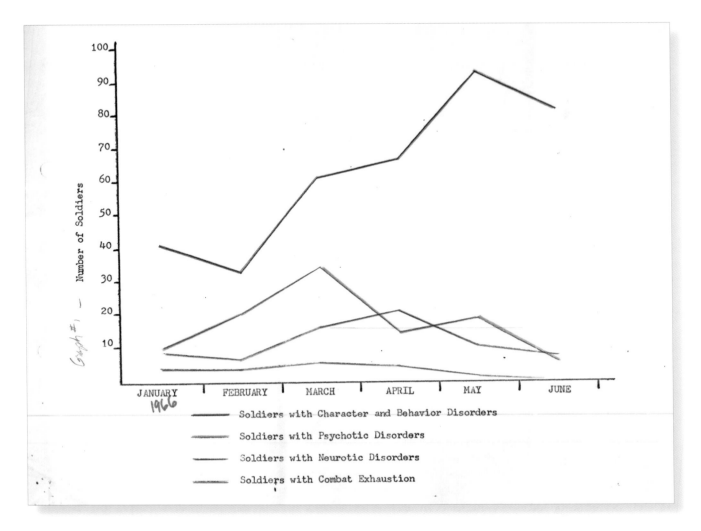

The type of psychiatric referrals seen in Viet Nam deserve special consideration. There were, of course, a small number of soldiers, less than 5% of all referrals, who presented with a well defined psychosis, usually a paranoid schizophrenic or a manic depressive reaction, and who presented no diagnostic or dispositional problem. In contrast to World War II or the Korean Conflict, combat exhaustion was rarely seen, and represented less than 2% of all referrals. [The author uses two criteria in the diagnosis of combat exhaustion: (1) actual exposure to combat, ie, under hostile fire; and (2) the presence of fatigue, whether produced by physical causes such as exertion, heat, dehydration diarrhea, and loss of sleep, or by psychological causes such as anxiety and insomnia.] Combat exhaustion was rarely seen because combat was usually short-lived as the VC [Viet Cong guerrillas] did not choose to "stand and fight" very often; adequate food and rest were usually available to our troops. Nevertheless, a tremendous psychological stress was always present, as no area was considered safe from ambush, terrorist activities, or sniper fire. Exhaustion states, however, were usually secondary to the extreme heat, dehydration, diarrhea, and toxic diseases. Uncomplicated cases of combat fatigue were usually treated at the battalion aid station and few were returned to the P&N Center. A high morale among the combat troops also contributed to the low rate of combat exhaustion and more generally to a low P&N casualty rate. Otherwise, the critical time period between the time a soldier arrived in Viet Nam and the time he was first seen for psychiatric evaluation peaked at 1–2 months. Of 491 soldiers referred for evaluation, it was our prediction that a very high percentage of high school dropouts would be referred for administrative separation, but this did not prove true. Only about

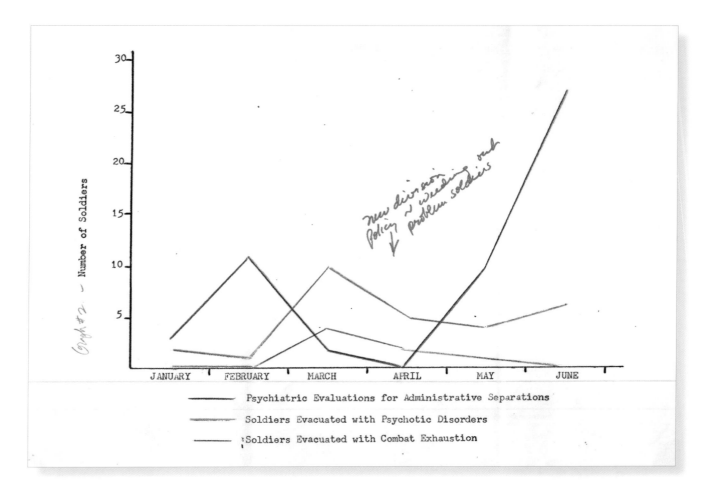

31% of the high school dropouts referred to the P&N Clinic were referred for administrative separations, and the remaining 69% of the high school dropouts were referred for other reasons.

The majority of soldiers referred to the KO Team presented either behavioral difficulties or somatic complaints of a specific nature. The somatic complaint was one that usually temporarily removed the soldier from the stresses he was experiencing in an honorable way, [that is], the complaint or symptom did not cause him to receive an Art. XV or courts-martial. For example, a soldier on guard duty may be referred with symptoms of narcolepsy or sleep-walking.
A soldier on a search-and-destroy mission where silence was sometimes life-saving may present symptoms of sleep-talking or nightmares in which he would shout out, thus endangering his whole unit. The symptom, therefore, not only rendered the soldier ineffective but also sometimes even made him a liability to his unit.

We wish to discuss in detail some of the symptoms seen in soldiers under stress in the combat zone in Viet Nam. For the sake of brevity and clarity the symptoms most often encountered in the soldier under stress in Viet Nam are divided into two categories: symptoms seen in nonwounded soldiers and symptoms seen in wounded soldiers. The symptoms are not listed in order of prevalence.

A. Stress Symptoms Seen in Nonwounded Soldiers:
    1. Somnambulism.
    2. Anxiety dreams with talking or shouting.
    3. Syncope and vertigo.
    4. "Narcolepsy" like complaints.
    5. "Seizures"—not proved to be grand mal or petit mal.
    6. Musculoskeletal type complaints, such as low back pain where the orthopedic examination is negative.

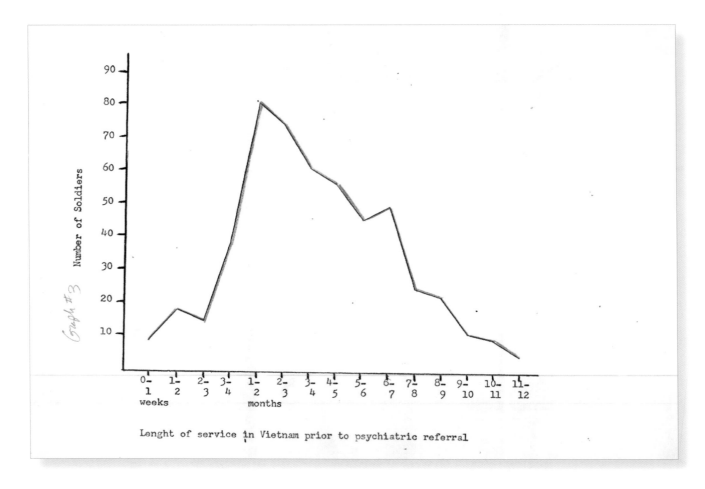

Graph #3

Lenght of service in Vietnam prior to psychiatric referral

7. Amnesia, especially following exposure to explosions (mortar, artillery, or mines) but having no concussion.
8. Blurred vision—when the ophthalmologist can find no visual defects.
9. Stuttering, especially following exposure to loud noises or automatic weapons fire.
10. "Aphonias" or other speech disturbances, such as speaking with a whisper.
11. Persistent nausea or abdominal pain in which no GI [gastrointestinal] disease could be demonstrated by the internal medicine service.
12. Headaches, atypical but severe, persistent and disabling, most often diagnosed as "tension headache."
13. Loss of hearing—in which ENT [ear, nose, and throat] examination could find no hearing loss.

B. Stress Symptoms Seen in Wounded Soldiers—The disabling symptoms of wounded soldiers usually developed after hospitalization, or if present

when hospitalized, the symptoms persisted or became more severe, requiring neuropsychiatric consultation:
1. Persistent anxiety dreams.
2. Pain in wounded extremity following complete healing.
3. Sensory defects in which the patient claimed hypesthesia and weakness of an extremity but the neurological examination was negative.

There was a very close liaison between the psychiatric staff and the medical and surgical specialties, since we both lived in one BOQ and worked together in the same clinic building. Consultations were frequently accomplished on an immediate and informal level, but even formal consultations were completed in 24–48 hours. There was a standard operating procedure for handling these psychiatric referrals. The soldier's symptoms were considered real by both the referring physician and psychiatrist. A physical examination and the appropriate X-rays and lab studies were ordered

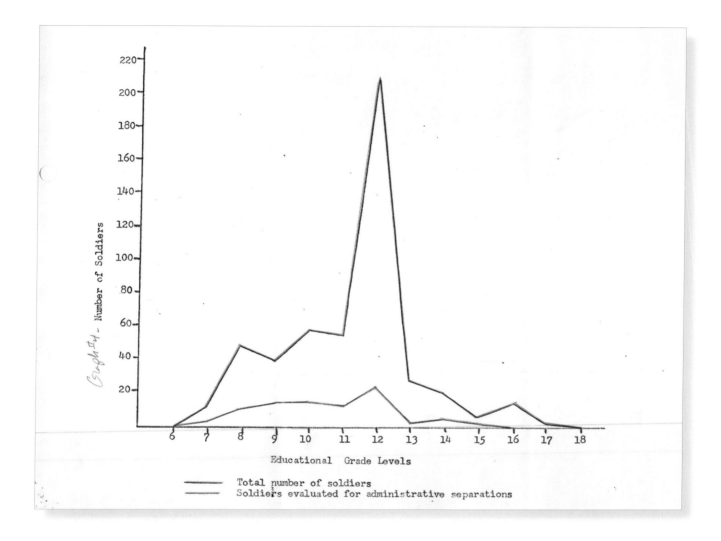

when necessary. When the referring physician was sure there was no organic etiology to the complaint, the soldier was directly questioned about his feelings about returning to duty (after he had been reassured there was no organic illness present). Frequently the soldier/patient felt relieved to know that "nothing serious was wrong" and desired to return to his unit. Occasionally the soldier ventilated concern to the nurse or doctor about returning to duty. In refractory cases or when tranquilizers were thought necessary, the physician referred the soldier for psychiatric evaluation. The soldier was allowed to ventilate feelings, especially fear of death or fear of derangement [sic] of his body image, but the contract between the consultant (psychiatrist/social worker), the consultee (soldier), and the referring agency (CO [commanding officer] or physician) was well-defined in one respect: The presenting symptom

would not be allowed to be used as a lever [for the soldier] to be relieved from duty or evacuated from Viet Nam. It took repeated contacts with the referring agencies by the KO Team personnel to keep the above communication concerning the intent of the consultation intact. The KO Team personnel would work to the best of their abilities to help the soldier with his problem, but the presenting symptom was rarely considered sufficient reason to evacuate the soldier from Viet Nam unless, of course, upon evaluation the soldier proved to be frankly psychotic. In most cases the soldiers gave up their symptoms and returned to duty asymptomatic or with less severity of symptoms. There were few recurrences. Occasionally mild sedatives were used, but tranquilizers were seldom prescribed. It was the staff's feeling that tranquilizers would tend to reinforce the soldier's concept of being ill.

Occasionally a soldier asked forthrightly to be relieved from combat because he was "too nervous." Some were vehement and demanding, some tearful, some agitated, and some emotionally labile. Too, some pleaded to be given a noncombatant assignment (often the request was to be a medic and work in the hospital). The staff did not allow evacuations from the combat zone or transfers within the combat zone unless it was medically indicated or militarily feasible. Due to our rigidity on evacuation policy our colleagues in the BOQ [bachelor officers' quarters] frequently referred to us as "tough guys" and whimsical but pointed remarks about "Catch 22" were aimed in our direction.

Indeed it was difficult to return to duty a soldier who had seen considerable combat, or had been wounded, or a soldier who had seen his best friend killed. After a period of grief, catharsis, or rest we found many of the soldiers ready for duty. In spite of mild to moderate anxiety, the soldiers for the most part did function effectively when returned. Frequently the members of the KO Team turned to each other for support when we returned a soldier to duty who may have narrowly escaped death or injury and was now reluctant to go back to combat. Without our own intra-group support a firm policy on evacuation could not have existed.

Another large group of referrals to the outpatient clinic were soldiers whose behavioral difficulties led to punitive or administrative action. The three most frequent behavioral problems were:

1. frequent or repeated AWOLs [absence without leave];
2. regressive behavior: excessive drinking, loss of pride in personal appearance; and
3. aggressive behavior: indiscriminate firing of weapons, insubordination, assault, and threats of violence to NCOs [noncommissioned officers] and commissioned officers.

In most of these administrative referrals the soldier usually acknowledged that he wanted either out of the unit or out of the Army. After a unit command consultation we decided whether to recommend administrative separation or to attempt further counseling with the consultee.

Consideration must be given to our administrative separation policies. Certain behaviors that would have been punished in CONUS were often condoned in combat, such as a soldier's being unshaven or having a dirty uniform or unpolished boots; one can understand this after experiencing the monsoon season in Viet Nam.

Most referrals to the P&N Clinic for administrative separation resulted from AWOL, insubordination, and aggressive or regressive behavior. The CO's lament was, "I have to fight a war. I am too busy with plans for our next operation to spend time with soldiers who don't work for me." The CO's point was reasonable; he really needed his time for fighting the war. The Commanders of support and logistical troops, however, did have more time to work with their problem soldiers and the MHCS representative. The marked increase of 208–209 cases in May and June 1966 was first thought to reflect the large numbers of replacements who had been drafted and sent to the Republic of Viet Nam. Further evaluation suggested that it represented a change in command policy in one of the local large tactical units. The policy in essence became to weed out any soldiers who got into difficulty [that] came to the attention of command.

During the first six months of 1966 we averaged about 300 referrals per month and a daily inpatient census of 10–12 patients. The therapeutic approach to hospitalized soldiers on the psychiatric ward included brief psychotherapy, both ventilative and supportive, tranquilizing drugs, and most important, the use of the milieu principle. Soldiers were admitted, given clean clothing, a shower, a warm meal, and sedation when appropriate. The soldier/patient was expected to keep his area clean and to assist ward personnel in maintaining an orderly ward. For example, the soldier/patient washed windows and policed the ward area inside and out. A patient NCOIC [noncommissioned officer in charge] was appointed to direct ward details and to manage the "buddy" system. The soldiers helped each other and exerted controls on their own behavior. The soldier not considered well enough to be off the ward alone was assisted by a convalescent patient to the mess hall, latrine, shower, or Red Cross lounge. Soldier/patients were required to stand for ward rounds and to display the same military courtesy to their attending physician that they would to their commanding officer. At all times the soldier was reminded that he was a part of the US Army in a combat situation and was expected to behave accordingly.

The practical reality in Vietnam was that the entire country was a hostile area, there were no traditional "front lines," and there were great distances between tactical units and hospital facilities. However, the goal of maintaining unit identity was generally feasible because of the helicopter. When a soldier was admitted to our psychiatric ward at the 935th, we requested the parent unit to make regular visits to him, to bring him his mail, and to pay him on the ward. The line commanders well understood the need to maintain contact with their men in the hospital and cooperated to the fullest with our visitation program. No soldier, therefore, could feel lost or separated from his unit when hospitalized, even though his unit was 250 miles away. The use of the above principles of milieu therapy, the "buddy" system, and frequent unit contacts greatly decreased the amount of acting-out behavior, and consequently the number of soldiers requiring medical evacuation was reduced. Thus in effect, we were able to apply the principles of combat psychiatry (eg, treating the soldier as close to the combat area as possible and returning him to duty as soon as possible were effectively applied) and it was possible to return to duty about 90% of all hospitalized soldiers referred to the Psychiatry and Neurology Treatment and Evacuation Center (935th KO team).

Appendix 12 INTERESTING REACTION TYPES ENCOUNTERED IN A WAR ZONE

UNPUBLISHED PAPER: CAPTAIN H SPENCER BLOCH (MD)
DIRECTOR OF THE PSYCHIATRY AND NEUROLOGY INPATIENT SERVICE
935TH PSYCHIATRIC DETACHMENT (AUGUST 1967–1968)

Although the main interest in orientation of military psychiatry since WWII [World War II] has been in the direction of community psychiatry, nevertheless it is probable that the most valuable and lasting contributions of psychiatrists in the military to understanding of psychological processes has come from the clinical studies from WWII. Works such as Grinker and Spiegel's *Men Under Stress* remain as comprehensive classics of reaction types and treatment of the effects of stress and strain on men. In fact, in the current war zone [Vietnam] psychiatrists are hard-pressed to find psychiatric casualty types which were not reported in *Men Under Stress*. Nevertheless, in an overview of a large number of psychiatric casualties seen and treated in Vietnam, certain reaction patterns or types of response to stress were noted that may help to elucidate further our understanding of human psychodynamics. Not withstanding that distinction made by Grinker and Spiegel between certain types of reactions which are seen in ground forces and are not seen in personnel who fly, one has the impression comparing present day material with that seen during WW II of an increasing tendency towards reaction patterns which capitalize upon essentially alloplastic defensive adaptational techniques as opposed to autoplastic ones. Certainly a large number of psychosomatic and psychophysiological responses, as well as anxiety states, are seen in Vietnam today. Nevertheless, one is impressed by the degree to which externalizing defenses and the paranoid positions are adopted in setting of stress there. The degree to which this is related to the nature of the stresses of people serving on the ground as opposed to the degree to which it may reflect alterations in personality structure are as yet unanswered questions. In another recent communication an overview of army Clinical psychiatry in Vietnam was presented with some representative case histories that were included to convey a spectrum of the nature of hospitalized psychiatric patients seen there. This paper presents several case histories which serve as prototypes of certain reaction patterns seen in Vietnam. The cases chosen are ones which demonstrate the point to be made quite graphically and are presented with illustrating the kind of phenomena that could be frequently seen in other patients in which these presenting symptomatology was not as dramatic or graphic. The purpose in presenting these cases is to add further data to our understanding of human response to stress and strain.

THE CONCEPT OF INFANTILE REGRESSION

Case #1: A 20 year-old single PFC rifleman with 13 months active duty service and 8 months in Vietnam, was apparently sitting on guard duty with his combat unit in the field one night. The unit was not actively engaged in fighting. At that time he was noted by his companions to become kind of "crazy." That is, he became confused, disoriented, unable to answer questions coherently, and was allegedly hallucinating, though this was not described in the referral note. No precipitant was discernible. He was taken to the medical clearing station and kept there overnight. The next morning he was mute and was flown to the psychiatric ward which was about 20 minutes away. He was admitted at that point, and on admission he was sucking his thumb constantly and alternately nodding and shaking his head. He seemed bewildered and appeared frightened. He would not talk initially and neither gentle nor forceful efforts by the ward corpsmen induced him to stop sucking his thumb, which he did incessantly. When [his] sadness was [confronted] he burst into tears and said in baby talk that his mommy had told him that his father was dead and that now he wanted to see his brother. Later he said "bumble bees sting . . . today." And he pointed to his ankle around which a bandage was wrapped and under which was found no evidence of any sting or other injury. The type of interest that he seemed to manifest in this and other body parts suggested that his body was very much hypercathected. His only other activity was to awkwardly write a few words on paper with his left hand in response to questions (for example his home of residence and "no" was written in response to questions about the presence of any psychotic manifestations in his thinking). All the while he sucked his right thumb.

Physical examination was within normal limits and he was put to sleep with Thorazine for approximately 24 hours after being told that he would be better when he awoke. Upon awakening he was asymptomatic and was progressively mobilized in the ward milieu during the second 24 hours of the hospital stay. He remained completely amnesic for the episode and wondered what had happened. He denied any drug usage, confirmed the fact that his father had been killed by an automobile when he was very young and that he did have one brother. He was right handed. He was returned to full duty at the beginning of his third hospital day and never again seen at the psychiatric facility.

Comment: Although there is a paucity of anamnestic material available in this case, it is included because it demonstrates so clearly reversion to literal infantile behavior and attitudes in a classic manner, presumably related to some internal or externally perceived distress. More frequently reversion to infantile or child-like attitude was more prominent1y viewed in stress situations than reversion to concomitant behavior, though that was also seen. The next case gives a demonstration of this latter point.

Case #2: Was a 27-year old Army physician, a Captain, who had been a battalion surgeon with 4 months of active duty service and 2 months in Vietnam. He was referred to the psychiatric ward by his division Psychiatrist after he had developed self-referential ideas and perhaps loosely formed, delusional, ideations in the setting of intensified fears of bodily injury or death.

He was the son of a meat cutter and dominating mother who he claimed always wanted him to achieve more. He was raised in lower middleclass Jewish surroundings in an urban area. He recalled a long-standing history of fears in his childhood including of dogs (he would cross the Street to avoid them), fears when showering in the bathroom with soap in his eyes (that someone would come in and hurt him), consciously recalled fears of injury to his penis, fears of going into his room at night (he would check under the bed in the dark), feeling that it was crazy but "I couldn't help it." He described a relative social isolation during his growing and college and medical school years in response to his fears. Despite this he remained conscientious, eager to always do a good job, and competent in his work as a physician. He was fearful about his assignment to Vietnam, and his fears became markedly activated with some realistic basis when he was assigned as a battalion surgeon. To combat extreme anxiety while he served in that capacity he took morphine once and 30–40 Librium on another occasion for insomnia and anxiety. He was hospitalized briefly then and then put to work in a clearing company hospital where he functioned reasonably well. He was then returned to his own battalion headquarters where he worked in a medical company and did well for several days. However, then, in a setting of having to go out into civilian villages with the Med Cap Team plus with the death of another battalion surgeon by hostile fire, his fears increased markedly, not only that he was going to be injured or killed, but that the people around him in command were trying to kill him by making him go out into the field this way. He began to think that a dream he had had of having communicated with God was, in fact, true; that he had to stop the war by no longer working and by letting the world know "what was really happening" in Vietnam. Also, as noted, he felt that people were trying to get him killed. In this setting he was referred to the psychiatric ward.

At admission he was frightened, sullen, withdrawn, suspicious, and thought he had been betrayed by people who had sent him there. He was not psychotic but operating from a stance of childish or infantile regression to the point of projecting and externalizing the basis of his distress. Over the course of the next several days, intensive individual psychotherapy was undertaken wherein he was urged to review his present day fears in light of his long-standing concerns about bodily injury or death. He described the intensity of his fright in his unit and his concomitant feeling of hopelessness. He specifically related to the fact that he could do nothing about his fear, could trust no one, in fact, he could not even trust himself at that point. Despite the seemingly overwhelming quality of his desire and necessity of fleeing the situation and adopting the paranoid defense, the part of himself that really stated in a very small voice that he really wanted to do a good job and didn't like to be the way he was, was not only heard by the therapeutic personnel but implicitly fostered, acknowledged, agreed with, and supported at the same time the intensity of his fears were accepted by the psychiatrist. After these clarifications had been made in an attempt to decondition his fear of not being able to control himself, that is, not be able to control his reaction (fear), he was readily mobilized to work in the hospital area as a physician and subsequently assigned to another hospital where he completed his tour of duty in an exemplary manner. At times of imminent danger from enemy attack he would contact the psychiatrist by mail it to briefly express his fears as well as his hopes of continuing to do a good job—which he did.

Comment: This case illustrates an important point, both I think in understanding and in management of reactions to stress. The presenting phenomenology in the case, and the impetus from the man's unit, was that he was experiencing a significant paranoid reaction, perhaps paranoid schizophrenia and that he should be evacuated from the war zone. Such a disposition and label would probably have influenced significantly and adversely this man's future career, his feelings about himself, and potentially his life.

When the phenomena were viewed as a kind of reversion to a type of infantile attitude at a time of fright, treated that way—as a child blaming others because he could not cope with the intensity of his fear—then the patient was readily able to reconstitute to his premorbid level of functioning and gain himself a modicum of self-esteem in the process. Needless to say, having the motivation to go on and conduct oneself appropriately and beneficially is important in the success of this type of management. But focusing back on the psychodynamic factors involved, this case shows reversion to infantile attitudes with concomitant behavior emerging in response to stress. Never quite disorganized, though becoming that way, and more ominous than the type of symptoms exhibited in case #1, because our general thinking is that the paranoid defense is more ominous than the hysterical one. This may or may not be true as we will see in the next case.

Case #3. I first saw JM, a 21 y.o., single, negro Pfc who worked as a stock clerk in a supply and service company (13 months in the Army and 8 months in RVN) when he was transferred to us from a surgical hospital following an overnight admission for "agitated, combative, and unmanageable behavior." He was reported by the referring physician (not a psychiatrist) to be a marijuana user, and it was alleged that he had smoked pot that evening and had developed delusions of death and persecution. He was unresponsive, sullen, and unwilling or unable to communicate when admitted to the surgical hospital. He was given Thorazine and Seconal overnight and transferred to us the next day. An MP [military police] escort was required in transit.

He was lethargic and drowsy when admitted to our ward, but he could be aroused quite readily and was oriented, a little defensive, but cooperative. When interviewed after the effects of the sedation had worn off, he adamantly denied recent or past marijuana usage. He explained his recent symptoms as a "nervous breakdown", though he professed amnesia for the events leading up to his hospitalization. He claimed that 3 weeks earlier while sitting tower guard with another EM [enlisted man] he had heard voices of other members of his family, though he couldn't distinguish what they were saying. These voices had not recurred but subsequent to hearing them he had experienced the onset of a generalized mistrust of people plus a pervasive suspiciousness with referential ideation but apparently no true delusions.

Background information was not particularly revealing, though he was guarded in imparting biographical data. He was the 4th of 5 children born to a couple who raised him, though 2 of his sisters were raised by a grandmother. He described himself as extroverted though moody during his growing years. He denied neurotic traits or difficulty in his interpersonal relationships. He had spent 8 months in reform school, allegedly for his first offense (breaking and entering). Upon graduation from high school he held one job in a knitting mill for 3 years before being drafted. He had two Article 15's during basic training when he wanted to get out of the service; however, after deciding to fulfill his service obligation he had no further administrative actions against him.

During his next two days in the hospital he remained asymptomatic without evidence of psychosis or severe neurosis. He eventually suggested that the episode resulted from a buildup of feelings of boredom and frustration associated with the routine, repetitious, and confining nature of his job in supply and his life in Tay Ninh. He said that he wanted out of the Army and to go home. He was discharged and went to the 90th Replacement Battalion to await transportation to his company area, only to be brought into our Emergency Room late the same night by MPs. He had been assaultive at the 90th Replacement Battalion and had been found wandering around looking for a certain buddy. The following morning he was asymptomatic and indicated that he had been drinking the night before, though he denied the use of marijuana. He was discharged and returned to his unit. The next day he was sent from the same surgical hospital with a note indicating that he had a 3–4 week history of bizarre behavior, hallucinations and delusions, and aggressive behavior. These symptoms included seeing himself as dead and being mourned by his family, praying at the feet of his buddy, thinking that his buddy was God, and imagining that his friends were physically attacking him and trying to kill him. The referring physician indicated that he was not fit to serve in an area where weapons were available. The KO team psychiatrist who admitted him from the clinic noted the man to be "slightly confused, rather loose and concrete, oriented, reading the Bible, and checking his penis while expressing, fears

of losing his "nature." However, once again his ward behavior was completely unremarkable except for a running dialogue he held with several other Negro patients. This involved having sold his soul to the Devil. This dialogue seemed primarily in the service of provoking another patient who was very much obsessed with good and evil as personified by God and the Devil. A diagnostic\therapeutic trial of Thorazine was begun (75mg q.i.d.) but PFC JM promptly became somnolent on this relatively small dose, so it was discontinued. A full battery of psychological testing was performed and resulted in perhaps the most normal profile we have seen in a ward patient. There was evidence of sociopathic and hypomanic features in his personality but no suggestion of psychosis.

After 6 days he was returned to duty with a certificate clearing him for administrative action. Because the concern of the referring physicians was justifiable it was recommended that the EM see the neighborhood division psychiatrist if necessary in the future, so that symptoms could be observed at their source. This had been suggested twice previously.

Apparently the next night the EM was found strangling a buddy in his bunk. He was admitted to a division clearing station facility, claiming not to remember what had happened. However, upon questioning he told a corpsman that he had been strangling another man. A few minutes later a former KO team psychiatrist who had known the patient on our ward before he joined the division came by, recognized the patient, and asked him what had happened. The patient avowed vehemently that he didn't know and couldn't recall. When confronted with the fact that he had just told a corpsman about trying to strangle a friend he became defensive and claimed that the corpsman had made it all up. The patient was returned to his unit for administrative action and placed in the stockade where he has presented no problem, although he did visit the Social Work Officer there once to express concerns about the Devil. The defense lawyer for the case claims that everyone involved, including the prosecuting attorney, is convinced that this man is mentally deranged, and they are all loathe to try the case in a Court Martial.

Comment: Let me say at the outset of my discussion that I don't know what this man's diagnosis is. It's not my intent to try to convince you one way or the other about it. The case is complicated by the fact that he may well have been a marijuana user. But I present it because it illustrates dramatically the type of patient that causes us so much trouble in diagnosis and disposition. I will make some general observations about them, some dynamic speculations, and a few comments about my experience in managing them.

From several cases that we've seen I have noted:
1) Many if not most of these men are Negro.
2) They almost always present as behavioral problems in their units of gradual, rather than acute, onset. This is often in the form of intransigent, disobedient, or resistive behavior. They either have been violent or their units fear aggressive outbursts from them.
3) Hallucinatory or delusional phenomena, when present, usually involve a communication with God and have some religious significance related to Good and Evil. Interestingly enough, when two or more of these types are on our ward at the same time they seem to understand these symptoms in each other without surprise or difficulty.
4) In interviewing them the primary psychotic-type manifestation in their thinking is the prominent use of projection as defense mechanism in conjunction with their anger. This projection is rarely well-organized; rather is pervasive and not accompanied by a great deal of denial. It does not have a bizarre quality. Rather, it appears to be an accentuation of a preexisting character trait, or more accurately the emergence in more vivid form of a latent character trait which has been mobilized under stress.

To conceptualize, I think that we are dealing with a group of action-oriented young men whose usual style for handling tension and frustration is discharge through physical activity. Their frustration tolerance is low, depression is not well-tolerated, and in civilian life both aggressive and sexual tensions are dissipated in the streets, so to speak.

Most of them are in non-combatant jobs, and their tension has at least three sources:
1) The tedium and boredom in their work without sufficient diversionary opportunities,
2) The ever-present fear of death, and particularly of mutilation, that is experienced by everyone in the combat zone,

3) The crowded, all-male living conditions, which predispose to activation of adolescent homosexual concerns.

Their psychological structure has little resiliency and few outlets for coping with these tensions other than discharge of them, and this is limited by the confining aspects of military structure. In this setting projection emerges as an adaptational mechanism to accommodate the pressure from the upsurge of these instinctual tensions. At this point they are often referred to psychiatric sources.

I do not feel that these men are borderline characters. They don't demonstrate any particular fluidity of defenses with a tendency to utilize a variety of defense mechanisms to accommodate the stress of everyday living. Nor do they usually show a typical pattern of psychotic regression under stress. Rather these men use projection to handle their anger and frustration, and any behavioral outbursts don't stem from the projection as much as from feelings of narcissistic entitlement to discharge their tension.

Nor do I think that these people are experiencing one of the forms of transient infantile regression seen quite frequently here. This latter group usually responds dramatically to a 24–48 hour period of sleep treatment with Thorazine.

In approaching these potential patients I suggest diagnosing their projection first; is it evidence of severe regression which they can't handle, or is it a less ominous character trait? Next, in as fearless a way as possible, confront the aggression to determine its relative danger. Then consider a brief (1-2 day) trial of Thorazine, keeping the man in his company area or at the division level if his unit is very scared of him, treating him similar to a combat reaction but using Thorazine in an attempt to leech out some of the anger. I believe that maintaining the expectation that the man perform his duties or take the administrative consequences is vital; for there are two dangers: (1) The first is that the man receives the communication that his sick behavior has tangible rewards. This motivates secondary-gain factors which perpetuate his symptoms. (2) The other danger is that the man receives the communication from us that he is in fact dangerous. That is—that he has been relieved of his responsibilities because he is a feared person. Such a message causes these men to unconsciously become frightened of their own uncontrollability, and they get worse (via panic). I feel that we have a more difficult time reconstituting them than workers at a more forward echelon, and I urge that vigorous but short-lived treatment always be tried before sending this type patient rearward to us. Once again, I present this material, not as a definitive explanation, but as observations and temporary conclusions for your consideration as we try to find the most effective ways of dealing with these difficult problems in diagnosis and management.

Comment: This case represents a not infrequently seen and perplexing group of patients who often appear much differently in their units than they do when they arrive at the hospital, which is often no more than 5 miles away. Some general observations about this latter group of patients will be made, but it is included as the 3rd of this triumvirate of cases because it contains both the kind of hysterical features suggested in the first case and also the use of projection in more ominous kinds of defenses in times of stress in settings that are not really quite clearly delineated. It was unclear in this group of cases whether we were primarily dealing with the emergence of projection that represented a kind of latent character trait that emerged under stress in a certain group of young men, and, as such, was more analogous to the situation of case #2, or whether we were primarily seeing transient psychotic reactions at times of stress in certain predisposed, characteriologically-disordered soldiers. My inclination would be to view these two phenomena on a spectrum with the more seriously disordered ones showing the capacity to disorganize briefly under certain stresses which will be delineated subsequently.

In line with the nature of the regressive phenomena being talked about in response to stress, namely a reversion to behavior (case #1), attitudes (case #2), or a combination in varying severity (case #3), the following case illustrates the reversion to a fantasy that represents an unresolved developmental conflict. In addition it bridges the gap again with adoption of both hysterical and paranoid phenomena, and points out some of the difficulties that professionals have in dealing with patients who know they are only separated by about 5 miles of physical distance.

Case #4: A 21-year-old Sp4 who had functioned effectively as a mortar man in a weapons platoon for 6 months began showing up at sick-call because of low back pain. When he continued to return to sick call after several negative physical examinations, he was referred to the division psychiatrist who cleared him and sent him back to duty. However, the night before returning to the field, while lying in a bunk he hallucinated a big man holding an open-mouthed snake coming after him. He ran out in fear, panicked, wild-eyed, and certain of the hallucination. He hallucinated the man and snake on several occasions and was seen again by the division psychiatrist who referred him to the psychiatric ward with the diagnosis of schizophrenic reaction.

On the night of his arrival on the psychiatric ward, he experienced one episode of hallucinating the man with the snake while going outside to the latrine. However, from that time on he remained symptom free without evidence of psychoses. Amnestic material revealed a stable pre-service adjustment, though he had a long-standing fear of snakes, and there seemed to be good evidence of unresolved castration fears. After several days he was returned to his unit via the division psychiatrist with a note elucidating the psychodynamics which had been uncovered and with the diagnosis of hysteria. At the divisional level his symptoms recurred almost immediately after learning that he would be sent to zone company area. He was treated at the division level for a week where, in addition to recurrence of hallucinations, he also experienced several bizarre episodes of dissociation and derealization in which he exhibited strange behavior for which he remained amnesic. He was sent back to psychiatric ward with a note indicating that, although the dynamics which had been postulated were interesting, they were not really relevant to this man's situation or to this case. The pertinent facts were that the enlisted man had functioned well until receiving a minor gunshot wound in the arm approximately one month before his back pain developed. Subsequent to that injury, he had been ineffective to the point where the above noted symptoms developed. The division psychiatrist indicated that the man was ineffective, psychotic, and should be treated though medical channels. The division psychiatrist's point was well taken, but also, the data that he added confirmed the postulated dynamic issues. They offered corroborative evidence of castration fears to his body image that had been activated. Once again, the patient showed no symptoms in the psychiatric ward setting and was eventually returned to the care of the division psychiatrist. At that point both psychiatrists agreed that the man should be transferred to a non-combat unit for a trial of duty. Accordingly he was transferred from infantry duty to work at the docks and remained symptom free for the remaining 6 months of his tour of duty.

Appendix 13 LETTERS OF COLONEL (RETIRED) MATTHEW D PARRISH

Lieutenant Colonel Matthew D Parrish, Medical Corps, served in Vietnam (July 1967–July 1968) as the third Neuropsychiatry Consultant to the Commanding General, US Army, Republic of Vietnam Surgeon. He was deployed during the period of the most intense fighting in Vietnam, which included that surrounding the enemy Tet offensives. Following his assignment in Vietnam, Parrish was assigned as Psychiatry and Neurology Consultant in the Army Office of the Surgeon General. He had served over 20 years as an Army officer before his assignment in Vietnam, including a tour in World War II as a bombardier, and one in Korea during the war as an Army psychiatrist. He received his psychiatric training at Walter Reed General Hospital in the early 1950s. The following are excerpts from correspondence with the author 17 years after his service in Vietnam.

EXCERTS FROM CORRESPONDENCE: LIEUTENANT COLONEL MATTHEW D PARRISH
THIRD NEUROPSYCHIATRY CONSULTANT TO THE COMMANDING GENERAL
(JULY 1967–JULY 1968)

From what I experienced, heard and read, I concluded that VN [Vietnam] was the easiest war of the century—shorter battles, better medicine, better food, better respite, entertainment, even weather, though some of this may be a matter of taste. Korea, in all those ways, was much tougher. Even Pentagon support seemed worse [during the Korean War].[1]

My personal records of Vietnam are rather poor with regard to most of the questions you ask. I did send tapes back to some people, . . . I published some articles in USARV [US Army Republic of Vietnam Medical Bulletin] and one in JAMA [Journal of the American Medical Association], but that one was on surgery.[2] I was officially advised in the combat zones of WW II [World War II], Korea, and Vietnam that I should keep no diaries or personal records (because of possible capture).[3] I hope you can teach the full literature and the history [of Army psychiatry in Vietnam] to those who, like me, had part-experiences [there]. Otherwise, those who served in one place and time will not see the meaning and relative importance of their own experience.[1]

The military historians in Long Binh told me that every major unit incountry was monitored by a military historian. Commanders were required to write up any engagement within three days of the event. The theory was that if the commander waited 30 days to write, he could get away with more lies—as Julius Caesar did. Yet there was no such monitoring of the psychiatric work of each major unit. It doesn't have to be "real research." A psychiatric team's reports would be a checkup on other reports and research. There seems to be fear in the upper echelons, however, that the local team might use such a report to make complaints or to persuade higher staff that some unreasonable action should be taken. In 1967–68 there were several studies on drug abuse in the psychiatric units of hospitals and divisions. I myself thought they should be transmitted to SGO [Surgeon General's Office] or WRAIR [Walter Reed Army Institute of Research] but the USARV surgeon's office, and I think even MACV [Military Assistance Command Vietnam], tried to suppress them at first. Eventually they encouraged some local reports to counter the unsavory statistics of the first study (by Sokol et al) which by then was demanded by SGO. The theater Neuropsychiatry Consultant always sent a monthly statistical report to SGO. That report was obtained in part from the psychiatric units, and in part from USARV. The USARV statistics also contained interesting statistics from Air Force and Navy which showed much higher psychiatric evacuation rates than the Army.

. . . It appeared to me after I got back to SGO that WRAIR would be a better place than SGO to "archive" the reports and journals produced in VN. SGO sometimes cleans out [old] papers.[1] Crude [psychiatric] counts were acceptable in Vietnam because Vietnam was fought as a management war. It set measurable goals and measured the progress toward those goals—counting bodies, friendly villages, shells, gallons, pills, calories, hours and dollars, not . . . technical skill, improvisation, persuasiveness, leadership, language fluency, transcultural understanding, political forces, group cohesion. Most loved was any measurement [that] could be expressed in dollars.[1]

The TET offensive [which took place while Parrish was in Vietnam], of course, was only incidentally directed at the troops in VN. It was primarily aimed, through the media, at the highest command echelon of the US military—the American people and their politicians. The Saigon chief of police, Mr. Loan, unwittingly cooperated by shooting that Charlie in the head with a .45 while on TV. Half the people in the US saw that man's head bounce with the bullet. Very spectacular. [General Westmoreland] unwittingly set up TET by announcing in January that victory was just around the corner. Soon after the 1968 Martin Luther King riots in Washington I was eating at the Division Commander's table near Pleiku. A California congressman was at the table. He expressed surprise to find that the damage in Saigon was so slight. When he took off from National Airport in Washington he had seen the whole length of H Street ablaze or smoking from downtown to the Anacostia River—much worse than TET in Saigon. Furthermore he had read in *Time Magazine* that TET had destroyed Peiku. But now he found that not a shot had been fired there. In May a *Time* correspondent interviewed me, so I asked him why *Time* had said Pleiku was destroyed. He said, "Oh, some colonel in MACV told us that." [I asked,] "Why didn't *Time* retract it in the next issue?" [His reply,] "Oh it wouldn't have been news then." Again, we cooperated nicely with the enemy. . . .[1]

But should the individual soldier be knowledgeable of the current history he is helping to create? In the traditional military of the past centuries the yeoman soldier was either kept dumb or he was fed the kind of propaganda that would keep him properly motivated against the enemy and for the Fatherland. . . . The poorly controlled media in the wars of our lifetimes have made something of a mess of that. Back in the mid-sixties Marshall McLuhan predicted that, solely because of TV, the US could not win the Vietnam War or any other prolonged conventional war. But by the time of the VN war every American soldier was high tech . . . [and the] Army trusted him pretty well. The PX [Post Exchange] sold the John Birch literature as well as *Ramparts* and other super liberal or even Marxist magazines. The US soldier was no illiterate yeoman. Some theories of military management consider that a disadvantage. But then didn't the psychiatrist need to understand the social and political situation that the soldiers (and he himself) faced?[4]

[Regarding] psychoactive drugs. At Letterman years ago Douglas Kelly (psychologist who examined Goering and others) reminded us that WW II in Europe was fought with gasoline and alcohol—even cognac. The Army in [Vietnam] made it easy for most troops to get all the alcohol they wanted—cheap. Neuroleptics were less addicting, probably relieved more anxiety, may have been no more impairing, probably set up no tardive dyskinesia in the time and dosage frame allotted them. Hospitals, civilian and military, should develop more skill in controlling behavior and even relieving anxiety without dangerous drugs. . . . [Neuroleptics and the assumption that medication is a cheaper alternative] had a profound effect on psychiatrists—making them into diagnosis and medication doctors. They control behavior and other symptoms by physical and chemical means, less often by psychological [ones]. . . . In VN, however, the 9th Infantry Division and some others utilized auxiliary corpsmen gleaned from the soldiers who had gotten 3 purple hearts and been excused from combat but who knew about re-motivating combat fatigue subjects.[1]

[The] training [of psychiatrists deployed in Vietnam] could have been better, but numbers were close to proper. Because of travel problems and Murphy's Law we were chronically one or two psychiatrists short.[3] [I]f the theater consultant can see the [newly deployed] psychiatrist on the day of his arrival in Vietnam, can orient him when he is ready to be 'imprinted," can walk him to his division Surgeon and CG and to his division psychiatry unit, then the new psychiatrist performs well for troops.[1]

I think "treating" a [soldier] patient meant for Gentry Harris [Army psychiatrist in Korea] a long psychoanalytically oriented relationship. [Preferable is] "managing" [refers to] the practical enmembering of patient into a functioning group. (If your squad accepts you, the Army will accept you. If it doesn't, you must get another squad to accept you or else get out of the Army.)[1]

The psychiatrist helps the soldier to "Stay committed to the welfare of his combat unit. . . ." In a good combat team . . . the welfare of the individual DEPENDS on the welfare of the unit. For an experienced combat soldier the most terrible fear comes from being assigned to a poor team. Even to work with a good team you are not used to is bad enough. The problem then is that your mind is not a part of the team mind. You are not sure what everyone else is up to. The psychiatrist helps to keep these soldier-unit covalent bonds from breaking.[4] Psychiatric residencies today do not emphasize community psychiatry or even group therapy—only individual psychology: humanistic psychoanalytic work, or dehumanized behavior mod[ification] (which need not be dehumanized).[1]

The Theater Consultants in psychiatry advised SGO that the Consultant should always be a full colonel because he or she could then most easily obtain the country-wide transportation so essential to doing true consultation. The LTCs [lieutenant colonels] had to get special standing orders [that] allowed them to ride on almost any passenger plane going their way. Sometimes they rode in a Caribou or a C-130 which was carrying migrating Vietnamese or perhaps just freight. Sometimes they rode as an extra passenger on a light plane or helicopter some colonel had requested for the day. But another great advantage is that a full colonel can more easily talk with generals—Division Commanders. . . . On the other hand, a Colonel is just as accepted as a [Lieutenant] Colonel when it comes to conferring with Corpsmen, and other soldiers as well as company commanders.[4]

My tour in Vietnam certainly gave me a lot of experience, learning and contacts. I thought that I had been trained about as well to do the job as anyone. I was irked however, that I was not allowed to finish and put together my work at WRAIR [before I was sent] and also that I had had two hardship tours already while many other had had none. A year later, having finished WRAIR, for better or for worse, I would have had much less objection. . . . My thought was that the Army should have a dozen persons who had been so trained. And I thought, perhaps erroneously, that VN could be a training ground . . . [but] apparently others thought . . . that it was best to keep using the same one or two experts over and over.[5]

But I found out that assignments of the [USARV] Consultant were not made on the basis of rank and probably not on the basis of skill or of proper career development but rather on the basis of what influential psychiatrists wanted to be assigned in Hawaii or to Letterman [General Hospital in San Francisco], or wanted to get out of DA staff work.[4]

It seemed to me that [some deployed psychiatrists] had a good time in Vietnam—professionally, personally, even politically. But I doubt if it would be smart for [them] to advertise that now. I think this is true of a lot of us. It's not a question of, "Did I benefit by going to Vietnam?" rather it is, "SHOULD I have benefited?"—given today's view of history.[4]

Source
Written comments from Matthew D. Parrish to Norman M. Camp; dated: (1) 24 July 1985: first installment of a lengthy response to early chapter drafts; (2) 23 February 1983 cover letter returning survey; (3) 21 February 1983 comments in survey; (4) 1 August 1985: second installment of the response; and (5) 17 August 1985: third and final installment of the response.

Appendix 14 COLONEL CLOTILDE D BOWEN, MC, END OF TOUR REPORT

Colonel Clotilde D Bowen, MC, served in Vietnam (July 1970–71) during the drawdown phase as the sixth Neuropsychiatry Consultant to the CG/USARV Surgeon—the senior Army psychiatrist in the theater. In her role as the Army's chief psychiatrist in Vietnam, Colonel Bowen oversaw the work of the deployed psychiatrists and allied mental health personnel. She was also responsible for planning and coordinating the Army's rapidly developing drug and race relations programs in Vietnam and often was called upon to brief congressmen, visiting foreign dignitaries and ranking officers, and news media about the eroding morale and mental health of the troops.

AVBJ-PS END OF TOUR REPORT: COLONEL BOWEN/DH/481
SIXTH NEUROPSYCHIATRY CONSULTANT TO THE COMMANDING GENERAL
(8 JUNE 1971)

1. **Organizational changes and impact on mission accomplishment:**

a. Early in FY 71, the psychiatrist in the Cam Ranh Bay area was detached from the South Beach MHCS and attached to the 483rd AF Hospital. The Air Force had two psychiatrists on TDY from out-of-country. Thus the attachment of the Army psychiatrist afforded needed additional help and aided in the successful return to duty, out-of-country evacuation and administration actions for Army patients. In August, the 483rd AF Hospital was the first to report an Army death due to heroin overdose proven by autopsy. In October 1970 this hospital was receiving the largest number of Army personnel with drug problems. The Cam Ranh MHCS was manned by a social work officer and psychology/social work specialists until April 1971 when the clinic was discontinued at DEROS of the two remaining personnel. With the continuing draw down of Army personnel in the Cam Ranh area, the psychiatrist was reassigned to the 935th KO Detachment in May 1971. When the 67th Medical Group Headquarters moved from the 95th Evacuation Hosptial premises to Camp Baxter in August 1970, the 98th KO team took over these buildings and remodeled them to suit a MHCS. They began to function more efficiently in October when a new, permanent commander arrived, Maj. Norman Camp.

b. In April 1971, the in-patient portion of psychiatric service and the neurology clinic of the 935th KO team were moved from the 93rd Evac Hospital to the 24th Evac Hospital on Long Binh when the former hospital closed. In addition the MHCS was moved to the old admission portion of time 93rd Evac Hospital while the 32nd Medical Depot took over the major portion of the 93rd buildings. This has resulted in the same type difficulties experienced a year ago when the 98th KO moved from Nha Trang to Da Nang. Much engineer work will be necessary before the EEG area in properly shielded.

c. Both the 4th and the 25th Infantry Divisions stood down in Nov and Dec respectively, freeing the MHCS staffs. Dr. Jeppsen from the 25th was reassigned to the 23rd (American) Infantry (Mobile). He was reassigned to the 935th KO team in June 1971, as a replacement. Dr. Cushman of the 4th Division covered the 3rd Field MHCS psychiatrist for 6 weeks while the latter enjoyed a 30 day extension leave, then was reassigned to the 101st ABN at Camp Eagle for the remainder of his tour. There was much disorder to these stand downs with loss of morale esprit de corps, and credibility among the enlisted mental health specialists who were reassigned, often times outside of their mental health specialist MOSs.

d. The MHCS of the 23rd Div at Chu Lai received both in-patients and out-patients from the 91st Evac Hospital and the 27th Surgical as well as from non-divisional support units. This was an excellent arrangement for all concerned.

2. Technical & professional advances:

a. In January 1971, the 935th KO team, augmented, opened a half-way house, called Cross Roads, at the 24th Evac Hospital. This is essentially a detoxification center for heroin drug addicts. As of June, 1971, it is being reorganized and staffed with personnel from other Long Binh Post activities under the direction of the post commander.

b. As early as September 1970, all division MHCS's were setting up beds of 6-25 for the treatment of heroin drug addicts. Starting with that month, all psychiatric activities began to include with their monthly reports, a list of EM by name, rank, unit, drugs used and amount. Many drug abusers were admitted to psychiatric words of MEDCOM Hospitals until late December 1970, when numerous Amnesty-Rehabilitation programs took over these functions.

c. The lack of psychiatric coverage at the lst/5th Mech Brigade near Quang Tri had resulted in the loss of at least 200 men-days per month. Through the 67th Medical Group and XXIV Corps Surgeon arrangements were made to have a psychiatrist and/or social worker from the 98th KO team in Da Nang visit the 1/5 Mech Brigade weekly. This arrangement was continued until the onset of heavy monsoon rains in October and November. The brigade surgeon, a board certified psychiatrist, assumed these responsibilities at this time.

d. Medical Technical Guidance, Drug Abuse, was written by Maj. Eric Nelson, C.O. of 935th KO Detachment with help of Medical Consultant as a 'crash' project early in September l970. Upon critical review by the NP Consultant it was revised and re-published on 15 October. This manual has been distributed to all physicians as they arrive in-country since January 1971, along with a short briefing on the RVN drug problem and its solution.

e. Revision of USARV Reg No. 40-34, pertaining to Mental Health & Neuropsychiatry, was published on 15 October 1970 with changes in the morbidity report form (USARV Form 55) and explicit instructions. Even with this revision it was evident that the entire psychiatric reporting system was poor: (1) personnel admitted to medical services for treatment of alcoholism, drug abuse, psychosomatic conditions, etc. are reported to MRO as neuropsychiatric disease. Thus, the NP report forwarded to the consultant does not give a true picture of psychiatric morbidity. In addition, services other than psychiatry have evacuated patients out-of-country with NP diagnoses.

f. Revision of USARV Supplement to AR 635-212 on 27 October 1970 by TWIX provided guidance for the psychiatric portion of the medical evaluation to be performed by general medical officers when a psychiatrist was not readily available. On 12 April 1971 this was made an Army wide policy by CGUSAMC Wash D.C.

g. NP Consultant worked with USA MEDCOMV DC/S P&0 in setting up better recording system for drug abuse. Worked with Medical Consultant & 9th Medical Lab to set up better processing of autopsies in suspected drug deaths and urinalysis for drugs. Worked USARV Special Personnel Actions Division and Information Office on defining drug programs and press releases concerning drugs.

3. Personnel, logistics, and other problems encountered:

a. On 1 July 1970 there were 20 psychiatrists in-country. Eighteen DEROS'ed during the year. At present there are 15, including a husband and wife. Ten will DEROS in June, July and August 1971, including the NP Consultant. Replacements for nine will not arrive until a week to 10 days after the last DEROS's in August.

b. One psychiatrist who was to DEROS in Jan 71 extended until August 1971. He is a flight surgeon and was transferred to the 23rd Division on 4 June 1971 as interim division surgeon. The psychiatrist assigned to the 3rd Brigade of the 1st Cav is reassigned to the formers' position at the 3rd Field Hospital.

c. Of the ten projected 3129's in August 1971, six are fully trained. The four D 3129's should be sent to the field as 3100's and the six partially-trained physicians already in-country placed in KO detachments.

d. Plans are in progress to integrate KO detachments into the 95th & 24th Evac Hospitals as psychiatric services, as a space saving maneuver.

4. **Recommendations for future action:**

a. Dissolve KO detachments and reassign personnel to two evacuation hospitals

b. Re-assignment of D 3129's already In-country to hospital psychiatric services under a fully-trained, preferably RA, chief of psychiatry.

c. Assignment of Social Work Consultant to Professional Services Division USAMEDCOMV.

d. No extensions beyond regular DEROS should be considered for psychiatric personnel. During the last seven months the person is entitled to a 30 day leave, a one week leave, and an R & R. Because of these frequent breaks and other psychological factors, work performed is less than satisfactory.

e. That reports from psychiatric services to NP Consultant be considered informational, at best. No statistical reports should be generated from these reports; they indicate trends only. The best way to track of psychiatric services is frequent liaison visits.

f. Consideration should be made to assign MHCS's to support units and/or combine MHCS's of division and support units in a geographical area. Support units usually have more psychiatric problems than divisions.

g. Psychiatric personnel should continue to be consultants to drug and alcohol programs rather than running programs. They should provide educational assistance to commanders, chaplains and other physicians involved in drug & human relations problems.

h. Efforts should be made to combine Human Relations & Drug-Alcohol Abuse programs, at least conceptually.

i. A means for better communication between command and staff of divisions and the division psychiatrist should be improvised. At present the Army has many morale, racial and E.M. problems which era in the purview of the psychiatrist and which the division surgeon does not accurately convey to command. Consideration should be made for psychiatrists to have equal status with surgeons in divisions.

CLOTILDE D BOWEN
COL, MC
Neuropsychiatric Consultant

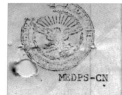

DEPARTMENT OF THE ARMY
OFFICE OF THE SURGEON GENERAL
WASHINGTON, D.C. 20315

MEDPS-CN

3 0 SEP 1969

Honorable Ogden R. Reid

House of Representatives

Dear Mr. Reid:

This is in response to your letter dated 16 September 1969 requesting
information on psychiatric care of military personnel.

It is not correct to state that there are no statutory provisions for
psychiatric care of military personnel with respect to 10 U.S.C. 55.
All active duty military personnel are eligible to receive psychiatric
care at existing military facilities when local military medical personnel have ascertained that a need for such care exists. In addition,
retired military personnel and military dependents may receive military
psychiatric care on a space available basis or through local civilian
facilities through the Office for Civilian Health and Medical Program
of the Uniformed Services (OCHAMPUS).

A copy of AR 40-216, "Medical Service Neuropsychiatry", is inclosed
for your information. This regulation is currently under revision.

Personality (character and behavior) disorders are not considered to
be either illnesses or diseases and therefore do not qualify an individual for medical separation or disability. Personality characteristics,
be they desirable or undesirable, are developed during one's formative
years, are essentially lifelong, and generally well ingrained by the
time an individual enters on active duty; they are never service-incurred.
One's personality structure, again for better or worse, is seldom
amenable to change through psychiatric intervention. Personality diagnoses (really descriptive adjectives pertaining to dominant characterological traits and recurring patterns) may often be applied to a majority of
the population, military or civilian. This is of little consequence,

MEDPS-CN
Honorable Ogden R. Reid

however, since we are not talking about disease or illness. Motivation is generally the major factor in determining whether or not such individuals successfully complete their obligated military service. The vast majority of individuals with characterological defects do, in fact, complete their Service obligation. The Army's method of dealing with unsuitable characterological types is not particularly unique. If a civilian employee is confronted with an individual whose personality characteristics make him an unsuitable or undesirable employee, his services are terminated (he is "fired"); he is not discharged for medical reasons, nor is he given a pension. Similarly, if a soldier's personality characteristics repeatedly bring him into conflict with the Army and attempts to motivate him toward more satisfactory service are non-productive, the Army has a way of "firing" him (administrative separation under the provisions of AR 635-212). In this case the final decision regarding the quality of his work and, therefore, the need for the termination of his services should and does rest with his employer, i.e., the Commanding Officer, and not with medical authority. Both psychiatric and medical evaluations are obtained prior to separation, however, to rule out the presence of any unfitting psychiatric (psychosis, neurosis) or medical condition.

There are approximately 330 psychiatrists currently on active duty, or about one psychiatrist per 4,500 active duty soldiers.

It is recognized that there is a large area of disagreement between the military psychiatrist and an ever-growing number of active duty soldiers and their civilian counterparts; the former maintaining the expectancy that a soldier should become a member of his military group and do his best to participate and further the group effort, the latter being more concerned with avoiding his military obligation by any and all means at the disposal of his ingenuity. This is seen as a reflection of the times and not as a manifestation of psychiatric illness.

I trust this information will be helpful to you in answering questions from your constituents.

Sincerely yours,

1 Incl
AR 40-216

HAL B. JENNINGS, JR.
Brigadier General, MC
Deputy Surgeon General

CF
The Surgeon General
OTSG Record Room
Dir, Prof Svc
RETURN: P&N Cons Br
ROOM 6B-044

2

Appendix 16 VIETNAM STUDY

Franklin Del Jones was assigned as an Army psychiatrist to the 3rd Field Hospital in Saigon (September 1966–January 1967) during the second year of the war. On 29 August 1977, Jones made a presentation in Honolulu, Hawaii, to the World Psychiatric Association, titled "Reactions to Stress: Combat Versus Combat Support Troops." Included were results of a field study Jones conducted at the 3rd Field Hospital. The study presented here provides the only systematically collected data comparing combat and non-combat personnel in Vietnam regarding psychiatric and behavior problems.

REACTIONS TO STRESS COMPARING COMBAT AND SUPPORT TROOPS
FRANKLIN DEL JONES, PSYCHIATRIST
3RD FIELD HOSPITAL, SAIGON (SEPTEMBER 1966–JANUARY 1967)

From September 1966 through December 1966, Jones saw 120 consecutive patients for whom enough data is available to classify their status as CT [combat troops] or CST [combat support troops] and to determine their symptomatology. Table [1] lists their demographic features and number of patients on whom the data is based.

Demographic variables tended to separate CT and CST only with regard to age (median for CT was 23 and CST was 29) and marital status (CT were 65% single, CST were 49% single). Both groups were about equally represented in percentages of officers and Blacks, and the median rank for enlisted in both groups was E-4 (corporal).

Table [2] taken from the records of 98 CST and 22 CT casualties and four in which status was not known (total 124 patients) seen by Jones at the Third Field Hospital, Saigon, From September through December 1966, reveals some of the symptomatology found in the 120 CT and CST subjects.

A surprising disparity is seen in numbers of patients having symptomatic alcoholism in CT and CST, only 1 in CT and 26 in CST, roughly 5% in CT and 25% in CST or a five-fold difference. Drug abuse was absent in CT and present in 5 of CST. Another surprise was the relatively high incidence of homosexuality in CST 9% but none in CT. Psychosis accounted for about 8% of CST but none in CT. Often there was an involvement of drugs or alcohol in these psychotic cases; at least two occurred in soldiers who had just smoked marijuana and two occurred in alcoholic soldiers. Character and behavior disorders (CBD) were found in about half the CT and over one-third of the CST, while anxiety and conversion symptoms occurred in about the same proportion, ie, half the CT and over one-third of the CST. Psychophysiologic symptoms (usually gastrointestinal or headaches) were present in about 20% of the CT and 15% of the CST.

In only 47 cases (20 CT, 27 CST) could the type of conflict be determined with some degree of certainty as seen in (Table [3]). Thirteen of 22 CT and five of 98 CST had a primary conflict over being in a combat zone. Security Clearances, usually based on previous psychiatric contact, were requested on 13 (1 CT, 12 CST), only one of which was recommended to be denied due to a severe personality disorder. Most of them had seen a psychiatrist years before for minor situational anxiety problems.

TABLE 1. Demographic Variables

DEMOGRAPHIC VARIABLE	COMBAT TROOPS (number of patients)	SUPPORT TROOPS (number of patients)
Median age	23 years old (20)	29 years old (93)
Percentage Caucasian	79% (19)	80% (94)
Percentage Single	65% (17)	49% (92)
Percentage Enlisted	84% (19)	88% (92)

TABLE 2. Symptomatology

SYMPTOM OR BEHAVIOR	COMBAT TROOPS (n=22)		SUPPORT TROOPS (n=98)	
	Primary Symptom*	Secondary Symptom**	Primary Symptom	Secondary Symptom
Alcoholism	1	0	19	7
Character and Behavior disorder	7	3	18	18
Anxiety	4	1	16	5
Homosexuality	0	0	8	1
Psychophysiologic Symptoms	3	1	7	5
Psychosis	0	0	6	2
Conversion Symptoms	5	1	5	2
Drug Abuse	0	0	4	1
Depression	0	0	6	2
Other	1	4	3	7
None (Security Clearance)	1	0	5	0
TOTAL	22	10	98	50

* Primary Symptom refers to the most prominent symptom or behavior bringing the soldier to psychiatric attention (one per case)

** Secondary Symptom refers to additional symptoms present in the soldier (one or more per case)

TABLE 3. Postulated Conflicts

TYPE OF CONFLICT	COMBAT TROOPS (n=20)	SUPPORT TROOPS (n=27)	UNKNOWN (n=1)
Being in a combat zone	13	5	
Marital problems	4	16	1
Family problems	1	5	
Job problems	2	1	
None (Security Clearance)	(1)	(12)	

When overlapping, about equally distributed symptoms are eliminated, the CST casualty stands out as being very much more likely to be alcoholic, homosexual and psychotic. These findings are in striking conformity with those of Tureen and Stein (1949) during World War II. Their report, one of the few contrasting combat with combat support troops, stated that soldiers with "constitutional psychopathic states" constituted 10% of admissions when the hospital operated in a rear base section (combat support) but only 1.8% in a forward base section (combat). These "constitutional psychopathic states" consisted primarily of "chronic alcoholism, sex perversion, criminalism [sic], inadequate personality and emotional instability."[1]

SUMMARY

Military psychiatry has essentially solved the problem of handling combat psychiatric casualties with a program of immediate, forward, simple treatment involving rest in an atmosphere of expectation that the soldier will soon return to combat. The problems of combat support troops, involving complex self-destructive behavioral responses to separation from loved ones and demoralization with loss of unit integrity, will require more complex solutions. Most important is restoration of unit identity, perhaps by keeping units cohesive from basic training to combat and perhaps by rotating entire units. Drastic disorders may require drastic remedies. Another attack point would be to make combat support experience more like the positive appeal of combat experience; ie, goal-oriented with little time for boredom. Finally, drug abuse or other such behavior, such as failure to take antimalarial tablets or failure to prevent frostbite [as seen during the Korean War], must not be allowed to become an "evacuation syndrome" removing the soldier from the combat zone.

REFERENCE

1. Tureen LL, Stein M. The base section psychiatric hospital. In: Hanson FR, ed. *Combat Psychiatry*. Washington, DC: U.S. Government Printing Office; 1949:105–134. [Also published as a Supplement to *Bulletin of US Army Medical Department*, 1949, 9.]

Appendix 17

MENTAL HYGIENE BULLETIN NO1   20 February 1968

SUGGESTIONS IN THE MANAGEMENT OF ALCOHOLISM

Management of alcoholics and excessive use of alcohol continues to plague commanders who have responsibility for all aspects of this problem except for its medical complications. For this reason we would like to offer some additional suggestions to supplement those outlined in a previous memorandum.

As noted previously, AA remains the most effective group treatment approach for alcoholics. The unit on Long Binh Post continues to meet on Monday evenings at 1900 hours at the 93d Evacuation Hospital Chapel. It is recommended that new members be brought to the first meeting by the unit's first sergeant or some superior. No other (preliminary) proceedures are necessary in making a referral to AA.

It has been our experience that when an alcoholic's drinking becomes uncontrolled, he needs strong and firm help from others to regain his ability to cope more successfully with his desire to drink. At such times, it is both appropriate and therapeutic for a commander to take such measures as:

      1) barring the alcoholic from all clubs under threat of administrative action.

      2) invalidating that part of his ration card having to do with alcoholic beaverages.

      3) requiring him to report to the ISG or some superior each day before work to make sure that he is sober and fit for duty.

      4) assigning the man sufficient duties to keep him busy and occupied.

      5) insuring attendance at AA if there is an AA unit available.

In conjunction with such steps, the dispensary physician or the batallion surgeon can collaborate with the commander's efforts by prescribing a mild tranquilizer such as librium (10 to 20 mg four times daily) for those alcoholics who are experiencing undue anxiety.

If measures of this type are undertaken by the commander with the conviction that there is value in inducing the alcoholic to stop drinking, and with willingness on his part to back up his orders with administrative or judicial action, then many of these men will regain some self-control over their drinking, as well as considerable self-esteem. If these measures fail, then it can be concluded that all appropriate rehabilitative measures have been tried. At that point administrative separation should be strongly considered without regard to grade, age, or length of service.

Appendix 18 EXCERPTS FROM THE BAKER/HOLLOWAY REPORTS

Between 22 February and 23 March 1971, Colonel Stewart L Baker Jr; Chief Psychiatry and Neurology Consultant, Office of the Surgeon General, US Army, conducted an official inspection tour of the primary drug treatment and rehabilitation programs in the Pacific Theater Command (PACOM), including South Vietnam. Two months later, between 28 April and 28 June, Colonel Harry C Holloway, research psychiatrist with the Army Medical Research and Development Command, conducted a more extensive tour, including the programs visited by Baker. Baker and Holloway ultimately produced the report CINCPAC [Commander in Chief, Pacific Area Command] Study for Evaluation of PACOM Drug Abuse Treatment/Rehabilitation Programs, which combined their findings in the Vietnam theater with those from visits to other US military installations in the Pacific theater.

CINCPAC STUDY FOR EVALUATION OF PACOM DRUG ABUSE TREATMENT/REHABILITATION PROGRAMS
1 SEPTEMBER 1971

VIETNAM: REPORT SUMMARY AND CONCLUSIONS

(1) Drug abuse in the US military forces represents a significant threat to effective combat readiness and jeopardizes the very survival of the traditional concept of the military as a vehicle of national policy.

(2) Efforts at drug use suppression and treatment/rehabilitation to date in Vietnam have failed.

(3) Any drug abuse control program must concentrate sufficient resources and be of such a massive scale that success can be reasonably predicted.

(4) In-country treatment and on-the-job rehabilitation provides the most feasible and effective method for dealing with the incidence of drug use.

(5) Whereas an individual identified as a drug user must be immediately removed from his unit (to guarantee reduction of prevalence, to decrease social contagion, and to prevent the disruption of organizational integrity and discipline), evacuation of all identified drug users from the command is unacceptable (both from the standpoint of military manpower management and from the viewpoint of minimizing the reinforcement/fixation of failure in the individual drug user).

(6) Chemical monitoring is absolutely essential to proper management of troops undergoing withdrawal (detoxification) and of rehabilitees being followed in field units.

(7) The entire population in Vietnam should be subjected to urine screening within each 90 days by means of mobile collection teams, and rehabilitees and counselors in units should be tested at least twice each week.

(8) Actual rehabilitation of the individual must take place on the job through the use of locally trained unit counselors and is ultimately the responsibility of the commanding officer.

VIETNAM: DETAIL OF BAKER'S OBSERVATIONS FOLLOWED BY SUMMARIES OF HOLLOWAY'S SUBSEQUENT FINDINGS

The following excerpts provide detail from Baker's report regarding his observations of drug treatment and rehabilitation programs in Vietnam. Each is followed by a summary of Holloway's observations [in *italics*] of the same programs roughly two months later. It should be noted that the programs described below were the primary Army programs in Vietnam at that time, but there were numerous smaller ones as well as programs of other service branches, most of which were visited by Holloway and also addressed in his report.

935th Neuropsychiatric Medical Specialty Detachment (KO)/24th Evacuation Hospital on Long Binh Post: 9 March 1971

. . . The 935th (KO) operates a 30 bed drug abuse rehabilitation center ["Crossroads"], which serves the Long Binh area [near Saigon]. Arrivals are screened by social work technicians, including ex-users, to evaluate motivations for admission. The patient, if accepted, is stripped, searched, and given a shower (necessarily cold water), then entered into the ward area, which is located inside a barbed wire enclosure. A staff of eighteen 91-Bs and 91-Fs, including two former users, man the unit. Methadone withdrawal technique is used, initially 30 mgm. per day, decreasing thru the first three days. Compazine is used for nausea and vomiting. Lomotil is used for diarrhea. By the 3rd day the patient is off drugs. The amnesty support provided is a one time opportunity. In the event of any relapse, the patient is refused readmission. The average stay is five days. Toxicology is provided by the 3rd Med Lab.

Drug free statistics appear to vary with the man's parent organization, perhaps a reflection of aftercare attitudes and practices:

- In one organization, 6 of 35 graduates have returned to drugs
- In another organization, 9 of 11 are back on drugs

During the month of February, there were 150 admissions, 64 of these left AMA [against medical advice] (less than 4 days in the program). Follow-up data indicate 40–50% of those completing the 5 day rehab program remain drug-free. The number of those leaving AMA who remain drug free is not known. In general there is great shame associated with being labeled a "junkie," and this is frequently one's experience on returning to his unit following detoxification. It is often noted that those who fail in the rehab program express strong criticism of it, alleging no care was given, minimizing the quality of the group encounter sessions, etc., as though a paranoid defense against further guilt.

. . . It is the impression of those involved in drug rehab efforts that a number of men volunteer for RVN [Republic of Vietnam] in part because of the easy access to drugs, and that some extend their tour in part because of this ready availability. Most volunteers for amnesty program attentions have less than 90 days before DEROS [date expected return from overseas]. Other motivations apparently propelling soldiers toward the center include a drug death in the unit, or the news of

an admission for drug overdose. Survey of admissions during the last 6 months indicates that most drug abusers start such behavior in RVN before the end of their 3rd month there. There is a formidable group or peer pressure which greets a new arrival and identifies his drug attitude. . . . One is expected to either declare himself by joining the drug practices of a core group or declare himself in opposition. This same pressure greets the amnesty program graduate, who is seen as "square" or a potential "stoolie" on return to his unit unless he rejoins his former associates in drug abuse behaviors.

Holloway observed later (13 May and 20 June) that this medically based treatment facility, which was housed in a former prisoner of war ward, limited its focus to detoxification and a group therapy. It was not staffed sufficiently to operate at full capacity and did not receive sufficient line command support in terms of resources and personnel.

USARV confinement facility ("LBJ") on Long Binh post—9 March 1971

The 935th (KO) supports the Long Binh stockade, where there are 375 prisoners with 45 days average stay there. Reportedly, most serious crimes seen in RVN are associated with drug abuse, particularly binoctal. A section of G-1 is collecting data on the long series of fraggings which have occurred within the past two years, and will forward this data to DCSPER, DA [Deputy Chief of Staff for Personnel, Department of the Army] in the future.

Holloway observed later (13 May) that there were a number of prisoners who required detoxification, and that medically supervised withdrawal and rehabilitation counseling was provided in confinement cells. Also, it was widely rumored that drugs were readily available within the facility, and ex-guards were regularly incarcerated for heroin offenses.

18th Surgical Hospital and the 1/5th Infantry Brigade (Mechanized) at Quang Tri near the DMZ— 10 March 1971

At the time of my visit the esprit de corps appeared high throughout the area, clearly reflecting the satisfaction and confidence with the military actions going on in nearby Laos. . . . The general morale appeared in clear contrast to that of units I visited later, far from the northern hub of activity. Lower morale seemed more characteristic of the units involved in passive defense activities, particularly in the south.

The 18th Surgical Hospital had provided a [heroin] rehab program since November 1970, offering amnesty and medical support. A general medical officer had directed this effort until late February 1971, when the staff in support of this program became somewhat depleted by requirements in support of the Laos incursion. Two social work technicians had carried the responsibility of the program almost alone for several weeks. Reflecting the movement of troops to the west, and decrease in staff, the number of patients seen in this program had declined from 85 patients (240 visits) in November, 1970, to 20 patients (90 visits) in February, 1971. During recent days the number of patients had begun to increase again. . . . Currently the drug rehabilitation program is entirely outpatient, employing Valium and Donnatal to assist withdrawal. No follow-up was attempted within the units. No ex-abusers were employed. The Laotian incursion had occurred quite suddenly, with little alerting of the troops. The quick move to Khe San and the border had interrupted personal pipelines for heroin supplies, so a number of soldiers experienced withdrawal reactions during the first day or two. Within several days, however, drug supplies were beginning to arrive in the Khe Sanh area, reportedly brought by the GI truck driver who hauled supplies, and withdrawal reactions were no longer observed [in the field]. . . .

The clinic staff felt drug usage was quite high particularly among supply and transportation personnel, estimating that approximately 80% of the group use heroin. The access to drugs was quite difficult to control in this group, since their duties provided them access to villages en route to various destinations. Several deaths due to heroin overdoses were described.

Holloway observed later (6 May and 20 May) that following Baker's visit an extensive heroin problem emerged within the 1/5th Infantry Brigade (Mechanized), forcing them to establish their own 10-bed treatment ward, which was staffed by four technicians and a partially trained psychiatrist. However, the detoxification process was not effective as heroin could not be kept off the ward. Follow-up efforts were spotty and no valid statistics were available. Trips to nearby fire bases verified that heroin was being used in the field and on patrol, and heroin use had infiltrated every level of the brigade structure including the medical battalion. Two

drug treatment "hootches" in company-sized units were also observed, but the lack of sufficient resources, particularly trained personnel, clearly limited their effectiveness.

101st Airborne Division in the Hue-Phu Bai area—10 March 1971

The Drug Center of Camp Eagle employs a ward area for initial admission and drug withdrawal. This unit is led by [a physician with] one year of psychiatric training. Morphine is used to medically support the patient during withdrawal. Both to facilitate referral of drug abusers and to develop follow-up support for ex-users, a number of Battalion Drug Teams have been developed. A Drug Team is composed of the Battalion Surgeon, Battalion Chaplain, and one or two enlisted members in Grade E-6 or below. [The team] is available on a 24 hour basis. Following return to duty, the drug rehab graduate may be seen daily at first, then less frequently. A recently initiated Assay of Intake at the Drug Center (n = 64) indicates that the average admission has a history of self-abuse with multiple drugs [although] heroin dependency was the reason for admission in 98% of the cases. [Of those] 48% stated they shot it by needle and the remainder described they chose to sniff it. There was no follow-up data available to determine the effect of the program.

Holloway observed later (6 May) that the program sought to withdraw 150 to 200 soldiers per month for heroin dependence, but because this took place under outpatient circumstances programmatic success was limited because drugs were readily accessible. The division had made systematic efforts to regulate the Vietnamese nationals within its compounds without measurable effects. In fact inspections of fire support bases demonstrated, as in other combat divisions, that heroin was available and being used in the field.

95th Evacuation Hospital and the 98th Neuropsychiatric Medical Specialty Detachment (KO) at Da Nang—11 March 1971

[The] account of the psychiatric team's operations indicated [that there was] no formal drug rehab program developed here; the referrals were all evaluated and treated within the outpatient area except when admission for treatment of withdrawal reaction was required. The focus on amnesty was not a major one, and the number of patients self-referred for this was not very large. In fact

... the staff expressed concern regarding the tradition of openness in the psychiatric referral system, and felt that this ... renders it vulnerable to manipulation.

Holloway observed later (5 May) that the Da Nang Area Support Command reported a high level of heroin dependence in all subordinate units. Whereas line officers complained that they were not receiving adequate support from medical facilities, the psychiatric team expressed the strong position that the drug abuse was primarily a neglected leadership/command problem.

23rd Infantry Division at Chu Lai—
12 March 1971

... Since September 1970, more than 200 persons had volunteered for the amnesty program at the Medical Battalion level. Slightly more than 50 of these were hospitalized there for withdrawal. In less than 4 days they were returned to duty, with recommendation that they find a buddy, preferably an NCO, to assist them in remaining off drugs. Each of the four medical companies has its own drug abuse program, separate from the medical battalion activity. Most amnesty cases undergo drug withdrawal at medical company and dispensary level.

Holloway observed later (6 May and 27 May) that the division's drug program mostly emphasized troop education and vigorous drug suppression/enforcement efforts, and there was no structured program for rehabilitation and follow-up of amnesty volunteers. Recent arrests of dispensary staff for drug possession demonstrated the difficulty of establishing a "drug-free environment" for withdrawal. Visits to fire support bases revealed little difference in drug use from the other divisions.

67th Evacuation Hospital in Qui Nhon—
13 March 1971

This hospital supports a port facility and supply area.

The drug abuse program employs methadone for withdrawal, three days hospitalization and then outpatient clinic appointments for three scheduled follow-up visits. In addition, a letter is regularly forwarded to the man's unit, requesting unit-based counseling, and the institution of a buddy system to respond to the patient's aftercare needs.

A number of severe marijuana cases have been hospitalized, with history of use of 15–20 joints daily for three to six months. These cases have strong organic brain syndrome characteristics.

... A number of cases are known in which the soldiers "crash" themselves with binoctal, a barbiturate, to come off heroin. This is obviously a dangerous practice.

Holloway observed later (8 June) that in terms of outcome, the heroin rehabilitation program here, consisting of traditional outpatient care with a few general medical beds allocated for inpatients, resulted in only 10% of referrals achieving withdrawal.

II Field Force Headquarters on Long Binh Post—
14 March 1971

Pioneer House was activated in August 1970 by General Davidson. It was clear following the Cambodian campaign that drug abuse was increasing at an alarming rate. [An earlier] directed drug program delivered by educational "teams" visiting the various areas did not appear to reach the troops effectively. An emergent leader in the person of an aggressive social work technician proposed a new format, a nonmilitary-nonmedical model, led by enlisted men, primarily by ex-drug abusers. Obtaining a trailer and locating it in the area, this small group of enlisted men began a hard-line, low professional profile program which concentrated on the hard drugs, especially heroin, and minimized marijuana. Personnel admitted to Pioneer House had it banged into their heads that heroin kills, and themes such as "where's your head? If it's off on smack, bad" were stressed. Ex-drug abusers were preferred as staff because of the concern about personal commitment ... of trained professionals, who might feel it was just another job. ... The program was intense and motivational.

Withdrawal was accomplished with thorazine and probanthine. Lately, Valium has also been employed. [M]ost admissions are for heroin abuse. An open door policy permitted admission of literally anyone who arrives.... Since amnesty was originally considered to call for anonymity, there were no records kept in the traditional medical form ... therefore, statistics were initially quite poor. An analysis of the last 100 graduates of the program, however, gives a somewhat surprising profile of the hard drug user, when compared to [civilian addicts]: his average age was 20; 25% of the time he's married; in 90% of the instances both parents are alive, and in

75% of the instances the parents are neither separated nor divorced; 50% of cases had no record of Article 15 [disciplinary action], and another 25% have had one Article 15; 60% of the admissions arrive within four months of their DEROS. . . . In summary, the profile of the potentially rehabilitatible drug user was described as: strung out on heroin, but you don't know it—he's doing his job.

. . . Pioneer House accepts a man back when he relapses to drug abuse. It is locally held that, as in problem drinking, often a truly rehabilitatible man will fail at least once.

. . . The modus operandi of the activity [12–15 patients]: for the first 48 hours no one may leave. . . . A medical technician stays with the new admission, checking blood pressure and pulse, to watch for a strong withdrawal reaction following a recent "hit." Much is made of the touching of patients during this withdrawal crisis, holding them, rubbing the back, in essence giving concern and love. Initially, the staff man will try to get a relationship going with the new admission, and then will emphasize that [his drug use is volitional and it is his responsibility to abstain]. The ex-user is skilled in helping the patient identify his motivational attitudes. The regimen of withdrawal was "cold turkey", with some medical support as described. The withdrawal symptoms become fairly strong 18-24 hours after admission, on the average. About 25% of cases have mild symptoms and 25% have quite severe symptoms. The rehab center is not considered to be a medical facility per se, so the hard reactions are taken to the hospital for management of the medical crisis. About the third day many participants begin to waver. Basically they want heroin. This is quite a vulnerable period. . . . Currently the practice is to return the patient to duty around the fifth day, with the request for another ex-user in the unit area to help him readjust there in a non-drug culture.

. . . Followup data is quite incomplete in this activity. There is evidence that 30% of the graduates are still drug free, another 30% have relapsed to drug use, and there is no information about the remaining 40%, many of whom have DEROS'd to CONUS [continental United States].

Holloway observed later (14 May) that ex-drug users on the staff had subverted the program by supplying drugs to the participants. As a consequence it had recently been restructured using a lieutenant and enlisted man with non-drug use backgrounds.

3rd Brigade, 1st Cavalry Division (AMBL) Bien Hoa—14 March 1971

The 1st Cavalry Division is about to be deactivated in Vietnam. A sizeable morale problem associates to the impact of unit stand-downs which causes large numbers of troops to be transferred as excess. . . . This is felt to aggravate the tendency toward drug abuse. A drug abuse ward was developed in October 1970, at the 1st Cav MHCS [mental hygiene consultation service], directed particularly toward heroin abuse. A medical officer in attendance provided for controlled withdrawal from drugs. At the present time admissions are increasing to this unit, reflecting predominantly men approaching their DEROS, and others being transferred to another divisional unit with worry about the new unit's attitude and drug supply. Most of these patients are described as fairly healthy persons who "wandered" into drugs, with better prognosis for recovery than the drug addict stereotype.

Holloway observed later (15 June) that because of rapidly rising heroin use levels the brigade established its own drug treatment center. It operates under the authority of the Brigade Surgeon and uses medical personnel exclusively, and it is housed in a group of buildings surrounded by a high fence to facilitate drug-free detoxification. Amnesty volunteers were segregated from the other soldiers undergoing treatment and rehabilitation for drug abuse. Also, because the Vietnamese living in the area adjacent to an outlying firebase were a ready source of heroin, the brigade established a "customs house," which was used to search troops arriving or leaving the base for drugs and contraband. Success measures for these initiatives were not available.

164th Combat Aviation Group south of Saigon in Can Tho in the Mekong River delta— 15 March 1971

[Project Rebuild] is an eight week program which ordinarily follows the individual's involvement in an outpatient group while awaiting admission: Week one—withdrawal ward; week two—rebuild platoon; week three—daily counseling; week four through eight—weekly counseling. Nothing is placed in the official medical record. Necessary records are kept in the Chaplain's office. This is a heavily invested, multidisciplinary, highly professional model [staffed by physicians, a social worker, a nurse, chaplains, medics, ex-users, full-time and part-time officers]. . .

Project Rebuild is a balanced, well considered program whose statistics are equal or better to those of other programs. Screening of individuals is vigorously pursued. The balance of credibility of the program is further evidenced in the training curriculum which emphasizes alcohol "highs" as well. There is a model of team leadership in each rebuild platoon, conjointly between medical officer, chaplain and platoon leader. Substitutions for hard drug use by marijuana, alcohol, or other practice are not supported. The concept of rehabilitation has more to do with increased understanding than with any sense of mastery or arrival, as from a medical illness. The client is educated to his drug problem much as Alcoholics Anonymous proposes that for him the drug will remain a special problem, requiring special and unrelenting vigilance and personal adaptations.

Holloway observed later (5 June) that despite strong command support and the application of the most well structured and professionally competent therapeutic techniques observed throughout Vietnam, follow-up statistics could verify only 15% effectiveness. Also, north of Can Tho at Vinh Long, a sister program was in operation under the auspices of 7/1st Air Cavalry unit and experienced similar results.

Cam Ran Bay and the 483rd AF Hospital—17 March 1971

[The 483rd AF Hospital] is an attractively located, though aging hospital. . . . The drug rehab program [which serves large numbers of Army patients] is carried through on the psychiatry ward, and involves requirement that the soldier turn himself in first to his CO [commanding officer], be sent to the hospital, be given a four day detoxification, and then returned to duty. [A] letter was sent to each man's CO following his discharge, requesting follow-up information, but after four months of no response this was terminated. It would appear that no aftercare structure has been possible from this location.

Holloway observed later (10 June) that since the 483rd AF Hospital had stopped treating Army patients in their program, Support Command was forced to establish its own drug rehabilitation facility, "Operation Guts." This program was an example of an exclusively command organized, supported, and maintained program that featured a well-planned physical facility and a detailed operational plan; but it lacked trained counselors and medical support. Personnel included a lieutenant colonel in charge, a 1st Lieutenant project officer, three NCOs, including one administrative sergeant with Alcoholics Anonymous experience, and a number of EM with a variety of MOSs [military occupational specialties] (including two medics and one ex-user). The staff was mainly characterized by enthusiasm and inexperience; they were developing their skills as care-givers on the spot. However, the program and related education and enforcement efforts failed to slow the extensive heroin use in the Cam Ranh Bay area.

Appendix 19 THE PROFESSIONAL CONSULTATION MODEL

The distribution for this document is uncertain, but apparently it was intended to integrate the 935th Psychiatric Detachment's outreach and consultation services with the primary care medical dispensaries, post chaplains, and other Army agencies in their catchment area, primarily the sprawling Long Binh Post and nearby units. It is in the form of a position paper and explains their rationale for emphasizing secondary preventive activities (the promotion of early detection of developing psychiatric conditions and behavior problems among soldiers and their management as outpatients) over primary preventive activities (efforts devoted to influencing the conditions under which soldiers live, work, and fight so as to reduce the incidence of maladjustment and the occurrence of new psychiatric conditions).

UNPUBLISHED: PSYCHIATRIC CONSULTATION IN THE WAR ZONE
CAPTAIN H SPENCER BLOCH (MD)
DIRECTOR OF THE PSYCHIATRY AND NEUROLOGY INPATIENT SERVICE
935TH PSYCHIATRIC DETACHMENT (AUGUST, 1967–1968)

I would like to present two ideas briefly:
Our experience and perspective have led us to two conclusions upon which our current program of psychiatric consultation is based. The first is that emotional reactions and symptoms are harder to prevent than they are to adapt to and live with. The second is that, in a war zone, one should do the least intervention that is necessary to enable a man to function effectively in his unit.

DISCUSSION
To elaborate on these points let me begin by mentioning that the general orienta-tion and emphasis of military psychiatrists since WW II has been in the area of preventive psychiatry. Practitioners of this approach feel that there are principles of preventive psychiatry that can be conveyed to the leaders of units, and when these principles are put into practice, somehow psychiatric symptomatology and illnesses can be significantly aborted within a unit. This has been the rationale for psychiatrists and other mental health [professionals] spending much of their working time visiting units, meeting and consulting with key people (COs and NCOs) and somehow, in the process, accomplishing the transmittal of concepts and actual plans that will effectively prevent psychiatric illness from developing within the unit.

Our own perspective and experience has led the staff of the 935th to a different conclusion and approach. Namely, we believe that everyone is probably better off if we leave unit leaders alone to conduct their mission in the best way they have been taught and have learned. What general principles of preventive psychiatry that may exist are known by most leaders and are generally common sense. The numbers and kinds of variables within and between units probably make it impossible to formulate any specific principles for preventive psychiatry anyway. Rather, we can best be of most help when specific problems arise. And we can best bring our knowledge and suggestions to bear through channels of professional consultation. In this way COs get their suggestions through their close associates and advisors, such as dispensary or battalion surgeons or unit chaplains. To this end we encourage such professional service people to consult with us about problems that have come their way from units they support. Often the natural reaction from the unit and then from the first professional who sees him (like the primary care physician or the chaplain) is that "This man needs help—more than I can give him—(ergo), please take him off our hands; he's ineffective and bothersome and sometimes frightening—or at least anxiety-provoking." This is a natural reaction, especially if a person is exhibiting behavior that is not readily understood.

Our general approach in consulting with such personnel is to guide them in helping the unit both to manage their behavior or symptoms and also to help the unit to become more tolerant and accepting of behavior that is somewhat aberrant. So that, rather than trying to prevent emotionally-induced symptomatology and behavior (which we think is impossible to do), we attempt to increase the unit's toleration for variation and idiosyncrasy. Certainly some people must be removed and hospitalized, and this is done when necessary, but usually it isn't. When we have combated the unit's panic about deviant behavior by not being overwhelmed by it ourselves and through aiming at an understanding of it, then we can help the unit do the same and help the individual get back closer to the norm.

From what has just been said it can be seen how our first premise (i.e., that it is usually easier to live with and manage psychopathology than to prevent it) relates to our second one (i.e., in the war zone where our interest is in supporting the unit's mission, we, of necessity, wish to do the least that is necessary to enable a man to function effectively in his unit—to make the fewest and most innocuous adjustments that are required to achieve compatibility and enhanced efficiency between the deviant man and his group). We don't mean to imply either laziness, dereliction of responsibility, or second class professionalism on the part of the advisors and treators. One doesn't stint, but rather one thinks small rather than in the more grandiose terms that psychiatrists often do in trying to remake a person's character structure. As you are well aware, the vast majority of patients that we see are operating with mechanisms they've been using for years to handle certain typed of situations and stresses. We don't want to alter this radically now. We just presume that most of these folks have gotten along adequately until the time when we see them, that something has shoved them over the line into ineffectiveness, and our interest is in determining what we can recommend to help them pull themselves back over that line into the realm of acceptable functioning. These principles govern our approach in advising people like you who are the closer confidants and advisers of unit leaders.

Index